Handbook of Preformulation

T0141280

Handbook of Preformulation

Chemical, Biological, and Botanical Drugs

Second Edition

Sarfaraz K. Niazi, PH.D., SI, FRSB, FPAMS, FACB

Adjunct Professor of Biopharmaceutical Sciences,
University of Illinois and University of Houston
Patent Agent, USPTO, Chicago, Illinois, U.S.A.

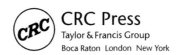

CRC Press
Taylor & Francis Group
Boca Raton London New York

CRC Press is an imprint of the
Taylor & Francis Group, an **informa** business

CRC Press
Taylor & Francis Group
6000 Broken Sound Parkway NW, Suite 300
Boca Raton, FL 33487-2742

First issued in paperback 2022

ISBN-13: 978-1-138-29755-5 (hbk)
ISBN-13: 978-1-03-233847-7 (pbk)
DOI: 10.1201/9781315099187

Library of Congress Cataloging-in-Publication Data

Names: Niazi, Sarfaraz, 1949- author.
Title: Handbook of preformulation : chemical, biological, and botanical drugs / Sarfaraz K. Niazi.
Description: Second edition. | Boca Raton, Florida : CRC Press, [2019] | Includes bibliographical references and index.
Identifiers: LCCN 2018056180| ISBN 9781138297555 (hardback : alk. paper) | ISBN 9781315099187 (ebook)
Subjects: LCSH: Pharmaceutical technology--Handbooks, manuals, etc. | Mixing--Handbooks, manuals, etc. | Drugs--Dosage forms--Handbooks, manuals, etc.
Classification: LCC RS199.F67 N53 2019 | DDC 615.1/9--dc23
LC record available at https://lccn.loc.gov/2018056180

Visit the Taylor & Francis Web site at
http://www.taylorandfrancis.com

and the CRC Press Web site at
http://www.crcpress.com

To Durdana, Aliyah, Noor, and Aminah, my grand preteens

Contents

Preface to the Second Edition...xvii
Other Selected Books by Author xxvii
Author xxix

1. Drug Discovery Trends..1
  1.1   Introduction 1
        1.1.1   Genome Editing 1
        1.1.2   Microbiome..2
        1.1.3   Antibiotics...3
        1.1.4   Artificial Intelligence...3
        1.1.5   Marijuana...3
        1.1.6   Target-Based Discovery 4
        1.1.7   High-Through Screening 4
        1.1.8   Rational Drug Design 5
        1.1.9   Target Family Knowledge..5
        1.1.10 DNA-Encoded Library Technology..............................6
        1.1.11 Phenotype..6
        1.1.12 Biologics...6
        1.1.13 Botanicals 7
  1.2   The Preformulation Focus...9
  1.3   Development Phases..9
        1.3.1   Stage 1: Lead Finding or Establishing Directions (1–2 Years)......9
        1.3.2   Stage 2: Candidate Drug Screening (1–10 Years).......................10
        1.3.3   Stage 3: Candidate Drug Selection (1–2 Years).........................11
        1.3.4   Stage 4: Preclinical Studies (1–2 Years) 12
        1.3.5   Stage 5: Phase I Clinical Studies (1–2 Years) 12
        1.3.6   Stage 6: Phase II and Phase III Studies and Launch
                (4–6 Years).. 13
        1.3.7   Stage 7: Postmarket Surveillance (3–5 Years)...........................13
  1.4   Phytomedicines 14
  1.5   Recombinant Drugs... 17
  Web References 18
  Bibliography... 18

2. Intellectual Property Considerations... 21
  2.1   Introduction 21
  2.2   Patenting Strategies 21
        2.2.1   Patenting Systems 23
        2.2.2   What Is a Patent? 24
        2.2.3   Patent Myths 25
        2.2.4   What Is Not Patentable?..26

2.3   Patent Search 27
       2.3.1   Internet Search Engines 30
       2.3.2   Information Portals 31
       2.3.3   Technical Databases..32
       2.3.4   Patent Search and Intellectual Property Services.......................32
       2.3.5   Patent Copies and Search Facilities 33
2.4   Components of a Patent Application..33
       2.4.1   Drawing(s) (§113) 36
       2.4.2   Specification (§112 ¶1) 36
       2.4.3   Paragraph 1 35 USC §112 Requirements....................................37
       2.4.4   Paragraph 2 35 USC §112 Requirement: Parts of a Claim 38
2.5   Understanding Claims..38
       2.5.1   Reading a Claim 38
       2.5.2   Punctuation of Claim...38
       2.5.3   Definiteness of Claim 38
       2.5.4   Narrowing of Claim...39
       2.5.5   Dependent Claims (§112 ¶3 ¶4) 39
       2.5.6   Multiple Dependent Claims (§112 ¶5) 39
       2.5.7   Dominant-Subservient Claims...39
       2.5.8   Means-Plus-Function Clauses §112 ¶6 40
       2.5.9   Process Claims..40
       2.5.10 Step-Plus-Function Clauses 40
       2.5.11 Ranges..40
       2.5.12 Negative Limitations...41
       2.5.13 Relative and Exemplary Terminology 41
       2.5.14 Markush Group 41
       2.5.15 Markush Alternates..41
       2.5.16 Jepson-Type Claims—Improvement Claims 41
       2.5.17 Mixed-Class Claims 41
       2.5.18 Product-by-Process Claims...42
       2.5.19 Patent Term Adjustment..42
       2.5.20 Patent and Trademark Office Delays: Guaranteed
                   Adjustment Basis 44
       2.5.21 Required Reduction Basis..45
2.6   Food and Drug Administration 45
Web References 51
Bibliography...51
Recommended Reading..51

3. The Scope of Preformulation Studies..55
3.1   Introduction 55
3.2   Preformulation Testing Criteria..55
3.3   Regulatory Requirements...56
       3.3.1   Small Molecules/General..56
       3.3.2   Phytomedicines...62
       3.3.3   Large-Molecule Drugs..64
       3.3.4   Recombinant DNA Products 65

3.4   Testing Systems 67
    3.4.1   Polymorph Screening 67
    3.4.2 pK_a, Partitioning, and Solubility 68
    3.4.3   Salt Screening 71
3.5   Solid-State Characterization 72
    3.5.1   Powder Properties 72
    3.5.2   Microscopy 74
    3.5.3   Thermal Analysis 75
    3.5.4   Molecular Spectroscopy 76
    3.5.5   X-Ray Diffraction 77
    3.5.6   Stability Testing 77
        3.5.6.1   Moisture Isotherm 78
        3.5.6.2   Excipient Compatibility 80
3.6   Transport Across Biological Membranes 80
    3.6.1   Drug Efflux and Multidrug-Resistance Studies 80
    3.6.2   In Vitro–In Vivo Correlation 81
    3.6.3   Caco-2 Cell Studies 81
Web References 82
Bibliography 82
Recommended Reading 83

4. **Dissociation, Partitioning, and Solubility** 93
4.1   Introduction 93
4.2   The Ionization Principle 94
    4.2.1   The Acid–Base Theory 94
        4.2.1.1   Bronsted–Lowry Theory 94
        4.2.1.2   Lewis Theory 97
        4.2.1.3   Henderson–Hasselbalch Equation 98
        4.2.1.4   The pH Scale 99
        4.2.1.5   Compendia Specification for pH Measurement 102
        4.2.1.6   Dissociation 103
4.3   Quantitative Structure–Activity Relationships 105
    4.3.1   Hansch Analysis 110
4.4   Partitioning 113
    4.4.1   Distribution Coefficient 114
    4.4.2   Partitioning Solvent 116
    4.4.3   Solubility 118
        4.4.3.1   Molecular Size 120
        4.4.3.2   Additives 120
        4.4.3.3   Temperature 120
4.5   Measurement Strategies 120
    4.5.1   Ion Pair Log P 121
        4.5.1.1   Manual Titration 125
        4.5.1.2   Spectroscopy 125
    4.5.2   Solubility Method 126
    4.5.3   Filter Probe Method 126
    4.5.4   Shake-Flask Method 126

     4.5.5   High-Pressure Liquid Chromatography 127
     4.5.6   Capillary Zone Electrophoresis 128
     4.5.7   Plate Method for Solubility Testing 128
Web References 131
Bibliography 131
Recommended Reading 131

5. Release, Dissolution, and Permeation 159
  5.1   Introduction 159
  5.2   Release 160
     5.2.1   Solubility Modulation 163
  5.3   Assay Systems 165
     5.3.1   Permeability Assays 166
     5.3.2   Parallel Artificial Membrane Permeability Analysis 168
     5.3.3   Caco-2 Drug Transport Assays 169
     5.3.4   Animal Model Testing 172
     5.3.5   In Vitro–In Vivo Correlation 172
          5.3.5.1   Internal Validation 174
  5.4   Waiver of In Vivo Bioavailability and Bioequivalence Studies
       for Immediate-Release Solid Oral Dosage Forms Based on a
       Biopharmaceutics Classification System: Guidance for Industry 175
  5.5   Using BDCS in Preformulation 189
Recommended Reading 192

6. Solid-State Properties 233
  6.1   Introduction 233
  6.2   Crystal Morphology 234
  6.3   Polymorphism 240
  6.4   High-Throughput Crystal Screening 245
     6.4.1   Crystalline Index of Refraction 247
  6.5   Solvates 247
     6.5.1   Hydrates 248
  6.6   Amorphous Forms 249
  6.7   Hygroscopicity 250
  6.8   Solubility 251
     6.8.1   Salt Form 252
     6.8.2   Melting Point 255
     6.8.3   Dissolution 255
  6.9   Study Methods 255
     6.9.1   Thermal Analysis 256
     6.9.2   Differential Scanning Calorimetry 256
     6.9.3   Hot-Stage Microscopy 258
     6.9.4   Thermogravimetric Analysis 258
     6.9.5   Solution Calorimetry 258
     6.9.6   Isothermal Microcalorimetry 259
     6.9.7   Infrared Spectroscopy 259
     6.9.8   X-Ray Powder Diffraction 261

6.9.9   Phase Solubility Analysis 264
6.9.10   Dynamic Vapor Sorption 265
6.9.11   Dissolution Testing..267
6.9.12   High-Performance Liquid Chromatography...........................268
Web References 269
Recommended Reading..269

7. Dosage Form Considerations in Preformulation 287
7.1   Introduction 287
7.2   Solid Dosage Form Considerations..291
      7.2.1   Particle Size Studies..292
      7.2.2   Particle Size Distribution...297
      7.2.3   Surface Area 299
      7.2.4   Porosity 301
      7.2.5   Instrumentation for Particle Size, Surface Area, and
               Porosity 302
      7.2.6   True Density...305
      7.2.7   Flow and Compaction of Powders 305
      7.2.8   Color..307
      7.2.9   Electrostaticity 308
      7.2.10   Caking...309
      7.2.11   Polymorphism 309
7.3   Solution Formulations 310
      7.3.1   Solubility...310
7.4   Emulsion Formulations 311
      7.4.1   Stability Considerations...314
      7.4.2   Oxidation...314
      7.4.3   Trace Metals..315
      7.4.4   Photostability 317
      7.4.5   Surface Activity 318
      7.4.6   Osmolality...319
7.5   Freeze-Dried Formulations 319
7.6   Suspensions 321
7.7   Topical 322
7.8   Pulmonary Delivery 322
7.9   General Compatibility...323
Web References 324
Recommended Reading..324

8. Chemical Drug Substance Characterization.............................329
8.1   Introduction 329
8.2   Scheme of Characterization 330
      8.2.1   Specifications..332
               8.2.1.1   Description 332
               8.2.1.2   Identification..332
               8.2.1.3   Chirality 332

8.2.2	Assay	....	333
	8.2.2.1	Impurities	334
8.2.3	Physicochemical Properties		334
	8.2.3.1	Particle Size	335
	8.2.3.2	Polymorphic Forms	335
	8.2.3.3	Microbiology	336
	8.2.3.4	Excipients	336
8.2.4	Stability Evaluation		338
	8.2.4.1	Hydrolysis	339
	8.2.4.2	Oxidation	342
8.2.5	Regulatory Consideration in Stability Testing		352
	8.2.5.1	Stress Testing	353
	8.2.5.2	Selection of Batches	353
	8.2.5.3	Container Closure System	354
	8.2.5.4	Specifications	354
	8.2.5.5	Testing Frequency	354
	8.2.5.6	Stability Commitment	356
	8.2.5.7	Statements/Labeling	358

8.3   Impurities 361
    8.3.1   Good Manufacturing Practice 366
    8.3.2   Quality Management 368
Web References 370
Recommended Reading 370

9. Characterization of Biopharmaceuticals 379
9.1   Background 379
    9.1.1   Developing Biosimilars 380
9.2   Protein Structure 382
    9.2.1   Building Elements 382
    9.2.2   Translation 382
    9.2.3   Peptide Bond 385
9.3   Motifs and Domains 387
9.4   Association and Aggregation 389
9.5   Posttranslational Modification 391
    9.5.1   Glycosylation 395
9.6   Protein Expression Variability 398
9.7   Preformulation Considerations 400
9.8   Preformulation Studies 404
    9.8.1   Stability 406
        9.8.1.1   Excipients 407
9.9   Packaging and Materials 422
    9.9.1   Dosage Form and Storage 422
    9.9.2   Cryopreservation 423
        9.9.2.1   Cryogranulation 423
        9.9.2.2   Spray Drying 423
        9.9.2.3   Undercooling 424
        9.9.2.4   Lyophilization 424

9.9.3		Characterization Methods	429
	9.9.3.1	Spectroscopy	429
	9.9.3.2	Electrophoresis	430
	9.9.3.3	Chromatography	431
	9.9.3.4	Mass Spectroscopy	433
	9.9.3.5	Process Validation	434
	9.9.3.6	Facility and Equipment Validation	435
	9.9.3.7	Analytical Methods	435
	9.9.3.8	Software Validation	436
	9.9.3.9	Cleaning Validation	436
	9.9.3.10	Expression System Characterization	436
9.9.4		Stability Considerations	436
	9.9.4.1	Proteolysis	437
	9.9.4.2	Deamidation	437
	9.9.4.3	Oxidation	438
	9.9.4.4	Carbamylation	440
	9.9.4.5	β-Elimination	441
	9.9.4.6	Racemization	442
	9.9.4.7	Cysteinyl Residues	442
	9.9.4.8	Hydrolysis	444
	9.9.4.9	Denaturation	444
	9.9.4.10	Aggregation	446
	9.9.4.11	Precipitation	446
9.9.5		Forced Degradation Studies	450
	9.9.5.1	Stress Testing	452
	9.9.5.2	Selection of Stress Conditions	453
9.9.6		Specifications	454
	9.9.6.1	Physicochemical Properties	455
9.9.7		Biological Activity	455
9.9.8		Immunochemical Properties	456
9.9.9		Purity, Impurities, and Contaminants	456
	9.9.9.1	Purity	456
	9.9.9.2	Impurities	457
	9.9.9.3	Contaminants	457
9.9.10		Quantity	458
9.9.11		Analytical Considerations	458
	9.9.11.1	Reference Standards and Reference Materials	458
	9.9.11.2	Validation of Analytical Procedures	458
9.9.12		Process Controls	458
9.9.13		Release Limits versus Shelf-Life Limits	459
9.9.14		Justification of Specifications	460
9.10		Physiochemical Characterization Tests	461
9.10.1		Structural Characterization and Confirmation	461
	9.10.1.1	Amino Acid Sequence	461
	9.10.1.2	Amino Acid Composition	461
	9.10.1.3	Terminal Amino Acid Sequence	461
	9.10.1.4	Peptide Map	461

9.10.2 Sulfhydryl Group(s) and Disulfide Bridges 461
9.10.3 Carbohydrate Structure 462
9.10.4 Physicochemical Properties 462
    9.10.4.1 Molecular Weight or Size 462
    9.10.4.2 Isoform Pattern 462
    9.10.4.3 Extinction Coefficient (or Molar Absorptivity) 462
    9.10.4.4 Electrophoretic Patterns 462
    9.10.4.5 Liquid Chromatographic Patterns 462
9.11 Spectroscopic Profiles 462
    9.11.1 Process-Related Impurities and Contaminants 463
    9.11.2 Product-Related Impurities, Including Degradation
           Products 463
        9.11.2.1 Truncated Forms 463
        9.11.2.2 Other Modified Forms 464
        9.11.2.3 Aggregates 464
9.12 Design of Preformulation Studies 464
Web References 465
Bibliography 465
Recommended Reading 468

10. Botanical Drugs 485
10.1 Introduction 485
10.2 Regulatory Status 486
    10.2.1 Characteristics of Phytomedicines 486
    10.2.2 Specifications 491
        10.2.2.1 Standardization 492
    10.2.3 Efficacy and Safety 493
    10.2.4 Regulatory Filing Procedure 494
        10.2.4.1 Plant Substance 494
        10.2.4.2 Product (Capsule, Tablet, and Intravenous
                 Formulation) 495
    10.2.5 Overview of Chemistry, Manufacturing, and Control
           Evidence Needed to Support Clinical Trials for Botanical
           Drugs 496
    10.2.6 Information on a Plant Product That Was the Subject of
           Prior Human Use 496
    10.2.7 Information on the Plant Product Proposed for Phase I/II
           Studies 497
        10.2.7.1 Plant Substance 497
        10.2.7.2 Plant Product 497
    10.2.8 Information on the Plant Product Proposed for Phase III
           Studies 498
        10.2.8.1 Plant Substance 498
        10.2.8.2 Plant Product 498
    10.2.9 Starting Material 499
        10.2.9.1 Control of Herbal Substances and of Herbal
                 Preparations 500

10.2.10   Control of Vitamins and Minerals (If Applicable)............... 501

10.2.10.1   Control of Excipients.. 501

10.2.11   Stability Testing.. 501

10.2.11.1   Testing Criteria.. 502

10.2.12   Herbal Substances.. 502

10.2.13   Herbal Preparations 504

Recommended Reading.. 506

Index.. 529

Preface to the Second Edition

The first edition of this book was published about 12 years ago; given the notable changes in science, driven by advanced instrumentation, augmented reality, and artificial intelligence, the pace of development of just about every industrial product has changed dramatically, but none has changed as much as the new drug discoveries and their development. So, a gap of decade in revising this book should be a big gap, demanding a complete updation of this book that has been a reference source for the development of scientists and teachers across the globe. While the second edition provides updated information on the science of preformulation, the fundamental principles that go in the preformulation phase of development remain the same, being dependent on the basic molecular structure. However, these discussions have also been updated, with special attention to an aspect that is rarely appreciated by the scientists—the legal framework of preformulation. The chapter on intellectual property has been updated and expanded to include the discussion of freedom to operate, to provide guidance on avoiding infringement of intellectual property rights, as the preformulation steps are taken, from the very beginning. As a patent law practitioner myself, I take these considerations seriously to help avoid costly litigation later in the development cycle that can be a very expensive setback.

I see this book as a continuation of the series of books that I have written, and they have all been published by CRC Press; the next in the sequence is the revision of my six-volume formulation book that has provided manufacturing-ready formulations for over 3000 products; and to follow that, I have written a handbook on bioequivalence testing to complete the cycle of regulatory filing for new products. Whereas the development of chemical drugs has become rather straightforward, the development of the biological drugs and the gene therapy products remains elusive. I have written several books in those fields also, and these have also been published by the CRC Press.

Preformulation studies constitute the delicate connection between the two major groups of scientists: those at the drug discovery end and those at the drug delivery end. Whereas scientific camaraderie, or perhaps stubbornness, at the two ends of new drug development has historic roots, it is the preformulation group of comrades that brings peace to the table. It is often humbling for the drug discovery group to bring out a novel molecule with a remarkable potential only to be shot down by the formulation group as a worthless exercise in taking it to a deliverable form. The preformulation group works with both ends and helps to reduce the overall cost and shrink the timeline of drug development. Whereas in some companies the dividing line between preformulation and formulation is often a gray zone, those who have understood the significance of keeping the two groups separate have reaped great rewards. This book is a practical manual for those involved in the preformulation stages of drug development, yet it would also be a good read for the drug discovery and drug development groups. The traditional scope of textbooks and manuals on this topic is expanded here to include biological drugs, particularly therapeutic proteins and botanical drugs or phytomedicines. The latter category is particularly significant, as it is fast becoming evident that such regulatory authorities as the U.S. Food and Drug Administration and the European Medicines Evaluation Agency will start approving them in the same system of approval as is ordinarily reserved for small- and large-molecule, well-characterized drugs.

The goals of preformulation studies are to choose the correct form of the drug substance, evaluate its physical and chemical properties, and generate a thorough understanding of the material's stability under the conditions that will lead to the development of a practical drug delivery system. Preformulation is a science that serves as a big umbrella for the fingerprinting of a drug substance or product, both at the early stage and at a later stage of development in pharmaceutical manufacturing. The preformulation phase is a critical learning time about candidate drugs. Typically, it begins during the lead optimization phase and continues through prenomination and into the early phases of development. Decisions made on the information generated during this phase can have a profound effect on the subsequent development of those compounds. Therefore, it is imperative that preformulation should be performed as carefully as possible to enable rational decision-making. The quantity and quality of the drugs available at this stage can affect the quantity and quality of the data generated—so can the equipment available and the expertise of the personnel conducting the investigations. In some companies, there are specialized preformulation teams, but in others, the information is generated by a number of scattered teams. Whichever way a company chooses to organize its preformulation information gathering, one of the most important practices to adopt is to keep close communication among the various groups involved.

The classic definitions and the management systems to conduct preformulation studies are discussed in the chapters; it would suffice for now to claim that there is a need to apply the most current knowledge and analytical sophistication available to deliver these goals. Over the past quarter of a century, the science of analysis and characterization has taken a giant leap and so have the options that are now available to scientists regarding the basic substances, as we enter the era of nanoparticles and intelligent delivery designs. A recent study authorized by the National Security Agency and conducted by Rand Corporation listed nano- and material science to be the leading sciences in the year 2015; this is an important indication of what is to come and that the science of drug discovery will be greatly affected by it. With new possibilities of materials and systems such as nano pumps, the evaluation of new drug entities will have to take a different perspective.

Crystalline structure studies form the core of preformulation studies, because molecules make crystals, crystals make particles, and particles make dosage forms. Novel research in crystallography of new entities involves the studies of amorphous forms to learn how local properties contribute to the chemical reactivity of these short-interacting forms. Solid solutions are better understood today, and studies on the effect of different solvents on the formation of solid solutions remain a challenging opportunity, which are made easy by computer simulation models. Predicting accurate behavior of amorphous forms will allow great opportunities in drug delivery. By understanding the effects of various cations and anions on crystal structure and properties, one can move toward the rational selection of counterions for salt formation and the design of stable salt forms. Neutral pharmaceuticals and excipients can and do form stable cocrystals. These cocrystals may possess superior physical properties, such as solubility, melting point, and compaction behavior. These studies seek to understand the forces that promote the formation of neutral cocrystals, in particular intermolecular hydrogen bonding. There is an increasingly strong driving force to predict the properties of a drug in its solid form, and this, in turn, drives the need to predict the three-dimensional structure. It is important to compute all reasonable low-energy conformers from a known chemical structure and place these conformers into ranked three-dimensional crystal structures. Studies of how particle shape influences packing properties and how this affects the translational stress into strain in the tableting process are useful. By studying such material constants as friction coefficients, Young's modulus, and viscoelasticity, one can obtain properties of the bulk powder. This then should be followed to study polydispersity (in particle size) and to validate the model with X-ray microtomography of glass powder. The controlled crystallization of organic molecules on surfaces controls the nucleation and deposition of drug crystals of chosen structure, as formed by manipulation of the substrate surface. This provides the groundwork for the development of self-assembled three-dimensional and chemical cage formulations. The idea is that by controlling the nature of the surface of the substrate, particular polymorphs may be encouraged to grow. In addition, the directing surface may prove to be a way of stabilizing more favorable, but higher-energy, polymorphs, such that solid form selection may be made on the basis of polymorph properties and not be limited to the thermodynamically most stable form. Self-assembled functional dosage forms could provide the next generation of pharmaceutical products, obviating the need for extreme conditions encountered during tableting. Areas of research include the manipulation of surfaces to allow coating and filling and the controlled crystallization and production of porous polymeric structures by using polymethyl methacrylate as a "proof of concept" polymer.

The availability of new scientific tools is not limited to the development of small molecules; large-molecule drugs, particularly therapeutic proteins, are now studied with greater accuracy than was possible when they were first approved a quarter of century ago. With almost certainty that biogeneric (or biosimilar or follow-on, depending on which side of the Atlantic you live on) products will be approved by the U.S. Food and Drug Administration, as the European Medicines Evaluation Agency is already approving them, there will be a great rush to develop tools to study the equivalence of protein products. Given the complexities involved in predicting the side effects related to three-dimensional and even four-dimensional structures, a lot of science is yet to be developed in executing the comparability protocols. The *Handbook of Preformulation: Pharmaceutical, Biological, and Natural Products* provides a broad discussion of testing of biological products at the preformulation level, and it is anticipated that many new techniques will become available in the near future.

Botanical drugs had long been set aside by the busy regulatory authorities, partly because of a lack of resources to monitor them and partly because they were so poorly understood that it was better to leave them alone. This is changing fast, as all regulatory authorities worldwide have announced the guidelines on the development and submission of marketing authorization applications for phytomedicines. These are likely to be treated somewhere between the small- and large-molecule categories; a detailed discussion of the new requirements for chemistry, manufacturing, and control package submission are presented in this book, with particular emphasis on the preformulation work that needs to be performed in the development of these drugs. There is a need to devote an entire volume to these studies.

Given the fast-changing backdrop in the studies that constitute preformulation, it is heartening to know that there are several excellent resources that can be tapped by scientists on a routine basis. The American Association of Pharmaceutical Scientists (www.aaps.org) offers, among many other useful sources of information, the Preformulation Focus Group, which was established in 1993 to bring together all American Association of Pharmaceutical Scientists members, with a common interest in the broad area of preformulation research. The ultimate goal of the group is to provide a forum for the exchange of ideas and development of strategies, thereby collectively improving our capabilities in this important area of research. The goals of the group are as follows:

- To provide a forum for information exchange of issues relating to solid- and liquid-state characterization of chemical entities, active pharmaceutical ingredients, excipients, and early-phase development of pharmaceutical dosage forms and delivery systems
- To promote and disseminate novel scientific advances in the areas of discovery and development of drug substances and products through themed meetings and workshops in pharmaceutical technologies or pharmaceutics and drug delivery sections
- To encourage and promote joint programs with other focus groups, academia, and regulatory agencies, for example, the Food and Drug Administration, the U.S. Pharmacopeia, and other national regulatory agencies worldwide
- To participate in the portals as the focus group newsletters, student chapters, conferences, volunteer activities, and the American Association of Pharmaceutical Scientists list serve
- To support nominations of preformulation scientists for the American Association of Pharmaceutical Scientists awards

The reader is highly encouraged to join the group and benefit from a ready knowledge base, particularly as the harmonization of the international standards of the technical packages of new drug applications is achieved. Besides these discussion groups, several journals publish relevant articles on preformulation, including the following:

- American Association of Pharmaceutical Scientists www.aaps.org
- www.admet.net is a newer web portal. It aims to keep researchers and business leaders up to date on what is happening in the dynamic fields of absorption, distribution, metabolism, excretion, and toxicology. Updated on a daily basis, the unique mix of exclusive interviews, specialist supplier listings, events, news, and new products makes this a one-stop shop for essential information. For reference, there are links to research centers, journals, books, reviews, and market reports.
- www.htscreening.net is the main web information portal that aims to keep researchers and business leaders up to date on what's happening in the dynamic field of biomolecular screening. Updated on a daily basis, the unique mix of exclusive interviews, specialist supplier listings, events, news,

and new products makes this a one-stop shop for essential information. For reference there are links to research centers, journals, books, reviews, and market reports.

- www.CombiChem.net is the main web information portal dedicated to combinatorial and medicinal chemistry. Updated on a daily basis, the unique mix of exclusive interviews, specialist supplier listings, events, news and new products makes this a one-stop shop for essential information. For reference there are links to research centers, journals, books, reviews, and market reports.
- The Drug Delivery Insight (www.espicom.com/ddi) offers a detailed review and takes the hard work out of staying in touch with the companies, products, alliances, and research activities shaping the industry.

The work of scientists has been substantially eased through the availability of search engines on the Internet. A search for "preformulation" yielded 338,000 hits in 0.39 seconds; for "pharmaceutical preformulation," the number was 233,000; both of these are 10 times greater than when the first edition of this book was published. The problems, therefore, arise regarding how to parse the data; a lot of redundant and superfluous information is available. It is for this reason that despite the wide availability of information, knowledge must be gained from such condensed sources as this book and other books written on the subject.

Another change in this edition takes a lead on how bibliographies and references are provided. Today, references and information are widely available, so instead of listing publications of importance, I have selected a few recent publications that are presented with abstract, to add to the current knowledge on the topic; I hope that the readers will appreciate this added value to the book.

Over the past two decades, a large number of highly sophisticated laboratories have emerged that offer excellent opportunities to outsource the preformulation work. Some of these include the following:

ABC Laboratories
Advanced Chemistry Development, Inc.
Agami
Agere Pharmaceuticals Inc.
Aizant Drug Research Solutions
Ajinomoto Althea, Inc.
Alcami
Alliance Contract Pharma
AllTranz
Almac Group
AMRI
Apredica
APS Altora Pharma Solutions, LLC
Aptuit
ARDL, Inc.

Argenta Limited

Ashland Specialty Ingredients

Avacta Analytical

Avantium Technologies BV

Averica Discovery

Avomeen Analytical Services

Azopharma

Baxter Biopharma Solutions

Bilcare, Inc.

Bio-Concept Laboratories

BioDuro

BioNimbus

Biorelevant.com

BioScreen Testing Services, Inc.

Biotechnology Consulting

Biotechpharma

Blue Stream Laboratories

Camargo Pharmaceutical Services

Capsugel, now a Lonza company

Carbogen Amcis AG

Cardinal Health

Catalent Pharma Solutions

Ceutical Laboratories, Inc.

Chemic Laboratories, Inc.

Chemir Analytical Services

CMC Pharmaceuticals, Inc.

CMIC CMO USA Corp.

Comprehensive CMC Outsourcing

Cook Pharmica, LLC

Corealis Pharma, Inc.

CoreRx, Inc.

Covance, Inc.

CPL

CRID Pharma

Dalton Pharma Services

deCode Chemistry & BioStructures

Dow Development Laboratories, LLC

Dow Pharmaceutical Sciences

DPT Laboratories

Ei LLC

Emerson Resources, Inc.

Eminent Services Corporation

Enco Pharmaceutical Development, Inc. (EPDI)

Encompass Pharma

Exelead

Exemplar Pharmaceuticals

ExxPharma Therapeutics

Formatech

Formex

Fortitech

Fresenius Kabi Product Partnering

Fresenius Product Partnering

Frontage Laboratories, Inc.

Fujifilm Diosynth Biotechnologies

Fulcrum Pharma Developments

Fulcrum Pharma Developments, Inc.

Galenix Innovations

Genzyme Pharmaceuticals

Gland Pharma Limited

Glatt Pharmaceutical Services

Grifols International, S.A.

Groupe Parima, Inc.

Halo Pharmaceutical, Inc.

Hovione

HTD Biosystems Inc.

Idifarma

IDT Australia Ltd.

InSymbiosis

Integrity Bio

Intertek

iuvo BioScience

Kemwell Biopharma

KP Pharmaceutical Technology

Kumar Organic Products

Latitude Pharmaceuticals, Inc.

LyoTechnica LLC

MedPharm Ltd.

Metrics Contract Services

Micron Technologies, Inc.

Mikart, Inc.

Murty Pharmaceuticals, Inc.

Naxpar Pharma

Nerviano Medical Sciences

Neurogen

Newport Scientific, Inc.

Nitto Avecia Pharma Services

Nupharm Group

OctoPlus N.V.

Olympus Biotech Corp.

Omnia Biologics

Orbus Pharma, Inc.

Particle Sciences, Inc.

Patheon

Penn Pharma

Penn Pharmaceutical Services, Ltd.

Phares AG

Pharmaceutical Consulting Services

Pharmaceutical Development & Manufacturing Service

PharmaDirections

PharmaFab

PharmaForm

Pharmaron, Inc.

Pharmatek Laboratories, Inc.

Pharmaterials Ltd.

PharmaZell, Inc.

PharmPro (Division of Fluid Air)

Pharmquest Corp.

Pierre Fabre Medicament

Pii

Piramal Pharma Solutions

ProJect Pharmaceutics GmbH

QS Pharma

Quality Assistance SA

Quality Chemical Laboratories (QCL)

Quay Pharma

Quintiles

Quotient Bioresearch Ltd.

Ricerca Biosciences

RiconPharma LLC

Roquette

RR Regulatory Solutions

Rubicon Research Pvt. Ltd.

SBS Pharma

SeránCascade

SICOR Biotech UAB

Singota Solutions

Sirius Analytical

Soluble Therapeutics, Inc.

Stason Pharmaceuticals, Inc.

Sterling Pharmaceutical Services, LLC

Suven Life Sciences Ltd.

Sypharma Pty Ltd.

Tedor Pharma Inc.

Temmler Pharma

Tergus Pharma

TetraGenX

Triclinic Labs, LLC

University of Iowa Pharmaceuticals

UPM Pharmaceuticals, Inc.

Velesco Pharmaceutical Services

Wolfe Laboratories

WuXi AppTec

Many of these fine companies have extended their courtesy to me in providing technical information, for which I am very grateful. In the previous edition, I had provided a URL link to these companies, but I realized that you should be able to locate them by name alone, to avoid any change in the web addresses.

The organization of this book was at first difficult, as I kept sifting away those materials that would classically constitute formulation work or be more closely related to drug discovery. However, preformulation studies, slotted in between these two, must, by necessity, overlap these disciplines to some degree. Starting with an overview of the drug discovery process in the first chapter, the book takes the reader to more specific topics, including the regulatory environment and the intellectual property requirements for both understanding how it is developed and avoiding a drug infringement. Classical studies of basic property evaluation of new drug substances for the three types of products—chemical, biological, and botanicals—are presented, along with examples of the newest trends in the use of newer techniques.

In writing this book, I have benefited greatly from those who have ventured this road before me and produced great published works. I have tried to acknowledge them in bibliographies; however, it is impossible for me to fully credit these authors and quote their written works for they may be embedded in the very language of preformulation sciences. However, despite much care, it is inevitable that errors remain; these are all mine, and I would appreciate it if the reader would bring them to my attention at niazi@niazi.com, so that I may correct them in future editions of the book.

The support of the editors and publisher was exemplary, as it has been in the previous books that I wrote for CRC Press (Informa Healthcare). The continuous support and encouragement of Jessica Poile and Hilary Lafoe and many others is deeply acknowledged.

Sarfaraz K. Niazi

Other Selected Books by Author

Niazi SK. *Textbook of Biopharmaceutics and Clinical Pharmacokinetics*. New York: John Wiley & Sons, 1979.

Niazi SK. *The Omega Connection*. Westmont, IL: Esquire Press, 1982.

Niazi SK. *Adsorption and Chelation Therapy*. Westmont, IL: Esquire Press, 1987.

Niazi SK. *Attacking the Sacred Cows: The Health Hazards of Milk*. Westmont, IL: Esquire Press, 1988.

Niazi SK. *Endorphins: The Body Opium*. Westmont, IL: Esquire Press, 1988.

Niazi SK. *Nutritional Myths: The Story No One Wants to Talk About*. Westmont, IL: Esquire Press.

Niazi SK. *Wellness Guide*. Lahore, Pakistan: Ferozsons Publishers, 2002.

Niazi SK. *Love Sonnets of Ghalib: Translations, Explication and Lexicon*, Lahore, Pakistan: Ferozsons Publishers, 2002.

Niazi SK. *Filing Patents Online*. Boca Raton, FL: CRC Press, 2003.

Niazi SK. Pharmacokinetic and Pharmacodynamic Modeling in Early Drug Development, in Smith CG and O'Donnell JT (eds.), *The Process of New Drug Discovery and Development* (2nd ed.). New York: CRC Press, 2004.

Niazi SK. *Handbook of Biogeneric Therapeutic Proteins: Manufacturing, Regulatory, Testing and Patent Issues*. Boca Raton, FL: CRC Press, 2005.

Niazi SK. *Handbook of Preformulation: Chemical, Biological and Botanical Drugs*. New York: Informa Healthcare, 2006.

Niazi SK. *Handbook of Bioequivalence Testing*. New York: Informa Healthcare, 2007.

Niazi SK. *Handbook of Pharmaceutical Manufacturing Formulations, Volume 1 Second Edition: Compressed Solids*. New York: Informa Healthcare, 2009.

Niazi SK. *Handbook of Pharmaceutical Manufacturing Formulations, Volume 2 Second Edition: Uncompressed Solids*. New York: Informa Healthcare, 2009.

Niazi SK. *Handbook of Pharmaceutical Manufacturing Formulations, Volume 3 Second Edition: Liquid Products*. New York: Informa Healthcare, 2009.

Niazi SK. *Handbook of Pharmaceutical Manufacturing Formulations, Volume 4 Second Edition: Semisolid Products*. New York: Informa Healthcare, 2009.

Niazi SK. *Handbook of Pharmaceutical Manufacturing Formulations, Volume 5 Second Edition: Over the Counter Products*. New York: Informa Healthcare, 2009.

Niazi SK. *Handbook of Pharmaceutical Manufacturing Formulations, Volume 6 Second Edition: Sterile Products*. New York: Informa Healthcare, 2009.

Niazi SK. *Textbook of Biopharmaceutics and Clinical Pharmacokinetics*. Hyderabad, India: The Book Syndicate, 2010.

Niazi SK. *Wine of Passion: Love Poems of Ghalib*. Lahore, Pakistan: Ferozsons Publishers, 2010.

Niazi SK. *Disposable Bioprocessing Systems*. Boca Raton, FL: CRC Press, 2012.

Niazi SK. *Handbook of Bioequivalence Testing*, 2nd ed. New York: Informa Healthcare, 2014.

Niazi SK. *There is No Wisdom: Selected Love Poems of Bedil*. Translations from Farsi D, Niazi SK and Tawoosi M. Lahore, Pakistan: Ferozsons Publishers, 2015.

Niazi SK. *Wine of Love: Complete Translations of Urdu Persian Love Poems of Ghalib*. Lahore, Pakistan: Ferozsons Publishers, 2015.

Niazi SK. *Biosimilars and Interchangeable Biologics: Tactical Elements.* CRC Press, 2015.
Niazi SK. *Biosimilars and Interchangeable Biologicals: Strategic Elements.* CRC Press, 2017.
Niazi SK, Brown JL. *Fundamentals of Modern Bioprocessing.* CRC Press, 2015.

Bibliography

Anton P, Silberglitt R, Schneider R. The Global Technology Revolution: Bio/Nano/ Materials Trends and their Synergies with Information Technology by 2015, Rand Corporation 2001. Santa Monica, CA (http://www.rand.org/pubs/monograph_ reports/MR1307/index.html).

Blumenthal M, Daniel E, Farnsworth N, Riggins C. *Botanical Medicine: Efficacy, Quality Assurance and Regulation.* Mary Ann Liebert, 2003.

Carpenter JF, Manning MC, eds. *Rational Design of Stable Protein Formulations: Theory and Practice (Pharmaceutical Biotechnology).* New York: Plenum Press, 2003.

Carstensen JT. *Pharmaceutical Preformulation.* Boca Raton, FL: CRC Press, 1998.

Florence AT, ed. *Materials Used in Pharmaceutical Formulation* (Critical Reports on Applied Chemistry, Vol. 6). Blackwell Science, 1984.

Gibson M. *Pharmaceutical Preformulation and Formulation: A Practical Guide from Candidate Drug Selection to Commercial Dosage Form.* Boca Raton, FL: CRC Press, 2001.

Hovgaard SF Jr. *Pharmaceutical Formulation Development of Peptides and Proteins.* Boca Raton, FL: CRC Press, 1999.

Niazi SK. *Filing Patents Online.* Boca Raton, FL: CRC Press, 2003.

Niazi SK. Pharmacokinetic and Pharmacodynamic Modeling in Early Drug Development, in Smith CG and O'Donnell JT (eds.), *The Process of New Drug Discovery and Development* (2nd ed.). New York: CRC Press, 2004.

Niazi SK. *Handbook of Biogeneric Therapeutic Proteins: Manufacturing, Regulatory, Testing and Patent Issues.* Boca Raton, FL: CRC Press, 2005.

Niazi SK. *Handbook of Preformulation: Chemical, Biological and Botanical Drugs.* New York: Informa Healthcare, 2006.

Niazi SK. *Handbook of Bioequivalence Testing.* New York: Informa Healthcare, 2007.

Niazi SK. *Handbook of Pharmaceutical Manufacturing Formulations, Volume 1 Second Edition: Compressed Solids.* New York: Informa Healthcare, 2009.

Niazi SK. *Handbook of Pharmaceutical Manufacturing Formulations, Volume 2 Second Edition: Uncompressed Solids.* New York: Informa Healthcare, 2009.

Niazi SK. *Handbook of Pharmaceutical Manufacturing Formulations, Volume 3 Second Edition: Liquid Products.* New York: Informa Healthcare, 2009.

Niazi SK. *Handbook of Pharmaceutical Manufacturing Formulations, Volume 4 Second Edition: Semisolid Products.* New York: Informa Healthcare, 2009.

Niazi SK. *Handbook of Pharmaceutical Manufacturing Formulations, Volume 5 Second Edition: Over the Counter Products.* New York: Informa Healthcare, 2009.

Niazi SK. *Handbook of Pharmaceutical Manufacturing Formulations, Volume 6 Second Edition: Sterile Products.* New York: Informa Healthcare, 2009.

Niazi SK. *Textbook of Biopharmaceutics and Clinical Pharmacokinetics.* Hyderabad, India: The Book Syndicate, 2010.

Niazi SK. *Biosimilars and Interchangeable Biologics: Tactical Elements.* CRC Press, 2015.

Niazi SK. *Biosimilars and Interchangeable Biologicals: Strategic Elements.* CRC Press, 2017.

Niazi SK, Brown JL. *Fundamentals of Modern Bioprocessing.* CRC Press, 2015.

Wells JI. *Pharmaceutical Preformulation: The Physicochemical Properties of Drug Substances.* Chichester, UK: Ellis Horwood, 1988.

Author

Sarfaraz K. Niazi, PhD, is adjunct professor of biopharmaceutical sciences at the University of Illinois and the University of Houston. He is the founder of Pharmaceutical Scientist, LLC, a consulting company, and Karyo Biologics and Adello Biologics, biosimilar development companies. Dr. Niazi has published more than 100 research papers, more than 50 books, and more than 500 blogs on scientific and literary topics and owns more than 100 patents. He is also a practitioner of patent law with the United States Patent and Trademark Office.

1

Drug Discovery Trends

There'll always be serendipity involved in discovery.

Jeff Bezos

1.1 Introduction

If the number of drugs approved by the U.S. Food and Drug Administration (FDA) can be taken as a measure of success, then there is a steady approval pace; over the past 4 years, 2015–2018, the FDA has already approved approximately 150 novel drugs and about 500 since the year 2000, bringing the total novel drugs approved to about 1500 since the year 1930. The new drugs under development are into thousands; for example, at least 500 new drugs are currently developed for neurological disorders that affect 100 million Americans.

Much has changed in the discovery of drugs over the past 50 years; the pace of change has accelerated exponentially since the first edition of this book was published. Microprocessor-driven instrumentation has revolutionized data-handling systems, robotic systems have eased large sample processing, and the integration of various physical and chemical sciences has resulted in the emergence of newer techniques. For example, high-throughput screening (HTS) is now an integral component of the drug discovery process that has evolved over the past decade from crude automation to the use of sophisticated computer-driven array systems using robotic devices. Improved physicochemical data on prospective new active entities (NAEs) provide a great stimulus to new drug development, as well as offer insights for the preformulation scientists to project the characteristics of the NAEs that would prove useful in their downstream processing. The downstream processes include hit-to-lead (HTL); lead optimization (LO); and in vitro absorption, distribution, metabolism, elimination, and toxicology (ADMET) studies, all driven by the peculiar characteristics of the NAE.

Figure 1.1 shows the most common types of drug discovery modalities, their costs, and the time it takes for the discovery.

1.1.1 Genome Editing

Targeted genome editing technology, based on the clustered regularly interspaced short palindromic repeats (CRISPR)-Cas9 system, offers a great promise for the future of medicine. Clustered regularly interspaced short palindromic repeats or CRISPR refers to the system consisting of two key molecules: an enzyme Cas9—"molecular scissors," able to cut the two strands of DNA at a specific location in the genome, and a piece of

A. Molecular target screen-based approach:

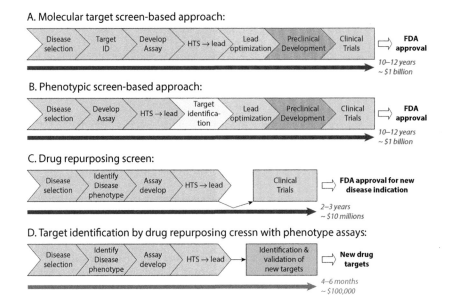

B. Phenotypic screen-based approach:

C. Drug repurposing screen:

D. Target identification by drug repurposing cressn with phenotype assays:

FIGURE 1.1 Comparison of phenotype screen and drug development using drug repurposing screen, with traditional process of drug discovery. (From https://www.ncbi.nlm.nih.gov/pmc/articles/PMC4531371/.)

predesigned RNA sequence—"guiding" RNA (gRNA), within a longer RNA scaffold. The role of the latter is to direct Cas9 "scissors" to the exact location in the DNA of interest and modify it as desired. The CRISPR/Cas9 gene editing approach has transformed the biomedical research field forever. Compared with its "predecessors," such as zinc finger nucleases (ZFNs) and transcription activator-like effector nucleases (TALENs), the CRISPR-Cas9 system is simpler, more precise, and relatively cheaper, making it an ideal vehicle for "playing with genome." On October 10, 2018, the FDA announced that it has lifted the clinical hold and accepted the Investigational New Drug (IND) application for CTX001 for the treatment of sickle cell disease (SCD), the first CRISPR product.

With a number of existing strategies to influence the immune systems, such as using checkpoint inhibitors, vaccines, and monoclonal antibodies, it is the chimeric antigen receptor (CAR) T-cell therapy where a patient's own immune cells (or cells from another donor) are removed and modified, so that they can recognize and attack the patient's particular cancer. The engineered CAR T-cells are then grown in the lab to reach billions in numbers, followed by infusion back into the patient's body. The CAR T-cell technology has already proved to be extremely promising in the case of hard-to-treat lymphoma and is considered an ultimate future of the immunotherapy field. The FDA has approved two CART products.

1.1.2 Microbiome

The microbiome trend is growing rapidly and can possibly become one of the major game-changers in the biopharmaceutical industry. Microbiota is the ecosystem of more than 100 trillion microorganisms living inside our body or on the skin, coexisting naturally with human organism and performing vital functions such as the synthesis of vitamins, digestion, and taking part in the development of the immune system. The versatility of genes of the microbiota—microbiome—attracts the increasing interest of research community and biotech companies, as they try to develop new therapies or even find novel antibiotics by using the understanding of how our own bacteria contribute to diseases, immune responses, and the overall condition of an organism.

1.1.3 Antibiotics

The efforts for the discovery of new antibiotics have changed significantly after a long silent period. Over the last several years, the main drivers for the revived interest are the new stimuli created by the government and private organizations. Examples in the United States include the Generating Antibiotic Incentives Now (GAIN) Act of 2012 and a more recent qualified infectious disease product (QIDP) designation for antibiotics and antifungals, which provides new candidates with priority review and five additional years of market exclusivity when approved. Further support could come from the 21st Century Cures Act, approved by the House in July 2015, which includes the Antibiotic Development to Advance Patient Treatment (ADAPT) Act that permits the FDA to approve antibacterial drugs to treat serious or life-threatening infections, based on small clinical trials.

The increasing need for new antibiotics and new incentives available for business stimulate new biotech startups to emerge. Some of the recent examples include Forge Therapeutics (small molecule inhibitors of LpxC, a zinc metalloenzyme in gram-negative bacteria), Cidara Therapeutics (immunotherapy platform to fight bacterial infections), Visterra (antibody–drug conjugate therapy), Tetraphase Pharmaceuticals, Macrolide Pharmaceuticals, Iterum Therapeutics, Spero Therapeutics, and Entasis Therapeutics.

1.1.4 Artificial Intelligence

Besides the mechanical approaches to drug discovery, the functional classification of what constitutes a drug has also changed exponentially, from gene-driven therapies to artificial intelligence (AI)-based treatment modalities. We have now entered an era that was impossible to visualize even a decade ago.

The AI and machine learning advances have already been in practical use for some time in many industries, including smart cars, natural language processing (NLP), image recognition, smart online search and recommendations, fraud detection, financial trading, weather forecasting, personal and data security, and chatbots, to name a few. However, the biopharmaceutical industry is just beginning to adopt the new computational technologies, though quite rapidly.

1.1.5 Marijuana

The legalization of marijuana in the United States and the use of marijuana for recreational use in Canada have sparked a growing interest of investors, who now turn their focus to the small—but rapidly expanding—medical marijuana industry. It is estimated that the global market for medical marijuana could reach $50 billion by 2025.

While United States is now the biggest market for medical-grade cannabis, Israel is pushing hard to position itself as a global player in this rapidly growing area of biopharmaceutical research. It is reported that about 120 research programs, including clinical trials looking at the effects of cannabis on autism, epilepsy, psoriasis, and tinnitus, are active in Israel.

The FDA has not approved marijuana as a safe and effective drug for any indication. The agency has, however, approved one specific drug product that contains the purified substance cannabidiol, one of more than 80 active chemicals in marijuana, for the treatment of seizures associated with Lennox-Gastaut syndrome or Dravet syndrome in patients 2 years of age and older. The FDA has also approved two drugs containing a synthetic version of a substance that is present in the marijuana plant and one other drug containing a synthetic substance that acts similarly to compounds from marijuana but is not present in marijuana. The FDA is aware that there is considerable interest in the use of marijuana to attempt to treat a number of medical conditions, including, for example, glaucoma, AIDS wasting syndrome, neuropathic pain, cancer, multiple sclerosis, chemotherapy-induced nausea, and certain seizure disorders.

1.1.6 Target-Based Discovery

A vital part of any small-molecule drug discovery program is hit exploration—the identification of those starting point molecules that would embark on a journey toward successful medications (however, they rarely survive this journey)—via numerous optimization, validation, and testing stages. The key element of hit exploration is the access to an expanded and chemically diverse space of drug such as molecules to choose candidates from, especially for probing novel target biology. Given that the existing compound collections at the hands of pharma were built in part based on the small-molecule designs targeting known biological targets, new biological targets require new designs and new ideas instead of recycling.

Target-based drug discovery has enabled a great expansion of chemotypes and pharmacophores available for the medicinal chemist during the past three decades. New techniques such as HTS, fragment-based screening (FBS), crystallography in combination with molecular modeling, and combinatorial and parallel chemistry have created a considerable diversity of chemical lead structures well beyond the known natural products and ligands used as chemical starting points for drug discovery in the past. Moreover, this wealth of chemotypes can now be used as a source for tool compounds to study unexplored biological space and find new drug targets or for phenotypic screening by using systems-based approaches to identify drug candidates in a target-agnostic manner.

1.1.7 High-Through Screening

Typically, the libraries are composed of the compounds synthesized over time by individual companies and influenced by a company's history; for example, Novartis has a large number of ergot compounds in its library, and Roche would have many benzodiazepines. However, as many companies work on similar targets or scaffolds, there must also be some overlap between the libraries. These libraries are a key component of the success of pharmaceutical companies; however, they have once been in danger of getting lost. At the time when combinatorial chemistry became possible in the 1980s, eventually allowing the rapid synthesis of millions of compounds, it was thought that all possible compounds could be made when needed by starting from individual scaffolds, and the historical libraries were neglected for a while. However, it became apparent in HTS that the hit rate, when using these combinatorial libraries, was distinctly lower than that with the historical libraries. One reason for this was that combinatorial libraries were strongly dependent on chemical parameters, such as the possibility to do chemistry with molecules attached on beads rather than on potential biological activity alone. This insight led to a revalorization of the collection of historical compounds that had been made for pharmacological activity. It also led some companies to maintain and expand their natural-compound libraries, as these can be seen as compounds selected for biological activity for hundreds of millions of years. Medically useful compounds from natural substances are described previously. Today, the realization that even the millions of compounds available cover only a small part of the biologically active compound universe makes it important to continue the efforts to diversify our libraries, as repeatedly few or no ligands are found in the existing libraries for some newly discovered targets.

A specific variant of HTS is FBS. It is based on the idea that smaller molecules (usually with molecular weights less than 250 Da) are better suited to sample the chemical space, because it is much less complex for small molecules than it is for the bigger ones. Hits are generally more frequent but may bind only weakly to the biological target, which requires growing them or combining them to produce a lead with a high affinity. So far, the only successful example of this relatively new technology is the BRAF V600E mutant kinase inhibitor vemurafenib. The underlying chemotype was discovered by FBS, using a panel of recombinant kinases. The 7-azaindole compound was subsequently optimized to the final inhibitor by conventional medicinal chemistry methods.

1.1.8 Rational Drug Design

The renin inhibitor aliskiren has been approved for the treatment of hypertension in 2007. Renin is an aspartic protease that catalyzes the rate-limiting step in the renin–angiotensin system. Aliskiren is the product of rational drug design, utilizing the inhibitory principle of pepstatin, a naturally occurring hexa-peptide that contains the unusual γ-amino acid statin. The statin-based inhibitory principle was grafted onto small peptide-like compounds derived from the natural renin substrate, and these compounds were further optimized to the final drug by using structural information.

1.1.9 Target Family Knowledge

Leveraging target family knowledge is another way of generating chemical starting points for targets that are members of larger protein families such as kinases, proteases, E3 ligases, and G-protein-coupled receptors. The BCR-ABL kinase inhibitor imatinib, which revolutionized the treatment of chronic myelogenous leukemia (CML), was discovered based on an aminopyrimidine lead compound that was originally identified in a screen for the inhibitors of protein kinase C. Chemical optimization toward BCR-ABL selectivity and oral bioavailability led to the final molecule.

1.1.10 DNA-Encoded Library Technology

An alternative approach to access new drug-like chemical space for hit exploration is to use DNA-encoded library technology (DELT). Owing to the "split-and-pool" nature of DELT synthesis, it becomes possible to make huge numbers of compounds in a cost- and time-efficient manner (millions to billions of compounds).

Despite its uncertainty of the mechanism of action, the interest in RNA targeting remains high. DNA stores the information for protein synthesis, and RNA carries out the instructions encoded in DNA, leading to protein synthesis in ribosomes. While a majority of drugs is directed at targeting proteins responsible for a disease, sometimes it is not enough to suppress the pathogenic processes. It seems like a smart strategy to start earlier in the process and influence RNA before proteins are even synthesized, therefore substantially influencing the translation process of genotype to unwanted phenotype (disease manifestation).

1.1.11 Phenotype

Many drugs are discovered using phenotypic screening than target-based approaches. Beyond just comparing phenotypic and target-based approaches, there is a clear trend toward more complex cellular assays, for example, going from immortal cell lines to primary cells, patient cells, co-cultures, and three-dimensional (3D) cultures. The experimental setup is also becoming increasingly sophisticated, going far beyond univariate readouts toward observing changes in subcellular compartments, single-cell analysis, and even cell imaging.

The simplest phenotypic screens employ cell lines and monitor a single parameter such as the cellular death or the production of a particular protein. High-content screening where changes in the expression of several proteins can be monitored simultaneously is also often used.

1.1.12 Biologics

Modern molecular biology techniques have also expanded the drug space beyond traditional synthetic small-molecular-weight compounds and have enabled the design, production, and development of biologic molecules such as drugs. Of the 624 drugs approved by the FDA over the past 20 years, 84 were biologics. However, their impact for the pharmaceutical industry has been even bigger than these numbers suggest, as most of the top-selling drugs are biologics. So far, these drugs were dominated by antibodies, soluble receptor constructs, immunoglobulin fusion proteins, and secreted naturally occurring proteins. The most prominent examples are tumor necrosis factor (TNF) alpha-blocking antibodies (infliximab and adalimumab) and the soluble TNF receptor fusion protein (etanercept) for the treatment of rheumatoid arthritis, the anti-CD20 antibody rituximab for non-Hodgkin's lymphoma, the antivascular endothelial growth factor A (VEGF-A) antibody bevacizumab for colorectal and other cancers, and the antihuman epidermal growth factor receptor 2 (HER2) antibody trastuzumab for the treatment of breast cancer. Beyond these "classical" drugs, the biologics space has grown over recent years, for example, by the introduction of antibody–small-molecular-weight-drug conjugates and bispecific antibodies, and is likely to continue to grow at a rapid pace over the coming years. The advantages of biologics are their high affinity for and specificity to their targets, but so far, they are mostly limited to secreted or cell surface targets.

1.1.13 Botanicals

It is likely that humans have used plants as medicine for as long as we have existed. Archeological excavations dated as early as 60,000 years ago have found remains of medicinal plants, such as opium poppies, ephedra, and cannabis. Since the beginning, humans have experimented with plants to learn how they can help us heal. In essence, humans have been involved for thousands of years in a vast "clinical trial" with medicinal plants. The wisdom that resulted from this global experiment is a large part of our history of healing and healthcare. In many early cultures, the knowledge of a plant's curative properties came through the practice of Shamanism, which is a kind of spirit medicine still practiced in many parts of the world. Some Shamans communicate with certain plants ("plant teachers") to access the knowledge about other plants and healing techniques. As the knowledge from Shamanism and other practical experimentation grew, herbalists began to catalog their knowledge of medicinal plants.

One of the oldest written records on medicinal plants, dated 1500 B.C., is the Egyptian Ebers Papyrus. In India, the Charaka Samhita, dated 700 B.C., documented the uses of more than 300 medicinal plants. Throughout much of history, humans believed that the "vital spirit" of the plant contributed to its therapeutic effect. But in the early 1800s, scientists isolated morphine from opium, which led to the belief (in the West at least) that a single, non-living compound in a plant was responsible for its healing properties. This, in turn, helped to create the biomedical model of pharmacotherapy that remains in medicine today. In this model, plants are seen simply as the source of a single chemical that targets a single receptor site or other part of the body and fixes the individual's health problem.

Eventually, most scientists believed that there was no need to use plants in drugs, because chemists could synthesize compounds that were more potent (and often more toxic) than the natural products offered by nature. Now, most pharmaceuticals are synthetic compounds. But note that the structure of the synthetic pharmaceuticals often resembles that of the natural molecules; 11% of the 252 drugs considered essential by the World Health Organization are exclusively derived from flowering plants.

The 1990s witnessed a swing back toward a more holistic perspective in medicine, with less reliance on potent drugs that often have serious side effects. This change contributed to a renewed interest in botanical medicines that generally have fewer risks than pharmaceutical drugs. In 1994, in response to the overwhelming public demand, the federal government passed the Dietary Supplement Health and Education Act (DSHEA). This act allowed botanical medicines to be sold as "dietary supplements" as long as the manufacturers did not make any health claims. (Note that this provision can be somewhat confusing and puts the burden on consumers to research the dietary supplements themselves.) In 2007, the Food and Drug Administration (FDA) announced a final rule establishing current good manufacturing practice requirements for dietary supplements. The final rule requires manufacturers to report all adverse events to the FDA, as well as to evaluate the identity, purity, quality, strength, and composition of its dietary supplements. This change places more accountability on the industry and should increase consumers' confidence in the quality of dietary supplements, according to the FDA.

Between 1990 and 1997, the use of botanical medicines in the United States increased by 380%. By 2010, the global retail sale of botanical dietary supplements amounted to more than $25 billion. Outside the United States, the World Health Organization reports that 75%–85% of the world's population continues to rely on botanical medicines dispensed by traditional healers for primary healthcare, as they have always done.

In 2004, the FDA established an industrial guideline for botanical drugs (Botanical Drug Guidance) as an effort to take the initiative in the botanical drug market. The first botanical drug approved by the FDA was Veregen® (MediGene, Inc.), a treatment for genital and perianal warts that is derived from green tea. A number of years later, the FDA approved another New Drug Application (NDA) for the drug Fulyzaq™ (Napo Pharmaceuticals), an indicator drug for human immunodeficiency virus (HIV)-associated diarrhea, extracted from the blood-red latex of the South American croton tree. GW Pharmaceuticals, an English company, developed Sativex (Oromucosal Spray), a marijuana extract efficacious for rigidity due to multiple sclerosis. GW Pharmaceuticals raised $11 million with Sativex. In Europe, they use the term herbal medicinal product (HMP) to encompass all drugs that contain one of more kind of herbal substances in the herbal preparation. The Chinese developed Traditional Chinese Medicine (TCM), a prescription of their traditional medicines, based on their own experiences of its usage, and eastern ideas.

There have been numerous attempts to bring botanical drugs to the market through FDA approval, including more than 500 pre-IND meetings and IND applications, with limited success in reaching the final NDA stage. In fact, only two NDAs have been approved by the FDA so far. The FDA requires "adequate and well-controlled" multicenter clinical studies on any new drug candidate to document and support its safety and efficacy and imposes the maximum level of scrutiny prior to approval. It is crucial for these efficacy studies to have a well-defined target population (according to the FDA protocol's eligibility criteria), proper experimental controls (such as placebo or active treatment), appropriate outcome measures (agreed upon by the FDA), independent monitoring, and accurate analysis. Consequently, the single most common reason that any new drug candidate, including botanical drugs, fails to reach the NDA step is the failure to present statistically significant evidence for having efficacies of clinical relevance. Unrealistic expectations are often set forth by drug sponsors with insufficient experience with a drug development program, for multiple reasons, and the resulting miscommunication could hinder the drug approval process. For one, the initial stages of IND development are relatively less strict, and this may falsely suggest to new drug sponsors that botanical drugs, compared with conventional synthetic drugs, are less rigorously evaluated by the FDA. Another reason for drug sponsors to have unrealistic expectations is the confusion that arises from the lack of internationally standardized regulatory requirements for botanicals. In other words, many non-U.S. botanical drug sponsors, especially those that have no experience in fielding a drug development operation in the United States, are not aware of the practical differences in regulations between the United States and a foreign market. As an anecdote, some sponsors do not reconcile the fact that "raw data" (chemistry, nonclinical safety testing, or clinical study databases), instead of data summaries or "expert" opinion, is required by U.S. regulations.

1.2 The Preformulation Focus

While the nature of drugs has changed rapidly, the science of preformulation remains traditional—to deliver, we must first know what we are delivering. The drugs developed today fall into three main categories: small molecules, large molecules, and botanical extracts. The preformulation work required for each category is quite different from the others. The classic small-molecule chemistry involves the measurement of solubility, pK_a, crystallinity, polymorphism, and so on. For large molecules, particularly proteins and peptides, often, the 3D structure or even interaction with formulation components requiring a four-dimensional (4D) evaluation of drugs in solution must be studied. Botanical extracts, the oldest class of drugs, are now the newest category for the preformulation scientist, as the regulatory authorities such as the U.S. FDA and the European Medicines Agency (EMA) have established guidelines for their approval. For botanical drugs (often called phytomedicines in Europe), the fingerprinting methods using thin-layer chromatography (TLC), infrared (IR), or mass spectrometry (MS) are more relevant.

The preformulation of botanical drugs presents a different set of understanding; the uncertainty of the chemical or biological structures involved, the use of extracts that are difficult to characterize, and the variability of the cultivar involved, all offer many scientific challenges. However, these challenges also offer many new opportunities for bringing in new science that will allow us to better understand how drugs work.

1.3 Development Phases

The development of NAEs undergoes a lengthy and expensive cycle that varies greatly depending on the type of drug developed. What follows is a typical development cycle.

1.3.1 Stage 1: Lead Finding or Establishing Directions (1–2 Years)

These are studies to understand how alteration of a biological function or mechanism would create a therapeutically useful entity or process. The strategic research of a particular company is usually guided by factors such as its inherent research competence and expertise, therapeutic areas of unmet medical need, and market potential. Market potential is the strongest motivation, and as a result, companies invest heavily in specific therapy areas. It is not difficult to label companies as cardiovascular, anticancer, endocrine, or other such focused companies. It takes years, often decades, to pool the scientific and clinical expertise that would provide the combination of elements necessary for efficient new discoveries. However, in recent years, many large companies have begun to look outside for new drug leads; smaller research companies have often proven more efficient. Outsourcing of research, even at the level of research lead compounds, is now a common place, and companies such as Abbott Laboratories have developed an expertise in securing new drugs from the outside vendors. The in-house expertise development is limited not only to scientific expertise to provide a specific direction but also at times to a specific type of product, such as biological drugs versus the small molecules, innovative drug delivery systems versus the traditional systems, and so on.

It is not uncommon for large companies to suddenly establish a direction through serendipitous discoveries. Alexander Fleming discovered penicillin as a result of "serendipity." Although many of the drugs that are in use today have been discovered in this way, it is a difficult route for the pharmaceutical industry to follow and breaks are few and far between. More recently, the discovery that phosphodiesterase type 5 inhibitor (originally tested as antihypertensive agents) can be a good candidate for male erectile dysfunction has changed the focus of research at Pfizer and, as a result, at several other companies.

1.3.2 Stage 2: Candidate Drug Screening (1–10 Years)

In the previous step (stage 1), a particular biological mechanism is identified or targeted; the phase that follows it involves the identification of chemicals or modalities that would interfere or interact with it and thereby identify what the industry calls "leads." This stage requires extensive screening for biological activity, a process that used to be tedious and slow; however, over the last decade, the use of techniques such as "combinatorial chemistry" and automated HTS has made it possible to identify a large number of synthetic or biosynthetic molecules.

Organizations may differ in library acquisition methods (e.g., synthesis vs. purchase), compound inclusion criteria, synthesis methodology, or how they mine their collections to uncover leads. The rationale, however, remains constant: to find new, patentable structures as efficiently as possible. Automated synthesis and HTS, pioneered during the 1990s, enabled companies to synthesize, test, and maintain compound libraries populated with hundreds of thousands—even millions—of unique compounds. Automation opened the door to new chemistry and a very large number of compounds, with a typical large pharmaceutical company possessing between 1 million and 10 million compounds in its various compound collections. The reliance on large libraries has now become an effort with diminishing returns. Now, outsourcing the lead compounds appears more plausible. This allows greater molecular diversity, expanding what may end up as a myopic view of a company. Companies such as Abbott Laboratories have done well in emphasizing chemical diversity. As combinatorial chemistry became more automated and specialized, companies created separate groups to handle synthesis, library acquisition, and compound management. Aventis, for example, maintains a 60-person combinatorial chemistry group in Tucson, Arizona, that feeds libraries of various sizes to the rest of the company. Other firms take a more traditional view, preferring not to segregate discovery-related chemical competencies. Like most large discovery organizations, Roche constructs libraries to target gene families and protein targets or to expand the chemical diversity of the company's compound collection. Roche's lead-generation strategy includes acquiring libraries from specialist compound suppliers, contracting with external partners for library synthesis, and developing libraries in-house. Roche's view on library size is in line with the current thinking, and Roche has gradually moved away from very large compound libraries. Roche uses all modern synthetic tools, including parallel synthesis, combinatorial chemistry, and solid-phase methods, principally (although not limited to) solid-phase reagents and scavengers in the latter. Resin-bound synthesis is also used but only in situations where the technique can offer an advantage such as when very large numbers of related structures are desired. In today's discovery paradigm, the prime focus is more toward activity than on numbers of compounds.

Today, the pendulum has swung back toward rational design. Large libraries, despite their waning appeal, are, however, still in demand from specialty synthesis vendors. The hit rate can be improved when refined compound libraries are created from an existing hit through designing libraries for a given chemotype or pharmacophore, which amounts to the second-generation combinatorial methods coupled with computational chemistry.

Many large companies do not purify individual compounds in 100,000-entry libraries, instead preferring to bias reaction pathways toward products that are reasonably pure. Eventually, when discovery chemists settle on focused panels of between 200 and 1000 compounds, they rely on a number of tools to help them clean up these smaller libraries. One method is solid-phase scavenger reagents, which can soak up substantial amounts of impurities and side products and even drive reactions toward completion by shifting equilibrium. Simple anion- or cation-exchange resins are popular for removing anionic or cationic species, respectively. Scavengers work well to remove major impurities from individual reactions, but top-tier libraries in the 200–1000 compounds range probably require more careful cleaning up. Newer techniques such as solution-phase mixture synthesis obviate the problems associated with solid-phase synthesis, since the kinetics are easier to study in homogeneous systems.

Genomics is emerging as a useful technique in the drug selection process and has begun to play a significant role in the identification of lead compounds.

The distinct phases of stage 2 include the following:

- *Research planning*: This may involve classical structure–activity correlation studies, rational drug design modeling, HTS of libraries obtained by combinatorial chemistry, leads from natural sources, and so on.
- *Obtaining test compounds or samples*: Laboratory-scale preparation, preparation of compounds or sample libraries, determination of in vitro or animal models to test activity, and setting up of HTS.
- *Screening*: Basic pharmacological and biochemical screening. This involves the selection of "hits" and identification of active compounds. It is at this stage that the patent application for the compound will normally be filed. However, the strategies on the timing of patent filing will be discussed later.
- Preformulation studies consist of all that it takes to characterize a drug substance to enable its formulation into a practical drug delivery system. The preformulation studies begin immediately after a drug molecule (at this stage a lead) has been recognized. The process of LO integrates preformulation studies to ensure that all optimal forms of the drug (e.g., salt and crystalline forms) have been identified.

1.3.3 Stage 3: Candidate Drug Selection (1–2 Years)

With a solid chemical lead on hand, companies can create compounds with more optimal characteristics—pharmacological and formulation compatible forms that lead to nomination candidates. Ideally, the nominated candidate would have the following features:

- A simple structure
- No chiral centers

- Fewer steps in synthesis
- Passes carcinogenicity, mutagenicity, and lethal dose 50 (LD50) level testing
- Nonhygroscopic
- Crystalline with sufficient solid-state stability
- Possible to be administered orally, with sufficient bioavailability
- No strong colors or odors
- Compatible with standard excipients

Obviously, not all conditions are met, but by every compound we keep this direction in mind, it is easier to sift through many possibilities offered. It requires testing a range of selected compounds in in vitro and in vivo animal studies, and thus, preformulation work gets combined with biopharmaceutic studies to identify product design issues.

One of the major factors that often slows down the preformulation studies is the availability of a sufficient quantity of a compound at this stage, especially if biopharmaceutic studies are conducted; as a result, methods that would utilize the smallest quantity of the substance need to be devised; this is amply emphasized throughout the testing phases in this book. Another factor that often slows down the work at this stage is the often-misplaced importance on validated test methods and documentation; while this is desired, the perennial shortage of manpower requires that some things take secondary importance.

1.3.4 Stage 4: Preclinical Studies (1–2 Years)

Preclinical trials (4–6 years):

- Pre-IND meetings with the FDA
- *Preclinical trials stage I*: Acute toxicity, detailed pharmacological studies (main effect, side effect, and the duration of effect), analytical methods for active substance, and stability studies
- *Preclinical trials stage II*: Pharmacokinetics (absorption, distribution, metabolism, and excretion), subchronic toxicity, teratogenicity, mutagenicity, the scale-up of synthesis, the development of the final dosage form, and the production of clinical samples (Chemistry, Manufacturing, and Control [CMC] section for the FDA)

1.3.5 Stage 5: Phase I Clinical Studies (1–2 Years)

This is the stage of proof of concept or phase I testing to understand how the candidate drug is absorbed and metabolized in healthy human volunteers before testing it in patients. Often small-scale studies are done in patients when the cost factors are high, to make sure that there is sufficient indication for the drug's utility. There are significant differences in regulatory filings at this stage; in the United States, a fully approved IND is required, whereas in Europe, these filings are not required. Also, once an IND has been filed with the U.S. FDA, any study conducted overseas comes under the purview of this IND. Some companies may therefore decide to conduct their phase I studies prior to filing INDs in the United States to circumvent the issue of informing the FDA of their work. However, where the safety may be an issue, the U.S. law prohibits testing of drugs outside of the United States, to overcome the barrage of testing done by the big pharma on new molecules in non-U.S. subjects, some with disastrous results. Incidentally, this restriction applies only to the U.S. companies; other companies can still do such studies without penalty.

1.3.6 Stage 6: Phase II and Phase III Studies and Launch (4–6 Years)

The longer-term safety and clinical studies come under phases II and III, wherein patients suffering from the disease are studied. In phase II studies, the goal is to perform studies on different dose ranges in perhaps a few hundred patients to evaluate the effectiveness of the drug and its common side effects. It is at this stage that commercial formulation is developed and its scale-up is optimized. This is necessary because whatever formulation goes into phase III trials becomes the final formulation. In phase III studies, several thousand patients may be involved. Most regulatory authorities require sufficient data to demonstrate the safety and efficacy, and almost always, it is a mutually agreed-upon limit to which the drug companies are required to conduct the studies. The EMA has started a program of technical consultation, wherein for a sizeable fee of around $150,000, companies can sit down with the review staff and fine-tune their protocols; the investment is worth the effort. Once the regulatory authorities declare an application to be approvable, a marketing authorization request is made, and trucks are loaded pending issuance of the letter of approval that may have cost companies hundreds of million dollars.

- Sequence of clinical trials (4–6 years):
  - *Phase I*: Tolerance in healthy volunteers, pharmacokinetics in man, and supplementary animal pharmacology
  - *Phase II*: First controlled trials on efficacy in patients, dose range studies, chronic toxicity, and carcinogenicity studies in animals
  - *Phase III*: Large-scale trial at several centers for the final establishment of therapeutic profile (indications, dosages and types of administration, contraindications, and side effects), proof of efficacy and safety in the long-term administration, the demonstration of therapeutic advantages in comparison with known drugs, and the clarification of interactions with other medication
- Registration, launch, and sales (2–3 years):
  - *Registration with health authorities*: Documentation of all relevant data; expert opinions on clinical trials and toxicology; preparation for launch; information for doctors, wholesalers, and pharmacists; training of sales staff; preparation of packaging and package inserts; and dispatch of samples
  - *Launch and sales*: Production and packaging of the final form and quality control

1.3.7 Stage 7: Postmarket Surveillance (3–5 Years)

Although the intent of larger phase III trials is to bring out any statistically driven side effects, it is impossible to predict them even with several thousand patients. Phase IV studies continue to collect clinical efficacy and toxicity data; the pharmacovigilance program required by the EMA is one such example. It is important to recognize that it is during this phase of studies that drugs are recalled. The most recent example of the recall of the cyclooxygenase (COX)-2 selective inhibitor medication Vioxx (generic drug name is rofecoxib) (Merck) in September 2004 shows the importance of this phase of study. Although the studies of phases I–III are expensive to conduct, a failed phase IV study can bankrupt companies.

Given the statistical reality that only one of the 5000 lead compounds reaches the market, the amortized cost over the entire development program has exceeded the billion-dollar mark for each new approval; however, for the molecule in question, it may range from $100 million to $300 million, depending on the complexity of the testing involved.

According to pharmaceutical research-based manufacturers (PhRMa), the representative body of the research-based pharmaceutical companies, in 2017, 20 top PhRMa member companies invested an estimated $100 billion in research to develop new treatments for diseases.

1.4 Phytomedicines

The search for and the exploitation of natural products and properties have been the mainstays of the biotechnology industries. However, natural product search and discovery are not synonymous with drug discovery. But, if we examine how novel natural product chemotypes along with interesting structures and biological activities continue to be reported, this becomes the mainstay of drug discovery, as it has been in the therapeutic areas, such as neurodegenerative disease, cardiovascular disease, most solid tumors, and immune-inflammatory diseases. Today, well over half of the drugs are either directly derived from biological sources or have been produced as a result of biodiversity evaluation. Antibiotics remain the largest sellers of all drugs. Significantly, however, the reported discovery of microbial metabolites with nonantibiotic activities has increased progressively over the past 30 years and now exceeds that of antibiotic compounds.

One prerequisite of natural product discovery that remains paramount is the range and novelty of molecular diversity. This diversity surpasses that of combinatorial chemical libraries and consequently provides unique lead compounds for drug and other developments. Newly discovered bioactive products do not usually become drugs per se but may enter a chemical transformation program in which the bioactivity and pharmacodynamic properties are modified to suit particular therapeutic needs. In recent years, most regulatory authorities worldwide have carved out a path to approve natural products, without having to identify the exact active ingredients of their specifications. The use of markers is suggested, and greater emphasis is placed on characterization of extracts. This means a greater involvement of the preformulation group in drug discovery for natural or botanical products. Recent efforts to harmonize standards are evident from the monographs developed by the American Herbal Pharmacopoeia. Another major effort is the European Scientific Cooperative on Phytotherapy (ESCOP). It was founded in June 1989 as an umbrella organization representing national phytotherapy associations across Europe, especially in their discussions with European medicine regulators. Since 1996, it has been a company in the United Kingdom. Its goals are to advance the scientific status of phytomedicines and to assist with the harmonization of their regulatory status at the European level; to develop a coordinated scientific framework to assess phytomedicines; to promote the acceptance of phytomedicines, especially within general medical practice; to support and initiate clinical and experimental research in phytotherapy; to improve and extend the international accumulation of scientific and practical knowledge in the field of phytotherapy; to support all appropriate measures that will secure optimum protection for those who use phytomedicines; and to produce reference monographs on the therapeutic use of plant drugs. The ESCOP has published a large number of monographs and has established uniform standards for several botanical drugs (Table 1.1).

The search for drugs through botanical sources has its roots in the realization that it is unlikely that some of the most successful drugs could have been discovered by

TABLE 1.1

List of Monographs of Phytomedicines Available from European Scientific Cooperative on Phytotherapy

Absinthii herba	Alexandrian senna pods
Aloe capensis	Aniseed
Anisi fructus	Arnica flower
Arnicae flos	Bearberry leaf
Blackcurrant leaf	Cape aloes
Caraway	*Carvi fructus*
Cascara	*Centaurii herba*
Centaury	*Crataegi folium cum flore*
Dandelion leaf	Dandelion root
Devil's claw	*Echinacea pallida radix*
Echinacea purpurea radix	*Eucalypti aetheroleum*
Eucalyptus oil	Fennel
Feverfew	Frangula bark
Frangulae cortex	Garlic bulb
Gentian root	*Gentianae radix*
Ginger	Golden rod
Hamamelidis folium	Hamamelis leaf
Harpagophyti radix	Hawthorn leaf and flower
Hippocastani semen	Hop strobiles
Horse-chestnut seed	*Hyperici herba*
Iceland moss	Ispaghula
Ispaghula husk	Java tea
Juniper berries	*Juniperi fructus*
Lichen islandicus	*Lini semen*
Linseed	*Lupuli flos*
Matricaria flower	*Matricariae flos*
Meliloti herba	Melilotus
Melissa leaf	*Melissae folium*
Menthae piperitae aetheroleum	*Menthae piperitae folium*

(Continued)

TABLE 1.1 (*Continued*)

List of Monographs of Phytomedicines Available from
European Scientific Cooperative on Phytotherapy

Myrrh	*Myrrha*
Nettle leaf and herb	Nettle root
Allii sativi bulbus	*Ononidis radix*
Orthosiphonis folium	Pale coneflower root
Passiflora	*Passiflorae herba*
Peppermint Leaf	Peppermint oil
Plantaginis ovatae semen	*Plantaginis ovatae testa*
Polygalae radix	Primula root
Primulae radix	*Psyllii semen*
Psyllium seed	Purple coneflower root
Restharrow root	*Rhamni purshiani cortex*
Rhei radix	Rhubarb root
Ribis nigri folium	Rosemary
Rosmarini folium cum flore	Sage leaf
Salicis cortex	*Salviae folium*
Senega root	Senna leaf
Sennae folium	*Sennae fructus acutifoliae*
Sennae fructus angustifolia	*Solidaginis virgaureae herba*
St. John's wort	*Tanaceti parthenii herba/folium*
Taraxaci folium	*Taraxaci radix*
Thyme	*Thymi herba*
Tinnevelly senna pods	*Urticae folium/herba*
Urticae radix	*Uvae ursi folium*
Valerian root	*Valerianae radix*
Willow bark	Wormwood
Zingiberis rhizoma	

any process of rational or semirational design. For example, the mode of action of the immunosuppressants cyclosporin A and rapamycin is that both bind to *cis-trans* prolyl isomerase, but only cyclosporine A is involved in further steps of signal transduction cascades through calcineurin; this would be too complex to design on an a priori basis. Similarly, two of the most successful antimalarial drugs quinine and chloroquinine exert their effect by inhibiting the host-encoded functions rather than the activities encoded by *Plasmodium falciparum*. Chloroquine resistance in *P. falciparum* resides in a 36-kDa nucleotide sequence, which contains genes of unknown function, along with 40% of the *P. falciparum* genome. In the search for new classes of antibiotics over the last 25 years, traditional approaches have also failed to deliver new drugs fast enough to keep up with the loss of effectiveness of existing drugs against the increasingly resistant pathogens (95% of *Staphylococcus aureus* are penicillin resistant and 60% are methicillin resistant, and there are cases of vancomycin resistance in China, Japan, Europe, and the United States). The development of resistance may be followed by compensatory mechanisms to adjust for reduced fitness, which may then lock the resistance mechanism. The search for antibiotics through random screening seems to have been abandoned in view of the poor performance in finding leads in favor of rational, target-based approaches. Molecular biology, robotics, miniaturization, massively parallel preparation and detection systems, and automatic data analysis now dominate the search for drug discovery leads.

Natural product extracts and bacterial culture collections do not necessarily work well together on drug discovery platforms. The separation, identification, characterization, scale-up, and purification of natural products for large-scale libraries suitable for these HTS are daunting, and rational arguments for the selection of organisms and/or natural product molecules are often absent, especially given the poor taxonomic characterization of strains in natural product bacterial strain collections.

Many of these screening systems are not sufficiently robust to handle complex mixtures of natural products from ill-defined biological systems and may be inhibited by interactions with uncontrolled physicochemical conditions, simple toxic chemicals, and known bioactive compounds. This has led to significant efforts in rational drug design, combinatorial chemistry, peptide libraries, antibody libraries, combinatorial biosynthesis, and other synthetic and semisynthetic methods to provide clean inputs to screens. However, natural products are still unsurpassed in their ability to provide novelty and complexity. In the chemical screening of natural products, complex mixtures of metabolites from growth and fermentation are separated, purified, and identified using high-pressure liquid chromatography, diode array ultraviolet (UV)/visible spectra, and MS. Novel chemical structures are passed on for screening, now uncontaminated, with background interference from the original complex mixture, and built up into high-quality, characterized natural product libraries. This strategy suffers from poorly characterized culture collections, which makes the choice of organisms for screening difficult, and from the inability to control the expression of metabolic potential.

1.5 Recombinant Drugs

Recombinant DNA techniques coupled with the typing of human genes now allow the development of a new class of drugs, ranging from the expression of proteins to individualized drugs that would show specific response in patients. Once a biotechnological target has been identified, decisions must be made regarding the choice of the expression organism and the screening procedures to evaluate efficiency. Rules of thumb include relying on proven organisms such as actinomycetes, using taxon-chemistry and taxon-property databases to predict antibiotic potential, and focusing on novel and overlooked taxa. An example of the last consideration is the study of cyanobacteria to isolate the HIV-inactivating protein cyanovirin-N. There is a strong view that biopharmaceutical leads are more likely to be detected in cell function assays than in the in vitro assays. In this context, the construction of surrogate host cells for in vivo drug screening is an interesting development. For example, the ability of *Saccharomyces cerevisiae* to express heterologous proteins makes it an attractive option; it is used in screens based on substitution assays, differential expression assays, and transactivation assays, which are proved to be an effective route for drug discovery.

Considerable effort has been and is being expended in the development of screening assays, particularly as a response to the need for the evaluation of large numbers of samples in HTS and the expectation that many new targets will be identified in the wake of genome sequencing projects. High-throughput screening involves the robotic handling of very large numbers of candidate samples, the registering of appropriate signals from the assay system, and data management and interpretation. However, the advent of HTS, whereby lead discoveries may be identified in a matter of days from libraries of 103–105 compounds, may be limited by the provision of sufficient quantities of the assay components. The development of surrogate hosts, such as enzyme inhibition, receptor binding, and cell function assays, provides possible means of alleviating such bottlenecks.

A large number of drugs manufactured through recombinant methods are coming off patents, creating markets for biogeneric medicines.

WEB REFERENCES

1. Eder J, Herrling PL, Trends in modern drug discovery. *Handb Exp Pharmacol.* 2016;232:3–22. https://www.ncbi.nlm.nih.gov/pubmed/26330257.
2. Top 7 trends in pharmaceutical research in 2018, April 25, 2018. https://www.biopharmatrend.com/post/60-top-7-trends-in-pharmaceuticalresearch-in-2018-and-beyond/.
3. Nielson, K, Emerging Trends in Healthcare and Drug Development.
4. Trends in Drug Development.
5. Drug Discovery Market 2017. Latest trend, Demand, Development Status, Size, Share & 2022 Global Industry Growth Analysis Report.
6. Better Market Intelligence. https://offer.alpha-sense.com/better-market-intelligence-whitepaper-pharma?utm_campaign=Better%20Market%20Intelligence%20With%20 Smart%20Search&utm_source=FiercePharma&utm_medium=Display&utm_ term=WPv1&utm_content=Roller.

BIBLIOGRAPHY

Ahn K. The worldwide trend of using botanical drugs and strategies for developing global drugs. *BMB Rep.* 2017;50(3):111–116.

Amoroso L, Haupt R, Garaventa A, Ponzoni M. Investigational drugs in phase II clinical trials for the treatment of neuroblastoma. *Expert Opin Investig Drugs.* 2017;26(11):1281–1293.

Awad A, Trenfield SJ, Goyanes A, Gaisford S, Basit AW. Reshaping drug development using 3D printing. *Drug Discov Today.* 2018;23(8):1547–1555.

Berry BJ, Smith AST, Young JE, Mack DL. Advances and current challenges associated with the use of human induced pluripotent stem cells in modeling neurodegenerative disease. *Cells Tissues Organs.* 2018:1–19.

Brunetti J, Falciani C, Bracci L, Pini A. Models of in-vivo bacterial infections for the development of antimicrobial peptide-based drugs. *Curr Top Med Chem.* 2017;17(5):613–619.

Cal PM, Matos MJ, Bernardes GJ. Trends in therapeutic drug conjugates for bacterial diseases: A patent review. *Expert Opin Ther Pat.* 2017;27(2):179–189.

Cuykx M, Rodrigues RM, Laukens K, Vanhaecke T, Covaci A. In vitro assessment of hepatotoxicity by metabolomics: A review. *Arch Toxicol.* 2018;92(10):3007–3029.

Dai X, Theobard R, Cheng H, Xing M, Zhang J. Fusion genes: A promising tool combating against cancer. *Biochim Biophys Acta Rev Cancer.* 2018;1869(2):149–160.

Delogu GL, Matos MJ. Coumarins as promising scaffold for the treatment of age-related diseases—An overview of the last five years. *Curr Top Med Chem.* 2017;17(29):3173–3189.

Dorval T, Chanrion B, Cattin ME, Stephan JP. Filling the drug discovery gap: Is high-content screening the missing link? *Curr Opin Pharmacol.* 2018;42:40–45.

Farmakiotis D, Kontoyiannis DP. Epidemiology of antifungal resistance in human pathogenic yeasts: Current viewpoint and practical recommendations for management. *Int J Antimicrob Agents.* 2017;50(3):318–324.

Gothai S, Muniandy K, Gnanaraj C, Ibrahim IAA, Shahzad N, Al-Ghamdi SS, Ayoub N et al. Pharmacological insights into antioxidants against colorectal cancer: A detailed review of the possible mechanisms. *Biomed Pharmacother.* 2018;107:1514–1522.

Haasen D, Schopfer U, Antczak C, Guy C, Fuchs F, Selzer P. How phenotypic screening influenced drug discovery: Lessons from five years of practice. *Assay Drug Dev Technol.* 2017;15(6):239–246.

Hollingsworth SA, Dror RO. Molecular dynamics simulation for all. *Neuron.* 2018;99(6):1129–1143.

Järbe TUC, Raghav JG. Tripping with synthetic cannabinoids ("Spice"): Anecdotal and experimental observations in animals and man. *Curr Top Behav Neurosci.* 2017;32:263–281.

Khan H, Rengasamy KRR, Pervaiz A, Nabavi SM, Atanasov AG, Kamal MA. Plant-derived mPGES-1 inhibitors or suppressors: A new emerging trend in the search for small molecules to combat inflammation. *Eur J Med Chem.* 2018;153:2–28.

Laubach JP, Paba Prada CE, Richardson PG, Longo DL. Daratumumab, elotuzumab, and the development of therapeutic monoclonal antibodies in multiple myeloma. *Clin Pharmacol Ther.* 2017;101(1):81–88.

Law BYK, Wu AG, Wang MJ, Zhu YZ. Chinese medicine: A hope for neurodegenerative diseases? *J Alzheimers Dis.* 2017;60(s1):S151–S160.

Li J, Qiao Y, Wu Z. Nanosystem trends in drug delivery using quality-by-design concept. *J Control Release.* 2017;256:9–18.

Li W, Pang IH, Pacheco MTF, Tian H. Ligandomics: A paradigm shift in biological drug discovery. *Drug Discov Today.* 2018;23(3):636–643.

Meyer RJ. Commentary on R&D trends away from general medicine/cardiovascular drugs: Can the FDA help reverse the trend? *Clin Pharmacol Ther.* 2017;102(2):186–188.

Mukherjee PK, Harwansh RK, Bahadur S, Banerjee S, Kar A, Chanda J, Biswas S, Ahmmed SM, Katiyar CK. Development of ayurveda—Tradition to trend. *J Ethnopharmacol.* 2017;197:10–24.

Nguyen MA, Flanagan T, Brewster M, Kesisoglou F, Beato S, Biewenga J, Crison J et al. A survey on IVIVC/IVIVR development in the pharmaceutical industry—Past experience and current perspectives. *Eur J Pharm Sci.* 2017;102:1–13.

Polini A, Mercato LLD, Barra A, Zhang YS, Calabi F, Gigli G. Towards the development of human immune-system-on-a-chip platforms. *Drug Discov Today.* 2018.

Rameshrad M, Razavi BM, Hosseinzadeh H. Saffron and its derivatives, crocin, crocetin and safranal: A patent review. *Expert Opin Ther Pat.* 2018;28(2):147–165.

Ran X, Gestwicki JE. Inhibitors of protein-protein interactions (PPIs): An analysis of scaffold choices and buried surface area. *Curr Opin Chem Biol.* 2018;44:75–86.

Rashidi MR, Soltani S. An overview of aldehyde oxidase: an enzyme of emerging importance in novel drug discovery. *Expert Opin Drug Discov.* 2017;12(3):305–316.

Robinson SD, Undheim EAB, Ueberheide B, King GF. Venom peptides as therapeutics: Advances, challenges and the future of venom-peptide discovery. *Expert Rev Proteomics*. 2017;14(10):931–939.

Sadick NS, Callender VD, Kircik LH, Kogan S. New insight into the pathophysiology of hair loss trigger a paradigm shift in the treatment approach. *J Drugs Dermatol*. 2017;16(11):s135–s140.

Sanger GJ, Andrews PLR. A history of drug discovery for treatment of nausea and vomiting and the implications for future research. *Front Pharmacol*. 2018;9:913.

Takura T. An evaluation of clinical economics and cases of cost-effectiveness. *Intern Med*. 2018;57(9):1191–1200.

Xiao K, Sun J. Elucidating structural and molecular mechanisms of β-arrestin-biased agonism at GPCRs via MS-based proteomics. *Cell Signal*. 2018;41:56–64.

2

Intellectual Property Considerations

Intellectual property has the shelf life of a banana.

Bill Gates

2.1 Introduction

The development of new pharmaceutical- or biotechnology-derived products undergoes a lengthy and expensive cycle, which is described adequately elsewhere in the book. Given the cost of development now hovering around the billion-dollar mark for each new drug, amortized over all other molecules under development, the only way to protect this investment is to create intellectual property claims not only to the active molecule but also, where possible, to each and every step of its production, processing, and testing. Almost 4% of the development cost is spent on filing and prosecuting patents. Preformulation scientists play an important role in creating intellectual property, because at this stage, the specifications of the new drug entity are defined, and often, newer lead compounds are substituted.

Typically, the research-based pharmaceutical companies spend about 15%–20% of their total sales revenue on developing new drugs, as compared with less than 4% for the industry as a whole; the cost of patent protection ranges between 1% and 3% of the R&D expenditure. Successful patenting, patent protection, and exploitation of expired patents involve a complex interaction among scientists and lawyers. Generally, the development teams should have a basic understanding of the patenting process to be able to make the best use of legal expertise in the field; the more complex the field is, the more the input from scientists becomes valuable. In this chapter, I describe the fundamentals of patenting that I consider important enough for scientists to understand well.

2.2 Patenting Strategies

Pharmaceutical and biotechnology scientists face several major challenges in designing their research:

- Does the research create a product that is prohibited by statute to be patented? This includes a thought process, a law of physics, an object of little utility, or another prohibited area of patentability. Obviously, the end goal is not always to secure a patent for a product; a proprietary process need not be patented if it is possible to keep it protected, something that is becoming very difficult to ensure, as the information flow becomes easier between individuals and around the world.

- Is the research likely to lead to a novel product or a process meaning something that has never existed before? Novel is not necessarily patentable, as we go through the legality of the patenting process; this is, however, one of the fundamental requirements.

- Is the novel research unobvious to those with ordinary skill in the art? This aspect of patenting is most confusing and often leads to the most rejections of patent applications. Researchers need to study existing art (what is called prior art) before designing experiments to ensure that they can create sufficient features in the invention to take it out of the obviousness arena. What is needed here is a demonstration that there was an inventive step, or in ordinary words, something was actually discovered that was not something that could have been discovered easily. A lot of experimentation goes into demonstrating unusual results to obviate the assertion of obviousness by the patent examiners.

- Can the claim made withstand court challenge? Even though these areas of interpretations are beyond what a scientist would be expected to have any expertise in, a keen understanding of the scope of claims is essential; a patent with too broad a claim is not necessarily a good patent, nor is a patent with too narrow a claim. The patent disclosure must support the claim adequately.

- Does the disclosure in the patent meet the legal requirements of patent allowance? In the United States, the patentee must disclose a best mode, the best formula, and the best approach to use the research outcome. There is no need to disclose an industrial model, but there should be a workable model. Keeping the information out of a patent can be a double-edge sword.

- Is it possible to create a sequel to a successful research product? It is not unusual for the companies to keep some portions of the research aside and out of a patent to be able to claim it later. This can be a dangerous practice. If prior art appears in the interim, then all research is lost and even one's own patent will be taken as a prior art.

- Is it possible to continue the patent coverage by designing products around an issued patent? This is most critical to the pharmaceutical and biotechnology industries. Good examples of this practice include changes in the formulation to improve the product, just like Abbott did when its patent on calcitriol expired; the company changed the specification on the level of oxygen in the solution. What it meant was that there would be no generic equivalent to Abbott's calcitriol, though the generic forms may not be any less active. Smith Kline Beecham's remarkable patenting of the combination of amoxicillin and clavulanic is a good example of intelligent patenting; you will find not only patents for a specific combination of the two antibiotics but also a score of different dosage forms; one patent is based only on the hardness of the tablet. This type of research requires a keen understanding of the patenting process.

- Is it possible to invent around a patent or a publication? When sildenafil citrate became a success and statins became the choice of treatment for lowering cholesterol, the drug companies rushed to make similar products; obviously, there were problems in prior art. What is already disclosed cannot be obviated. The researchers are then faced with a challenge to find solutions novel enough to be patented; some degree of reverse engineering is required. However, as we see the results, they did succeed. But, with each patent issued, the field narrows as to what can be patented. Scientists often get bogged down with the science and do not realize that to receive a patent on an invention, there is no need to explain how it works. In fact, there need not even be an explanation about how it came into existence. Just the fact that there is a working example is sufficient. In many instances, even a working example is not required. A new drug may be subject to the Food and Drug Administration's (FDA's) comments before the United States Patent and Trademark Office allows the claims; however, it is not required of the patent office. On the other hand, the patent office need not accept the approval by the regulatory authorities as a proof of the utility, a key requirement for patentability.

Obviously, a productive researcher contributes to the company's profits. To achieve marketability and profitability from the research, the product must be either patentable or of a type that could not be reverse-engineered if proprietary techniques are relied upon. The challenges to scientists are great, with expanding technology and stiffer competition to produce new products. One way to meet these challenges head on is to understand the art and the science of patenting. Keeping abreast of the knowledge is critical, and scientists are strongly urged to hone their skills in the use of computers to search the literature.

2.2.1 Patenting Systems

A patent is a grant of exclusive rights given by the government for a limited time with respect to a new and useful invention—rights to prevent others from making or selling the invention in a limited territory, as defined by the patent-issuing authority. A patent is not a right to sell the invention. The word "patent" means "open," and the words "letters patent" mean an announcement made to all that the inventor has been awarded the rights to the invention. Open here means without having to break any seal, as was the custom in the decrees issued in the past by the sovereign governments. Note that "letters patent" are not restricted to inventions, as even today, these are issued to appoint judges in the United Kingdom. Historically, patents were issued on elaborate stationary, as they still are to some extent. The point about the rights to exercise an invention, vis-à-vis to prevent others from practicing, needs further elaboration. The new chemical entity (NCE) patent for sildenafil citrate expired in March 2003; the use and composition patents listed for sildenafil citrate in the Orange Book (FDA) extended to 2012 and 2019; 17 U.S. patents were issued to Pfizer on the various aspects of sildenafil citrate. A total of 44 patents making claims for sildenafil citrate covered its use in Tourette's syndrome, its chewing gum formulations that require chewing the gum for not less than 2 minutes, and other uses.

The example of erythropoietin demonstrates how the patent laws can create great difficulties for biogeneric offerings. A classic example of exploiting patenting systems is the patent on interferon, held by both Roche and Biogen; when the patent was filed, the patent office declared interference, meaning that similar inventions were submitted by two companies. Both Roche and Biogen fought it for decades while agreeing to cross license when the patent was pending; decades later, when the patent was issued, they agreed to cross license as well, resulting in an unprecedented protection of more than 35 years; this will likely be challenged in the courts.

2.2.2 What Is a Patent?

It is noteworthy that patents are awarded for things or "res" that must have some use; there need not be any rationale provided as to why an invention works; obviously, it must meet all statutory requirements to be eligible for patenting. The patent laws are extremely complex, often inexplicably irrational, and in almost all instances questionable in their enforcement.

The following definitions and terms are commonly used in describing patent laws:

- *Invention*: An invention is the conception of a new and useful article, machine, composition, or process.
- *Patent application*: A document describing an invention in detail, which is to be submitted to a patent office with the aim of obtaining a patent on the invention.
- *Patent*: Right of ownership granted by the government to a person that gives the owner the right to exclude others from making, selling, or using the claimed invention.
- *Reduction to practice*: An in-depth description of how the invention works, described in concrete terms.
- *Prior art*: The existing or public knowledge available before the date of an invention or more than 1 year prior to the first patent application date.
- *Utility*: This is the most common type of patent. It includes inventions that operate in a new and useful manner.
- *Design*: The emphasis of this type of patent is on the design of the invention and not on its functionality. What are important with this type of patent are the invention's unique ornamental and aesthetic properties.
- *Plant*: This type of patent includes new varieties of asexually reproduced plants.
- *Actual reduction to practice*: Constructing the machine or article, synthesizing the composition, or performing the method and testing sufficiently to demonstrate that the invention works for its intended purpose. Testing is NOT required if one with ordinary skills in the art would recognize that it will work.
- *Constructive reduction to practice*: Filing U.S. patent application—in compliance with the first paragraph of §112.
- *Diligence*: Working on reducing the invention to practice, or else, it is considered abandoned.

2.2.3 Patent Myths

The patenting of inventions is a complex process that has historically been confusing, particularly to the inventors who may not be practitioners of patent law. For example:

- Patents are valuable only if they can be used to protect a profit stream by excluding others from making, using, or selling whatever is covered by the patent's claims.
- A patent does not mean that the invention works as verified by the government; that is left for the licensors to evaluate. It is suspected that as many as 10% of all issued patents are invalid for being nonfunctional, as claimed.
- A Provisional Application is not "just describing the idea," "it is a complete application except for the required claim(s)." You may not change anything in the body of the application when you file the regular application if you want to take priority advantage.
- You cannot get a patent for an idea or mere suggestion. Patents are granted to people who (claim to) "invent or discover any new and useful process, machine, manufacture, or composition of matter, or any new and useful improvement thereof," to quote the essence of the U.S. statute governing patents. A complete and enabling disclosure is also required.
- A patent can be enforceable from the time it is issued till it expires, not necessarily 20 years. New rules provide some guarantee that the enforceable term of a utility patent will be at least 17 years and that some royalties may be collectable when a patent is published before it is issued. Design patents are good only for 14 years and cover only the ornamental appearance of the item and not its structure or functionality.
- A patent does not give the owner the exclusive right to make, use, and sell the invention; it gives its owner the right to EXCLUDE others from making, using, and selling exactly what is covered by the owner's patent claims. A holder of a prior patent with broader claims may prevent the inventor whose patent has narrower claims from using the inventor's own patent. A patent right is exclusory only.
- A U.S. patent is enforceable only in the United States. It can be used to stop others from importing what the patent covers into the United States, but people in other countries are free to make, use, and sell the invention anywhere else in the world where the inventor does not have a patent. This is the reason why one must consider filing a Patent Cooperative Treaty and follow it up with either individual state filings or consortium filing, such as the European Patent Office.
- A patent does not protect an invention, because only a patent in conjunction with a legal opinion of infringement will give the owner(s) of the patent the right to sue in a civil case against the alleged infringer. The U.S. government does not enforce patents (however, the Customs Service can help block infringing imports), and infringement of a patent is not a crime. The responsibility and all expenses for enforcing the rights granted by a patent (and securing Customs Service help) lie with the patent owner(s).

- Filing for a patent is not the only way to protect an invention. When properly used, the United States Patent and Trademark Office's Disclosure Document Program ($10), non-disclosure agreements (free), and provisional applications for patent ($80), along with maintaining good records and diligent pursuit, can keep your patenting rights intact until you do file.
- A patent attorney or agent is not needed to file your patent; an inventor may choose to go pro se (on his own). However, given the complexity of the law, advice from professionals always proves invaluable.

Of great importance to the pharmaceutical industry is the Drug Price Competition and Patent Restoration Act of 1984, commonly known as the Hatch-Waxman Act, which provided for extensions of patent terms for human drugs, food additives, and medical devices. The commercialization of this act had been delayed by regulatory procedures in the FDA, making registration easier for competitors when patent protection expires, and allowing that testing for regulatory approval involving a patented drug did not amount to patent infringement.

There are three principal requirements for an invention to be patented as set out in the European Patent Convention:

- That the invention must be new;
- That it must involve an inventive step; and
- That it must be capable of industrial application.

The same three requirements must be met in one form or another in the United States, Japan, and indeed in practically every country that has a patent system at all. Some countries and conventions exclude certain inventions, but these exclusions may be forbidden under the Trade-Related Aspects of Intellectual Property Rights section (TRIPS) of the World Trade Organization's regulations.

2.2.4 What Is Not Patentable?

There are certain specific exceptions to patentability, which apply whether or not the invention is capable of industrial application. Artistic works and esthetic creations are not patentable and are also generally not industrially applicable. Also, scientific theories and mathematical methods, the presentation of information, business methods, and computer programs are unpatentable; however, they may very well be applied in industry.

Animal and plant varieties are not patentable in countries adhering to the European Patent Commission; however, in the United States, plants may be protected either by normal utility patents or by special plant patents for plant varieties. In the United Kingdom and certain other European countries, new plant varieties, although not patentable, can be protected by plant breeders' rights granted under the International Union for the Protection of New Varieties of Plants (UPOV) convention. Transgenic plants and animals are in principle patentable only if they do not constitute a variety that might create a difficult and uncertain situation. A further exception applies to offensive, immoral, or antisocial inventions, which need not just be an article prohibited by the law. If it is abhorrent to society, it is unpatentable; however, it may be legal.

A portable nuclear device would be such an example. Also excluded are the inventions contrary to well-established natural laws, for example, a perpetual motion machine; however, the European Patent Commission does not spell it out like this.

2.3 Patent Search

The patent offices worldwide have opened their databases to the public; there is no better place to start the search for patentability than with these free databases; the same databases that provide additional services and literature search are packaged by other vendors. The United States Patent and Trademark Office (1) has created one of the world's largest electronic databases that includes every patent issued; recently, published applications are also available in the database. Scientists are strongly urged to develop expert skills in interacting with the database of the United States Patent and Trademark Office. The search at United States Patent and Trademark Office can be most beneficial if the scientist learns how to use the patent classification system. (Tutorials are available on the United States Patent and Trademark Office website; alternately, please consult *Filing Patents Online: A Professional Guide* by Sarfaraz K. Niazi, CRC Press 2002).

The U.S. Patent Office Classification 435 includes the following subcategories related to therapeutic proteins:

Class 435: Chemistry: Molecular Biology and Microbiology provides for methods of purifying, propagating, or attenuating a microorganism; for example, a virus, bacteria, etc., except for propagating a microorganism in an animal for the purpose of producing antibody-containing sera. Class 435 provides for methods of propagating animal organs, tissues, or cells, for example, blood and sperm, and culture media. Class 435 is the generic home for the processes of (*i*) analyzing or testing that involve a fermentation step or (*ii*) qualitative or quantitative testing for fermentability or fermentative power.

435: Chemistry: Molecular Biology and Microbiology, see appropriate subclasses for processes in which a material containing an enzyme or microorganism is used to perform a qualitative or quantitative measurement or test; for compositions or test strips for either of the stated processes; for the processes of making such compositions or test strips; for the processes of using micro-organisms or enzymes to synthesize a chemical product; for the processes of treating a material with microorganisms or enzymes to separate, liberate, or purify a pre-existing substance or to destroy hazardous or toxic wastes; for processes of propagating microorganisms; for processes of genetically altering a microorganism; for processes of tissue, organ, blood, sperm, or microbial maintenance; for processes of malting or mashing; for microorganisms, per se, and subcellular parts thereof; for recombinant vectors and their preparation; for enzymes, per se, compositions containing enzymes not otherwise provided for and processes of preparing and purifying enzymes; for compositions for microbial propagation; for apparatus for any of the processes of the class; for composting apparatus; and subclasses 4+ for in vitro processes in which there is a direct or indirect, qualitative or quantitative, measurement or test of a material that contains an enzyme or a microorganism (for the purposes of Class 435, microorganisms include bacteria, actinomycetales, cyanobacteria [unicellular algae], fungi, protozoa, animal cells, plant cells, and virus). Class 424 definition contains controlling statements on the class lines.

93.2: Genetically modified microorganisms, such as a cell and a virus (e.g., transformed, fused, hybrid, and the like): This subclass is indented under subclass 93.1. Subject matter involving a microorganism, cell, or virus, which (i) is a product of recombination, transformation, or transfection with a vector or a foreign or exogenous gene or (ii) is a product of homologous recombination if it is directed rather than spontaneous or (iii) is a product of fused or hybrid cell formation. (1) Note. Examples of subject matter included in this and the indented subclass are compositions containing microorganisms, cells, or viruses resulting from (i) a process in which the cellular matter of two or more fusing partners is combined, producing a cell, which initially contains the genes of both the fusing partners or (ii) a process in which a cell is treated with an immortalizing agent, which results in a cell that proliferates in long-term culture or (iii) a process involving recombinant DNA methodology. (2) Note. Excluded from this subclass are the products of unidentified or noninduced mutations; products of microbial conjugation, wherein specific genetic material is not identified and controlled; and products of natural, spontaneous, or arbitrary conjugation or recombination events. These products are not considered genetically modified for this subclass and therefore will be classified as unmodified microorganisms, cells, or viruses.

93.21: Eukaryotic cell: This subclass is indented under subclass 93.2. Subject matter involving a eukaryotic cell, such as an animal cell, plant cell, fungus, protozoa, and higher algae, which has been genetically modified. (1) Note. A eukaryotic cell has a nucleus defined by a nuclear membrane wherein the nucleus contains chromosomes that comprise the genome of the cell.

93.3: Intentional mixture of two or more microorganisms, cells, or viruses of different genera: This subclass is indented under subclass 93.1. Subject matter involving a mixture consisting of two or more different microbial, cellular, or viral genera. (1) Note. A mixture of *Escherichia coli* and *Pseudomonas* or a mixture of *Aspergillus* and *Bacillus* would be considered proper for this subclass, while a mixture of *Bacillus cereus* and *Bacillus brevis* would be classified under *Bacillus* rather than in this subclass, as they are both in the genus *Bacillus*. (2) Note. Rumen, intestinal, vaginal, and other microflora mixtures are mixtures appropriate for this subclass unless mixture constituents are disclosed and are found to be contrary to the subclass definition.

133.1: Structurally modified antibody, immunoglobulin, or fragment thereof (e.g., chimeric, humanized, complementarity determining region-grafted, mutated, and the like): This subclass is indented under subclass 130.1. Subject matter involving an antibody, immunoglobulin, or fragment thereof that is purposely altered with respect to its amino acid sequence or glycosylation or with respect to its composition of heavy and light chains or immunoglobulin regions or domains, as compared with that found in nature, or wherein the antibody, immunoglobulin, or fragment thereof is part of a larger, synthetic protein. (1) Note. Structurally modified antibodies may be made by chemical alteration or recombination of existing antibodies or by various cloning techniques involving recombinant DNA or hybridoma technology. (2) Note. Structurally modified antibodies may be chimeric (i.e., comprising amino acid sequences derived from two or more nonidentical immunoglobulin molecules, such as interspecies combinations, and so on). (3) Note. Structurally modified antibodies may have domain deletions or substitutions (e.g., deletions of particular constant-region domains or substitutions of constant-region domains from other classes of immunoglobulins). (4) Note. Structurally modified antibodies may have deletions of particular glycosylated amino acids or may have their glycosylation otherwise altered, which may alter their function. (5) Note. While the expression of cloned antibody genes in cells of species other than from which they originated may result in altered glycosylation of the product, compared with that found in nature, this subclass and indented subclasses are not meant to encompass such antibodies or fragments thereof, unless such cloning is a deliberate attempt to alter their glycosylation. However, such antibodies or fragments thereof may still be classified here or in indented subclasses if they are structurally modified in other ways (e.g., if they are single chain and the like). (6) Note. It is suggested that the patents of this subclass and indented subclasses be cross-referenced to the appropriate subclass(es) that provide for the binding specificities of these antibodies, if disclosed.

141.1: Monoclonal antibody or fragment thereof (i.e., produced by any cloning technology): This subclass is indented under subclass 130.1. Subject matter involving an antibody or fragment thereof produced by a clone of cells or cell line, derived from a single antibody-producing cell or antibody fragment-producing cell, wherein the said antibody or fragment thereof is identical to all other antibodies or fragments thereof produced by that clone of cells or cell line. (1) Note. This and the indented subclasses provide for bioaffecting and body-treating compositions of antibodies or fragments thereof, as well as bioaffecting and body-treating methods of using the said compositions, said antibodies, or said fragments, which are produced by any cloning technology that yields identical molecules (e.g., hybridoma technology, recombinant DNA technology, and so on). (2) Note. Monoclonal antibodies, per se, are considered compounds and are provided for elsewhere. See the search notes that follow. (3) Note. Monoclonal antibodies are sometimes termed monoclonal receptors or immunological binding partners.

1.49 and 1.53, for methods of using radiolabeled monoclonal antibodies or compositions thereof for bioaffecting or body-treating purposes and said compositions, per se.

9.1+ for methods of using monoclonal antibodies or compositions thereof for in vivo testing or diagnosis and said compositions, per se.

178.1+ for bioaffecting or body-treating methods of using monoclonal antibodies or fragments thereof that are conjugated to or complexed with nonimmunoglobulin material; bioaffecting or body-treating methods of using compositions of monoclonal antibodies or fragments thereof, which are conjugated to or complexed with nonimmunoglobulin material; and said compositions, per se.

199.1: Recombinant virus encoding one or more heterologous proteins or fragments thereof: This subclass is indented under subclass 184.1. Subject matter involving a virus into whose genome one or more nucleic acid sequences encoding one or more heterologous proteins or fragments thereof are integrated. (1) Note. A heterologous protein is one derived from another species (e.g., another viral species). (2) Note. Such genetically modified viruses may be used as multivalent vaccines.

200.1: Recombinant or stably transformed bacterium encoding one or more heterologous proteins or fragments thereof: This subclass is indented under subclass 184.1. Subject matter involving a bacterium into whose genome one or more nucleic acid sequences encoding one or more heterologous proteins or fragments thereof are integrated or involving a bacterium that carries stable, replicative plasmids that include one or more nucleic acid sequences encoding one or more heterologous proteins or fragments thereof. (1) Note. A heterologous protein is one derived from another species (e.g., another bacterial species). (2) Note. Such genetically modified bacteria may be used as multivalent vaccines.

201.1: Combination of viral and bacterial antigens (e.g., multivalent viral and bacterial vaccines, and so on): This subclass is indented under subclass 184.1. Subject matter involving a combination of viral and bacterial antigens, such as that found in a multivalent viral and bacterial vaccine.

202.1: Combination of antigens from multiple viral species (e.g., multivalent viral vaccine, and so on): This subclass is indented under subclass 184.1. Subject matter involving a combination of antigens from multiple viral species, such as that found in a multivalent viral vaccine. (1) Note. A combination of antigens from multiple variants of the same viral species should be classified with that viral species.

203.1: Combination of antigens from multiple bacterial species (e.g., multivalent bacterial vaccine, and so on): This subclass is indented under subclass 184.1. Subject matter involving a combination of antigens from multiple bacterial species, such as that found in a multivalent bacterial vaccine. (1) Note. A combination of antigens from multiple variants of the same bacterial species should be classified with that bacterial species.

801: Involving Antibody or Fragment thereof Produced by Recombinant DNA Technology: This subclass is indented under the class definition. Subject matter involves an antibody or fragment thereof produced by recombinant DNA technology.

A search under CCL/"435/69.1" yields 8898 patents, including the earliest patents, wherein insulin was produced by genetically modified fungi from the University of Minnesota, and the two classic patents from Stanford and Columbia.

Second to the United States Patent and Trademark Office, the largest database is accessed through the European Patent Office, where one should conduct a similar classification search, as suggested previously for the United States Patent and Trademark Office (2). The World Intellectual Property Organization (3) offers many useful features, including complete details of the Patent Cooperative Treaty and its gazette.

2.3.1 Internet Search Engines

Though intended for the lay public, the Internet can turn up remarkable information, particularly as it pertains to prior art. The following sites are recommended:

www.searchenginecolossus.com/
www.searchengineguide.com/
www.google.com/
www.lycos.com/
www.yahoo.com/
www.altavista.com/
www.alltheweb.com/
www.webcrawler.com/
www.excite.com/
www.infoseek.com/
www.msn.com/
www.infospace.com/

2.3.2 Information Portals

http://lcweb.loc.gov	The Library of Congress is the best place to start, as it is the world's largest library.
www.firstgov.gov/	Gateway to all government information.
http://spireproject.com/	A guide to what is coming online.
http://scout.cs.wisc.edu/	The Scout Report is one of the Internet's longest-running weekly publications, offering a selection of new and newly discovered online resources.
http://infomine.ucr.edu/Main.html	A University of California Library service on what is available on the Internet in the sciences.
www.ipl.org/ref/RR/	Internet Public Library. An annotated collection of high-quality Internet resources for providing accurate, factual information on a particular topic or topics.
www.invent.org/	A highly artistic website on the patenting process with much support for independent inventors.
www.access.gpo.gov/getcfr.html	This page describes the HTML coding necessary to link directly to the documents contained in the *Code of Federal Regulation* (CFR) databases resident on Government Printing Office's wide area information system servers.
http://vlib.org/	The WWW Virtual Library.
www.invent1.org/	Minnesota Inventors Congress; inventor resources and the oldest convention center.
www.innovationcentre.ca	The Canadian Innovation Center.
www.sul.stanford.edu/depts/swain/patent/pattop.html	Selected resources for patents, inventions, and technology transfer selected by Stanford University.
www.bl.uk/	The 150-million volume British Library is a good source; search here with the key word "patent."
www.rand.org/radius	The most comprehensive listing of federally funded research projects, free to federal employees.
www.knowledgeexpress.com/Knowledge	Express provides business development and competitive intelligence resources—including intellectual property, technology transfer, and corporate partnering opportunities—to organizations involved with science and technology research and new inventions.
http://searchlight.cdlib.org/cgi-bin/searchlight	Publicly available databases and other resources.
http://productnews.com	New product information on thousands of products weekly.
www.techexpo.com	Aimed at manufacturers and inventors.
www.pubcrawler.ie/	Health and medical information.

(Continued)

http://medlineplus.gov/	National Library of Medicine consumer site on health.
http://clinicaltrials.gov/	Information on all U.S. clinical trials underway, and you can branch out to learn about how to do clinical trials.
www.pubmedcentral.nih.gov/	A major archive of free online life science journals.
http://highwire.stanford.edu/lists/freeart.dtl	Free online journals in science, technology, and medicine.
www.healthfinder.gov/	Reliable health information from government agencies.
www.cdc.gov/	The Centers for Disease Control and Prevention.
www.fda.gov	Food and Drug Administration regulations.
www.nal.usda.gov/fnic/	USDA food and nutrient information center.
www.mdtmag.com	Medical design technology for devices.
www.medscape.com/	Medical information from WebMD.
http://bmn.com	Biomedical information portal.
www.intelihealth.com	Consumer healthcare information from Harvard.
www.bmj.com	British Medical Journal; prestige medical issues.
www.devicelink.com/	Medical devices.
www.ornl.gov/hgmis/	The human genome project.

2.3.3 Technical Databases

The National Institutes of Health (NIH; Ref. 5) offers over 12 million research papers, mainly in the biomedical sciences that are available through the National Library of Medicine. This free database allows downloads of abstracts in an ASCII format for direct placement into programs such as Microsoft Word to develop a comprehensive bibliography.

Derwent (6) is one of the most widely used databases, from which the United States Patent and Trademark Office examiners benefit as well.

Dialog (7) is another large database that allows you to search without having to register an account; you pay as you go along, using your credit card. You cannot do this if you are searching for trademarks.

Delphion (formerly IBM Intellectual Property database; Ref. 8) allows for more in-depth search of patents and access to many consolidated databases. It is a low-cost solution.

American Chemical Society offers large databases (9). This is one of the premier scientific databases where you will be able to get original papers faxed to you if you need them urgently.

Nerac (10): Numerous online databases.

2.3.4 Patent Search and Intellectual Property Services

- Patent Cafe (11): a hangout for patent product vendors.
- Investor's Digest (12): Resources for inventors. Very active site.

- The Massachusetts Institute of Technology (MIT) (13): It has provided an elaborate and detailed website for invention development; it is worth a detailed look.

2.3.5 Patent Copies and Search Facilities

- Micropatent (14): This is perhaps the most comprehensive service available at a very reasonable cost and is an easy website to navigate. This is a highly recommended site.
- Questel (15)
- Faxpat (16)
- Patentec (17)
- Lexis-Nexus (18)
- Mayall (19)

2.4 Components of a Patent Application

A patent specification (not specifications) is a legal document that gets published as the patent, if granted. Great care and detail go into writing this document in defining the scope of invention, deciding what is claimed, and wording the claims (which are part of specification) such that they can withstand challenges.

Deciding on what is "invented" is the job of the research scientist, but the decision is made in light of prior art; for example, if there is a discovery of a new group of chemicals, the breadth of the group should be ascertained in light of the prior art available, what can be reasonably predicted regarding the structure of chemicals, and the ability to synthesize representative chemicals, if not all. Where a completely new molecular structure has been invented, a broad scope, including all kinds of derivatives of the basic structure that the inventor thinks may be useful, is possible. It is surprising how many times scientists who are sure of the novelty of a structure, composition, or application find out otherwise when a thorough search is made of the possible prior art. It is worth realizing that with the availability of databases in electronic format, the Internet, and generally a faster access to remove publications (even brochures for promotion in remote countries), what a thorough search would reveal; know that the patent examiners have access to these same channels of information and even more. The author has been humbled more than once by what the patent examiner can dig out. So, scientists are advised not to jump the gun in making very broad claims, until advised so by the patent attorneys, after conducting a thorough patent search. Obviously, the scope is narrowed down gradually as more and more prior art emerges. The goal is not to narrow it down to a point where it loses its commercial importance. The scope of protection, which is commercially important to achieve, varies from one field to another. In extreme situations, it is sufficient to have a scope that includes a singular compound, if that is what the company wishes to market. The strength in this approach comes from the regulatory control of pharmaceutical products. Once a company receives marketing authorization from the FDA, at a great expense, imitators would like only to reproduce the invention, which they cannot do through the course of the patent term and any extensions granted by the FDA. So, while there may be other molecules, perhaps better ones, available, imitators are unlikely to invest in their development, as they are unprotected and there is no guarantee that the FDA will approve them. So, in the field of a new drug development, a single chemical entity does have substantial value. Such is not the case in other industries where regulatory costs are not involved, such as in the chemical industry.

Once a decision is made about what is invented, how much to claim, and what specifically to claim, the process of drafting the specification begins. One method is to draft the main claim, defining the scope of the invention in the form of the statement of invention, which is the heart of the patent specification, and then, the rest of the specification and claims will be drafted.

Specification begins with a title. Newcomers to the field of patenting would be amazed or perhaps amused at the choice of patent titles and even the language used to describe an invention. Historically, inventors kept the titles vague to keep the searchers (who then did manual searches) from finding out about their inventions. Today, as most patent offices have gone electronic, this is no long an issue; nevertheless, the practice continues.

Patent applications have fixed formats that often vary between patent offices but nevertheless require a similar information submission: a background, summary, details of invention, and so on. The patent application must be comprehensive to demonstrate novelty and the inventive step in light of prior art. It should be understood that the purpose is not to fool the patent examiner into allowance but to protect the invention from the competitors who will challenge it, should it be worth anything. A full disclosure is required to keep the infringers out, to decrease the chance of their success in knocking out a patent. Additional statements are included, defining the features of the invention for use as a basis for specific claims, for example, stating "In one aspect the invention provides...." "In another aspect the invention provides...." The described widgets are new and form part of the invention. Attorneys have their word preferences, and standard statements to fill the specification are written quickly.

After the statements of invention, there is a description to indicate the preferred parts of the scope, and one or more formulae may be given, defining narrower subgeneric scopes. This section fulfills the requirement of the adequacy of description. The specification must also describe how the invention is to be carried out, an essential part of a patent application. This is a critical stage in deciding how and what to disclose. As discussed earlier, often at this stage, a decision may be made not to file a patent application, for the disclosure will inevitably cause the invention to escape from the hands of inventors, and if there were no certain ways to determine infringement, this would make patenting useless. It is also not a smart move to be deceptive when it comes to describing how the invention works; many a patent application has been declared invalid after the companies have made significant investments in marketing the invention, because a competitor was able to demonstrate that the inventors hid certain critical facts. It must be understood that the disclosures need not be for a commercial model of the invention and thus need not include many fine details generally required for a large-scale production of the invention, such as in-process specifications, certain handling conditions, the grade of excipients used, and so on, which may be material to produce a product fit for a particular purpose, such as human consumption. As long as the competitor can manufacture the article, not necessarily for the commercial production, using the details provided, the requirement of sufficiency of disclosure is met. This becomes more important in the discovery of NCEs, where chemical synthesis can be described adequately, but not necessarily for the grade of material required; for example, the impurity profile of an NCE (FDA) is critical for the purpose of a New Drug Application (NDA: FDA). Manufacturers often are able to produce a product that would meet the FDA's requirement for quality, yet not report this method in the patent, which would allow the competitor to manufacture the product only with impurities. The reason that companies are able to get away with this trick is that the patent claims a chemical compound, not necessarily what would be suitable for ingestion by humans. Obviously, if the molecule turns out to be a blockbuster, many will imitate the process and may challenge the patent; case law on this aspect is silent. It is well known as a result that once an NCE comes to the end of its patent cycle, new sources of an active pharmaceutical ingredient (API) are developed with greater difficulty than what would be anticipated from the disclosures in the patent.

Next is an indication of what the invention is useful for, a part of the specification usually called the utility statement. In the case of mechanical inventions, it is often obvious, whereas for chemical inventions, it requires explanation, along with any peculiar or particular advantages. It is important to know that there is no requirement to explain how and why the invention works; thus, it is best not to offer any hypothesis about the invention. However, if a theory must be given, one should leave room for a change of mind later, for example, by wording as, "while we do not intend to be bound to any particular theory, it is believed that...." In a chemical case, a number of examples are given, with detailed instructions for the preparation of at least one of the compounds within the scope and for the use of the compounds.

After these is the heart of the patent, the claims. There is no limitation on how many claims are made; however, redundant and superfluous claims are frowned upon by the examiners and should be avoided. It is important to know that all dependent claims are narrower in scope and written exclusively for the purpose of protecting the invention, or any part of it, should the broader claim or claims be knocked out in court proceedings.

Other parts of a patent application, such as priority dates, affidavit requirements, assignment, and appointment of attorney or agents, are best left to the patent practitioners and the company's legal department to worry about; however, there may be some interaction with the inventor in filling out certification documents. The filing of an application is followed by numerous communications and office actions from the patent office, the responses to which are drafted in full consultation with the scientists and their approval for the accuracy of information and its interpretation. A word of caution is needed here. In the United States, there is a clause of "estoppel," under which admissions made in the specification or in responses to office action about what was actually taught by the prior art may be binding upon the applicant. A wrong statement about the acceptance of an article as prior art may be reversed later. Court proceedings will have the entire text of correspondence available for examination, and the "file wrapper" becomes part of the patent. The safest rule is to admit nothing and say as little as possible about the prior art. Of course, all relevant prior arts known to the applicant or his attorney must be brought to the attention of the United States Patent and Trademark Office, but this does not mean that it has to be mentioned in the specification.

There must be at least one claim in each patent application. Claims define the scope of the subject matter for which protection is sought. A competitor does not infringe and cannot be stopped unless he makes, sells, or offers for sale; imports; or does something that falls within the scope of at least one claim of the granted patent; in other words, if the infringing object "reads onto claim," then it is an infringement. How claims are interpreted keeps the courts filled with opportunities to create case laws. Claims are always read in light of the published specification, and thus, the issue of prior art comes up again; had there been a mistake in allowing a claim in the light of prior art, the claim will be thrown out, and in some cases, the entire patent is rendered invalid.

All claims fall into one of the two broad categories: they claim either a product (a mechanical device, a machine, a composition of matter, and the like) or a process (a method of making, using, or testing something). For chemical patents, this may include the chemical per se as a useful intermediate, a composition in a pharmaceutical product, a specific form (optical isomer, crystal form, and so on), or for direct use. The process claims would include the processes of synthesis, isolation, or purification, as the case may be; the methods of use may be the first use or a subsequent use, such as a method of medical treatment or diagnosis or testing and analysis methods.

2.4.1 Drawing(s) (§113)

When necessary, drawings must be submitted, most likely in mechanical or electrical applications and some chemical applications. Filing date is not assigned if drawings are not provided at the Office of Initial Patent Examination (OIPE's) level of evaluation. Examiner may require drawings, but filing date is not affected. Drawings MUST show all of the claimed elements; drawings may be added later by amendment if already described in the specification or claim as originally filed; no need for manufacturing drawings (such as tolerances or in-process controls).

2.4.2 Specification (§112 ¶1)

The written description, the manner, the and process of making and using, in such full, clear, concise, and exact terms, as to enable any person skilled (with ordinary skills) in the art to which it pertains, or with which it is most nearly connected, to make and use the invention and setting forth the best mode contemplated by the inventor for carrying out his invention. There are three requirements of disclosure that are dealt with in the following:

Description

- Must describe what is claimed clearly.
- Focus is on the claimed invention only.
- Scope commensurate with scope of claim(s): disclosure of a single species may or may not support a generic claim.

- Critical or essential element MUST be recited in claims.
- The vantage point is one of ordinary skill in the art.
- Inventors may be their own lexicographers by so stating; however, the term cannot be used in a contrary manner to what is commonly acceptable.
- Theory need not be set forth; if the theory is wrong, the error is not fatal (unless the theory is claimed invention).
- Manner of invention (how the invention was made) is not important.

Enablement

- To one of the ordinary skills to make and use.
- Without undue experimentation.
- Not necessarily for commercial production.
- This requirement is different from §101's requirement of being useful.
- Claim not reciting essential matter may be rejected for a lack of enablement or for failing to claim the subject matter, which the applicant considers as the invention.
- Publications after filing date may not be used to support enablement but may be used to defeat enablement (such as by examiner).
- Scope of enablement must be commensurate with the scope of claims(s).
- Amount of disclosure required depends on the state of the art and predictability—the more is known and the greater is the predictability; the less is the required disclosure.

Best Mode

- What inventors consider as the best mode is not what anyone or everyone else considers and not what is objectively the best.
- After an application is filed, it need not and cannot be updated by amendment (as it will be considered new matter), even in a division or continuation, but can be updated in continuation-in-part if it pertains to a new claim made.
- It must be disclosed, though not necessarily identified as such. Embodiment disclosed is automatically considered as the best mode; several embodiments may be disclosed without identifying which one is the best.

2.4.3 Paragraph 1 35 USC §112 Requirements

Description, enablement, and best mode must exist in each claim as filed, or else, it renders claims invalid if contested. All of these are intended to be understood by a person of ordinary skills in the art, not a layperson. Any one or more of the following can satisfy each of these three requirements: specification, drawing(s), and claims, as originally filed. Unclaimed inventions need not satisfy this requirement.

2.4.4 Paragraph 2 35 USC §112 Requirement: Parts of a Claim

- Preamble sets the scope of the invention's technical environment and class (composition, process, apparatus, and the like: a method of..., apparatus for..., a composition...). It is not limiting if it merely states the purpose of the invention; however, if it breathes life and meaning into the claim (such as if it is essential to tell what is claimed or if the body of claim refers to it as an antecedent support), it can become limiting.

- Transitional phrase connects the body of the claim to the preamble: comprising, consisting of, consisting essentially of, and the like. Three types: (i) open-ended: comprising, including, containing, characterized by, and the like; (ii) closed: consisting of, also composed of, having, being, and so on—some of these can be interpreted differently; and (iii) partially closed: consisting essentially of..., wherein it allows only those additional elements that do not affect the basic and novel characteristics of invention. No synergism. The applicant has a burden of proof to show that additional elements in prior art would materially change the characteristics of the invention. If ABCD is known and ABC is claimed, the absence of D must be demonstrated to materially affect the invention.

- Body is a list of elements, such as ingredients of a composition and components of the apparatus; all elements must be interconnected. (There must a reason why a component is recited, not just to list it.)

2.5 Understanding Claims

The heart of a patent is within the boundaries defined by the claims.

2.5.1 Reading a Claim

Determination of infringement is done by reading (or matching) the claim to prior art to prove the validity of the claim. A device or process to indicate infringement or own specification satisfies the §112 requirements. Claim does not read on prior art with elements ABCD if the claim is ABC and closed (consisting of), but it reads if the transitional phrase is open, such as "comprising," and may or may not read if it is "consisting essentially of."

2.5.2 Punctuation of Claim

A claim is written as one sentence; it contains a comma after preamble and a colon after introducing another element; and each element gets its own paragraph. There is a semicolon at the end of each paragraph and between the last two elements. If more than one period is used, this would be rejected as an indefinite claim (¶2 §112).

2.5.3 Definiteness of Claim

Without proper antecedent basis, a claim is rendered indefinite. "A" or "an" introduces an element for the first time, except in a means-plus-function format. "Said" or "the" refers back to previously introduced elements or limitations or refers to the inherent properties (not required to be recited for antecedent purpose; for example, "the surface of said element" when "surface" is not defined earlier). Inferential claiming where interconnectivity of elements is not certain does not tell if the element is part of combination or not.

2.5.4 Narrowing of Claim

Narrowed by adding an element or limitation to a previously recited element; narrow claim can be dependent or independent. Adding a step narrows method claims. Adding an element to a closed (such as Markush Group) claim broadens, not narrows the claim.

2.5.5 Dependent Claims (§112 ¶3 ¶4)

- Claim can be dependent or independent; a dependent claim incorporates by reference all the limitations of the claims to which it refers and is always narrower; it must depend on a preceding claim and not on a following claim (numbering of claims is readjusted during prosecution).
- "Further comprising" or "further including" are used to narrow a claim by adding another element or step.
- Claims are narrowed by further defining an element or the relationship between elements. Transitional element "wherein" is used to add limitation. Narrowing can be both adding an element and further defining its relationship.
- Defining a step further narrows a method claim.

2.5.6 Multiple Dependent Claims (§112 ¶5)

- A claim referring to more than one previously set forth claim, but only in the alternative ("or") narrows the claim on which it depends.
- Cannot serve as a basis for another multiple dependent claim; may refer to other dependent claims, and a dependent claim may depend on a multiple dependent claims.
- Incorporates by reference all the limitations of the particular claim in relationship to which it is being considered (individually and not collectively).
- It takes the place of writing several dependent claims—in its spirit.
- A flat special fee is charged at the time of filing application if multiple dependent claim or claims are included.

2.5.7 Dominant-Subservient Claims

Dominant claims involve subcombination or genus, while combination means subsurvient species. Two members (species) are needed to have genus, which is illustrated by the selection of species; genus is an inherent commonality among embodiments (species).

2.5.8 Means-Plus-Function Clauses §112 ¶6

A claim defines an element by its function, not what it is. It is a means for performing a function and is interpreted by the literal function recited and corresponding structure or materials described in specification and equivalents thereof. It does not cover all structures for performing the recited function. A claim reciting only a single means-plus-function clause without any other element is impossible. It must have the phrase, "means for," which then must be modified by functional language but not modified by the recitation of structure sufficient to accomplish the specific function. If specification does not adequately disclose the structure corresponding to the "means" claimed, the claims fail to comply with paragraph 2 of the patent law requirement for "particularly pointing out and distinctly claiming" the invention. If disclosure is implicit (for those skilled in the art), an amendment may be required or stated on record what structure performs the function. *Equivalents*: Examiner must explain rationale; prior art must perform, not excluded by explicit definition in the specification for an equivalent, prior art supported by the following:

- Identical function, substantially same way, substantially same results
- Art-recognized interchangeability
- Insubstantial differences
- Structural equivalency

2.5.9 Process Claims

These include a method for making a product, comprising the steps of... and a method of using a specified or known material, comprising the steps of...; recitation of at least one step is required, and a single-step method claim is proper.

2.5.10 Step-Plus-Function Clauses

- Functional method claims recite a particular result but not the specified act— that is, techniques used to achieve results: adjusting pH, raising temperature, reducing friction, and so on.
- No recital of acts in support required.
- Typically introduced by words such as "whereby," "so that," and "for."
- Addition of a functional description alone is not sufficient to differentiate claim—rejected under §102.
- Functional language without recitation of structure, which performs the function, may render the claim broader (rather than narrower)—rejected under §112 ¶1.

2.5.11 Ranges

Commonly used for temperature, pressure, time, and dimensional limitations. "Up to" means from zero to the top limit; "at least" means not less than (does not set upper limit, which must be fully disclosed in specification); specification must support eventual ranges. A dependent claim cannot broaden the range. Range within range is indefinite in a claim but acceptable in specification.

2.5.12 Negative Limitations

Permissible if boundaries are set forth definitely, such as free of an impurity or a particular element or incapable of performing a certain function. Absence of structures cannot be claimed—holes, channels, and the like—as structural elements.

2.5.13 Relative and Exemplary Terminology

Imprecise language may satisfy definiteness requirement (for one of ordinary skill). "So dimensioned" or "so spaced" can be definite if it is as accurate as the subject would permit; "about" is clear and flexible but rendered indefinite if specification or prior art does not provide indication about the dimensions anticipated. "Essentially," "substantially," and "effective amount" are definite if one with ordinary skills would understand. Exemplary terminology is always indefinite: such as, of like material, similar—all are rejected.

2.5.14 Markush Group

Closed form comprises two forms one wherein P is a material selected from a group consisting of A, B, C, and D; or wherein P is A, B, C, or D. Members must belong to a recognized class and possess properties in common, as disclosed in the specification, and these properties are mainly responsible for their function, or the grouping is clear from their nature or the prior art that all members possess the property. Adding members broadens claim. Prior art with one of the members anticipates the claim.

2.5.15 Markush Alternates

"Or" terminology is used if choices are related: one or several pieces; made entirely or part of; red, blue, or white. If choices are unrelated, the use of "or" will lead to indefinite interpretation. "Optionally" is used if definite or if there are no ambiguities in the scope of the claim as a result of the choices offered.

2.5.16 Jepson-Type Claims—Improvement Claims

Preamble defines what is conventional; transitional phrase, "wherein the improvement comprises;" body builds on preamble; can add element or modify element in preamble. Preamble is limiting.

2.5.17 Mixed-Class Claims

Mixed elements are improper: methods claims should have no structural elements; apparatus claims should have no step elements. Limitations can be mixed, such as method step may include a structural limitation, and an apparatus may include a process limitation.

2.5.18 Product-by-Process Claims

A product claim that defines the claimed product in terms of the process by which it is made: A product made by the process comprising of steps... Patentability based on product itself and NOT on the method of production. If the product is the same (as prior art), using another process does not make it patentable. If examiner shows that the product appears to be the same or similar, the burden shifts to the applicant; the United States Patent and Trademark Office bears lesser burden of proof in making out a case of prima facie obviousness. One-step method claims are acceptable, but claims where body consists of single "means" elements are not acceptable.

2.5.19 Patent Term Adjustment

The United States Congress passed legislation known as the Hatch-Waxman Act in 1984. It weakened patent law for pharmaceuticals, making it easier for generic copies to enter the market based on the innovator's safety and effectiveness data. Under the act, pharmaceutical research companies lost nearly all of their rights to defend their unexpired patents before generic copies entered the market. Patent holders can sue to defend their unexpired patents *only* when a generic drug manufacturer submits a filing to the FDA, seeking to bring the generic copy to the market. The act also created a 30-month stay procedure to allow patent holders the opportunity to obtain a court ruling on whether the generic copy infringes their patent. Thirty-month stays do not extend patents—they are triggered *before* the patent expires and provide a period of time during which patent infringement cases can be resolved.

Patent lawsuits based on the act are rare, because generally, challenges to patents on prescription medicines are rare. The FDA reports that of 8,259 generic applications filed between 1984 and 2001, only 6% raised a patent issue, the necessary condition for patent litigation. According to the Federal Trade Commission, more than one-quarter of patent challenges studied did not result in a lawsuit by the innovator company. Since enactment of the law, generic company share of prescription medicine use has increased from 19% of prescription units in 1984 to 50% today.

The average effective patent life for prescription medicines under the Hatch-Waxman Act is 11–12 years, compared with an average of 18.5 years for other products.

With effect from August 18, 2003, the FDA revised its regulations as follows:

It permits only one 30-month stay in the approval process for a generic drug pending resolution of patent litigation. Past regulations acquiesced to the delayed launch of generic versions beyond 30 months, when there were multiple, consecutive patent challenges that were made against the launch of the generic versions, even if the challenges were frivolous.

It clarifies the types of patents that may be listed in the "Orange Book," which is the FDA's official register of approved pharmaceutical products that provides notice to generic drug makers of name brand patent rights. Patents that cover drug packaging or other minor matters not related to effectiveness may no longer be listed. Patents that pertain to active ingredients, drug formulations/compositions, and approved uses of a drug are to be listed. A more detailed, signed attestation will be required to accompany a patent submission. False statements in the attestation can lead to criminal charges.

For patents that are granted after the drug application is filed, the brand name drug maker has 30 days to list the patent(s) from the grant date.

To seek approval for a generic drug, the generic drug maker must certify to the FDA that (i) there are no Orange Book-listed patents for the brand name drug or (ii) the patent(s) has (have) either expired or (iii) will expire by the time approval is sought or (iv) the listed patent(s) is (are) invalid or will not be infringed. If the latter, the notice of the certification is given to the patent owner and to the brand name drug maker, with an explanation as to why the patent(s) is (are) invalid or not infringed. If the patent owner does not bring a patent infringement suit against the generic drug maker within 45 days, the FDA may approve the generic version. Otherwise, the approval process is stayed for the shorter of 30 months or till the date when a court concludes the patent(s) is (are) either invalid or not infringed.

It requires generic manufacturers to demonstrate to the FDA that their generic drug is therapeutically equivalent to an approved brand name drug; that is, it is equivalence in terms of safety, strength, quality, purity, performance, intended use, and other characteristics. It reviews drug applications for generics more quickly. The FDA is hiring 40 generic drug experts to expedite the approval process and to institute targeted research to expand the range of generic drugs available to consumers.

It has improved the review process for generic drugs by instituting internal reforms. The reforms include making early communications with generic drug manufacturers who submit applications and guiding generic manufacturers in preparing and submitting quality, complete applications.

The recent decision in the U.S. patent infringement case Madey versus Duke is very important to academic researchers and the industry. Duke University had challenged the general assumption that academic research using a patented device or method cannot constitute infringement. The subject matter was a laser device, which had originally been developed and patented by Duke University. When the inventor left the university to pursue commercial applications for the laser, Duke University continued to use their model for research purposes. Duke claimed that it was entitled to continue using the laser for noncommercial purposes under the experimental use exception in the U.S. patent law. However, the court held that Duke University's use of the laser "unmistakably" furthered its commercial goals, including facilitating the education of students. The court further held that research using the laser had helped the university to obtain research grants. The equivalent provision in English law is section 60(5)(b) of the Patents Act 1977, which states that an act relating to the subject matter of a patent that is done for "experimental purposes" will not constitute infringement. The provision does not set out whether the exemption is available to those whose experimental purposes have a commercial element. There is no U.K. equivalent, however, of the U.S. exemption, which permits the unauthorized use of a patented device or method by a person seeking the FDA's approval to market a new product. The exemption applies only while the application is pending but extends to the use of patented devices or drugs in clinical trials, their sale for use in trials, demonstrations at trade shows, and the reporting of clinical data to potential investors.

The United States Patent and Trademark Office prescribes specific regulations regarding patent term adjustment (PTA):

- Application filed prior to June 8, 1995: 17 years from the date of issuance, regardless of the length of prosecution.

- Application filed June 8, 1995–May 28, 2000: The Uruguay Round Agreements Act (URAA): 20 years from the filing date but with up to 5 years' extension for delays resulting from secrecy orders, interferences, and/or successful appears.
- Application pending or patent in force on June 8, 1995: 17 years from the issue date or the period between the issue date and the 20th anniversary of the filing date, whichever is greater.
- Application filed on or after May 29, 2000: American Inventors Protection Act (AIPA) may be entitled to PTA in a continuing application, including continued prosecuting application (CPA), request for continued examination (RCE) filed after May 29, 2000, in an application filed before May 29, 2000, does NOT provide PTA eligibility; Patent Cooperative Treaty's eligibility depends on its filing date, not on its national-stage entry date (Patent Cooperative Treaty must be filed on or after May 29, 2000, to be eligible for PTA).
- PTA: Termination date (20th anniversary from filing date) is extended by the number of days that Patent and Trademark Office delays minus the number of days that the applicant delays.

2.5.20 Patent and Trademark Office Delays: Guaranteed Adjustment Basis

Guaranteed adjustment basis (GAB)1: Patent and Trademark Office's failure to take certain actions within 14 months from filing date and 4 months from other events: Patent and Trademark Office must mail an examination notification (first office action, including Quayle action or notice of allowability, restriction requirement, and request for information, but not Office of Initial Patent Examination (OIPE) notice of incompleteness of application or other such notices) to applicant within 14 months of the filing date; the Patent and Trademark Office must also respond within 4 months to the applicant's reply to an office action or applicant's opening appeal brief. It must act within 4 months of a board of patent appeals and interferences (BPAI) or court decision, where allowable claims remain in the application. The Patent and Trademark Office must issue the patent within 4 months of date on which the issue fee is paid and all outstanding requirements are satisfied.

GAB2: The Patent and Trademark Office delays due to interference, secrecy order, or successful appellate review (where BPAI or court reverses the determination of the patentability of at least one claim [allowance by examiner after a remand from BPAI is not a final decision]). GAB2 was also the basis of PTA under URAA, but for a maximum of 5 years, AIPA removes 5-year limit.

GAB3: The Patent and Trademark Office fails to issue a patent within 3 years, excluding the time consumed in RCE, secrecy order, interference, or appellate review (whether successful or not); the time consumed by applicant-requested delays (e.g., suspension of action up to 6 months for "good and sufficient cause," up to a 3-month delay request at the time of filing RCE or CPA, and up to 3-year deferral of examination requested by applicant). Filing an RCE for an application filed on or after May 29, 2000, cuts off any additional PTA owing to failure to issue patent within years, but it does NOT eliminate PTA in GAB1 and GAB2.

2.5.21 Required Reduction Basis

Applicant's delay for failure to engage in reasonable effort to conclude the prosecution of the application is subtracted from GAB1–3: failure to reply within 3 months to any notice from the office making any rejection, objection, argument, or other requests (even though the applicant pays for and receives extension), days in excess of 3 months are deducted; reinstatement of deduction of up to 3 months can be made by applicant, showing that "in spite of all due care, the applicant was unable to reply," due perhaps to testing to demonstrate unexpected results, death of applicant's sole practitioner, or a natural disaster. (Do not confuse the 3 months' concession with 3 months required to respond.) Additional required reduction bases (RRBs) are generated because of suspension of action under Rule 1.103, deferral of issuance under Rule 1.3114, abandonment or late payment of issue fee, petition to revise more than 2 months after the notice of abandonment, conversion of provisional to nonprovisional, preliminary amendment within 1 month of office action that requires supplemental office action (i.e., a response is sent when an office action is to come within 1 month)*, inadvertent omission in reply to office action*, supplemental reply not requested by examiner*, submission filed after BPAI or court decision within 1 month of office action that requires supplemental office action*, submission filed after the notice of allowance*, and filing a continuing application to continue prosecution. Note that in instances marked with an asterisk (*), information disclosure statement submission will not create reduction if information is received from foreign patent office within the last 30 days (i.e., the applicant responds within 30 days of receiving such information).

Summary: Patent term begins on the day of patent issuance; terminal disclaimer date ends patent term; failure to pay a postissuance maintenance fee ends patent term (notice: no such fee is required for design and plant patents); term extension beyond statutory period is only through private congressional legislation or by showing government agency delays (e.g., the FDA); 20-year term begins from the earliest ancestral application from which priority is claimed (does not include provisional application or a foreign application for term running purpose); design applications excluded from URAA and AIPA, as they have a fixed 14-year term from issue.

2.6 Food and Drug Administration

A listing of drugs for which the patent term had been extended by the U.S. FDA is available at the website mentioned in Ref. 20. The longest patent term extension given by the U.S. FDA to any drug belongs to U.S. Patent 3,737,433 for 2494 days.

The point in the development program at which a patent application is filed will vary somewhat from company to company but will normally be at an early stage in the process, when the substance has been made and been shown to be active in early screening. For a patent with a nominal term of 20 years from filing, the effective term during which the patentee has exclusive rights to a marketed product is only 8–12 years. This explains the importance attached by the pharmaceutical industry to provisions to extend the patent term, whether directly, as in the United States and Japan, or indirectly by way of the supplementary protection certificate (SPC), as in Europe, in order to compensate for this loss of effective patent term. It also explains the importance to the industry of the minimum 20-year term guaranteed by the TRIPS agreement. The SPC for medicinal and plant protection products by the U.K. Patent Office does not extend the entire scope of the patent on which it is based but is limited to the product covered by the marketing authorization and for any medicinal use of the product that has been authorized before the expiration of the certificate. Thus, sales of the product for nonmedicinal uses do not infringe, but the SPC would be infringed by sales of a medicinal product by a third party, even if that party had a marketing authorization for a different indication. Apart from this, the SPC confers the same rights as the basic patent and is subject to the same limitations and obligations to allow existing licenses under the basic patent to continue under the SPC. The scope of protection given by a U.S. patent during the Hatch-Waxman extension period is essentially the same.

Here are some of the most commonly questions asked and answered by the FDA:

1. What is the difference between patents and exclusivity?

   Patents and exclusivity work in a similar fashion but are distinct from one another and governed by different statutes. Patents are a property right granted by the United States Patent and Trademark Office anytime during the development of a drug and can encompass a wide range of claims. Exclusivity refers to certain delays and prohibitions on the approval of competitor drugs available under the statute that attaches upon the approval of a drug or of certain supplements. An NDA or abbreviated new drug application (ANDA) holder is eligible for exclusivity if statutory requirements are met. See 21 CFR 314.108, 316.31, and 316.34 and sections 505A, 505E, and 505(j)(5)(B)(iv) of the Food, Drug, and Cosmetic Act (FD&C) Act. Periods of exclusivity and patent terms may or may not run concurrently. Exclusivity was designed to promote a balance between new drug innovation and greater public access to drugs that result from generic drug competition.

2. How long is a patent term?

   Patent terms are set by statute. Currently, the term of a new patent is 20 years from the date on which the application for the patent was filed in the United States. Many other factors can affect the duration of a patent.

3. How long does an exclusivity period last?

   It depends on what type of exclusivity is at issue.

   Orphan Drug Exclusivity (ODE)—7 years

   New Chemical Entity Exclusivity (NCE)—5 years

   Generating Antibiotic Incentives Now (GAIN) Exclusivity—5 years added to certain exclusivities

   New Clinical Investigation Exclusivity—3 years

   Pediatric Exclusivity (PED)—6 months added to existing patents/exclusivity

   Patent Challenge (PC)—180 days (this exclusivity is for ANDAs only)

   Competitive Generic Therapy (CGT)—180 days (this exclusivity is for ANDAs only)

   See 21 CFR 314.108, 316.31, and 316.34 and sections 505A, 505E, 505(j)(5) (B)(iv), and 505(j)(5)(B)(v) of the FD&C Act.

4. Why does the exclusivity expire before the patent?

Patent before exclusivity?

Why does a particular drug product only have patents?

Only have exclusivity?

Have neither?

Patents and exclusivity apply to drugs in different ways. Patents can be issued or expire at any time, regardless of the drug's approval status. Exclusivity attaches upon the approval of a drug product if the statutory requirements are met. Some drugs have both patent and exclusivity protection, while others have just one or neither. Patents and exclusivity may or may not run concurrently and may or may not cover the same aspects of the drug product. Patents and exclusivities that have expired are removed from the Orange Book.

5. What information related to pediatric exclusivity is listed in the Orange Book?

When pediatric exclusivity is obtained, a 6-month period of exclusivity is added to all existing patents and exclusivity on all applications held by the sponsor for that active moiety. Pediatric exclusivity does not stand alone but attaches to existing exclusivity. When pediatric exclusivity attaches, in the patent column of the Orange Book, the patent is shown twice—once with the original patent expiration date and a second time reflecting the 6-month period of pediatric exclusivity linked to that particular patent. Related information can be found on the web page Qualifying for Pediatric Exclusivity Under Section 505A of the Federal Food, Drug, and Cosmetic Act: Frequently Asked Questions on Pediatric Exclusivity (505A), The Pediatric "Rule," and their Interaction.

6. Where can I find patent and exclusivity regulations in the Code of Federal Regulations (CFR)?

See 21 CFR 314.50 Content and format of an NDA

See 21 CFR 314.52 Notice of certification of invalidity, unenforceability, or noninfringement of a patent

See 21 CFR 314.53 Submission of patent information

See 21 CFR 314.54 Procedure for submission of a 505(b)(2) application requiring investigations for approval of a new indication for, or other change from, a listed drug

See 21 CFR 314.60 Amendments to an unapproved NDA, supplement, or resubmission

See 21 CFR 314.70 Supplements and other changes to an approved NDA

See 21 CFR 314.94 Content and format of an ANDA

See 21 CFR 314.95 Notice of certification of invalidity, unenforceability, or noninfringement of a patent

See 21 CFR 314.96 Amendments to an unapproved ANDA

See 21 CFR 314.97 Supplements and other changes to an ANDA

See 21 CFR 314.101 Filing an NDA and receiving an ANDA

See 21 CFR 314.107 Date of approval of a 505(b)(2) application or ANDA

See 21 CFR 314.108 New drug product exclusivity

See 21 CFR 316.31 Scope of orphan-drug exclusive approval

See 21 CFR 316.34 FDA recognition of exclusive approval

Code of Federal Regulations on the Government Publishing Office website.

7. How is an NDA holder notified if their application has received a period of exclusivity?

No letters are sent to the application holder to indicate that a period of exclusivity has attached to his or her application. The posting of exclusivity information in the Orange Book is the official vehicle for dissemination of this information.

8. When should an NDA holder submit patent information?

Patent information is required to be submitted with all NDAs and certain supplemental applications (sNDAs) on Form FDA 3542a at the time of submission of the NDA or sNDA. Patent information for listing in the Orange Book must be submitted on Form FDA 3542 within 30 days following the approval of an NDA or supplemental application. For patents issued after the approval of the NDA or supplement, the NDA holder must submit the required patent information within 30 days of the issuance of the patent for it to be considered timely filed. If the NDA holder timely submits the required patent information, but the FDA notifies the NDA holder that its Form FDA 3542 is incomplete or shows that the patent is not eligible for listing, the NDA holder must submit an acceptable Form FDA 3542 within 15 days of the FDA's notification to be considered timely filed as of the date of the original submission of patent information. New patent information may still be submitted after 30 days of the issuance of the patent, but such information is not considered timely filed.

9. What is a patent submission date?

A patent submission date is the date on which the FDA receives patent information from the NDA holder. See 21 CFR 314.53(d)(ii)(5).

10. Why doesn't the Orange Book include patent submission dates for most records?

The FDA began patent submission date data collection in 2013. The October 2016 final rule "Abbreviated New Drug Applications and 505(b)(2) Applications" states, "FDA intends to list the date of submission of patents and patent information in the Orange Book on a prospective basis beginning as soon as is practicable after the effective date of this rule." The Orange Book will now publish patent submission dates for all new records, going forward.

11. How can an NDA holder request a patent submission date error correction?

The NDA holders should email error correction requests, including justification for the request to: orangebook@fda.hhs.gov.

Requests will be considered on a case-by-case basis and, if accurate, will be updated in the Orange Book as soon as is practicable.

12. How should an NDA holder correct or request the removal of patent information?

An NDA holder must submit a correction or change to the previously submitted patent information on a new Form FDA 3542. For changes to descriptions of approved methods of use, see question 14.

If an NDA holder determines that a patent or patent claim no longer meets the requirements for listing, the NDA holder must promptly notify the FDA to amend the patent information or withdraw the patent or patent information and request that the patent or patent information be removed from the list. The NDA holder seeking to withdraw a patent must submit to its NDA a statement containing the NDA number to which the request applies, each product(s) approved in the NDA to which the request applies, and the patent number and identify the submission as "Time Sensitive Patent Information." If the NDA holder is required by court order to amend patent information or withdraw a patent from the list, it must submit an amendment to its NDA that includes a copy of the order, within 14 days of the date the order was entered. In addition, the NDA holder must submit a correction to the expiration date of the patent on Form FDA 3542 within 30 days after the grant of patent term extension.

13. Should an NDA holder submit patent information when seeking approval of a supplement?

An NDA holder must submit patent information when it seeks approval of a supplement to add or change the dosage form or route of administration, to add or change the strength, or to change the drug product from prescription use to over-the-counter use.

For supplements that seek approval for other changes (e.g., to change the formulation, to add a new indication or other condition of use, and to make any other patented change regarding the drug substance, drug product, or any method of use), the requirements for submitting patent information depend on whether the existing patent information in the Orange Book for the original NDA continues to claim the changed product:

If one or more patents for which information was properly submitted for the product approved in the original NDA claim the changed product, then the applicant is not required to resubmit this patent information, and the FDA will continue to list the patent information.

If one or more patents for which information was properly submitted for the product approved in the original NDA no longer claim the changed product, the applicant must submit a request to remove the listed patent information at the time of the approval of the supplement.

If one or more patents for which information was not previously submitted claim the changed product, the applicant must submit the patent information required under 314.53(c). The NDA holder also must submit patent information for any supplement if the description of the patented method of use in the Orange Book would change on the approval of the supplement.

14. When may an NDA holder amend the description of the approved method(s) of use claimed by the patent?

An amendment to the description of approved method(s) of use claimed by the patent will be considered timely if it is submitted within 30 days of

(1) patent issuance, (2) approval of a corresponding change to product labeling, or (3) a decision by the U.S. Patent and Trademark Office or a federal court that is specific to the patent and alters the construction of a method-of-use claim(s) of the patent (and the amendment contains a copy of the decision). Outside of these circumstances and except as provided in the patent listing dispute regulation (21 CFR 314.53(f)(1)), an amendment to the description of the approved method(s) of use claimed by the patent will not be considered timely filed.

If the amendment to the description of the approved method(s) of use claimed by the patent is filed within an acceptable time frame but is incomplete or shows that the patent is not eligible for listing, the NDA holder must submit an acceptable Form FDA 3542 within 15 days of the FDA's notification to be considered timely filed as of the date of the submission of amended patent information.

15. What actions must a pending ANDA or 505(b)(2) applicant take if patent information is untimely filed?

    If patent information is untimely filed, generally a previously submitted ANDA or 505(b)(2) applicant is not required to submit a patent certification or statement to address the patent or patent information that is late-listed with respect to the pending ANDA or 505(b)(2) application.

16. Is there a specific format in which patent information needs to be submitted to the agency?

    If the NDA applicant is submitting patent information with an original NDA, an amendment, or a supplement prior to approval, use Form FDA 3542a. If the NDA holder is submitting information on a patent that claims an approved drug or an approved method of using the drug after approval of an NDA or supplement, use Form FDA 3542. The agency will not list or publish patent information in the Orange Book if it is not provided on Form FDA 3542.

17. To which submissions does the final rule apply?

    The effective date of the final rule on "Abbreviated New Drug Applications and 505(b)(2) Applications" applies to any submission received by the FDA on or made after December 5, 2016, the effective date of the rule, including any changes to the previously submitted patent information.

18. Does previously submitted patent information have to be resubmitted on the new Forms FDA 3542 and 3542a?

    No. While any patent information submitted after the effective date of the final rule must be submitted in a manner consistent with the final rule, including use of the new forms, NDA holders and applicants are not required to resubmit patent information previously submitted on a prior version of the form.

19. Who do I contact with specific questions regarding what patents are eligible for listing in the Orange Book?

The FDA's patent listing role is ministerial. Generally, we will not respond to specific questions regarding the eligibility of patents for listing.

WEB REFERENCES

1. http://www.uspto.gov
2. http://ep.espacenet.com;http://register.epoline.org/espacenet/ep/en/srch-reg.htm
3. http://ipdl.wipo.int/
4. http://www.ic.gc.ca/opic-cipo/cpd/eng/search/basic.html
5. http://www4.ncbi.nlm.nih.gov/PubMed
6. http://www.derwent.com
7. http://www.dialog.com
8. http://www.delphion.com/
9. http://stneasy.cas.org/html/english/login1.html
10. http://www.nerac.com
11. http://www.patentcafe.com
12. http://www.inventorsdigest.com/
13. http://web.mit.edu/invent/
14. http://www.1790.com/0/patentweb9809.html
15. http://www.questel.orbit.com/
16. http://www.faxpat.com
17. http://www.patentec.com
18. http://www.lexis-nexis.com
19. http://www.mayallj.freeserve.co.uk/
20. http://www.uspto.gov/web/offices/pac/dapp/opla/term/156.html

BIBLIOGRAPHY

Grubb PW. *Patents for Chemicals, Pharmaceuticals and Biotechnology: Fundamentals of Global Law, Practice and Strategy (Hardcover)*, 4th ed. Oxford, UK: Oxford University Press, 2005.

Niazi S. *Filing Patents On Line*. Boca Raton, FL: CRC Press, 2003.

United States Patent and Trade Mark Office Manual of Patent Examination Practices. http://www.uspto.gov/web/offices/pac/mpep/mpep.html.

Voet MA. *The Generic Challenge: Understanding Patents, FDA and Pharmaceutical Life-Cycle Management*. Boca Raton, FL: Brown Walker Press, 2005.

RECOMMENDED READING

Eiberle, M. K. and A. Jungbauer (2010). "Technical refolding of proteins: Do we have freedom to operate?" *Biotechnol J* 5(6):547–559.

Expression as inclusion bodies in Escherichia coli is a widely used method for the large-scale production of therapeutic proteins that do not require post-translational modifications. High expression yields and simple recovery steps of inclusion bodies from the host cells are attractive features industrially. However, the value of an inclusion body-based process is dominated by the solubilization and refolding technologies. Scale-invariant technologies that are economical and applicable for a wide range of proteins are requested by industry. The main challenge is to convert the denatured protein into its native conformation at high yields. Refolding competes with misfolding and aggregation. Thus, the yield of native monomer depends strongly on the initial protein concentrations in the refolding solution. Reasonable yields are attained at low concentrations (≤ 0.1 mg/mL). However, large buffer tanks and time-consuming concentration steps are required. We attempt to answer the question of the extent to which refolding of proteins is protected by patents. Low-molecular mass additives have been developed to improve refolding yields through the stabilization of the protein in solution and shielding hydrophobic patches. Progress has been made in the field of high-pressure renaturation and on-column refolding. Mixing times of the denatured protein in the refolding buffer have been reduced using newly developed devices and the introduction of specific mixers. Concepts of continuous refolding have been introduced to reduce tank sizes and increase yields. Some of the patents covering refolding of proteins will soon expire or have already expired. This gives more freedom to operate.

Kowalski, S. P. et al. (2002). "Transgenic crops, biotechnology and ownership rights: What scientists need to know." *Plant J* 31(4):407–421.

Ownership of intellectual and tangible property (IP/TP) rights in agricultural biotechnology (ag-biotech) and transgenic plants has become critically important. For scientists in all institutions, whether industrialized or developing country, public or private sector, an understanding of IP/TP rights is fundamental in both research and development. Transgenic plants and ag-biotech products embody numerous components and processes, each of which may have IP/TP rights attached. To identify these rights, a transgenic plant or ag-biotech product must be dissected into its essential components and processes, with each "piece" analyzed under the IP/TP "microscope." This product deconstruction is an integral step in product clearance (PC) analysis leading to freedom to operate (FTO). To facilitate a PC analysis, the following points are important: (1) knowing what one has and where it's from, (2) organizing material transfer agreements and licenses, (3) researching scientific and patent databases and relevant literature, (4) instituting a laboratory notebook policy, (5) keeping track of ownership of germplasm and plant genetic resources, and (6) promoting ongoing IP/TP management, awareness and training. However, an FTO opinion does not solve the IP/TP issues of releasing a transgenic plant or ag-biotech product; rather, it is a management tool for assessing the risks of litigation. When transferring transgenic plants or ag-biotech to developing nations, scientists from industrialized countries have the heightened responsibility of verifying that IP/TP issues are fully addressed and documented. Successful technology transfer goes beyond research, development and licensing; it is an holistic package leading to long-term partnerships in international development. Managing IP/TP requires capacity-building in scientists and technology transfer offices, in both industrialized and developing countries.

Ma, J. K. et al. (2005). "Plant-derived pharmaceuticals—The road forward." *Trends Plant Sci* 10(12):580–585.

Plant-derived pharmaceuticals are poised to become the next major commercial development in biotechnology. The advantages they offer in terms of production scale and economy, product safety, ease of storage and distribution cannot be matched by any current commercial system; they also provide the most promising opportunity to supply low-cost drugs and vaccines to the developing world. However, despite the promised benefits, the commercialization of plant-derived pharmaceutical products is overshadowed by the uncertain regulatory terrain, particularly with regard to the adaptation of good manufacturing practice regulations to field-grown plants. The success of such products also depends on careful negotiation of the intellectual property landscape, particularly the achievement of freedom-to-operate licenses for use in developing countries.

Miralpeix, B. et al. (2014). "Strategic patent analysis in plant biotechnology: Terpenoid indole alkaloid metabolic engineering as a case study." *Plant Biotechnol J* 12(2):117–134.

The do-it-yourself patent search is a useful alternative to professional patent analysis particularly in the context of publicly funded projects where funds for IP activities may be limited. As a case study, we analyzed patents related to the engineering of terpenoid indole alkaloid (TIA) metabolism in plants. We developed a focused search strategy to remove redundancy and reduce the workload without missing important and relevant patents. This resulted in the identification of approximately 50 key patents associated with TIA metabolic engineering in plants, which could form the basis of a more detailed freedom-to-operate analysis. The structural elements of this search strategy could easily be transferred to other contexts, making it a useful generic model for publicly funded research projects.

Rommens, C. M. (2010). "Barriers and paths to market for genetically engineered crops." *Plant Biotechnol J* 8(2):101–111.

Each year, billions of dollars are invested in efforts to improve crops through genetic engineering (GE). These activities have resulted in a surge of publications and patents on technologies and genes: a momentum in basic research that, unfortunately, is not sustained throughout the subsequent phases of product development. After more than two decades of intensive research, the market for transgenic crops is still dominated by applications of just a handful of methods and genes. This discrepancy between research and development reflects difficulties in understanding and overcoming seven main barriers-to-entry: (1) trait efficacy in the field, (2) critical product concepts, (3) freedom-to-operate, (4) industry support, (5) identity preservation and stewardship, (6) regulatory approval and (7) retail and consumer acceptance. In this review, I describe the various roadblocks to market for transgenic crops and also discuss methods and approaches on how to overcome these, especially in the United States.

Schwartz, J. and C. Macomber (2017). "So, you think you have an idea: A practical risk reduction-conceptual model for academic translational research." *Bioengineering* (Basel) 4(2):29.

Translational research for new drugs, medical devices, and diagnostics encompasses aspects of both basic science and clinical research, requiring multidisciplinary skills and resources that are not all readily available in either a basic laboratory or clinical setting alone. We propose that, to be successful, "translational" research ought to be understood as a defined process from basic science through manufacturing, regulatory, clinical testing all the way to market. The authors outline a process which has worked well for them to identify and commercialize academic innovation. The academic environment places a high value on novelty and less value on whether, among other things, data are reproducible, scalable, reimbursable, or have commercial freedom to operate. In other words, when investors, strategic companies, or other later stage stakeholders evaluate academic efforts at translational research the relative lack of attention to clinical, regulatory, reimbursement, and manufacturing and intellectual property freedom to operate almost universally results in more questions and doubts about the potential of the proposed product, thereby inhibiting further interest. This contrasts with industry-based R & D, which often emphasizes manufacturing, regulatory and commercial factors. Academics do not so much choose to ignore those necessary and standard elements of translation development, but rather, they are not built into the culture or incentive structure of the university environment. Acknowledging and addressing this mismatch of approach and lack of common language in a systematic way facilitates a more effective "translation" handoffs of academic project concepts into meaningful clinical solutions help translational researchers more efficiently develop and progress new and better medical products which address validated needs. The authors provide an overview and framework for academic researchers to use which will help them define the elements of a market-driven translational program (1) problem identification and validation; (2) defining the conceptual model of disease; and (3) risk evaluation and mitigation strategies.

Sommer, A. (2012). "'Freedom to operate'. Patent legal aspects in the preparation of biosimilars." *Pharm Unserer Zeit* 41(6):481–484.

Webb, M. S. et al. (2007). "Liposomal drug delivery: Recent patents and emerging opportunities." *Recent Pat Drug Deliv Formul* 1(3):185–194.

It is challenging to develop innovative, as well as commercially viable, lipid-based drug delivery systems for the treatment of cancer because of the breadth of existing intellectual property that limits freedom-to-operate. For example, novel compositions can be described in which an NCE is associated with a lipid based carrier, but if the loading method or components of the lipid compositions are proprietary then the ability to develop novel compositions will require access to the appropriate intellectual property. We believe it is useful to present a review of the patent literature describing novel liposomal drug delivery systems given by parenteral administration to humans for the treatment of serious medical conditions such as cancer. This review is intended to: (i) identify and describe novel approaches that have recently been protected by US or international patents and patent applications; and (ii) identify founding technology in the field which is recently off-patent, thus presenting emerging opportunities for the development of new therapeutic options for patients. Issued patents, and selected patent applications, having publication dates in 2005 or 2006 were retrieved from searches of the US, European, German, Japanese, INPADOC and WIPO PCT databases. Liposomal delivery systems patented for systemic administration in the treatment of human medical conditions were reviewed in detail.

3

The Scope of Preformulation Studies

I didn't know of any homophile movements pre-Stonewall.

Sean Maher

3.1 Introduction

A detailed understanding of the properties of the drug substance is essential to minimize formulation problems in later stages of drug development, reduce drug development costs, and decrease the product's time to market (i.e., from drug substance to drug product). The goals of preformulation studies are to choose the correct form of the drug substance, evaluate its physical properties, and generate a thorough understanding of the material's stability under the conditions that will lead to development of an optimal drug delivery system. This chapter examines the continuously evolving scope of preformulation studies. These changes are driven by three forces: the regulatory requirements, the market requirements, and the technological development. However, prior to reviewing the various requirements that determine the scope of preformulation studies, it is important to review how the drug discovery models are rapidly changing and why there is a need for not just one but several levels of preformulation studies.

New drugs are discovered through serendipity, by chemical synthesis, by extraction from natural sources, or more recently through biotechnology processes. The drug discovery is rarely a linear process, and the many probes involved often run concurrently. Chapter 1 described in detail the various phases and stages of development. Although the industry has developed its own jargon about preclinical phases and clinical phases, the entire process of development goes through a highly orchestrated undertaking that requires very close association among all groups.

3.2 Preformulation Testing Criteria

The classical preformulation studies include the physicochemical characterization of the solid and solution properties of compounds that would be useful in formulating the drug into a suitable delivery system. It is in this critical decision-making about what constitutes the "suitable" that many a lead compound falls through. A good pharmacological and toxicological profile alone does not suffice. The drug delivery system must be able to take the molecules to the site of action at a cost and convenience commensurate with the treatment trends. An excellent remedy for headache that requires intravenous injection would not go past this stage; on the other hand, for those drugs that have no alternatives, such as in cancer treatment or other diseases in which the patient is hospitalized and critically ill, any dosage form would be acceptable if the cost and reimbursement issues do not impair the commercial projections of sales. Besides delivering the drug, the dosage form must provide a stable environment through a reasonable shelf life, preferably at room temperature and sufficient bioavailability, without any food or other drug interactions. Now, it is clearly seen as to why decision-making can be very difficult at the preformulation stages of drug development.

Although most preformulation studies start during the lead optimization (LO) phase, the involvement of some studies begins much earlier, even at the lead identification stage, to rule out undesirable features, such as chirality (though at times it can be the desired target), polymorphism, hygroscopicity, and extreme stability problems. The LO takes about 2 years to complete, and this narrows the choice to no more than about 3–4 compounds, based on the fine balance of pharmacology, toxicity, and biopharmaceutic compatibility. An optimally available oral drug would be a jackpot. Given the small quantity of sample available at this stage, agreements must be reached between the preformulation and drug discovery group to obviate redundant testing. The drug discovery group may take on nuclear magnetic resonance (NMR), mass spectra, and elemental analysis, whereas the preformulation group may use almost two-thirds of the supply (generally less than 10 mg) to perform Karl Fischer, pK_a, log P/log D, initial solubility, crystal structure, hygroscopicity, stability in solution and high-performance liquid chromatography (HPLC), and other spectroscopic data. For salt forms, additional testing of dynamic vapor sorption (DVS); X-ray; differential scanning calorimetry (DSC); solubility/stability tests; polymorphism studies using DSC/differential thermal analysis (DTA)/hot-stage microscopy (HSM); crystal habit using microscopy, both light and scanning electron microscopies (SEM); and stability using temperature and humidity stress to rule out hydrate or solvate status, often using circular dichroism, require a larger sample quantity, around 100 mg.

3.3 Regulatory Requirements

3.3.1 Small Molecules/General

Regulatory agencies are continuously pushing the quality systems that appear in the early phases of drug development. The International Conference on Harmonization (ICH) offers several guidelines for the characterization of the drug substance (Table 3.1).

The physicochemical and biological properties of the drug substance, specifically designed into the drug substance (e.g., by crystal engineering), that can influence the performance of the drug product and its manufacturability should be identified and discussed. Examples of the physicochemical and biological properties that might need to be examined include solubility, water content, particle size, crystal properties, biological activity, and permeability. These properties could be interrelated and might need to be considered in combination. Some of these properties can change with time and require time studies.

TABLE 3.1

International Conference on Harmonization (ICH) Guidelines for the Characterization of the Drug Substance

Category	Title	Type	Date
International Council on Harmonisation—Quality	Q1A(R2) Stability Testing of New Drug Substances and Products (PDF—58 KB)	Final guidance	11/01/03
International Council on Harmonisation—Quality	Q1B Photostability Testing of New Drug Substances and Products (PDF—339 KB)	Final guidance	11/01/96
International Council on Harmonisation—Quality	Q1C Stability Testing for New Dosage Forms (PDF—101 KB)	Final guidance	05/09/97
International Council on Harmonisation—Quality	Q1D Bracketing and Matrixing Designs for Stability Testing of New Drug Substances and Products (PDF—31 KB)	Final guidance	01/01/03
International Council on Harmonisation—Quality	Q1E Evaluation of Stability Data (PDF—221 KB)	Final guidance	06/01/04
International Council on Harmonisation—Quality	Q2(R1) Validation of Analytical Procedures: Text and Methodology (PDF—190 KB)		
International Council on Harmonisation—Quality	Q2A Text on Validation of Analytical Procedures (PDF—25 KB)	Final guidance	03/01/95
International Council on Harmonisation—Quality	Q2B Validation of Analytical Procedures: Methodology (PDF—132 KB)	Final guidance	05/19/97
International Council on Harmonisation—Quality	Q3A(R) Impurities in New Drug Substances (PDF—55 KB)	Final guidance	06/06/08
International Council on Harmonisation—Quality	Q3B(R) Impurities in New Drug Products (Revision 2) (PDF—171 KB)	Final guidance	08/04/06
International Council on Harmonisation—Quality	Q3C Impurities: Residual Solvents (PDF—41 KB)	Final guidance	12/24/97
International Council on Harmonisation—Quality	Q3C Tables and List (PDF—185 KB)	Final guidance	07/24/17
International Council on Harmonisation—Quality	Q3C Impurities: Residual Solvents: Maintenance Procedures for the Guidance for Industry Q3C (PDF—531 KB)	Procedures/recommendations	07/24/17
International Council on Harmonisation—Quality	Q3C Appendix 4 (PDF—120 KB)	Draft guidance	03/18/98
International Council on Harmonisation—Quality	Q3C Appendix 5 (PDF—216 KB)	Draft guidance	03/18/98
International Council on Harmonisation—Quality	Q3C Appendix 6 (PDF—128 KB)	Draft guidance	03/18/98
International Council on Harmonisation—Quality	Q4B Evaluation and Recommendation of Pharmacopoeial Texts for Use in the International Conference on Harmonisation Regions (PDF—55 KB)	Final guidance	02/20/07
International Council on Harmonisation—Quality	Q4B: Annex I: Residue on Ignition/Sulphated Ash General Chapter (PDF—58 KB)	Final guidance	09/18/17

(Continued)

TABLE 3.1 (*Continued*)

International Conference on Harmonization (ICH) Guidelines for the Characterization of the Drug Substance

Category	Title	Type	Date
International Council on Harmonisation—Quality	Q4B: Annex 2: Test for Extractable Volume of Parenteral Preparations General Chapter (PDF—69 KB)	Final guidance	09/18/17
International Council on Harmonisation—Quality	Q4B: Annex 3: Test for Particulate Contamination: Subvisible Particles General Chapter (PDF—993 KB)	Final guidance	09/18/17
International Council on Harmonisation—Quality	Q4B: Annex 4A: Microbiological Examination of Non-Sterile Products: Microbial Enumeration Tests General Chapter (PDF—69 KB)	Final guidance	09/18/17
International Council on Harmonisation—Quality	Q4B: Annex 4B: Microbiological Examination of Non-Sterile Products: Tests for Specified Micro-organisms General Chapter (PDF—69 KB)	Final guidance	09/18/17
International Council on Harmonisation—Quality	Q4B: Annex 4C: Microbiological Examination of Non-Sterile Products: Acceptance Criteria for Pharmaceutical Preparations and Substances for Pharmaceutical Use General Chapter (PDF—57 KB)	Final guidance	09/18/17
International Council on Harmonisation—Quality	Q4B: Annex 5: Disintegration Test General Chapter (PDF—69 KB)	Final guidance	09/18/17
International Council on Harmonisation—Quality	Q4B: Annex 6: Uniformity of Dosage Units General Chapter (PDF—53 KB)	Final guidance	06/13/14
International Council on Harmonisation—Quality	Q4B: Annex 7(R2): Dissolution Test General Chapter (PDF—102 KB)	Final guidance	06/23/11
International Council on Harmonisation—Quality	Q4B: Annex 8: Sterility Test General Chapter (PDF—68 KB)	Final guidance	09/18/17
International Council on Harmonisation—Quality	Q4B: Annex 9: Tablet Friability General Chapter (PDF—68 KB)	Final guidance	09/18/17
International Council on Harmonisation—Quality	Q4B: Annex 10: Polyacrylamide Gel Electrophoresis General Chapter (PDF—57 KB)	Final guidance	09/18/17
International Council on Harmonisation—Quality	Q4B Annex 11: Capillary Electrophoresis General Chapter (PDF—93 KB)	Final guidance	09/02/10
International Council on Harmonisation—Quality	Q4B Annex 12: Analytical Sieving General Chapter (PDF—87 KB)	Final guidance	09/01/10
International Council on Harmonisation—Quality	Q4B Annex 13: Bulk Density and Tapped Density of Powders General Chapter (PDF—94 KB)	Final guidance	05/24/13
International Council on Harmonisation—Quality	Q4B Annex 14: Bacterial Endotoxins Test General Chapter (PDF—96 KB)	Final guidance	10/15/13
			(*Continued*)

TABLE 3.1 (*Continued*)

International Conference on Harmonization (ICH) Guidelines for the Characterization of the Drug Substance

Category	Title	Type	Date
International Council on Harmonisation—Quality	Q5A Viral Safety Evaluation of Biotechnology Products Derived from Cell Lines of Human or Animal Origin (PDF—71 KB)	Final guidance	09/01/98
International Council on Harmonisation—Quality	Q5B Quality of Biotechnological Products: Analysis of the Expression Construct in Cells Used for Production of r-DNA Derived Protein Products (PDF—109 KB)	Final guidance	02/01/96
International Council on Harmonisation—Quality	Q5C Quality of Biotechnological Products: Stability Testing of Biotechnological/Biological Products (PDF—70 KB)	Final guidance	07/01/96
International Council on Harmonisation—Quality	Q5D Quality of Biotechnological/Biological Products: Derivation and Characterization of Cell Substrates Used for Production of Biotechnological/Biological Products; Availability (PDF—52 KB)	Final guidance	09/21/98
International Council on Harmonisation—Quality	Q5E Comparability of Biotechnological/Biological Products Subject to Changes in Their Manufacturing Process (PDF—58 KB)	Final guidance	06/01/05
International Council on Harmonisation—Quality	Q6A Specifications: Test Procedures and Acceptance Criteria for New Drug Substances and New Drug Products: Chemical Substances	Final guidance	12/29/00
International Council on Harmonisation—Quality	Q6B Specifications: Test Procedures and Acceptance Criteria for Biotechnological/Biological Products (PDF—54 KB)	Final guidance	08/01/99
International Council on Harmonisation—Quality	Q7 Good Manufacturing Practice Guidance for Active Pharmaceutical Ingredients Guidance for Industry (PDF—253 KB)	Final guidance	09/30/16
International Council on Harmonisation—Quality	Q8(R2) Pharmaceutical Development (PDF—402 KB)	Final guidance	11/20/09
International Council on Harmonisation—Quality	Q9 Quality Risk Management (PDF—113 KB)	Final Guidance	06/01/06
International Council on Harmonisation—Quality	Q10 Pharmaceutical Quality System (PDF—274 KB)	Final guidance	04/07/09
International Council on Harmonisation—Quality	Q8, Q9, and Q10 Questions and Answers (PDF—185 KB)	Final guidance	11/01/11
International Council on Harmonisation—Quality	Q8, Q9, & Q10 Questions and Answers—Appendix: Q&As from Training Sessions (Q8, Q9, & Q10 Points to Consider)	Final guidance	07/25/12
International Council on Harmonisation—Quality	Q11 Development and Manufacture of Drug Substances (PDF—708 KB)	Final guidance	11/19/12

(Continued)

TABLE 3.1 (*Continued*)

International Conference on Harmonization (ICH) Guidelines for the Characterization of the Drug Substance

Category	Title	Type	Date
International Council on Harmonisation—Quality	Q3D Elemental Impurities (PDF—685 KB)	Final guidance	09/09/15
International Council on Harmonisation—Quality	Q11 Development and Manufacture of Drug Substances—Questions and Answers (Chemical Entities and Biotechnological/Biological Entities) (PDF—843 KB)	Final guidance	02/23/18
International Council on Harmonisation—Quality	Q7 Good Manufacturing Practice Guidance for Active Pharmaceutical Ingredients Questions and Answers Guidance for Industry (PDF—218 KB)	Final guidance	04/19/18
International Council for Harmonisation—Quality	Q12 Technical and Regulatory Considerations for Pharmaceutical Product Lifecycle Management Core Guideline Guidance for Industry (PDF—451 KB)	Draft guidance	05/30/18
International Council for Harmonisation—Quality	Q12 Technical and Regulatory Considerations for Pharmaceutical Product Lifecycle Management Annex (PDF—223 KB)	Draft guidance	05/30/18
International Council on Harmonisation—Quality	Q3D(R1) Elemental Impurities (PDF—177 KB)	Draft guidance	07/13/18

To evaluate the potential effect of the physicochemical properties of the drug substance on the performance of the drug product, studies on drug product might be warranted. For example, the ICH *Q6A Specifications: Test Procedures and Acceptance Criteria for New Drug Substances and New Drug Products: Chemical Substances* describes some of the circumstances in which drug product studies are recommended. The knowledge gained from the studies investigating the potential effect of drug substance properties on drug product performance can be used, as appropriate, to justify elements of the drug substance specification.

One purpose of these comprehensive guidelines is to prepare for compliance with process analytical technology (PAT), a recent initiative of the Food and Drug Administration (FDA; Ref. 1). Process analytical technology is intended to encourage drug makers to build quality into their development processes, so that they can anticipate the impact of changes on a final formulation. Although PAT is voluntary, the initiative is designed to promote a better understanding, among drug manufacturers, of the mechanics of their processes, so that they can avoid failures and minimize the amount of testing required at the end of production. Preformulation studies support PAT by providing more information on an active pharmaceutical ingredient's (API's) characteristics to facilitate downstream efficiency and success. Drug manufacturers can eventually submit their documents to a special PAT group within the FDA, which can expedite regulatory approval. Preformulation studies also support reference standard characterization. The regulations of the FDA require that the drug manufacturers establish a primary reference standard at a certain stage in drug development, whereby a compound is characterized as thoroughly and precisely as possible. Subsequent tests and analyses must be based on samples that meet this standard.

The FDA considers PAT to be a system for designing, analyzing, and controlling manufacturing through timely measurements (i.e., during processing) of critical quality and performance attributes of raw and in-process materials and processes, with the goal of ensuring final product quality. It is important to note that the term *analytical* in PAT is viewed broadly to include chemical, physical, microbiological, mathematical, and risk analysis conducted in an integrated manner. The goal of PAT is to enhance the understanding and control the manufacturing process, which is consistent with our current drug quality system: *quality cannot be tested into products; it should be built in or should be by design.* Consequently, the tools and principles described in this guidance should be used for gaining the process understanding and can also be used to meet the regulatory requirements for validating and controlling the manufacturing process.

Quality is built into pharmaceutical products through a comprehensive understanding of the following:

- The intended therapeutic objectives; patient population; route of administration; and pharmacological, toxicological, and pharmacokinetic characteristics of a drug.
- The chemical, physical, and biopharmaceutic characteristics of a drug.
- Design of a product and selection of product components and packaging based on drug attributes listed previously.
- The design of the manufacturing processes by using principles of engineering, material science, and quality assurance to ensure acceptable and reproducible product quality and performance throughout a product's shelf life.

Effective innovation in development, manufacture, and quality assurance would be expected to answer the following questions:

- What are the mechanisms of degradation, drug release, and absorption?
- What are the effects of product components on quality?
- What sources of variability are critical?
- How does the process manage variability?

This guidance facilitates innovation in development, manufacture, and quality assurance by focusing on process understanding. These concepts are applicable to all manufacturing situations.

3.3.2 Phytomedicines

In January 2004, the U.S. FDA issued a guideline for botanical products and a revised draft in 2016. The information discussed in section VII.A.1 of the guideline pertains to the initiation of characterization of the drug substance. Also, it should be provided for all products. It is important for the safe conduct of clinical trials to ensure the proper identity of botanical raw materials used in the trials. As there is no history of experience in the United States with botanical raw materials marketed only outside the United States, a certificate of authenticity of the plant and plant parts should be provided for such materials. A trained professional who is competent to determine authenticity should sign this certificate. This information should also be provided, if available, for a botanical raw material marketed in the United States.

The general method of preparation (e.g., pulverization, decoction, expression, aqueous extraction, and ethanolic extraction) is provided under §312. 23(a)(7)(iv)(a). This is especially important where more than one process exists in the literature on which the safety of the botanical drug substance is based.

The European Medicines Agency (EMA) provides the following guidelines for herbal (botanical, as listed in United States) products:

- Patient Leaflet template concerning advice on the preparation of herbal teas as (traditional) herbal medicinal products by end-users
- Public statement on the interpretation of the term 'external use' for use in the field of traditional herbal medicinal products
- Public statement on CPMP List of Herbal Drugs with serious risks, dated 1992
- HMPC statement on environmental risk assessment of herbal medicinal products

A comprehensive specification for each herbal drug must be submitted, even if the starting material is a herbal drug preparation. This also applies if the applicant is not the manufacturer of the preparation. In the case of fatty or essential oils used as active substances of herbal medicinal products, a specification for the herbal drug is required, unless fully justified. The scientific names of the parent plant and its part(s) also need to be stated.

If no monograph for the herbal drug is given in a Pharmacopoeia referred to in Directives 75/318/European Economic Community (EEC) and 81/852/EEC, Annex 1, a comprehensive specification for the herbal drug must be supplied and should be set out in the same way, where practicable, as the monographs on herbal drugs in the European Pharmacopoeia. This should include the botanical name and authority and the common name, if used for labeling purposes. Information on the site of collection, the time of harvesting and stage of growth, treatment during growth with pesticides, and so on, as well as the drying and storage conditions should be included, if possible. The comprehensive specification should be established on the basis of recent scientific data. In the case of herbal drugs with constituents of known therapeutic activity, assays of their content (with test procedure) are required. The content must be included as a range, so as to ensure reproducibility of the quality of the finished product. In the case of herbal drugs where constituents of known therapeutic activity are not known, assays of marker substances (with test procedure) are required. The choice of the markers should be justified.

As a general rule, herbal drugs must be tested for microbiological quality and for residues of pesticides and fumigation agents; toxic metals, likely contaminants and adulterants; and others, unless otherwise justified. Radioactive contamination should be tested for if there are reasons for concerns. Specifications and descriptions of the analytical procedures must be submitted, together with the limits applied. Analytical procedures not given in a Pharmacopoeia should be validated in accordance with the ICH guideline "Validation of analytical procedures: methodology" (CPMP/ICH/281/95) and the registration of veterinary products (VICH) guideline (CVMP/VICH/591/98).

If the herbal medicinal product does not contain the herbal drug itself but a preparation, the comprehensive specification for the herbal drug must be followed by a description and validation of the manufacturing process for the herbal drug preparation. The information may be supplied either as part of the marketing authorization application or with the help of the European Drug Master File procedure.

For each herbal drug preparation, a comprehensive specification must be submitted. This must be established based on the recent scientific data and must give particulars of the characteristics, identification tests, and purity tests. This has to be done, for example, by the appropriate chromatographic methods. If deemed necessary by the results of the analysis of the starting material, tests on microbiological quality, residues of pesticides, fumigation agents, solvents, and toxic metals must be carried out. Radioactivity should be tested if there are reasons for concerns. Quantitative determination (assay) of markers or of substances with known therapeutic activity is required. The content must be indicated with the lowest possible tolerance. The test methods must be described in detail.

If preparations from herbal drugs with constituents of known therapeutic activity are standardized (i.e., adjusted to a defined content of constituents with known therapeutic activity), the mode of achievement of the standardization must be stated. If another substance is used for these purposes, it is necessary to specify the quantity, as a range, that can be added.

This section should be in accordance with the "Note for guidance on stability testing of new active substances and medicinal products" (CPMP/ICH/380/95 and CVMP/VICH/899/99) and the "Note for guidance on stability testing of existing active substances and related finished products" (CPMP/QWP/556/96 and EMA/CVMP/846/99).

Because the herbal drug or the herbal drug preparation in its entirety is regarded as the active substance, a mere determination of the stability of the constituents with known therapeutic activity will not suffice. It must also be shown, as far as possible, for example, by means of appropriate fingerprint chromatograms, that other substances present in the herbal drug or in the herbal drug preparation are likewise stable and that their proportional content remains constant.

If an herbal medicinal product contains several herbal drugs or preparations of several herbal drugs and if it is not possible to determine the stability of each active substance, the stability of the medicinal product should be determined by appropriate fingerprint chromatograms, appropriate overall methods of assay, and physical and sensory tests or by other appropriate tests. The appropriateness of the tests should be justified by the applicant.

In the case of an herbal medicinal product containing a herbal drug or herbal drug preparation with constituents of known therapeutic activity, the variation in content during the proposed shelf life should not exceed $\pm 5\%$ of the initial assay value, unless justified. In the case of a herbal medicinal product containing a herbal drug or herbal drug preparation, where constituents with known therapeutic activity are unknown, a variation in content during the proposed shelf life of $\pm 10\%$ of the initial assay value can be accepted, if justified by the applicant. These criteria also apply to the stability testing of active substances in a similar manner.

3.3.3 Large-Molecule Drugs

A biopharmaceutical drug can go into development before anyone knows much about how it works. The protein may be identified through genomics or proteomics activities or through more traditional medical research. It may initially be associated with a particular disease process or a certain metabolic event. In any case, its mechanism of action—as well as many of its structural characteristics and biochemical properties—may be unknown. One of the more challenging aspects of developing protein pharmaceuticals is dealing with and overcoming the inherent physical and chemical instabilities of proteins. This inherent instability has the potential to alter the state of the protein from the desired (native) form to an undesirable form (upon storage), compromising patient safety and drug efficacy. Marketing concerns come up earlier in the development of protein drugs. Route of administration is determined by the target product profile and if the product will treat a chronic or acute disorder, if it will need specific targeting—a broad or narrow therapeutic window—or if it will be administered at home or in the clinic or hospital. For example, marketing considerations arise early in product development for monoclonal antibodies (MAbs). Typically, MAbs are needed at high doses (hundreds of milligrams per dose) and are normally delivered intravenously. The drive to reduce healthcare costs has created a need to administer MAb therapeutics more conveniently, at home, subcutaneously. Thus, MAbs must be available at high concentrations (~200 mg/mL) in the vial. At these high concentrations, MAb-containing solutions are viscous, making them difficult to administer conveniently. Hence, a preformulation activity that needs to be considered is a concentration study investigating the solubility behavior, the effect of concentration on viscosity, and the increased potential for aggregation. These studies have the potential to strongly influence the target product profile and the design of the clinical trial.

All these questions can affect the optimal formulation of a drug. For example, an early formulation question is whether the product will be lyophilized (freeze-dried) or sold as a liquid. The advantages of a liquid include time-saving, lower cost, and ease of use for patients and clinicians, all of which are good sales points. But stability questions often make freeze-drying necessary for protein and peptide pharmaceuticals. Freeze-dried drugs have a longer shelf life and better stability for shipping and storage, even if they cost more and take longer to make.

The seemingly endless variation of polypeptides makes them interesting as potential therapeutics, but it also makes them a challenge to develop into products. Each protein is unique, and just because variation from protein to protein affects biologic production and purification, it is central to the formulation development process. Methods developed for one biopharmaceutical are not always directly applicable to others. Similarly, it is quite likely that a formulation developed for one biopharmaceutical may not provide the same level of stability for a different biopharmaceutical.

While there are numerous ways for a protein to lose its stability, the three most commonly encountered modes of denaturation and degradation are aggregation, oxidation, and deamidation. The commonly accepted strategy for rational formulation development relies on identifying mechanisms of denaturation and degradation, in order to develop effective countermeasures. Once the specifics of any particular degradation pathway are understood, a more informed choice regarding excipients and formulation can be made, accelerating the product development.

International disagreement over preservatives in food and drugs may present a problem at the preformulation stage. The U.S., European Union, and Japanese compendia standards differ regarding the timing of antimicrobial tests and the preservatives and excipients that are allowed. Japan, for example, does not accept phenol, a preservative used commonly in the United States. So, at this early stage, companies must decide if and where their products will be distributed outside the United States. The European Union is known to have the toughest acceptance criteria for preservatives. The ICH is working toward a common standard, but many formulators have criticized its slow progress. This is applicable if preformulation studies would conduct compatibility studies.

In the development of proteins, physical stability is of prime importance. Four important preformulation stress tests are the shake test (agitation), surfactant test, freeze–thaw test, and heating experiment. Each formulation configuration is shaken in a vial to determine whether it forms aggregates. Then, a surfactant (usually a polysorbate detergent, such as Tween) may be selected to prevent the formation of precipitants by making it harder for proteins to aggregate. Most proteins are stable around $2°C–8°C$, but few are stable at room temperature. Heating experiments help scientists examine degradation at temperature extremes by heating them to $30°C$ (about $86°F$) and maybe even to $45°C$ (about $113°F$). At high temperatures, different mechanisms of protein denaturation may arise.

3.3.4 Recombinant DNA Products

The U.S. FDA provides a detailed description of the characterization of the substances obtained by recombinant DNA technique. In addition, several guidelines of the ICH and other guidelines of the U.S. FDA provide additional information on stability testing of biological products. What follows in the successive paragraphs is an outline of what constitutes the required minimum studies. A drug substance is defined by the U.S. FDA as the unformulated active substance that may be subsequently formulated with excipients to produce the drug product.

A clear description of the drug substance should be provided. This description may include, but is not be limited to, any of the following: chemical structure, primary and subunit structure, molecular weight (MV), molecular formula, established U.S. Adapted Names, antibody class/subclass (if appropriate), and so on.

A description and the results of all the analytical testing performed on the manufacturer's reference standard lot and qualifying lots to characterize the drug substance should be included. Information from specific tests regarding the identity, purity, stability, and consistency of the manufacture of the drug substance should be provided. Examples of analyses for which information may be submitted include, but are not necessarily limited to, the following:

- Amino acid analysis
- Amino acid sequencing, entire sequence or amino- and carboxy-terminal sequences
- Peptide mapping
- Determination of disulfide linkage
- Sodium dodecyl sulfate-polyacrylamide gel electrophoresis (SDS-PAGE) (reduced and nonreduced)
- Isoelectric focusing
- Conventional chromatography and HPLC, for example, reverse-phase, size-exclusion, and ion-exchange
- Mass spectroscopy (MS)
- Assays to detect product-related proteins, including deamidated, oxidized, cleaved, and aggregated forms and other variants, for example, amino acid substitutions and adducts/derivatives
- Assays to detect residual host proteins, DNA, and reagents
- Immunochemical analyses
- Assays to quantitate bioburden and endotoxin

Additional physicochemical characterization may be required for products undergoing posttranslational modifications, for example, glycosylation, sulfation, phosphorylation, and formylation. Additional physicochemical characterization may also be required for products derivatized with other agents, including other proteins, toxins, drugs, radionuclides, and chemicals. The information submitted should include the degree of derivatization or conjugation, the amount of unmodified product, the removal of free materials (e.g., toxins, radionuclides, linkers, and others), and the stability of the modified product. All test methods should be fully described and the results provided. The application should also include the actual data, such as legible copies of chromatograms, photographs of SDS-PAGE or agarose gel, spectra, and the like.

A description and results of all relevant in vivo and in vitro biological testing performed on the manufacturer's reference standard lot to show the potency and activity(ies) of the drug substance should be provided. Results of relevant testing performed on lots other than the reference standard lot, which might have been used in establishing the biological activity of the product, should also be included. The description and validation of the bioassays should include the methods and standards used, the inter- and intra-assay variability, and the acceptable limits of the assay.

A description of the storage conditions, study protocols, and results supporting the stability of the drug substance should be submitted in this section. (ICH document Stability Testing of Biotechnological/Biological Products or other FDA documents, such as Guideline for Submitting Documentation for the Stability of Human Drug and Biologics, for specific information.) Data from tests to monitor the biological activity and degradation products, such as aggregated, deamidated, oxidized, and cleaved forms, should be included, as appropriate. Data supporting any proposed storage of intermediate(s) should also be provided.

3.4 Testing Systems

The significant downturn in the number of drugs approved by the U.S. FDA has prompted newer models of drug discovery that promise to produce a larger number of possible leads. All promising leads must be put through some level of preformulation testing, creating a large burden on preformulation groups to produce results in shorter times. The technologic developments in analytical methodologies allow greater understanding of drug substances, and most companies would rather quickly adopt these new techniques, particularly if they automate the testing methods. Some of the most recent introductions of new techniques include liquid chromatography (LC) or gas chromatography (GC)-MS/MS systems, use of Sirius GLpK_a and lipophilicity and pION pSOL instruments, CheqSol® (chasing equilibrium solubility) measurements, nanocrystal technology, and the modulating role of solubilizers on drug efflux by P-glycoprotein (Pgp). The in silico prediction of the effect of solubilizers on Pgp are some of the newer goals of preformulation studies. There are scores of new innovations in dissolution instrumentation, drug substance stability study, and identification of degradation products. One test at the preformulation level pertains to the biological transportability of the new drug substance; much of this information is gained from differential solubility analysis. Many methods such as the Caco-2 cells model are now routinely used to provide initial estimates about the biological activity potential of new compounds. All the changing regulatory requirements and technological developments place a significant burden on the preformulation team to stay alert and stay abreast of the technology.

3.4.1 Polymorph Screening

Some of the most significant information comes from identifying the optimal crystal form and the corresponding behavior in different humidity conditions. This information will have implications for a drug's stability and solubility and will guide decisions concerning the appropriate dosage form or formulation and how it is packaged, handled, and stored. If the compound is a crystal, the next step is to identify its shape or the different shapes it can take. This information is crucial for several reasons, the most obvious of which is to ensure uniform synthesis, manufacturing, and testing of the compound within a formulation.

Drug manufacturers need to confirm that each batch of API has the same crystalline structure and that this crystal form remains constant throughout the formulation and life of the drug product (particularly for solid oral dosage forms, powders, creams, ointments, and suspensions). The crystalline structure can also place physical constraints on the ability to manufacture a particular dosage form. For example, needle-shaped crystals tend to entangle and often do not flow well in manufacturing equipment. This can cause formulation of "hot spots," with high concentrations of the API in some areas and deficits in others. If the compound comes in different crystal shapes, then formulators will prefer the shape that is most conducive to the physical manufacture of the desired dosage form—other things being equal. For example, if drug manufacturers prefer a tablet or capsule, we may recommend that they synthesize more spherically shaped crystals rather than flat plates or needles. The crystalline structure also affects a compound's stability and solubility, which again have important implications for formulating, manufacturing, packaging, and storing pharmaceutical products and API. A trade-off may often present itself when selecting a crystal form. For example, crystalline structures that are more desirable from the standpoint of synthesis or formulation manufacture may be less advantageous when considering stability or solubility.

3.4.2 pK_a, Partitioning, and Solubility

Critical variables that should be considered when making formulation decisions are pK_a, lipophilicity, and solubility. The pK_a and lipophilicity can be measured using Sirius GLpK_a, and a pION pSOL instrument is used to measure the intrinsic solubility of the compound. The pK_a value is the pH at which acidic or basic groups attached to molecules exist as 50% ionized and 50% nonionized in aqueous solution. The pK_a value provides valuable data on the interaction of an ionizable drug with charged biological membranes and receptor sites and information on where the drug may be absorbed in the digestive tract. Knowing the pK_a also enables the scientist to know how much to alter the pH to drive a compound to its fully ionized or nonionized form for analytical and other purposes, such as formulation, solubility, and stability. Formulators need to know where a drug will dissolve in the digestive tract and whether that corresponds to the optimal region for absorption, especially if they are planning to create a dosage form that will be taken orally. If the drug dissolves too early, it may reprecipitate in a form that is absorbed poorly. But if a drug does not dissolve until after it travels through the stomach or small intestine, it is not likely to get absorbed. In the first case, scientists may want to create a formulation that slows the dissolution, and in the second case, they may want to create a formulation that speeds it up. Another option would be to formulate a dosage that could be administered by injection. Often, it is preferred to use a traditional, manual test process to evaluate solubility. For example, one may place samples into three buffer solutions at different pH, shake them mechanically overnight, and then measure how much of the compound has dissolved into the solutions. The measure of the intrinsic solubility of a compound (i.e., the fundamental solubility at which the compound is completely unionized) is useful for formulators in many ways. Working over a pH range from 2 to 11, the pSOL instrument can typically determine the intrinsic solubility across a range of 5–50 mg/mL. The use of the Sirius GLpK_a to create lipophilicity profiles is very useful. Drugs that can be taken orally must fall into a fairly narrow window between extreme lipophilicity and extreme hydrophilicity. Many drugs cross biological lipid membranes by passive transport, and there is an optimum value of lipophilicity for each type of membrane. For example, drugs that are highly lipophilic may be easily transported or absorbed but may get trapped inside fat-storage regions, where they will be ineffective. On the other hand, a drug that is extremely hydrophilic may not penetrate the membrane and, therefore, has no pharmacological effect. Hence, formulators often find lipophilicity profiles very valuable.

Poorly soluble compounds represent an estimated 60% of compounds in development and many major marketed drugs. It is important to measure and predict solubility and permeability accurately at an early stage and interpret these data to help assess the potential for development of candidates. This requires developing an effective strategy to select the most appropriate tools to examine and improve solubility in each phase of development and optimization of solid-state approaches to enhance solubility, including the use of polymorphs, co-crystals, and amorphous solids.

Poor solubility can hinder—or even prevent—drug development. Yet, the volume and level of poorly soluble compounds are increasing dramatically, leaving gaps in development pipelines. Currently, only 8% of new drug candidates have both high solubility and permeability. It is important to know the solubility of drugs, as it helps in the identification of potential screening and bioavailability issues. It is valuable in planning chemistry changes during biopharmaceutical evaluation, is important for the confirmation of bioavailability issues, and is also useful in the early development of formulations. In drug development, solubility knowledge is needed for biopharmaceutical classification, biowaivers, and bioequivalence; it is also required for formulation optimization and salt selection. In manufacture, solubility also affects the optimization of the manufacturing processes.

With this trend of increasingly insoluble drugs stretching resources, many companies are now reevaluating their strategy. They know that there are many available technologies to measure, predict, and improve solubility and several new emerging techniques. Studies that encompass this scope would include how membrane permeation of drugs can be enhanced by means of solubilizing agents, how the solid state is characterized and modified to improve solubility and drug performance, how salt screening and selection can impact dissolution rate and oral absorption, the application of nanocrystal technology to increase dissolution rate, and the analysis of the use of pharmaceutical co-crystals in enhancing drug properties.

There are several new emerging methods to measure the solubility of ionizable drugs, such as using the method called CheqSol. CheqSol is a software product that processes data and controls Sirius's existing GLpK_a, PCA200, and D-PAS instrumentation. Not only does CheqSol measure equilibrium and kinetic solubility rapidly and accurately, but it also provides insights into compound behavior that will be of value for the better understanding of drug bioavailability, modeling of precipitation processes, and investigating changes of crystalline form in suspensions. Pharmaceutical scientists need to know the solubility of drug molecules during drug discovery, as well as in confirmation of bioavailability issues, human formulation design, and biopharmaceutical classification, which is required by the FDA. CheqSol is much faster than shake-flask methods, and it measures both the equilibrium and the turbidimetric (or kinetic) solubilities in the same experiment. CheqSol works by monitoring the pH, as hydrochloric acid (HCl) or potassium hydroxide (KOH) solutions are carefully added to a 10-mL solution of the ionized drug until it precipitates, as detected by an abrupt decrease in the amount of light transmitted through the solution. The concentration at this point is equivalent to a kinetic solubility. Chasing equilibrium then begins—HCl and KOH are added sequentially to force the solution to become supersaturated or subsaturated, and the state of saturation is determined from subsequent small changes in the pH reading. The concentration of unionized species at the crossing points, when the pH change is zero and the sample is neither super- nor subsaturated, is equal to the intrinsic solubility. For "chasers," such as diclofenac, that supersaturate and chase equilibrium, CheqSol often finds an equilibrium solubility result within 20 minutes and confirms it several times during a 60-minute experiment. For "nonchasers," such as chlorpromazine, that do not chase equilibrium, the pH after precipitation follows the precipitation Bjerrum curve, and the software calculates the result from the shape of the curve.

Predicting aqueous solubility with in silico tools is a key drug property. It is, however, difficult to measure accurately, especially for poorly soluble compounds, and thus, numerous in silico models have been developed for their prediction. Some in silico models can predict aqueous solubility of simple, uncharged organic chemicals reasonably well; however, solubility prediction for charged species and drug-like chemicals is not very accurate. However, extrapolating solubility data to intestinal absorption from pharmacokinetic and physicochemical data, elucidating crucial parameters for absorption, and assessing the potential for improvement of bioavailability are important at the preformulation stages.

Solubilizers (e.g., organic solvents, detergents, and Pluronics) are often used to solubilize drugs in the aqueous solution, without considering their effects on biological systems, such as (i) lipid membranes and (ii) multidrug resistance (MDR) efflux transporters (e.g., Pgp and MDR1).

The modulatory role of solubilizers on drug efflux by Pgp and in silico prediction of the effect of solubilizers on Pgp are some of the newer goals of preformulation studies.

Liposomal solubilization is an effective approach for the delivery of potent, insoluble drug candidates. However, careful consideration of the various lipid and drug properties, along with an emphasis on manufacturing conditions, is needed for the successful development of a marketable formulation.

Increasing dissolution rates by using nanocrystal technologies is becoming common. The NanoCrystal Technology was developed by Elan Corporation (Dublin 2, Ireland). For poorly water-soluble compounds, Elan's proprietary NanoCrystal technology can enable formulation and improve compound activity and final product characteristics. The NanoCrystal technology can be incorporated into all dosage forms, including solid, liquid, fast-melt, pulsed release, and controlled-release dosage forms, both parenterally and orally. Poor water solubility correlates with slow dissolution rate, and decreasing particle size increases the surface area, which leads to an increase in dissolution rate. This can be accomplished predictably and efficiently by using NanoCrystal technology (4). NanoCrystal particles are small particles of the drug substance, typically less than 1000 nm in diameter, which are produced by milling the drug substance, using a proprietary wet milling technique (Figure 3.1). The NanoCrystal particles of the drug are stabilized against agglomeration by surface adsorption of selected GRAS (generally regarded as safe) stabilizers. The result is an aqueous dispersion of the drug substance that behaves like a solution—a NanoCrystal colloidal dispersion, which can be processed into finished dosage forms for all routes of administration.

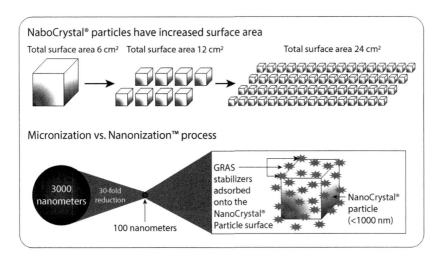

FIGURE 3.1 The NanoCrystal® technology. (Courtesy of Elan Corporation, Dublin 2, Ireland.)

Nanonization is a formulation technology that can be universally applied to all drugs—each drug can be transferred to drug nanocrystals. The main production technologies available to produce drug nanocrystals have their advantages and limitations. The reduction of solid particles to nanoparticles is achieved by high-pressure homogenization.

3.4.3 Salt Screening

Recent trends in combinatorial chemistry have resulted in the synthesis of large-MW lipophilic drugs. Converting the free acid/base form to a salt is an important option to explore when trying to improve solubility and oral bioavailability. Of the 21 new molecular entities approved by the FDA in 2003, 10 were salt forms. Selection of the right counterion with optimum physiochemical characteristics is crucial to drug development. Consideration of the new compound's physical–chemical properties, processability under various manufacturing conditions, and bioavailability must be made. A complete range of characterization tools for a complete salt screen would include the following:

- X-ray powder diffraction analysis (XRD)
- Thermal analysis (DSC, thermogravimetric analyzer [TGA], and thermo-mechanical analyzer [TMA])
- Microscopy (light and polarized)
- DVS—moisture absorption and desorption
- Density (intrinsic and bulk)
- NMR analysis
- Solubility analysis in various media
- Dissolution (including intrinsic dissolution testing)
- Particle size analysis (optical, laser light, and light obscuration)

Scheme 3.1 describes a salt-screening decision-making tree.

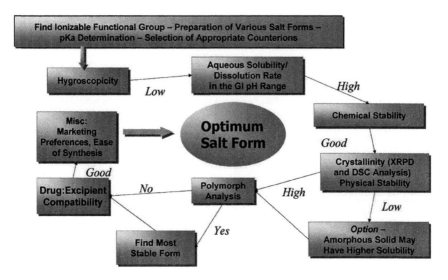

SCHEME 3.1   Salt selection tree. (Courtesy of Cardinal Health, Dublin, OH.)

3.5 Solid-State Characterization

3.5.1 Powder Properties

Powders are masses of solid particles or granules surrounded by air (or other fluid), and it is the solid plus fluid combination that significantly affects the bulk properties of the powder. It is perhaps the most complicating characteristic, because the amount of fluid can be highly variable.

Powders are probably the least predictable of all materials in relation to flow ability because of the large number of factors that can change their rheological properties. Physical characteristics of the particles, such as size, shape, angularity, size variability, and hardness, will affect flow properties. External factors, such as humidity, conveying environment, vibration, and perhaps most importantly, aeration, will compound the problem. The more common variables would include the following:

- Powder or particle variables:
    - Particle size
    - Size distribution
    - Shape
    - Surface texture
    - Cohesivity
    - Surface coating
    - Particle interaction
    - Wear or attrition characteristic

- Propensity to electrostatic charge
- Hardness
- Stiffness
- Strength
- Fracture toughness
- External factors influencing powder behavior:
  - Flow rate
  - Compaction condition
  - Vibration
  - Temperature
  - Humidity
  - Electrostatic charge
  - Aeration
  - Transportation experience
  - Container surface effects
  - Storage time

Another characteristic of powders is that they are often inherently unstable in relation to their flow performance. This instability is most obvious when a free-flowing material ceases to flow. This transition may be initiated by the formation of a bridge in a bin, by adhesion to surfaces, or by any event that may promote compaction of the powder. The tendency to switch in this way varies greatly from one powder to another but can even be pronounced between batches of the same material.

Therefore, the nature of powders is such that an adverse combination of environmental factors can cause an otherwise-free-flowing powder to block or flow with difficulty. Conversely, a very cohesive powder may be processed satisfactorily if the handling conditions are optimized.

Given the complex nature of powders, it is not surprising that processing difficulties are very common. Being able to predict flow performance would bring about many operational advantages, such as reducing stoppages and improving product quality. To achieve this, we need to know how a given powder is affected by the variables mentioned earlier and also to have a reliable indicator of the potential instability of the powder. Predicting flow ability performance in a particular plant therefore requires knowledge of the handling and processing conditions, as well as the flow ability characteristics of the material under these conditions. It means that the process conditions relevant to flow ability need to be determined. These might include the level of static and dynamic head produced in a storage bin or hopper; the amount of aeration that occurs; and the opportunity to adsorb moisture, become electrostatically charged, or be consolidated due to vibration. Another factor that can affect powder flow is an increase in the amount of finer particles as a result of attrition. All or at least the most important of these factors then need to be quantified regarding how they affect the flow ability.

Slight compaction, a small vibration, or the smallest amount of aeration can significantly affect the flow ability. This is the main reason why traditional methods of flow ability measurement have not been suitable as a basis for repetitive testing. In all traditional techniques, the packing condition and the air content are largely unknown quantities, and so, the results will vary accordingly. When making an assessment, it is essential to know what was tested and the condition of the powder when tested. In addition to the packing problem, traditional flow ability measurements are prone to operator error, have poor repeatability, and, for the most part, are very time-consuming. An automated test and analysis system that takes only minutes, is very repeatable, and is independent of the operator is needed.

The most important innovation required in relation to traditional techniques is a way of classifying powders, so that flow ability performance of each powder can be measured and recorded, along with its processing experience. Eventually, such a database of information could remove much of the uncertainty from processing and provide a reference base for the development of new powders. It would allow each production machine to be classified in terms of the powders that could be processed efficiently.

Ideally, the classification of powders would provide more than just flow ability data, such as flow rate and compaction indices. It would also include data describing the robustness and stability of the powder, for example, vulnerability to segregation, attrition, and vibration. Given this, the two key issues of powder processing could be addressed. First, will the powder flow satisfactorily—does it have flowability properties that suit the process? And second, is the powder robust—will it be adversely affected by being processed?

Freeman Technology and the FT4 Powder Rheometer offer real benefits to all users of powders. These include the following:

- The more efficient use of powder-handling systems by reducing stoppages and optimizing throughput
- Improved product quality by introducing quality conformance checks at all stages of production
- Overall—improved competitiveness

3.5.2 Microscopy

Significant advances have been made in the field of microscopy over the past decade, allowing the study of nanocrystals and elemental analysis using small samples. Some of the spectroscropic and microscopic methods available include the following:

- Energy-dispersive X-ray spectrometry (EDS) for quick and easy elemental analysis of samples in the SEM. It has a minimum detection limit of 0.1% by weight.
- Wavelength-dispersive X-ray spectrometry (WDS) for a more detailed elemental analysis of samples in the SEM. JEOL Four-Crystal Spectrometer attached to the JSM-35C SEM can be used for 1-μm spot analysis, digital and analog line scans, and X-ray image mapping. It provides elements' detection from Be to U and has a minimum detection limit of 0.01% by weight, fully quantitative results are by extended φ–ρ–z.
- Inductively coupled plasma-atomic emission spectroscopy (ICP) provides trace-level and bulk elemental analyses of solid and liquid samples.

Using Varian Analytical Instruments Liberty 100 air pass ICP, minimum detection limits better than 1 ppb by weight (element-/line-dependent), bulk solid acid digestion (for powders, residue, ingots, and so on) and liquid analyses can be performed. Analysis of all elements from Li to U (excluding N, O, F, S, and noble gases), 0.75-m Czerny Turner monochromator with holographic grating allows high-intensity spectra up to four peak orders, with 0.006-nm resolution through a wavelength range of 189–900 nm.

- Surface analysis (AES/XPS): Electron spectroscopy for elemental analysis of surfaces, sensitive to as low as two atomic layers. Physical electronics model PHI-570 Auger Electron Spectroscopy/X-ray Photoelectron Spectroscopy System is a double-pass cylindrical mirror energy analyzer with dual anode (Mg/Al) X-ray source and has a rapid sample introduction probe. It can detect elements at the first 5–10 atomic layers of sample and detect all elements, except H and He.

- Scanning electron microscopy for high-resolution and high-magnification photographs. It can also perform elemental analysis with EDS and WDS attachments. JEOL JSM6320F and JSM-35C research-grade SEM can provide imaging from 10× to 400,000×. Using analytical electron microscopy, very-high-magnification images with excellent depth of focus can be obtained. This is especially important when rough-surface structures are being examined. In addition, information about the chemical composition at the microlevel and the phase composition of the sample under study can be obtained directly. Using SEM, such as the Fraunhofer Institut Für Fertigungstechnik und Angewandte Material for Schung, it is possible to magnify structures up to 500,000 times with high depth of focus. A finely focused electron beam allows structures down to 0.001 mm to be resolved. The acceleration voltage of the electron beam directed at the sample surface can be varied between 300 V and 30 kV. The emitted secondary and backscattered electrons give information about the topology of the sample. Backscattering electrons can also be used to produce material-contrast images.

- X-ray diffraction (XRD) for phase analysis, crystallographic information, residual stress, texture analysis, and reflectometry on powders, bulk, or thin films. Philips X'Pert PRO and a second Philips dual diffractometer system with automated PC control, independent $\theta/2\theta$, sample spinner, and 21 sample changer can be used for crystallography and Rietveld analysis of samples—flat, irregular, thin films, or in glass capillaries.

- Fourier transform-infrared spectroscopy (FT-IR) is useful for identifying organic and inorganic compounds by comparison with library references. Perkin Elmer System 2000 offers near-IR, mid-IR, far-IR: 15,000–15,030 cm, transmittance (T), specular reflectance (SR; Ref. 6) and diffuse reflectance (DR), horizontal and vertical attenuated total reflectance (ATR) microscope (>10 μm spot, 10,000–10,580 cm)$^{-1}$.

3.5.3 Thermal Analysis

Material characterization requires the measurement of molecular and macroscopic properties. Thermal analysis techniques determine calorimetric and mechanical properties, such as heat capacity, mechanical modulus, sample mass, and dimensional changes in temperature ranges between −150°C and 1600°C. Thermal analysis utilizes DSC, TGA, TMA, and dynamic mechanical analysis instrumentation supplemented by software products, accessories, consumables, and documentation. Applications are frequently found in research and quality control environments. They cover the characterization of materials, process development, and evaluation, as well as safety investigations. All METTLER TOLEDO thermal analysis products belong to the latest-generation STARe family. The associated METTLER TOLEDO FP900 series includes instruments for the rapid determination of physical properties, such as melting, boiling, dropping, and softening points.

Microthermal analysis is a recently introduced thermoanalytical technique that combines the principles of scanning probe microscopy with thermal analysis via replacement of the probe tip with a thermistor. This allows samples to be spatially scanned in terms of both topography and thermal conductivity, whereby placing the probe on a specific region of a sample and heating, it is possible to perform localized thermal analysis experiments on those regions.

3.5.4 Molecular Spectroscopy

The foundations for fluorescence correlation spectroscopy (FCS) were already laid in the early 1970s, but this technique did not become widely used until single-molecule detection was established almost 20 years later with the use of diffraction-limited confocal volume element. The analysis of molecular noise from the GHz to the Hz region facilitates measurements over a large dynamic range covering photophysics, conformational transitions, and interactions, as well as transport properties of fluorescent biomolecules. From the Poissonian nature of the noise spectrum, the absolute number of molecules is obtainable. Originally used for the analysis of molecular interactions in solutions, the strength of FCS lies also in its applicability to molecular processes at either the surface or interior of single cells. Examples of the analysis of surface kinetics, including on and off rates of ligand–receptor interactions, will be given. The possibility of obtaining this type of information by FCS will be of particular interest for cell-based drug screening.

Recrystallization, grinding, compaction, and freeze-drying are used frequently in the pharmaceutical industry to obtain a desirable crystalline form of bulk powder and excipients. These processes affect not only the surface area but also the crystalline disorder of the powder materials. Because both these parameters may affect the bioavailability of a drug through the rate of dissolution, it is necessary to control the conditions under which the pharmaceutical drug powders are produced. The extent of disorder in a crystalline solid may induce the hygroscopicity of the drug, in addition to the flow, mechanical properties, and chemical stability. Because the qualities of a pharmaceutical preparation depend on the characteristics of the bulk powders and excipients, controlling the production process is important. An amorphous solid-state powder may determine the bioavailability of a slightly water-soluble drug, because the property affects solubility and, hence, absorption of the drug in the gastrointestinal tract. However, the amorphous form has problems regarding stability and hygroscopicity, resulting in transformation to a more stable crystalline form during preservation.

Therefore, in order to control the quality of pharmaceutical solid dosage products, techniques for the evaluation of crystallinity of the bulk powders and/or excipients are needed. Methods such as XRD, DSC, FT-Raman spectroscopy, and microcalorimetry are currently the most widely used to evaluate crystallinity.

Near-infrared (NIR) spectroscopy is becoming an important technique for pharmaceutical analysis. This spectroscopy is simple and easy because no sample preparation is required, and samples are not destroyed. In the pharmaceutical industry, NIR spectroscopy has been used to determine several pharmaceutical properties, and a growing literature exists in this area. A variety of chemoinfometric and statistical techniques have been used to extract pharmaceutical information from raw spectroscopic data. Calibration models generated by multiple linear regression (MLR) analysis, principal component analysis, and partial least squares regression analysis have been used to evaluate various parameters.

3.5.5 X-Ray Diffraction

The determination of the average morphology is often a "bottleneck" in elucidating other important behaviors of large quantities of crystalline powders used in pharmaceutical development and processing.

X-rays are electromagnetic radiation of wavelength about 1 Å (10^{-10} m), which is about the same size as an atom. They occur in that portion of the electromagnetic spectrum between gamma rays and the ultraviolet rays. The discovery of X-rays in 1895 enabled scientists to probe crystalline structure at the atomic level. X-ray diffraction has been in use in two main areas: for the fingerprint characterization of crystalline materials and for the determination of their structure. Each crystalline solid has its unique characteristic X-ray powder pattern, which may be used as a "fingerprint" for its identification. Once the material has been identified, X-ray crystallography may be used to determine its structure, that is, how the atoms pack together in the crystalline state and what are the interatomic distance and angle. X-ray diffraction is one of the most important characterization tools used in solid-state chemistry and materials science. The size and the shape of the unit cell for any compound can be most easily determined by using the diffraction of X-rays.

It is possible to use XRD techniques to estimate the average shape and "habit" of organic crystalline material using a single crystal. The relative intensities of the peaks in an XRD pattern from a sample exhibiting a "standard" preferred orientation correlate with the shape of the crystallites present. Models have been developed to yield a quantitative "enhancement" factor for each face. The combined simple forms morphology (CSM) of the material can be produced by indexing the observed faces and modifying the simulated Bravais–Friedel–Donnay–Harker (BFDH) morphology (7). The average shape of crystallites can be estimated from the CSM by multiplying each face by its enhancement factor.

3.5.6 Stability Testing

The regulatory authorities clearly define the protocols for the testing of drug products for stability during the shelf life. However, testing of drug substances at the preformulation level for stability evaluation offers several advantages and opportunities once the drug substances enter the formulation stage. First, it provides a clear idea about which types of dosage forms can be used. A highly unstable protein drug cannot be placed in anything but a highly preserved and protected parenteral form, as an example. The development of stability testing protocols starts with the development of stability-indicating methods, the details of which can be readily found in any pharmaceutical analysis text or through the website of the U.S. FDA. The Q1A R2 (Stability Testing of New Drug Substances and Products) is a good starting place (8). Similar guidelines are provided for biotechnology and botanical products.

3.5.6.1 Moisture Isotherm

The crystalline structure can significantly affect a compound's tendency to absorb moisture, which can impact sample handling for analytical testing, formulation, stability, and product shelf life in the areas of varying humidity. For example, if a compound attracts water as it is exposed to rising humidity levels, each kilogram of material will contain more water and less of the compound as the humidity level increases. This could carry over to the formulation, where, as a consequence of the higher moisture content in the API, a subpotent formulation could be manufactured. Hence, drug manufacturers need this information in order to adequately control humidity and ensure uniform moisture to compound ratios across batches. They also need the information to design specific formulations and packaging that will maintain the stability of a finished product when it is shipped and stored in different environments. A compound may remain stable in the controlled humidity and temperature of a lab or manufacturing facility but may degrade if it acquires water when trucked across country or stored on a pharmacy shelf. For example, compound A may exist in two salt forms—a nonhygroscopic monohydrochloride form and a hygroscopic dihydrochloride form. The client needs to use the dihydrochloride form for a solid oral dosage. Increasing moisture levels in the formulation leads to localized areas of high concentrations of hydrochloric acid in the vicinity of the API molecules. The decision must then be made whether to develop a capsule formulation or a tablet formulation, as each has its own unique set of manufacturing and packaging challenges. While the basic generation of a capsule formulation may be the quickest route, initially, the need for extensive coating and or packaging may slow the entire process. These measures would be required to protect the product from moisture, as the generation of hydrochloric acid in the formulation could result in partial digestion of the capsule shell. For a tablet formulation, the application of a moisture impermeable coating may be a simpler process, and more options may be available to package the material in a protective environment. Knowing this information at the beginning of the process may save the client a considerable time, while providing some early direct on to the development of an appropriate and successful formulation. Experimental data can generate a lot of information regarding the characteristic behavior of the molecule. In addition to understanding the hygroscopicity of the compound, drug manufacturers should know whether their compound's vapor sorption is "reproducible" as humidity levels go up and down. One of our most useful instruments is the vapor sorption analyzer, which, among other things, subjects samples to increases and decreases in relative humidity (RH).

These studies involve weighing out a small sample and exposing it to a very dry atmosphere at low or high temperatures. Once the sample dries to a prespecified level, the humidity is raised in increments, for example, from 5% to 95%, while keeping the temperature constant. By weighing the sample at each increment, one can determine how much moisture the compound acquires at a given percentage of RH. This is very important information for predicting the stability and shelf life. We can then determine whether vapor desorption is reproducible by weighing the sample as we decrease the humidity in the same increments. The kinetics of absorption can also be studied by subjecting samples to the same incremental humidity changes but by varying the times spent by different samples at each percentage of RH. In addition, the percentage of RH at which a transition occurs between an amorphous structure and a crystalline structure can be determined. An API may be more stable, more processable, or more soluble (giving the impression of different pharmacological activity) in one form or another and hence must be formulated, packaged, and handled to maintain that form. In general, four possible basic vapor sorption profiles are observed—the compound can be found to be nonhygroscopic, vapor sorption is reproducible, vapor sorption curves demonstrate a degree of hysteresis, or the vapor sorption is nonreproducible because of deliquescence, development of nonreversible hydrates, or other reasons.

Vapor sorption is reproducible when the rate at which a compound acquires moisture during humidity increases is matched by the rate at which it loses moisture during humidity decreases. If the rates are the same, then scientists can control the moisture-compound ratio simply by controlling the humidity levels, without having to consider the specific history of the material. Hence, if a batch of material has a certain water-compound ratio in facility A and acquires more water as it is moved across a humid environment to facility B, one can restore the original ratio by insuring that B's humidity level is the same as A's (and waiting for an adequate amount of time). If vapor sorption is not reproducible, then one will need to know how the absorption rate differs from the desorption rate and the precise humidity conditions that the material undergoes as it is transported from A to B, as the history of the material will affect the amount of moisture present in the material. Of course, whether vapor sorption is reproducible or not, it takes time to raise or lower the water content under certain humidity and temperature conditions. What is considered to be an adequate time can be ascertained experimentally by preformulation studies of the kinetics of vapor sorption for a particular compound, which focus not only on the amount of water absorbed or released but also on the time it takes for the processes to occur.

While the moisture content of the sample at any given RH is dependent on the history of the sample, all the moisture gained by the sample in the adsorption phase is eventually lost in the desorption phase.

While most experiments conducted using the vapor sorption analyzer involve monitoring weight changes at constant temperatures and varying humidity levels, the instrument can also be used to measure changes in weight when incrementally altering temperature, while maintaining a constant humidity.

Other methods and instruments to test the effects of temperature include the DSC and the TGA. The DSC measures the amount of energy (as heat) absorbed or released as a sample is heated, cooled, or held at constant temperature. These measurements provide information on effects such as glass transition, crystallization, and melting point and provide quantitative insight into the composition of a sample. When the sample is heated, inorganic salts first split off their water of crystallization, and then, other volatile components evaporate. The weight loss indicates the amount of water or volatile components in the sample. The TGA also helps formulators understand the decomposition behavior. Although some similar information can be obtained with the vapor sorption analyzer, the TGA is a specialized instrument that allows users to measure effects at much higher temperatures. They can even set the starting and ending temperatures and control the speed at which the temperature rises or falls.

3.5.6.2 Excipient Compatibility

Whereas the choice of excipients starts with the stages of formulation, some excipients are historically used in specific drug formulations; for example, if the newly discovered drug is a cephalosporin for use as an intravenous product, compatibility with arginine or sodium carbonate would be advised, as these are the most commonly used active excipients used for solubilization. Similarly, for drugs that are likely to be compressed, compatibility with common ingredients of compression and disintegration are the plausible choices at this stage. The relative emphasis on excipient interaction would depend on how the company research is planned; in many situations, the preformulation group is more closely aligned with the drug discovery group, and many of these studies are left to the formulation group.

3.6 Transport Across Biological Membranes

3.6.1 Drug Efflux and Multidrug-Resistance Studies

The problem of MDR has gained increasing importance in recent years, particularly in the fields of tumor therapy and treatment of bacterial and fungal infections. One of the major mechanisms responsible for the development of MDR is the overexpression of drug efflux pumps. These membrane-bound, ATP-driven transport proteins efflux a wide variety of natural product toxins and chemotherapeutic drugs out of the cells and give rise to decreased intracellular accumulation of these compounds. Thus, inhibition of efflux pumps is a versatile approach for overcoming MDR, and several compounds are in clinical phase III studies. The main target is Pgp, which is responsible for MDR in tumor cells, and transport systems in *Staphylococcus aureus*, *Pseudomonas aeruginosa*, and *Escherichia coli*. Owing to the fact that three-dimensional (3D) structures of the proteins at atomic resolution were not available, drug development was performed solely on the basis of ligand design. However, electron microscopy studies, as well as X-ray structures, of three bacterial efflux pumps may open the door to target-based drug design in the near future.

The lipophilicity of drug molecules (represented as the logarithm of the *n*-octanol/water partition coefficient) often strongly correlates with their pharmacological and toxic activities. It is therefore not surprising that there is considerable interest in developing mathematical models capable of accurately predicting their value for new drug candidates. The key importance of lipophilicity in biostudies is discussed for β-blockers. Examples of their lipophilicity-dependent pharmacological properties, including pharmacokinetic, pharmacodynamic, and clinical aspects, are reviewed. Comprehensive lipophilicity compilations of β-blockers are not available so far. Log *P* calculations with 10 programs for 30 clinically relevant β-blockers are presented for the first time in this review.

Modulators and inhibitors of multidrug efflux transporters, such as Pgp, are used to reduce or inhibit MDR, which leads to a failure of the chemotherapy of, for example, cancers, epilepsy, bacterial, parasitic, and fungal diseases. Binding and transport of first-, second-, and third-generation modulators and inhibitors of Pgp take into account the properties of the drug (H-bonding potential, dimensions, and pK_a values) and of the membrane.

Gram-positive lactic acid bacteria possess several MDRs that excrete out of the cell a wide variety of mainly cationic lipophilic cytotoxic compounds, as well as many clinically relevant antibiotics. These MDRs are either proton/drug antiporters belonging to the major facilitator superfamily of secondary transporters or ATP-dependent primary transporters belonging to the ATP-binding cassette superfamily of transport proteins.

It is increasingly recognized that efflux transporters play an important role, not only in chemo protection, for example, MDR, but also in the absorption, distribution, and elimination of drugs. The modulation of drug transporters through inhibition or induction can lead to significant drug–drug interactions by affecting intestinal absorption, renal secretion, and biliary excretion, thereby changing the systemic or target tissue exposure of the drug. Few clinically significant drug interactions that affect efficacy and safety are due to a single mechanism. and there is a considerable overlap of substrates, inhibitors, and inducers of efflux transporters and drug-metabolizing enzymes, such as CYP3A. In addition, genetic polymorphisms of efflux transporters have been correlated with human disease and variability of drug exposure.

3.6.2 In Vitro–In Vivo Correlation

The in vitro–in vivo correlation (IVIVC) is an extremely useful exercise at the preformulation level that determines how scale up and postapproval changes or Biowaiver principles would be exploited. Conceptually, IVIVC describes a relationship between the in vitro dissolution or release versus the in vivo absorption. This relationship is an important item of research in the development of drug delivery systems. In vitro dissolution testing serves as a guidance tool to the formulator regarding the product design and in quality control. Especially, it is of specific importance for modified-release dosage forms, which are intended for the purpose of prolonging, sustaining, or extending the release of drugs. By applying mathematical principles, such as linear system analysis and moment analysis, the data describing in vitro and in vivo processes can be obtained. Developing a predictable IVIVC depends on the complexity of the delivery system, its formulation composition, method of manufacture, physicochemical properties of the drug, and the dissolution method. Several sophisticated commercial dissolution methods are available, along with the software to develop IVIVC models; these will be discussed elsewhere in the book.

3.6.3 Caco-2 Cell Studies

Caco-2 monolayer, a model for human drug intestinal permeability, is of great interest. Kinetics of intestinal drug absorption, permeation enhancement, chemical moiety, structure–permeability relationships, dissolution testing, in vitro–in vivo correlation, and bioequivalence are studied using Caco-2. The Caco-2 cell line is heterogeneous and is derived from a human colorectal adenocarcinoma. Caco-2 cells are used as in vitro permeability models to predict human intestinal absorption, because they exhibit many features of absorptive intestinal cells. This includes their ability to spontaneously differentiate into polarized enterocytes that express high levels of brush-border hydrolases and form well-developed junctional complexes. Consequently, it becomes possible to determine whether passage is transcellular or paracellular, based on a compound's transport rate. Caco-2 cells also express a variety of transport systems, including dipeptide transporters and Pgp. Owing to these features, drug permeability in Caco-2 cells cor-relates well with human oral absorption, making Caco-2 an ideal in vitro permeability model. Additional information can be gained on metabolism and potential drug–drug interactions, as the drug undergoes transcellular diffusion through the Caco-2 transport model. The Millipore MultiScreen Caco-2 assay system is a reliable 96-well platform for predicting human oral absorption of drug compounds (using Caco-2 cells or other cell lines whose drug transport properties have been well characterized).

WEB REFERENCES

1. https://www.fda.gov/downloads/Drugs/Guidances/UCM458484.pdf
2. https://www.ema.europa.eu/en/human-regulatory/research-development/scientific -guidelines/multidisciplinary/multidisciplinary-herbal-medicinal-products

BIBLIOGRAPHY

Baertschi SW, Clapham D, Foti C, Kleinman MH, Kristensen S, Reed RA, Templeton AC, Tønnesen HH. Implications of In-Use Photostability: Proposed Guidance for Photostability Testing and Labeling to Support the Administration of Photosensitive Pharmaceutical Products, Part 2: Topical Drug Product. *J Pharm Sci.* 2015;104(9):2688–2701.

Baghel S, Cathcart H, O'Reilly NJ. Polymeric Amorphous Solid Dispersions: A Review of Amorphization, Crystallization, Stabilization, Solid-State Characterization, and Aqueous Solubilization of Biopharmaceutical Classification System Class II Drugs. *J Pharm Sci.* 2016;105(9):2527–2544.

Bergström CA, Holm R, Jørgensen SA, Andersson SB, Artursson P, Beato S, Borde A et al. Early Pharmaceutical Profiling Topredict Oral Drug Absorption: Current Status and Unmet needs. *Eur J Pharm Sci.* 2014;57:173–199.

Bhuptani RS, Deshpande KM, Patravale VB. Transungual Permeation: Current Insights. *Drug Deliv Transl Res.* 2016;6(4):426–439.

Chadha R, Bhandari S. Drug-excipient Compatibility Screening—Role of Thermoanalytical and Spectroscopic Techniques. *J Pharm Biomed Anal.* 2014;87:82–97.

Darji MA, Lalge RM, Marathe SP, Mulay TD, Fatima T, Alshammari A, Lee HK, Repka MA, Narasimha Murthy S. Excipient Stability in Oral Solid Dosage Forms: A Review. *AAPS Pharm Sci Tech.* 2018;19(1):12–26.

Egart M, Janković B, Srčič S. Application of Instrumented Nanoindentation in Preformulation Studies of Pharmaceutical Active Ingredients and Excipients. *Acta Pharm.* 2016;66(3):303–330.

Erxleben A. Application of Vibrational Spectroscopy to Study Solid-State Transformations of Pharmaceuticals. *Curr Pharm Des.* 2016;22(32):4883–4911.

Gajdziok J, Vraníková B. Enhancing of Drug Bioavailability Using Liquid Solid System Formulation. *Ceska Slov Farm.* 2015;64(3):55–66.

Hofmann M, Gieseler H. Predictive Screening Tools Used in High-Concentration Protein Formulation Development. *J Pharm Sci.* 2018;107(3):772–777.

Knopp MM, Löbmann K, Elder DP, Rades T, Holm R. Recent Advances and Potential Applications of Modulated Differential Scanning Calorimetry (mDSC) in Drug Development. *Eur J Pharm Sci.* 2016;87:164–173.

Paudel A, Raijada D, Rantanen J. Raman Spectroscopy in Pharmaceutical Product Design. *Adv Drug Deliv Rev.* 2015;89:3–20.

Razinkov VI, Treuheit MJ, Becker GW. Accelerated Formulation Development Ofmonoclonal Antibodies (mAbs) and mAb-based Modalities: Review of Methods and Tools. *J Biomol Screen*. 2015;20(4):468–483.

Talaczynska A, Dzitko J, Cielecka-Piontek J. Benefits and Limitations of Polymorphic and Amorphous Forms of Active Pharmaceutical Ingredients. *Curr Pharm Des.* 2016;22(32):4975–4980.

Yalkowsky SH, Alantary D. Estimation of Melting Points of Organics. *J Pharm Sci.* 2018;107(5):1211–1227.

RECOMMENDED READING

Allen, L. V., Jr. (2008). "Dosage form design and development." *Clin Ther* 30(11): 2102–2111.

BACKGROUND: Drugs must be properly formulated for administration to patients, regardless of age. Pediatric patients provide some additional challenges to the formulator in terms of compliance and therapeutic efficacy. Due to the lack of sufficient drug products for the pediatric population, the pharmaceutical industry and compounding pharmacies must develop and provide appropriate medications designed for children. OBJECTIVE: The purpose of this article was to review the physical, chemical, and biological characteristics of drug substances and pharmaceutical ingredients to be used in preparing a drug product. In addition, stability, appearance, palatability, flavoring, sweetening, coloring, preservation, packaging, and storage are discussed. METHODS: Information for the current article was gathered from a literature review; from presentations at professional and technical meetings; and from lectures, books, and publications of the author, as well as from his professional experience. Professional society meetings and standards-setting bodies were also used as a resource. RESULTS: The proper design and formulation of a dosage form requires consideration of the physical, chemical, and biological characteristics of all of the drug substances and pharmaceutical ingredients (excipients) to be used in fabricating the product. The drug and pharmaceutical materials utilized must be compatible and produce a drug product that is stable, efficacious, palatable, easy to administer, and well tolerated. Preformulation factors include physical properties such as particle size, crystalline structure, melting point, solubility, partition coefficient, dissolution, membrane permeability, dissociation constants, and drug stability. CONCLUSIONS: Successful development of a formulation includes multiple considerations involving the drug, excipients, compliance, storage, packaging, and stability, as well as patient considerations of taste, appearance, and palatability.

Baertschi, S. W. et al. (2015). "Implications of in-use photostability: Proposed guidance for photostability testing and labeling to support the administration of photosensitive pharmaceutical products, Part 2: Topical drug product." *J Pharm Sci* 104(9):2688–2701.

Although essential guidance to cover the photostability testing of pharmaceuticals for manufacturing and storage is well-established, there continues to be a significant gap in guidance regarding testing to support the effective administration of photosensitive drug products. Continuing from Part 1, (Baertschi SW, Clapham D, Foti C, Jansen PJ, Kristensen S, Reed RA, Templeton AC, Tonnesen HH. *J Pharm Sci*. 2013;102:3888–3899) where the focus was drug products administered by injection, this commentary proposes guidance for testing topical drug products in order to support administration. As with the previous commentary, the approach taken is to examine "worst case" photoexposure scenarios in comparison with ICH testing conditions to provide practical guidance for the safe and effective administration of photosensitive topical drug products.

Baghel, S. et al. (2016). "Polymeric amorphous solid dispersions: A review of amorphization, crystallization, stabilization, solid-state characterization, and aqueous solubilization of biopharmaceutical classification system Class II drugs." *J Pharm Sci* 105(9):2527–2544.

Poor water solubility of many drugs has emerged as one of the major challenges in the pharmaceutical world. Polymer-based amorphous solid dispersions have been considered as the major advancement in overcoming limited aqueous solubility and oral absorption issues. The principle drawback of this approach is that they can lack necessary stability and revert to the crystalline form on storage. Significant upfront development is, therefore, required to generate stable amorphous formulations. A thorough understanding of the processes occurring at a molecular level is imperative for the rational design of amorphous solid dispersion products. This review attempts to address the critical molecular and thermodynamic aspects governing the physicochemical properties of such systems. A brief introduction to Biopharmaceutical Classification System, solid dispersions, glass transition, and solubility advantage of amorphous drugs is provided. The objective of this review is to weigh the current understanding of solid dispersion chemistry and to critically review the theoretical, technical, and molecular aspects of solid dispersions (amorphization and crystallization) and potential advantage of polymers (stabilization and solubilization) as inert, hydrophilic, pharmaceutical carrier matrices. In addition, different preformulation tools for the rational selection of polymers, state-of-the-art techniques for preparation and characterization of polymeric amorphous solid dispersions, and drug supersaturation in gastric media are also discussed.

Bergstrom, C. A. et al. (2014). "Early pharmaceutical profiling to predict oral drug absorption: Current status and unmet needs." *Eur J Pharm Sci* 57:173–199.

Preformulation measurements are used to estimate the fraction absorbed in vivo for orally administered compounds and thereby allow an early evaluation of the need for enabling formulations. As part of the Oral Biopharmaceutical Tools (OrBiTo) project, this review provides a summary of the pharmaceutical profiling methods available, with focus on in silico and in vitro models typically used to forecast active pharmaceutical ingredient's (APIs) in vivo performance after oral administration. An overview of the composition of human, animal and simulated gastrointestinal (GI) fluids is provided and state-of-the art methodologies to study API properties impacting on oral absorption are reviewed. Assays performed during early development, i.e. physicochemical characterization, dissolution profiles under physiological conditions, permeability assays and the impact of excipients on these properties are discussed in detail and future demands on pharmaceutical profiling are identified. It is expected that innovative computational and experimental methods that better describe molecular processes involved in vivo during dissolution and absorption of APIs will be developed in the OrBiTo. These methods will provide early insights into successful pathways (medicinal chemistry or formulation strategy) and are anticipated to increase the number of new APIs with good oral absorption being discovered.

Bharate, S. S. and R. A. Vishwakarma (2013). "Impact of preformulation on drug development." *Expert Opin Drug Deliv* 10(9):1239–1257.

INTRODUCTION: Preformulation assists scientists in screening lead candidates based on their physicochemical and biopharmaceutical properties. This data is useful for selection of new chemical entities (NCEs) for preclinical efficacy/toxicity studies which is a major section under investigational new drug application. A strong collaboration between discovery and formulation group is essential for selecting right NCEs in order to reduce attrition rate in the late stage development. AREAS COVERED: This article describes the significance of preformulation research in drug discovery and development. Various crucial preformulation parameters with case studies have been discussed. EXPERT OPINION: Physicochemical and biopharmaceutical characterization of NCEs is a decisive parameter during product development. Early prediction of these properties helps in selecting suitable physical form (salt, polymorph, etc.) of the candidate. Based on pharmacokinetic and efficacy/toxicity studies, suitable formulation for Phase I clinical studies can be developed. Overall these activities contribute in streamlining efficacy/toxicology evaluation, allowing pharmacologically effective and developable molecules to reach the clinic and eventually to the market. In this review, the magnitude of understanding preformulation properties of NCEs and their utility in product development has been elaborated with case studies.

Bhuptani, R. S. et al. (2016). "Transungual permeation: Current insights." *Drug Deliv Transl Res* 6(4):426–439.

Nail disorders are beyond cosmetic concern; besides discomfort in the performance of daily chores, they disturb patients psychologically and affect their quality of life. Fungal nail infection (onychomycosis) is the most prevalent nail-related disorder affecting a major population worldwide. Overcoming the impenetrable nail barrier is the toughest challenge for the development of efficacious topical ungual formulation. Sophisticated techniques such as iontophoresis and photodynamic therapy have been proven to improve transungual permeation. This article provides an updated and concise discussion regarding the conventional approach and upcoming novel approaches focused to alter the nail barrier. A comprehensive description regarding preformulation screening techniques for the identification of potential ungual enhancers is also described in this review while highlighting the current pitfalls for the development of ungual delivery.

Chadha, R. and S. Bhandari (2014). "Drug-excipient compatibility screening—Role of thermoanalytical and spectroscopic techniques." *J Pharm Biomed Anal* 87:82–97.

Estimation of drug-excipient interactions is a crucial step in preformulation studies of drug development to achieve consistent stability, bioavailability and manufacturability of solid dosage forms. The advent of thermoanalytical and spectroscopic methods like DSC, isothermal microcalorimetry, HSM, SEM, FT-IR, solid state NMR and PXRD into pre-formulation studies have contributed significantly to early prediction, monitoring and characterization of the active pharmaceutical ingredient incompatibility with pharmaceutical excipients to avoid expensive material wastage and considerably reduce the time required to arrive at an appropriate formulation.

Concomitant use of several thermal and spectroscopic techniques allows an in-depth understanding of physical or chemical drug-excipient interactions and aids in selection of the most appropriate excipients in dosage form design. The present review focuses on the techniques for compatibility screening of active pharmaceutical ingredient with their potential merits and demerits. Further, the review highlights the applicability of these techniques using specific drug-excipient compatibility case studies.

Darji, M. A. et al. (2018). "Excipient stability in oral solid dosage forms: A review." *AAPS Pharm Sci Tech* 19(1):12–26.

The choice of excipients constitutes a major part of preformulation and formulation studies during the preparation of pharmaceutical dosage forms. The physical, mechanical, and chemical properties of excipients affect various formulation parameters, such as disintegration, dissolution, and shelf life, and significantly influence the final product. Therefore, several studies have been performed to evaluate the effect of drug-excipient interactions on the overall formulation. This article reviews the information available on the physical and chemical instabilities of excipients and their incompatibilities with the active pharmaceutical ingredient in solid oral dosage forms, during various drug-manufacturing processes. The impact of these interactions on the drug formulation process has been discussed in detail. Examples of various excipients used in solid oral dosage forms have been included to elaborate on different drug-excipient interactions.

Egart, M. et al. (2016). "Application of instrumented nanoindentation in preformulation studies of pharmaceutical active ingredients and excipients." *Acta Pharm* 66(3):303–330.

Nanoindentation allows quantitative determination of a material's response to stress such as elastic and plastic deformation or fracture tendency. Key instruments that have enabled great advances in nanomechanical studies are the instrumented nanoindenter and atomic force microscopy. The versatility of these instruments lies in their capability to measure local mechanical response, in very small volumes and depths, while monitoring time, displacement and force with high accuracy and precision. This review highlights the application of nanoindentation for mechanical characterization of pharmaceutical materials in the preformulation phase (primary investigation of crystalline active ingredients and excipients). With nanoindentation, mechanical response can be assessed with respect to crystal structure. The technique is valuable for mechanical screening of a material at an early development phase in order to predict and better control the processes in which a material is exposed to stress such as milling and compression.

Erxleben, A. (2016). "Application of vibrational spectroscopy to study solid-state transformations of pharmaceuticals." *Curr Pharm Des* 22(32):4883–4911.

Understanding the properties, stability and transformations of the solid-state forms of an active pharmaceutical ingredient (API) in the development pipeline is of crucial importance for process-development, formulation development and FDA approval. Investigation of the polymorphism and polymorphic stability is a routine part of the preformulation studies. Vibrational spectroscopy allows the real-time in situ monitoring of phase transformations and probes intermolecular interactions between API molecules, between API and polymer in amorphous solid dispersions or between

API and coformer in cocrystals or coamorphous systems and thus plays a major role in efforts to gain a predictive understanding of the relative stability of solid-state forms and formulations. Infrared (IR), near-infrared (NIR) and Raman spectroscopies, alone or in combination with other analytical methods, are important tools for studying transformations between different crystalline forms, between the crystalline and amorphous form, between hydrate and anhydrous form and for investigating solid-state cocrystal formation. The development of simple-to-use and cost-effective instruments on the one hand and recent technological advances such as access to the low-frequency Raman range down to 5 cm-1, on the other, have led to an exponential growth of the literature in the field. This review discusses the application of IR, NIR and Raman spectroscopies in the study of solid-state transformations with a focus on the literature published over the last eight years.

Gajdziok, J. and B. Vranikova (2015). "Enhancing of drug bioavailability using liquisolid system formulation." *Ceska Slov Farm* 64(3):55–66.

One of the modern technologies of how to ensure sufficient bioavailability of drugs with limited water solubility is represented by the preparation of liquisolid systems. The functional principle of these formulations is the sorption of a drug in a liquid phase to a porous carrier (aluminometasilicates, microcrystalline cellulose, etc.). After addition of further excipients, in particular a coating material (colloidal silica), a powder is formed with the properties suitable for conversion to conventional solid unit dosage forms for oral administration (tablets, capsules). The drug is subsequently administered to the GIT already in a dissolved state, and moreover, the high surface area of the excipients and their surface hydrophilization by the solvent used, facilitates its contact with and release to the dissolution medium and GI fluids. This technology, due to its ease of preparation, represents an interesting alternative to the currently used methods of bioavailability improvement. The article follows up, by describing the specific aspects influencing the preparation of liquid systems, on the already published papers about the bioavailability of drugs and the possibilities of its technological improvement. Key words: liquisolid systems bioavailability porous carrier coating material preformulation studies.

Hageman, M. J. (2010). "Preformulation designed to enable discovery and assess developability." *Comb Chem High Throughput Screen* 13(2):90–100.

Physicochemical properties of drug molecules impact many aspects of both in vivo and in vitro behavior. Poor physicochemical properties can often create a significant impediment to establishing reliable SAR, establishing proof of principle type studies using in vivo models, and eventually leading to added performance variability and costs throughout the development life cycle; in the worst case scenario, even preventing execution of the desired development plan. Understanding the fundamental physicochemical properties provides the basis to dissect and deconvolute experimental observations in such a way that modification or mitigation of poor molecular properties can be impacted at the design phase, insuring design and selection of a molecule which has a high probability of making it through the arduous development cycle. This review will discuss the key physicochemical properties and how they can be assessed and how they are implicated in both discovery enablement and in final product developability of the selected candidate.

Hofmann, M. and H. Gieseler (2018). "Predictive screening tools used in high-concentration protein formulation development." *J Pharm Sci* 107(3):772–777.

This review examines the use of predictive screening approaches in high-concentration protein formulation development. In addition to the normal challenges associated with protein formulation development, for high-concentration formulations, solubility, viscosity, and physical protein degradation play major roles. To overcome these challenges, multiple formulation conditions need to be evaluated such that it is desirable to have predictive but also low-volume and high-throughput methods in order to identify optimal formulation conditions very early in development without time- and material-consuming setups. Many screening techniques have been reported for use in high-concentration formulation development, but not all fulfill the requirements mentioned previously. This review summarizes the advantages and disadvantages of different screening approaches currently used in formulation development and the correlation of predictive data to protein solubility, viscosity, and stability at high protein concentrations.

Kawakami, K. (2012). "Modification of physicochemical characteristics of active pharmaceutical ingredients and application of supersaturatable dosage forms for improving bioavailability of poorly absorbed drugs." *Adv Drug Deliv Rev* 64(6):480–495.

New chemical entities are required to possess physicochemical characteristics that result in acceptable oral absorption. However, many promising candidates need physicochemical modification or application of special formulation technology. This review discusses strategies for overcoming physicochemical problems during the development at the preformulation and formulation stages with emphasis on overcoming the most typical problem, low solubility. Solubility of active pharmaceutical ingredients can be improved by employing metastable states, salt forms, or cocrystals. Since the usefulness of salt forms is well recognized, it is the normal strategy to select the most suitable salt form through extensive screening in the current developmental study. Promising formulation technologies used to overcome the low solubility problem include liquid-filled capsules, self-emulsifying formulations, solid dispersions, and nanosuspensions. Current knowledge for each formulation is discussed from both theoretical and practical viewpoints, and their advantages and disadvantages are presented.

Kerns, E. H. et al. (2008). "In vitro solubility assays in drug discovery." *Curr Drug Metab* 9(9):879–885.

The solubility of a compound depends on its structure and solution conditions. Structure determines the lipophilicity, hydrogen bonding, molecular volume, crystal energy and ionizability, which determine solubility. Solution conditions are affected by pH, co-solvents, additives, ionic strength, time and temperature. Many drug discovery experiments are conducted under "kinetic" solubility conditions. In drug discovery, solubility has a major impact on bioassays, formulation for in vivo dosing, and intestinal absorption. A good goal for the solubility of drug discovery compounds is >60 ug/mL. Equilibrium solubility assays can be conducted in moderate throughput, by incubating excess solid with buffer and agitating for several days, prior to filtration and HPLC quantitation. Kinetic solubility assays are performed in high throughput with shorter incubation times and high throughput analyses using plate readers.

The most frequently used of these are the nephelometric assay and direct UV assay, which begin by adding a small volume of DMSO stock solution of each test compound to buffer. In nephelometry, this solution is serially diluted across a microtitre plate and undissolved particles are detected via light scattering. In direct UV, undissolved particles are separated by filtration, after which the dissolved material is quantitated using UV absorption. Equilibrium solubility is useful for preformulation. Kinetic solubility is useful for rapid compound assessment, guiding optimization via structure modification, and diagnosing bioassays. It is often useful to customize solubility experiments using conditions that answer specific research questions of drug discovery teams, such as compound selection and vehicle development for pharmacology and PK studies.

Knopp, M. M. et al. (2016). "Recent advances and potential applications of modulated differential scanning calorimetry (mDSC) in drug development." *Eur J Pharm Sci* 87:164–173.

Differential scanning calorimetry (DSC) is frequently the thermal analysis technique of choice within preformulation and formulation sciences because of its ability to provide detailed information about both the physical and energetic properties of a substance and/or formulation. However, conventional DSC has shortcomings with respect to weak transitions and overlapping events, which could be solved by the use of the more sophisticated modulated DSC (mDSC). mDSC has multiple potential applications within the pharmaceutical field and the present review provides an up-to-date overview of these applications. It is aimed to serve as a broad introduction to newcomers, and also as a valuable reference for those already practising in the field. Complex mDSC was introduced more than two decades ago and has been an important tool for the quantification of amorphous materials and development of freeze-dried formulations. However, as discussed in the present review, a number of other potential applications could also be relevant for the pharmaceutical scientist.

Lagrange, F. (2010). "Current perspectives on the repackaging and stability of solid oral doses." *Ann Pharm Fr* 68(6):332–358.

Which are the guidelines and scientific aspects for repackaged oral solid medications in France in 2010 whereas it develops? The transient or definitive displacement of the solid oral form from the original atmosphere to enter a repackaging process, some-times automated, is likely to play a primary role in the controversy. However, the solid oral dose is to be repackaged in materials with defined quality. Considering these data, a review of the literature for determination of conditions for repackaged drug stability according to different international guidelines is presented in this paper. Attention is also paid to the defined conditions ensuring the conservation and handling of these drugs throughout the repackaging process. However, there is lack of scientific pub-lished stability data. Nevertheless, recent alternatives may be proposed to overcome the complexity of studying stability in such conditions. Then, the comparison of the moisture barrier properties of the respective package, a galenic model of hygroscopic molecules, or light sensitive molecules or stability data obtained during the industrial preformulation phase could also secure the list of drugs to be reconditioned. Similarly, a wise precaution will be to get stability data for the industrial blisters and unit doses undergoing the real conditions of the medication use process in hospitals and other healthcare settings. By now, reduction of dispensing errors and improvement of the compliance aid put a different perspective on the problem of repackaged drugs. To date, the pharmacist is advised to carry out its analysis of the risks.

Narayan, P. (2011). "Overview of drug product development." *Curr Protoc Pharmacol* Chapter 7: Unit 7.3.1–29.

The process for developing drug delivery systems has evolved over the past two decades with more scientific rigor, involving a collaboration of various fields, i.e., biology, chemistry, engineering, and pharmaceutics. Drug products, also commonly known in the pharmaceutical industry as formulations or "dosage forms," are used for administering the active pharmaceutical ingredient (API) for purposes of assessing safety in preclinical models, early- to late-phase human clinical trials, and for routine clinical/commercial use. This overview discusses approaches for creating small-molecule API dosage forms, from preformulation to commercial manufacturing.

Paudel, A. et al. (2015). "Raman spectroscopy in pharmaceutical product design." *Adv Drug Deliv Rev* 89:3–20.

Almost 100 years after the discovery of the Raman scattering phenomenon, related analytical techniques have emerged as important tools in biomedical sciences. Raman spectroscopy and microscopy are frontier, non-invasive analytical techniques amenable for diverse biomedical areas, ranging from molecular-based drug discovery, design of innovative drug delivery systems and quality control of finished products. This review presents concise accounts of various conventional and emerging Raman instrumentations including associated hyphenated tools of pharmaceutical interest. Moreover, relevant application cases of Raman spectroscopy in early and late phase pharmaceutical development, process analysis and micro-structural analysis of drug delivery systems are introduced. Finally, potential areas of future advancement and application of Raman spectroscopic techniques are discussed.

Razinkov, V. I. et al. (2015). "Accelerated formulation development of monoclonal antibodies (mAbs) and mAb-based modalities: Review of methods and tools." *J Biomol Screen* 20(4):468–483.

More therapeutic monoclonal antibodies and antibody-based modalities are in development today than ever before, and a faster and more accurate drug discovery process will ensure that the number of candidates coming to the biopharmaceutical pipeline will increase in the future. The process of drug product development and, specifically, formulation development is a critical bottleneck on the way from candidate selection to fully commercialized medicines. This article reviews the latest advances in methods of formulation screening, which allow not only the high-throughput selection of the most suitable formulation but also the prediction of stability properties under manufacturing and long-term storage conditions. We describe how the combination of automation technologies and high-throughput assays creates the opportunity to streamline the formulation development process starting from early preformulation screening through to commercial formulation development. The application of quality by design (QbD) concepts and modern statistical tools are also shown here to be very effective in accelerated formulation development of both typical antibodies and complex modalities derived from them.

Talaczynska, A. et al. (2016). "Benefits and limitations of polymorphic and amorphous forms of active pharmaceutical ingredients." *Curr Pharm Des* 22(32):4975–4980.

Active pharmaceutical ingredients (APIs) can exist in different polymorphic forms as well as in amorphous state. Polymorphic and amorphous forms of APIs can differ in physicochemical properties which in turn can significantly influence their therapeutic safety and effectiveness of the treatment. This review focuses on benefits and limitations of polymorphic and amorphous forms of APIs used in preformulation and formulation studies. Authors present their work on safety precautions for the use of polymorphic and amorphous forms of APIs, analytical techniques used for their identification as well as methods of their preparation especially in regard to limitations of labile APIs.

Yalkowsky, S. H. and D. Alantary (2018). "Estimation of melting points of organics." *J Pharm Sci* 107(5):1211–1227.

Unified physicochemical property estimation relationships is a system of empirical and theoretical relationships that relate 20 physicochemical properties of organic molecules to each other and to chemical structure. Melting point is a key parameter in the unified physicochemical property estimation relationships scheme because it is a determinant of several other properties including vapor pressure, and solubility. This review describes the first-principals calculation of the melting points of organic compounds from structure. The calculation is based on the fact that the melting point, Tm, is equal to the ratio of the heat of melting, DeltaHm, to the entropy of melting, DeltaSm. The heat of melting is shown to be an additive constitutive property. However, the entropy of melting is not entirely group additive. It is primarily dependent on molecular geometry, including parameters which reflect the degree of restriction of molecular motion in the crystal to that of the liquid. Symmetry, eccentricity, chirality, flexibility, and hydrogen bonding, each affect molecular freedom in different ways and thus make different contributions to the total entropy of fusion. The relationships of these entropy determining parameters to chemical structure are used to develop a reasonably accurate means of predicting the melting points over 2000 compounds.

4

Dissociation, Partitioning, and Solubility

Every problem that is interesting is also soluble.

David Deutsch

4.1 Introduction

For a newly discovered molecule to become an active drug, it must traverse through a multitude of physiologic barriers, both aqueous and nonaqueous; these barriers exist to protect our body from the noxious agents that can be toxic to our body. The system by which Nature chose to protect us is based on the solubility of compounds. A compound highly soluble in water or highly insoluble in water would not be able to penetrate the deeper tissues and is thus rendered ineffective. Neutral compounds without any polarizable centers often prove to be inert pharmacologically; for example, fluorinated hydrocarbons, such as perfluorodecalin, which is a hexane structure with full fluorination. Fluorine is so highly electronegative that it pulls the electrons from the parent structure, making it an inert compound. Interactions at the site of action are often electrically driven, and as a result, it is more likely that we will discover a compound that has weak acid or base properties as an active entity. This necessitates studies that would yield information on how well the compound will distribute throughout the body tissues, and the lipophilic–hydrophilic balance of the molecular structure becomes the focus of studies at an early stage in preformulation.

Compounds that ionize in the aqueous phase are rendered water-soluble, because they can polarize the medium and can create solute–solvent electrostatic bonding to increase their solubility. The ionization of a compound depends on the strength of binding of the ionizable group to the core of the molecule, a property determined by the value of the dissociation constant. Once ionized, the molecule acquires new solubility characteristics; when placed between aqueous and nonaqueous phases, the distribution between these two phases, generally called partitioning, will change. It is this partitioning behavior of drugs that makes them useful as drugs. Without a significant degree of partition between aqueous and nonaqueous phases of body tissues, no molecule can become active. This ionization also determines the quantity of a solute that is eventually contained in a medium, aqueous or nonaqueous—the solubility of compound. So, what starts with dissociation affects both partitioning and the solubility of the compound, the two most important parameters that will determine if a newly discovered molecule will end up as an active drug or not. This chapter describes these three interrelated properties that form the first step in any preformulation evaluation.

4.2 The Ionization Principle

Chemical moieties are known to attract to each other, and under appropriate conditions, they disassociate. When this process is driven by the electrical charges on the components of the moiety, this phenomenon is known as ionization. The physicochemical properties of dissociated species differ significantly from the undissociated species and form a basis not only of the physicochemical stability but also of the physiological activity of molecules and ions. A detailed description of ionization principle is provided here as a refresher for scientists and to emphasize the relative importance of this property.

4.2.1 The Acid–Base Theory

For hundreds of years, substances that behaved like vinegar have been classified as acids, while those that have properties like the ash from a wood fire have been referred to as alkalis or bases. The name "acid" comes from the Latin word *acidus*, which means "sour," and refers to the sharp odor and sour taste of many acids. Vinegar tastes sour because it is a dilute solution of acetic acid in water; lemon juice is sour because it contains citric acid; milk turns sour when it is spoilt because of the formation of lactic acid; and the sour odor of rotten meat can be attributed to carboxylic acids, such as butyric acid, formed when fat spoils.

Arrhenius was the first person to give a definition of an acid and a base in 1887. According to him, an acid is one that gives rise to excess of H^+ in aqueous solution, whereas a base gives rise to excess of OH^- in solution. This was modified by Bronsted and Lowry in 1923 such that a proton donor was defined as an acid and a proton acceptor was defined as a base. They also introduced the familiar concept of the conjugate acid–base pair. The final refinement to the acid–base theory was completed by Lewis in 1923, who extended the concept that acid is an acceptor of electron pairs, while base is a donor of electron pairs.

4.2.1.1 Bronsted–Lowry Theory

According to this theory, all acid–base reactions involve the transfer of an H^+ ion, or a proton. Water reacts with itself, for example, by transferring an H^+ ion from one molecule to another to form an H_3O^+ ion and an OH^- ion.

$$H_2O \ + \ H_2O \ \longrightarrow \ H_3O^+ \ + \ OH^-$$

$$+ \ H^+$$

$$- \ H^-$$

(4.1)

According to this theory, an acid is a "proton donor" and a base is a "proton acceptor." Acids are often divided into categories, such as "strong" and "weak." One measure of the strength of an acid is the acid-dissociation equilibrium constant, K_a, of the acid.

$$K_a = \frac{[H_3O^+][A^-]}{[HA]} \qquad (4.2)$$

When K_a is relatively large, we have a strong acid, which is mostly present in an ionized form:

HCl: $K_a = 1 \times 10^3$ (here, the ratio of ionized to unionized species is 1000–1).

When K_a is small, we have a weak acid, which is mostly present in an unionized form:

CH_3CO_2H: $K_a = 1.8 \times 10^{-5}$ (here, the ratio of ionized to unionized species is 0.000018–1).

When K_a is very small, we have a very weak acid, such as water:

H_2O: $K_a = 1.8 \times 10^{-16}$ (barely ionized)

As shown, the range of ratio of ionized and unionizes species can be very large; to manage it mathematically, the values of K_a and the ionized forms are expressed in a logarithmic form, since 1909 (suggested by Sorenson).

$$pH = -\log[H_3O^+] \qquad (4.3)$$

$$pOH = -\log[OH^-] \qquad (4.4)$$

The "p" in pH and pOH is an operator that indicates that the negative of the logarithm should be calculated for any quantity to which it is attached. Thus, pK_a is the negative of the logarithm of the acid-dissociation equilibrium constant.

$$pK_a = -\log K_a \qquad (4.5)$$

The only disadvantage of using pK_a as a measure of the relative strengths of acids is the fact that large numbers now describe weak acids and small (negative) numbers describe strong acids.

HCl: $pK_a = -3$

CH_3CO_2H: $pK_a = 4.7$

H_2O: $pK_a = 15.7$

An important feature of the Bronsted theory is the relationship that it creates between acids and bases. Every Bronsted acid has a conjugate base, and vice versa.

$$\begin{array}{ccccccc} HCl & + & H_2O & \longrightarrow & H_3O^+ & + & Cl^- \\ Acid & + & Base & & Acid & + & Base \end{array} \tag{4.6}$$

$$\begin{array}{ccccccc} NH_3 & + & H_2O & \longrightarrow & NH_4^+ & + & OH^- \\ Base & + & Acid & & Acid & + & Base \end{array} \tag{4.7}$$

Just as the magnitude of K_a is a measure of the strength of an acid, the value of K_b reflects the strength of its conjugate base. Consider what happens when we multiply the K_a expression for a generic acid (HA) by the K_b expression for its conjugate base (A^-).

$$\frac{[H_3O^+][A^-]}{[HA]} \times \frac{[HA][OH^-]}{[A^-]} = [H_3O^+][OH^-] \tag{4.8}$$

Now, if we replace each term in this equation by the appropriate equilibrium constant, we get the following equation:

$$K_a K_b = K_w = 1 \times 10^{-14} \tag{4.9}$$

Because the product of K_a and K_b is a relatively small number, either the acid or its conjugate base can be "strong." But if one is strong, the other must be weak. Thus, a strong acid must have a weak conjugate base.

$$\underset{\substack{Strong \\ acid}}{HCl} + H_2O \rightarrow H_3O^+ + \underset{\substack{Weak \\ base}}{Cl^-} \tag{4.10}$$

A strong base, on the other hand, must have a weak conjugate acid.

$$\underset{\substack{Strong \\ base}}{NH_4^+ + OH^-} \longrightarrow \underset{\substack{Weak \\ acid}}{NH_3 + H_2O} \tag{4.11}$$

Water has a limiting effect on the strength of acids and bases. All strong acids behave the same in water; 1 M solutions of the strong acids all behave as 1 M solutions of the H_3O^+ ion, and very weak acids do not act as acids in water. However, the acid–base reactions can take place in any solvent, and ionization in water is not a requirement to meet the definition. Figure 4.1 shows the inverse relationship that exists between pK_a and pK_b values of typical acids and bases.

The strongest acids appear on the left side of the figure, and the strongest bases on the right side of the figure. Any base can deprotonate any acid on the left side of it, a weaker base. Acetic acid, a weak acid will ionize (or get deprotonated) water, methanol, or ammonia. However, methanol will not deprotonate in water, but it will deprotonate in ammonia.

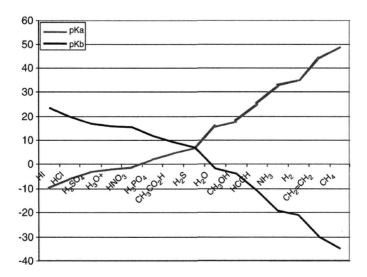

FIGURE 4.1 Typical Bronsted acids and their conjugate bases.

4.2.1.2 Lewis Theory

The theory of acids and bases, the Bronsted–Lowry theory, was dependent on the presence of proton (H^+) to show acidic or basic properties, which may not always be the case; hence, in 1923, G. N. Lewis introduced a theory of acids and bases with a more general definition of acid–base reactions by examining what happens when an H^+ ion combines with an OH^- ion to form water.

$$H^+ \quad {}^{++}_{++}\ddot{O}\!-\!H^- \longrightarrow H\!-\!{}^{++}_{++}\ddot{O}\!-\!H \tag{4.12}$$

In this observation, the H^+ ion picks up (or accepts) a pair of electrons from the OH^- ion to form a new covalent bond. As a result, any substance that can act as an acceptor of electron pair is a Lewis acid (such as the H^+ ion).

The pair of electrons that went into the new covalent bond was donated by the OH^- ion. Lewis therefore argued that any substance that can act as a donor of electron pair is a Lewis base (such as the H^- ion).

Whereas the Lewis acid–base theory does not contradict Bronsted theory, as "bases" in the Bronsted theory must have a pair of nonbonding electrons in order to accept a proton, it expands the family of compounds that can be called "acids": any compound that has one or more empty valence-shell orbital and provides an explanation for the instantaneous reaction of boron triflouride (BF_3) with ammonia (NH_3). The nonbonding electrons on the nitrogen in NH_3 are donated into an empty orbital on the boron to form a new covalent bond, as shown in Eq. 4.13.

$$(4.13)$$

It also explains why Cu^{2+} ions pick up NH_3 to form the four-coordinate $Cu(NH_3)_4^{2+}$ ion.

$$Cu^{2+} \text{ (aq)} + 4NH_3 \text{ (aq)} \rightarrow Cu(NH_3)_4^{2+} \text{ (aq)} \qquad (4.14)$$

In this case, a pair of nonbonding electrons from each of the four NH_3 molecules is donated into an empty orbital on the Cu^{2+} ion to form a covalent Cu–N bond.

$$(4.15)$$

$$(4.16)$$

The flow of electrons from a Lewis base to a Lewis acid is often indicated with a curved arrow.

4.2.1.3 Henderson–Hasselbalch Equation

The Henderson–Hasselbach equation defines the relationship between ionization and pH (Eq. 4.17). This equation relates the pK_a to the pH of the solution and the relative concentrations of the dissociated and undissociated parts of a weak acid.

$$pH = pK_a + \log[A^-]/[HA] \qquad (4.17)$$

or

$$pH = pK_a + \log[\text{salt}]/[\text{acid}] \qquad (4.18)$$

where $[A^-]$ is the concentration of the dissociated species, and $[HA]$ is the concentration of the undissociated species.

This equation can be manipulated into the form given by Eq. 4.19 to yield the percentage of a compound that will be ionized at any particular pH.

$$\text{Percent ionized} = \frac{100}{1 + 10^{[\text{charge}(\text{pH} - pK_a)]}} \qquad (4.19)$$

One simple point to note about Eq. 4.19 is the 50% dissociation (or ionization), pK_a = pH. It should also be noted that, usually, pK_a values are preferred for bases instead of the pK_b values ($pK_w = pK_a + pK_b$).

4.2.1.4 The pH Scale

The pH concept was introduced in 1909 by the Danish chemist S. P. L. Sorenson. The pH is defined by the negative logarithm of the hydrogen ion activity:

$$\text{pH} = -\log a_H \qquad (4.20)$$

where a_H is the activity of the hydrogen ion.

The pH scale is derived from the characteristics of the autodissociation of water. Pure water has a low conductivity and is only slightly ionized:

$$2H_2O = H_3O^+ + OH^- \text{ or } H_2O = H^+ + OH^- \qquad (4.21)$$

The concentration of H^+ and OH^- ions, which are equal, is 1×10^{-7} ions/L. The equilibrium constant (or ion product) for the dissociation of water, K_w, is

$$K_w \{H^+\}\{OH^-\} = 1.01 \times 10^{-14} \text{ at } 25°C \qquad (4.22)$$

By taking log of both sides, we get:

$$-\log \{H^+\} + -\log \{OH^-\} = 14 \qquad (4.23)$$

Using the standard abbreviation p for $\{-\log 10\}$, we get:

$$\text{pH} + \text{pOH} = 14 \qquad (4.24)$$

This equation sets the pH scale to 0–14, which gives a convenient way to express 14 orders of magnitude of [H^+]. Any solution with pH >7 contains excessive hydroxyl ions and is alkaline; those with pH <7 are acidic and contain excessive hydrogen ions. Figure 4.2 shows pH values of common fluids.

It should be noted that the previous definitions of pH are based on an assumption that the solution is behaving in an ideal nature, meaning that the thermodynamic activity is equal to concentration (e.g., what happens when the dilution is infinite). However, as the concentration increases, ionic attraction and incomplete hydration results in a decrease in the effective concentration (or the activity). This activity is defined as the "apparent concentration" of an ionic species, which is due to the attraction that ions exert on one another, and the incomplete hydration of ions in

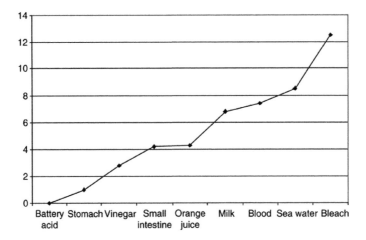

FIGURE 4.2 pH of common fluids.

the solutions that are too concentrated. The lower the concentration, the less is the interaction. At infinite dilution, activity coefficients approach unity.

The activity of a species X is equal to the product of its concentration and its activity coefficient, f_x:

$$\{X\} = f_x[X] \tag{4.25}$$

The pH from an electrode relates to $\{H^+\}$, and not $[H^+]$; though the value of ionic strength is less than 0.01, these terms have values that are very close between pH 2 and 10. A pH electrode consists of a pH sensor, which varies in proportion to the $\{H^+\}$ of the solution, and a reference electrode, which provides a stable constant voltage. The output is in mV, which needs to be converted to pH units (Figure 4.3).

A plot of electrode potential against pH at different temperature shows the effect of temperature on activity and should be corrected (Figure 4.4).

This results in the following equation, correlating the reference potential:

$$E_{obs} = \text{constant} + \text{slope} \cdot \text{pH} \tag{4.26}$$

$$E_{obs} = E_c + N_f \log \{H^+\} \tag{4.27}$$

where E_c is the reference potential and N_f is the Nernstian slope factor $= 2.3RT/nF = 59.1$ at 25°C, where R is the gas constant, T is the absolute temperature in Kelvin, F is the Faraday's constant, and n is the valance factor.

The slope factor is temperature-dependent, and thus, the pH is derived from:

$$\text{pH} = \text{pH}_{std} - (E - E_{std})/\text{slope} \tag{4.28}$$

At pH 7, where $\{H^+\} = \{OH^-\}$, the voltage from the electrode is zero. This is called the isopotential point (Figure 4.4). In theory, this point is temperature-independent. The International Union for Physical and Applied Chemistry (IUPAC) (1) operational

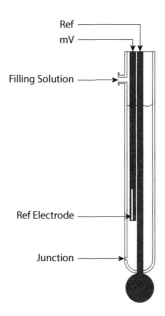

FIGURE 4.3 pH probe design.

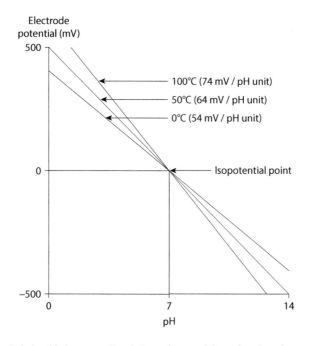

FIGURE 4.4 Relationship between pH and electrode potential as a function of temperature.

pH scale is defined as the pH relative to a standard buffer, measured using a hydrogen electrode. In practice, a pH electrode is calibrated with standard buffers of pH 7.00 and pH 4 or 9 to determine the isoelectric point and slope, respectively. Conventional pH meters will read accurately over a range of 2.5–11, and beyond these ranges, accuracy cannot be assured. However, recently, instruments that carry out calibration to allow correction for nonideal electrode behavior, allowing accurate measurements between ranges of pH 1 and 13, have become available.

4.2.1.5 Compendia Specification for pH Measurement

For compendial purposes, pH is defined as the value given by a suitable, properly standardized, potentiometric instrument (pH meter) capable of reproducing pH values to 0.02 pH unit by using an indicator electrode sensitive to hydrogen ion activity, the glass electrode, and a suitable reference electrode. The instrument should be capable of sensing the potential across the electrode pair and, for pH standardization purposes, applying an adjustable potential to the circuit by manipulation of "standardization," "zero," asymmetry, or "calibration" control. It should be able to control the change in millivolts per unit change in pH reading through a "temperature" and/or "slope" control.

Measurements are made at 25 ± 2, unless otherwise specified in the individual monograph. The pH scale is defined by the equation:

$$pH = pHs + (E - ES)/k, \tag{4.29}$$

where E and ES are the measured potentials, where the galvanic cell contains the solution under test, represented by pH, and the appropriate buffer solution for standardization, represented by pH, respectively. The value of k is the change in potential per unit change in pH and is theoretically $[0.05916 + 0.000198\,(t - 25°)]$ V at any temperature, t. This operational pH scale is established by assigning rounded pH values to the buffer solutions for standardization from the corresponding National Institute of Standards and Technology (NIST) molal solutions.

It should be emphasized that the definitions of pH, the pH scale, and the values assigned to the buffer solutions for standardization are for the purpose of establishing a practical, operational system, so that results may be compared between laboratories. The pH values thus measured do not correspond exactly to those obtained by the definition, $pH = -\log_a H^+$. As long as the solution being measured is sufficiently similar in composition to the buffer used for standardization, the operational pH corresponds fairly closely to the theoretical pH. Although no claim is made with respect to the suitability of the system for measuring hydrogen ion activity or concentration, the values obtained are closely related to the activity of the hydrogen ion in aqueous solutions.

Where a pH meter is standardized by use of an aqueous buffer and then used to measure the "pH" of a nonaqueous solution or suspension, the ionization constant of the acid or base, the dielectric constant of the medium, the liquid-junction potential (which may give rise to errors of approximately 1 pH unit), and the hydrogen ion response of the glass electrode are all changed. For these reasons, the values so obtained with solutions that are only partially aqueous in character can be regarded only as apparent pH values.

Because of variations in the nature and operation of the available pH meters, it is not practicable to give universally applicable directions for the potentiometric determinations of pH. The general principles to be followed in carrying out the instructions provided for each instrument by its manufacturer are set forth in the following paragraphs. Examine the electrodes and, if present, the salt bridge prior to use. If necessary, replenish the salt bridge solution and observe other precautions indicated by the instrument or the electrode manufacturer. Commercially available buffer solutions for pH meter standardization, standardized by methods traceable to the NIST (2) and labeled with a pH value accurate to 0.01 pH unit, may be used. Solutions prepared from the American Chemical Society reagent grade materials or other suitable materials, in the stated quantities, may be used, provided the pH of the resultant solution is the same as that of the solution prepared from the NIST-certified material.

To standardize the pH meter, select two buffer solutions for standardization whose difference in pH does not exceed 4 units and such that the expected pH of the material under test falls between them. Fill the cell with one of the buffer solutions for standardization at the temperature at which the test material is to be measured. Set the control "temperature" at the temperature of the solution and adjust the calibration control to make the observed pH value identical with that tabulated. Rinse the electrodes and the cell with several portions of the second buffer solution for standardization and then fill the cell with it, at the same temperature as the material to be measured. The pH of the second buffer solution is within ±0.07 pH unit of the tabulated value. If a larger deviation is noted, examine the electrodes and, if they are faulty, replace them. Adjust the "slope" or "temperature" control to make the observed pH value identical with that tabulated. Repeat the standardization until both buffer solutions for standardization give observed pH values within 0.02 pH unit of the tabulated value, without further adjustment of the control. When the system functions satisfactorily, rinse the electrodes and cell several times with a few portions of the test material, fill the cell with the test material, and read the pH value. Use carbon dioxide-free water for solution or dilution of test material in pH determinations. In all pH measurements, allow a sufficient time for stabilization.

Where approximate pH values suffice, indicators and test papers may be suitable for use, instead of pH meters.

4.2.1.6 Dissociation

At a given temperature, the thermodynamic ionization constants are independent of concentration, and at a pH value equal to pK_a, the activities of the ionized and neutral forms are equal. In many measurement techniques, we measure concentration rather than activity, such as in the use of spectroscopic methods. In such instances,

$$K_c a = [H^+][A^-]/[HA] \qquad (4.30)$$

where values in brackets are the observed concentrations from spectroscopic measurements based on the Beer–Lambert law. The "thermodynamic" ionization coefficient is related to the "concentration" ionization coefficient by:

$$K_a = K_c a \cdot (f_A f_H / f_{HA}) \qquad (4.31)$$

where f is the activity coefficient.

The pK_a values are also temperature-dependent, often in a nonlinear and unpredictable way. Samples measured by potentiometry are therefore held at a constant temperature bath, and therefore, pK_a value should be quoted at a specific temperature. Often, a temperature of 25°C is chosen to reflect room temperature whereas this may be quite different from the body temperature. Percent ionization at different temperatures can be calculated as:

$$\text{Percent ionized} = \frac{100}{1 + 10^{(\text{charge}(\text{pH} - \text{p}K_a))}} \tag{4.32}$$

where charge is 1 for bases and −1 for acids. Percent ionization is 50% when the pH equals pK_a (Figures 4.5 and 4.6).

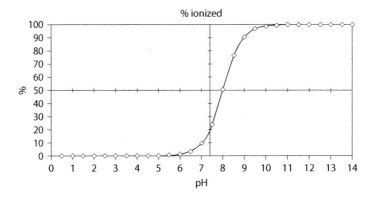

FIGURE 4.5   Percent ionization of an acid with pK_a of 8.0.

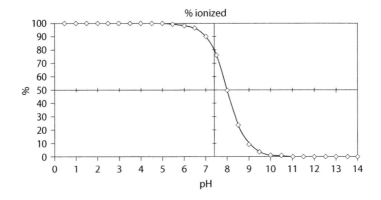

FIGURE 4.6   Percent ionization of a base with pK_a of 8.0.

4.3 Quantitative Structure–Activity Relationships

The relationship between chemical structure, lipophilicity, and its disposition in vivo has been studied extensively. This includes solubility, absorption potential, membrane permeability, plasma protein binding, volume of distribution, and renal and hepatic clearance. Activities used in quantitative structure–activity relationships (QSAR) include chemical measurements and biological assays. Currently, QSARs are applied in many disciplines, with many pertaining to drug design and environmental risk assessment.

The QSAR studies date back to the nineteenth century. In 1863, A. F. A. Cros at the University of Strasbourg observed that toxicity of alcohols to mammals increased as the water solubility of the alcohols decreased. In the 1890s, Hans Horst Meyer of the University of Marburg and Charles Ernest Overton of the University of Zurich, working independently, noted that the toxicity of organic compounds depended on their lipophilicity.

Little additional development of QSAR occurred until the work of Louis Hammett (1894–1987), who correlated the electronic properties of organic acids and bases with their equilibrium constants and reactivity. Consider the dissociation of benzoic acid:

$$\text{—COOH} \underset{K=6.27\times10^{-5}}{\rightleftharpoons} \text{—COO}^- + \text{H}^+ \tag{4.33}$$

Hammett observed that adding substituents to the aromatic ring of benzoic acid had an orderly and quantitative effect on the dissociation constant. For example,

$$\text{O}_2\text{N—} \text{—COOH} \underset{K=32.1\times10^{-5}}{\rightleftharpoons} \text{O}_2\text{N—} \text{—COO}^- + \text{H}^+ \tag{4.34}$$

a nitro group in the meta position increases the dissociation constant, because the nitro group withdraws electron, thereby stabilizing the negative charge that develops. Now, consider the effect of a nitro group in the para position:

$$\text{O}_2\text{N—} \text{—COOH} \underset{K=37.0\times10^{-5}}{\rightleftharpoons} \text{O}_2\text{N—} \text{—COO}^- + \text{H}^+ \tag{4.35}$$

The equilibrium constant is even larger than that for the nitro group in the meta position, indicating even greater withdrawal of electrons. Now, consider the case in which an ethyl group is in the para position:

$$\text{CH}_3\text{CH}_2\text{—} \text{—COOH} \underset{K=4.47\times10^{-5}}{\rightleftharpoons} \text{CH}_3\text{CH}_2\text{—} \text{—COO}^- + \text{H}^+ \tag{4.36}$$

In this case, the dissociation constant is lower than that for the unsubstituted compound, indicating that the ethyl group donates electrons, thereby destabilizing the negative charge that arises on dissociation.

Hammett also observed that substituents have a similar effect on the dissociation of other organic acids and bases. Consider the dissociation of phenylacetic acids:

$$\text{C}_6\text{H}_5-\text{CH}_2\text{COOH} \underset{K=5.20\times10^{-5}}{\rightleftharpoons} \text{C}_6\text{H}_5-\text{CH}_2\text{COO}^- + \text{H}^+ \qquad (4.37)$$

$$\text{O}_2\text{N}-\text{C}_6\text{H}_4-\text{CH}_2\text{COOH} \underset{K=10.7\times10^{-5}}{\rightleftharpoons} \text{O}_2\text{N}-\text{C}_6\text{H}_4-\text{CH}_2\text{COO}^- + \text{H}^+ \qquad (4.38)$$

$$\text{O}_2\text{N}-\text{C}_6\text{H}_4-\text{CH}_2\text{COOH} \underset{K=14.1\times10^{-5}}{\rightleftharpoons} \text{O}_2\text{N}-\text{C}_6\text{H}_4-\text{CH}_2\text{COO}^- + \text{H}^+ \qquad (4.39)$$

$$\text{CH}_3\text{CH}_2-\text{C}_6\text{H}_4-\text{CH}_2\text{COOH} \underset{K=4.27\times10^{-5}}{\rightleftharpoons} \text{CH}_3\text{CH}_2-\text{C}_6\text{H}_4-\text{CH}_2\text{COO}^- + \text{H}^+ \qquad (4.40)$$

Withdrawal of electrons by the nitro group increases dissociation, with the effect being less for the meta than for the para substituent, just as was observed with benzoic acid. The electron-donating ethyl group decreases the equilibrium constant, as expected.

The data for these equilibria are graphed in Figure 4.7.

K_0 or K_0' represents equilibrium constants for unsubstituted compounds and K or K_0 for substituted compounds. Values for the abscissa are calculated from the dissociation constants of the unsubstituted and substituted benzoic acid. Values for the ordinate are obtained from another organic acid or base with identical patterns of substitution, in this case phenylacetic acid.

Because this relationship is linear, the following equation can be written:

$$\log \frac{K}{K_0} = \rho \log \frac{K'}{K_0'} \qquad (4.41)$$

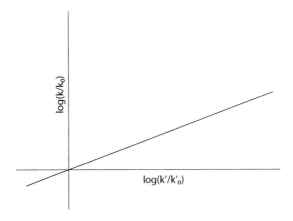

FIGURE 4.7   Example of a graph for a linear free-energy relationship.

where ρ is the slope of the line. The values for the abscissa in Figure 4.7 are always those for benzoic acid and are given the symbol σ. Therefore, we can write:

$$\log \frac{K}{K_0} = \rho\sigma \qquad (4.42)$$

where ρ, the slope of the line, is a proportionality constant pertaining to a given equilibrium. It relates the effect of substituents on this equilibrium to the effect of those substituents on the benzoic acid equilibrium. That is, if the effect of substituents on this equilibrium is proportionally greater than that on the benzoic acid equilibrium, then $\rho > 1$; if the effect is less than that on the benzoic acid equilibrium, then $\rho < 1$. By definition, ρ for benzoic acid is equal to one.

σ is a descriptor of the substituents. The magnitude of σ gives the relative strength of the electron-withdrawal and -donating properties of the substituents. σ is positive if the substituent is electron-withdrawing and negative if it is electron-donating.

These relationships, as developed by Hammett, are termed linear free-energy relationships, which relate free energy to an equilibrium constant:

$$\Delta G = -RT \ln K \qquad (4.43)$$

The free energy is proportional to the logarithm of the equilibrium constant. These linear free-energy relationships are termed "extrathermodynamic." Although they can be stated in terms of thermodynamic parameters, no thermodynamic principle states that the relationships should be true.

To develop a better understanding of these relationships, Table 4.1 gives some values of ρ.

In the aniline and phenol equilibria, the hydrogen ion dissociates and removes one atom from the phenyl ring, whereas in the benzoic acid equilibrium, two atoms are removed. Thus, substituents are able to exert a greater effect on the dissociation in aniline and phenol than in benzoic acid, and the value of ρ is >1.

TABLE 4.1

ρ Values of Various Substituents

Structure	ρ
⬡—NH_3^+	$\rho = 2.90$
⬡—OH	$\rho = 2.23$
⬡—CH_2COOH	$\rho = 0.49$
⬡—CH_2CH_2COOH	$\rho = 0.21$

TABLE 4.2

σ Values at Meta and Para
Substitution Positions

Substituent	σ_m	σ_p
−H	0.0	0.0
−NO$_2$	0.71	0.78
−Cl	0.37	0.23
−OCH$_3$	0.12	−0.27

In phenylacetic and phenylpropionic acids, the hydrogen ion dissociates and removes three and four atoms, respectively, from the phenyl ring. Substituents exert a lesser effect on the equilibrium in this case than on the benzoic acid equilibrium, and ρ is <1. Examples of σ for substituents in the meta and para positions are given in Table 4.2.

By definition, σ for hydrogen is 0. The positive values of σ for the nitro group indicate that it withdraws electrons. In understanding the magnitudes of the σ values for the nitro group in meta versus para positions, consider the mechanisms of electron withdrawal or donation. For a nitro group in the meta position, withdrawal of electrons is due to an inductive effect produced by the electronegativity of the constituent atoms. If only induction were operative, one would expect the electron withdrawal effect of a nitro group in the para position to be less than that in the meta position. The larger value for a para-substituted nitro group results from the combination of both inductive and resonance effects. The resonance structures for para-nitrobenzoate are shown below:

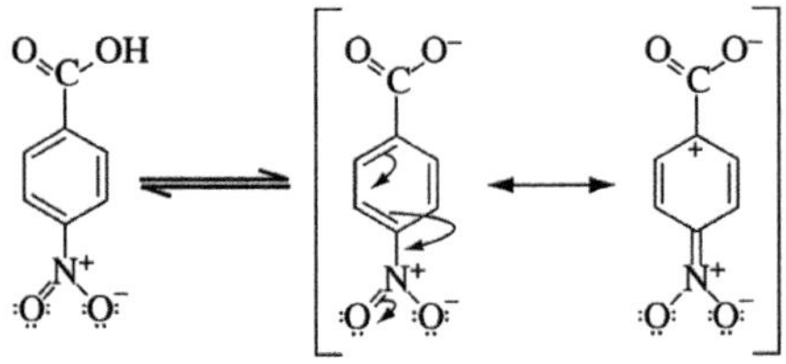

(4.44)

For chlorine, the electronegativity of the atom produces an inductive effect on electron withdrawal, with the magnitude of the effect in the para position being less than that in the meta position. For chlorine, only the inductive effect is possible. The methoxy group can donate or withdraw electrons, depending on the position of substitution. In the meta position, the electronegativity of the oxygen produces an inductive effect on withdrawal of electrons. In the para position, only a small inductive effect is expected. Moreover, an electron-donating resonance effect, as illustrated in Eq. 4.45, occurs for the methoxy group in the para position, giving an overall electron-donating effect.

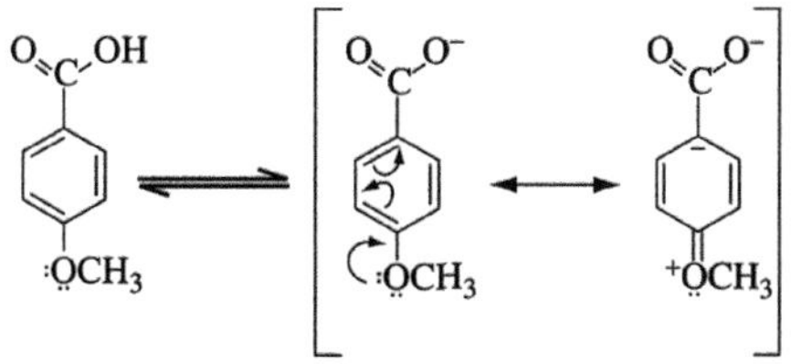

$$(4.45)$$

The σ values for numerous substituents available in the literature are shown in Table 4.3.

TABLE 4.3

Hammett σ Constants[a]

Group	σ_{meta}	σ_{para}	σ_I	σ_v	π	E_s	MR
H	0.00	0.00	0.00	0.00	0.00	0.00	1.03
CH_3	−0.07	−0.17	−0.04	0.52	0.56	−1.24	5.65
C_2H_5	−0.07	−0.15	−0.05	0.56	1.02	−1.31	10.30
$n\text{-}C_3H_7$	−0.07	−0.13	−0.03	0.68	1.55	−1.60	14.96
$i\text{-}C_3H_7$	−0.07	−0.15	−0.03	0.76	1.53	−1.71	14.96
$n\text{-}C_4H_9$	−0.08	−0.16	−0.04	0.68	2.13	−1.63	19.61
$t\text{-}C_4H_9$	−0.10	−0.20	−0.07	1.24	1.98	−2.78	19.62
$H_2C=CH$[b]	0.05	−0.02	0.09	2.11	0.82		10.99
C_6H_5[b]	0.06	−0.01	0.10	2.15	1.96	−3.82	25.36
CH_2Cl	0.11	0.12	0.15	0.60	0.17	−1.48	10.49
CF_3	0.43	0.54	0.42	0.91	0.88	−2.40	5.02
CN	0.56	0.66	0.53	0.40	−0.57	−0.51	6.33
CHO	0.35	0.42	0.25		−0.65		6.88
$COCH_3$	0.38	0.50	0.29	0.50	−0.55		11.18
CO_2H[b]	0.37	0.45	0.39	1.45	−0.32		6.93
$Si(CH_3)_3$	−0.04	−0.07	−0.13	1.40	2.59		24.96
F	0.34	0.06	0.52	0.27	0.14	−0.46	0.92
Cl	0.37	0.23	0.47	0.55	0.71	−0.97	6.03
Br	0.39	0.23	0.50	0.65	0.86	−1.16	8.88
I	0.35	0.18	0.39	0.78	1.12	−1.40	13.94
OH	0.12	−0.37	0.29	0.32	−0.67	−0.55	2.85
OCH_3	0.12	−0.27	0.27	0.36	−0.02	−0.55	7.87
OCH_2CH_3	0.10	−0.24	0.27	0.48	0.38		12.47
SH	0.25	0.15	0.26	0.60	0.39	−1.07	9.22
SCH_3	0.15	0.00	0.23	0.64	0.61	−1.07	13.82
NO_2[b]	0.71	0.78	0.76	1.39	−0.28	−2.52	7.36

(*Continued*)

TABLE 4.3 (*Continued*)

Hammett σ Constants[a]

Group	σ_{meta}	σ_{para}	σ_I	σ_v	π	E_s	MR
NO	0.62	0.91	0.37		−0.12		5.20
NH$_2$	−0.16	−0.66	0.12		−1.23	−0.61	5.42
NHCHO	0.19	0.00	0.27		−0.98		10.31
NHCOCH$_3$	0.07	−0.15	0.26		−0.37		16.53
N(CH$_3$)$_2$	−0.15	−0.83	0.06	0.43	0.18		15.55
N(CH$_3$)$_3^+$	0.88	0.82	0.93	1.22	−5.96		21.20

[a] σ_{meta} and σ_{para} are the Hammett constants; σ_I is the inductive σ constant; σ_v is the Charton's v (size) values; π is the hydrophobicity parameter; E_s is the Taft size parameter; and MR is the molar refractivity (polarizability) parameter.

[b] The group is in the most sterically hindered conformation.

Abbreviation: MR, molar refractivity.

In some cases, the σ values are generally applicable to much different equilibrium. In other cases, the σ values have been derived for specific equilibria, which is particularly true when one considers the σ values for ortho substituents. A good example of the application of Hammett's electronic descriptors in a QSAR relating the inhibition of bacterial growth is in the series of sulfonamides,

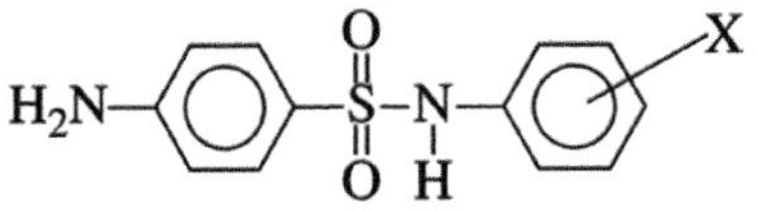

where X represents various substituents. A QSAR was developed based on the values of the substituents,

$$\log\left(\frac{1}{C}\right) = 1.05\sigma - 1.28 \tag{4.46}$$

where C is the minimum concentration of compound that inhibited the growth of *Escherichia coli*. From this relationship, it is seen that electron-withdrawing substituents favor inhibition of growth.

4.3.1 Hansch Analysis

The QSARs based on Hammett's relationship utilize electronic properties as the descriptors of structures. Difficulties were encountered when investigators attempted to apply Hammett-type relationships to biological systems, indicating that other structural descriptors were necessary. Robert Muir, a botanist at Pomona College, studied the biological activity of compounds that resembled indoleacetic acid and phenoxyacetic acid, which function as plant growth regulators. In attempting to correlate the structures of these compounds with their activities, he consulted his colleague in chemistry, Corwin Hansch, while using Hammett σ parameters to account for the electronic effect of substituents that did not lead to meaningful QSAR. However, Hansch recognized the importance of lipophilicity, expressed as the octanol–water partition coefficient, on biological activity. This parameter is now recognized to provide a measure of the bioavailability of compounds, which will determine, in part, the amount of the compound that gets to the target site.

Relationships were developed to correlate a structural parameter (i.e., lipophilicity) with activity. In some cases, a univariate relationship correlating structure and activity was adequate. The form of the equation is:

$$\log\left(\frac{1}{C}\right) = a\log P + b \tag{4.47}$$

where C is the molar concentration of the compound that produces a standard response (e.g., LD50 and ED50). With other data, it was observed that correlations were improved by combining Hammett's electronic parameters and Hansch's measure of lipophilicity, using an equation, such as:

$$\log\left(\frac{1}{C}\right) = k_1\pi + k_2\sigma + k_3 \tag{4.48}$$

where σ is the Hammett substituent parameter and π is defined analogously to σ. That is,

$$\pi = \log\left(\frac{P_x}{P_H}\right) \tag{4.49}$$

The significance of the slopes in univariate QSAR that involve the correlation of log P with toxicity has been considered. For example, an analysis of data in which the lysis of erythrocytes (hemolysis) by various neutral organic compounds (e.g., alcohols, carboxylic acids, amines, phenols, esters, and so on) was studied yielded the following general equation:

$$\log\left(\frac{1}{C}\right) = 0.93(\pm 0.17)\log P + 0.09(\pm 0.23) \tag{4.50}$$

Note that the slope of this equation is approximately one and that the intercept is approximately zero. Many other QSARs that involve nonspecific toxicity also show correlations of log P with toxicity, with a slope near one. However, a number of QSARs involving neutral organic compounds have slopes considerably less than one. The reasons for this phenomenon are not entirely clear. One analysis of the problem involves a consideration of the meaning of hydrophobicity at the molecular level. That is, hydrophobicity can be considered to be due largely to the free energy change associated with the desolvation of a compound as it moves from an aqueous phase to the biological phase, with which it interacts to produce toxicity (e.g., entering a membrane, binding to a protein, and so on). It appears that the slope of the regression equation is related to the desolvation of the compound that occurs when it interacts at its target site. When the slope of the equation is approximately one, the environment of the biological phase appears to be similar to that of octanol; partitioning of a compound from water into octanol would require complete desolvation of the compound. For some of the examples of QSAR with a slope less than one, the measured effect is a result of binding of ligands to proteins or DNA.

While most of the QSAR observations involve linear relationships between log P and toxicity, there are other relationships, such as parabolic, seen between biological response and hydrophobicity. One interpretation to account for this observation is that many membranes may have to be traversed for compounds to get to the target site, and compounds with the greatest hydrophobicity will become localized in the membranes they encounter initially, thereby slowing their transit to the target site.

Another factor that alters QSAR involves steric effects. For studies that involve reactivity of organic compounds, a steric parameter, E_s, was defined by Taft as:

$$E_s = \log\left(\frac{K_x}{K_H}\right)_A \tag{4.51}$$

where k is the rate constant for the acid hydrolysis of esters of the type:

$$
\begin{array}{c}
\quad\quad\quad O \\
\quad\quad\quad \parallel \\
X - CH_2 - C - OR
\end{array}
$$

The transition state for this hydrolysis can be represented as:

$$
\begin{array}{c}
\quad\quad\quad OH \\
\quad\quad\quad | \\
X - CH_2 - \; C \; - OR \\
\quad\quad\quad | \\
\quad\quad\quad HOH
\end{array}
$$

Assuming that the electronic effects of substituent X can be ignored, the size of X will affect the transition state and, hence, the rate of the reaction. By definition, $E_s = 0$ for X = H. Table 4.3 lists values of E_s for other substituents.

Another parameter related to molecular volume and steric effects is the molar refractivity (MR). Experimentally, it is obtained from the equation:

$$MR = \frac{n^2 - 1}{n^2 + 2} \cdot \frac{MW}{d} \tag{4.52}$$

where n is the index of refraction, d is the density, and MW is the molecular weight.

Steric effects can be particularly difficult to define in complex biological systems. Quantitative structure–activity relationships in biological systems have been developed by using parameters such as E_s and MR. In addition, factors such as van der Waals radii, standard bond angles and lengths, and conformational flexibility have been applied as a way to define the space occupied by molecules. However, it is often difficult to define a single parameter that can account for all these factors. A more recent treatment of steric effects that is applied to biological systems is the comparative molecular field analysis (CoMFA). This approach, which examines and superimposes the conformations of molecules of interest, is an extension of the ligand-based drug design.

One of the largest QSAR database is offered by the Pomona College (3); for advanced search functions, the user needs a license from Biobyte (4). These large databases represent large values for preformulation and drug discovery groups; most of the development in this area came about during the past few years, with the availability of high-speed computational devices.

4.4 Partitioning

The partition coefficient is a measure of the extent a substance partitions between two phases, generally an oil phase and an aqueous phase. This ratio is often expressed as log P (logarithm of partition ratio). Both pK_a and log P measurements are useful parameters for understanding the behavior of drug molecules at the preformulation stage. The pK_a will determine the species of molecules, which is likely to be present at the site of action, and how quickly or completely would the species cross a large number of transport barriers in the body, regardless of the route of administration. Factors such as absorption, excretion, and penetration of a drug in the central nervous system (CNS) are also related to the log P value of a drug, and in certain cases, predictions can be made; these are important in assessing the endogenous toxicity of compounds and their activity.

Partition coefficient (P) is a ratio of the concentration in two immiscible solvents:

$$P = [\text{organic}]/[\text{aqueous}] \tag{4.53}$$

where the values in brackets describe measured concentrations.

$$\log P = \log_{10} (\text{partition coefficient}) \tag{4.54}$$

In practical terms, the uncharged or neutral molecule exists for bases >2 pK_a units above the pK_a and for acids >2 pK_a units below the pK_a. In practice, the log P will vary according to the conditions under which it is measured and the choice of the partitioning solvent.

It is worth noting that this is a logarithmic scale; therefore, log $P = 0$ means that the compound is equally soluble in water and in the partitioning solvent. If the compound has a log $P = 5$, then the compound is 100,000 times more soluble in the partitioning solvent. A log $P = -2$ means that the compound is 100 times more soluble in water; that is, it is quite hydrophilic.

Log P values have been studied in approximately 100 organic liquid–water systems. As it is virtually impossible to determine lop P in a realistic biological medium, the octanol–water system has been adopted widely as a model of the lipid phase. While there has been much debate about the suitability of this system, it is the most widely used in pharmaceutical studies. Octanol and water are immiscible, but some water does dissolve in octanol in a hydrated state. This hydrated state contains 16 octanol aggregates, with the hydroxyl head groups surrounded by trapped aqueous solution. Lipophilic (unionized) species dissolve in the aliphatic regions.

Generally, compounds with log P values between one and three show good absorption, whereas those with log Ps greater than six or less than three often have poor transport characteristics. Highly nonpolar molecules have a preference to reside in the lipophilic regions of membranes, and highly polar compounds show poor bioavailability because of their inability to penetrate membrane barriers. Thus, there is a parabolic relationship between log P and transport; that is, candidate drugs that exhibit a balance between these two properties will probably show the best oral bioavailability.

4.4.1 Distribution Coefficient

The partition coefficient refers to the intrinsic lipophilicity of the drug, in the context of the equilibrium of unionized drug between the aqueous and organic phases. If the drug has more than one ionization center, the distribution of species present will depend on the pH. The concentration of the ionized drug in the aqueous phase will therefore have an effect on the overall observed partition coefficient. This leads to the definition of the distribution coefficient (log D) of a compound that takes into account the dissociation of weak acids and bases.

As in the aqueous phase, the total concentration may comprise both ionized and unionized forms, the distribution is given as:

$$\text{Distribution coefficient, } D = [\text{unionized}]_{(o)}/[\text{unionized}]_{(aq)} + [\text{ionized}]_{(aq)} \quad (4.55)$$

$$\log D = \log 10 \text{ (distribution coefficient)} \quad (4.56)$$

Log D is related to log P and the pK_a by the following equations:

$$\log D_{(pH)} = \log P - \log[1 + 10^{(pH - pKa)}]_{\text{for acids}} \quad (4.57)$$

$$\log D_{(pH)} = \log P - \log[1 + 10^{(pHa - pH)}]_{\text{for bases}} \quad (4.58)$$

Log D is the log distribution coefficient at a particular pH. This is not constant and will vary according to the protogenic nature of the molecule. Log D at pH 7.4 is often quoted to give an indication of the lipophilicity of a drug at the pH of blood plasma. Figures 4.8 through 4.10 show the distribution profiles of various acids and bases.

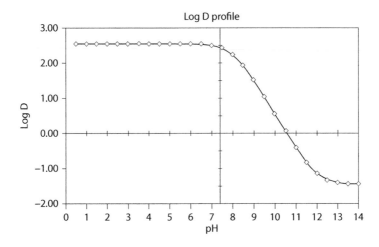

FIGURE 4.8 Log D profile of an acid with pK_a of 8.

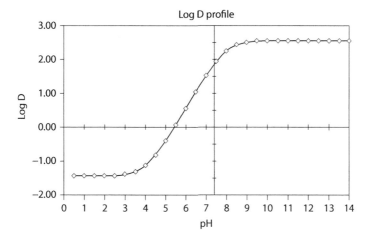

FIGURE 4.9 Log *D* profile of a base with pK_a of 8.

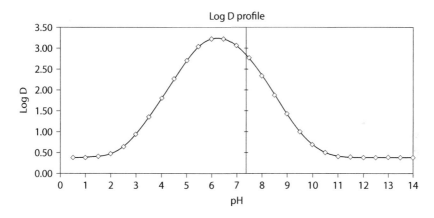

FIGURE 4.10 Log *D* profile of a zwitterion (base) with pK_a of 5.6 and 7.0 for acid and base, respectively.

It is important to understand that the species that partition are neutral molecules, or act like one, because of ion-pairing, resulting in transport of ionic species, complicating the calculations of log *P* and log *D*. However, instruments such as the Sirius PCA200 and G-pK_a can isolate the ion-pairing effect that requires several titrations. It is note-worthy that ion pairing also affects the readings taken using spectrophotometers. As a result, comparisons of values obtained from different methods may not corroborate, because of the differences in the concentrations or the differences in the use of the counterion involved. Generally, a 0.1 M solution of a background electrolyte is used, which is close to the biological level of 0.16 M. The type of electrolyte can make much difference, for example, 0.15 M potassium chloride in place of sodium chloride to obviate the "sodium effect" on the electrode at high pH, with similar profile as obtained using sodium chloride. Choice of a proper background electrolyte can be very important in many instances, especially where some significance to biological systems is desired.

Log D membrane, or log D_{mem}, is another way of measuring the lipophilicity of a compound, which is less frequently used than the octanol–water partition system. Log D_{mem} utilizes liposomes prepared from the synthetic phospholipids dimyristoylphosphatidyl-choline (DMPC), and although the system is more physiologically relevant than octanol, it suffers from a lack of predictability. This method requires 1 mg of the compound, whereby a solution of the compound is equilibrated with a solution of DMPC liposomes at 37°C for 2 hours. The free and liposome-bound compounds are then separated by centrifugation, and the solutions are analyzed by high-performance liquid chromatography (HPLC). Log D_{mem} is then calculated as the log of the ratio of the concentration of the compound in the liposome phase to that of the compound in the aqueous phase.

More recently, computer methods have been devised to calculate these values. The molecule is broken down into fragments of known lipophilicity, and the log P is calculated using various computer routines. Alternatively, there are atom-based methods, and lipophilicity is measured, and the calculated log Ps (c log Ps) agreement is reasonably good.

4.4.2 Partitioning Solvent

The choice of the partitioning solvent can have significant effects on the results obtained and also on its relevance to biological systems. The most commonly used solvent is octan-1-ol, which simulates the phospholipid membrane. To simulate the blood–brain barrier and skin penetration, octanol, chloroform, cyclohexane, and propylene glycol dipelargonate (PGDP) are more suitable. The log P values measured in these solvents show differences principally due to hydrogen-bonding effects. Octanol can donate and accept hydrogen bonds, making it amphiprotic; cyclohexane is inert; chloroform is a proton donor; and PGDP is an electron acceptor that can only accept electrons. Despite scores of very good publications and hundreds of studies on the choice of the solvent to be used, the choice remains very fluid. Differences in the log P values between different solvents of solvent mixture systems have often proven useful in QSAR studies. The differences in the partitioning value between PGDP–water and octanol–water or between octanol–water and alkali–water point to differences in hydrogen-bonding capacity that affects skin penetration. Compounds with high log P values and low H-bonding capacity can readily get past ester/phosphate groups in the skin membranes.

Partitioning experiments have been carried out using liposomes, where neutral log P values from liposomes tend to be very similar to those measured in octanol, but the log P values of the ion pair differ. The "surface ion pair" log P is found to be much higher in bases, zwitterions, and amphophiles. The values for acids tend to be similar to the values for octanol. This reflects the increased potential for partitioning of molecules with basic groups into membranes. Quantitative structure–activity relationship studies have found improved correlations with liposome-derived "surface ion pair" log P values.

The measurement of partitioning is practical only if the compound shows some solubility; insoluble compounds are difficult to characterize and often prove less valuable anyway. A relationship between log P and the observed biology is frequently found in a series where structural modifications do not significantly affect the pK_a values. The classical work of Hansch showed that these relationships were often parabolic;

hence, the relationship often leads to an optimum value for the log P for a desired activity or selective distribution. Relationships of this type include:

$$\text{Linear: Activity} = m \log P + k' \tag{4.59}$$

$$\text{Parabolic: Activity} = m \log P - c(\log P)2 - k \tag{4.60}$$

$$\text{Rectilinear: Activity} = m \log P - c(\log P + 1) - k \tag{4.61}$$

where m, k, and c are the constants generated using regression analysis to correlate the observed biological data with the measured partition coefficients. The mathematical techniques most commonly used to develop this correlation involve the use of multivariate analysis, principal component analysis, and partial least squares regression. Standard textbooks of statistics should be consulted to learn more about the applications and limitations of each of these approaches to data analysis.

The use of the organic solvents to model complex bilipids is very simplistic. While there have been some successes in modeling the response of compounds, large differences in the activity between molecules of different structures or the activity between enantiomers cannot be easily understood. In these cases, it is very useful to combine physical measurements with molecular modeling, molecular property, and spectroscopic data and use multivariate analysis. For both CNS penetration and gastric absorption, the relationship appears to be parabolic, with an optimum log P value of around 2 ± 1. Evidence for this comes from a wide variety of experiments in the literature, from brain concentration of radiolabeled compounds to behavioral studies.

Other methods of analysis used include molecular properties, such as charged partial surface area (PSA) and the study of the effects of hydrogen bonding on drug absorption.

Besides projecting the solubility, the log P value has several important applications, providing greater insight into how the molecule crosses various biological barriers and hence proves effective as a prospective new lead compound. In general, where passive absorption is assumed, log P can be related to various fixed-value ranges (Figure 4.11).

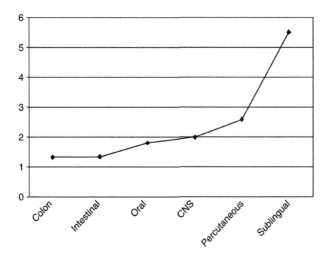

FIGURE 4.11 Optimal log P values for absorption from different parts of the gastrointestinal tract.

Generally, a low log P (less than 0) is desirable for injectable products, whereas a medium (0–3) range is suitable for oral administration; transdermal administration requires a higher value (3–4), but once the range of four to seven is reached, we risk the accumulation of the drug in the body fat that can prove toxic owing to the accumulation of drug in multiple dosing situations. The renal clearance of drugs with log D (measured at pH 7.4) greater than zero will decrease renal clearance and increase metabolic clearance; the pK_a of drugs also plays an important role here, as highly ionized drugs are kept out of cells and thus out of systemic toxicity; generally, a pK_a of six to eight will be most optimal for transport across various biological membranes.

When making a choice, generally, a drug with lowest log P will be desirable; however, it might be required to make a choice between a high- versus a low-MW molecule; it is known that high-MW drugs are generally more allergenic. The goal should be to achieve a minimum hydrophobicity, using a combination of log P, pK_a, and molecular size. The principle of minimum hydrophobicity keeps the drugs that might produce side effects such as depression out of the CNS, which means that most molecules should have a log P lower than two; this technique was used in the design of the new generation of nonsedative antihistamines. A very high lipophilicity should also be avoided because of the adverse effects on protein binding and on drug absorption, including solubility.

The ideal drug candidate, going into human studies, should have already been designed with the idea of keeping lipophilicity as low as possible, provided this can be done without the loss of affinity to the target receptor.

4.4.3 Solubility

The discussions of pK_a, log P, and log D above all pertain to the endpoint analysis of the solubility of a drug candidate. A correlation exists between log P of neutral immiscible liquids and their solubility in water; however, for solids, solubility also depends on the energy required to break the crystal lattice, where log P is related to solubility. It is therefore possible to have compounds with high log P values, which are still soluble on account of their low melting point. Similarly, it is possible to have a low-log P compound with a high melting point, which is very insoluble.

There are instances that when titrating a basic compound, there appears a precipitation; in such cases, the solubility of the free base may be calculated by using the equation:

$$St_x = S_0 \cdot [1 + 10^{pKa-pHx}] \tag{4.62}$$

where St_x is the solubility at pH_x, and S_0 is the solubility of the free base.

It is this parameter that ultimately determines the activity, toxicity, stability, dosage form, and the route of administration. The U.S. Pharmacopeia classifies drugs based on their solubility (Table 4.4).

High solubility is defined as the highest dose strength that is soluble in 250 mL or less of aqueous media across the physiological pH range. Poorly soluble drugs can be defined as those with an aqueous solubility of less than 100 µg/mL. If a drug is poorly soluble, then it will dissolve only slowly, perhaps leading to incomplete absorption.

TABLE 4.4

The U.S. Pharmacopeia Solubility Classification

Descriptive Term	Parts of Solvent Required for One Part of Solute
Very soluble	Less than 1
Freely soluble	From 1 to 10
Soluble	From 10 to 30
Sparingly soluble	From 30 to 100
Slightly soluble	From 100 to 1000
Very slightly soluble	From 1000 to 10,000
Practically insoluble or insoluble	10,000 and over

Some general observations about the behavior of solutes in solution systems include the following:

- Electrolytes dissolve in conducting solvents.
- Hydrogen-containing solutes capable of forming hydrogen bonds dissolve in solvents capable of accepting hydrogen bonds, and vice versa.
- Solutes having significant dipole moments dissolve in solvents having significant dipole moments.
- Solutes with low or zero dipole moments dissolve in solvents with low or zero dipole moments.

There are always exceptions to these rules, but a good rule of thumb "like dissolves like" mostly applies. Therefore, solvents fall into three classes:

- Protic solvents, such as methanol and formamide, which are hydrogen-bond donors
- Dipolar aprotic solvents (e.g., acetonitrile nitrobenzene) with dielectric constants greater than 15 but that cannot form hydrogen bonds with the solute
- Aprotic solvents in which the dielectric constant is weak and the solvent is nonpolar, for example, pentane and benzene

If the solubility of a compound is accompanied by degradation, the estimation of solubility becomes difficult and must be quoted with the degradant found. Many candidate drugs are ionizable compounds, and thus, there are a number of parameters that determine the solubility of a compound. These parameters include, for example, molecular size and substituent groups on the molecule, degree of ionization, ionic strength, salt form, temperature, crystal properties, and complexation.

As compound supply is likely to be limited, only a few solvent systems can be investigated during initial solubility studies. Typically, the solubility of the compounds in water, 0.9% w/v saline, 0.1 M HCl, and 0.1 M NaOH will be determined. If there is sufficient compound, then the solubility in other systems may be considered (e.g., cosolvents, such as polyethylene glycol 400 [PEG 400] and propylene glycol). In addition, the solubility in oils and surfactants systems (e.g., Tween 80) may be considered. Automated instruments allow ready measure of solubility, such as by using the pION's pSOL (5), whereas as little as 0.1 mg of the compound is sufficient to establish a complete solubility profile.

4.4.3.1 Molecular Size

Large organic molecules have a lesser aqueous solubility than smaller molecules. This is due to interactions between the nonpolar groups and water; that is, solubility is dependent on the number of solvent molecules that can pack around the solute molecule.

4.4.3.2 Additives

Additives might increase or decrease the solubility of a solute in a given solvent. In the case of salt, those that increase the solubility are said to "salt in" the solute, and those that decrease the solubility are said to "salt out" the solute. The effect of the additive depends very much on the influence it has on the structure of the water or its ability to compete with solvent water molecules. Both effects are described by the empirically derived Setschenow equation:

$$\log^{S0/S} = kM \tag{4.63}$$

This equation describes the relationship between the aqueous solubility of the sparingly soluble salts (S_0) and the empirical Setschenow salting-out constant $k = 0.217/S_0$. This relationship and the Setschenow equation are valid only at low concentrations of added salt. As the concentration of the added salt increases, the apparent k value is not constant but is dependent on the solubility and the rate of change of solubility with added salt concentration. It was concluded that the Setschenow treatment is generally inappropriate for the description and analysis of common ion equilibria.

Another aspect of the effect of electrolytes on the solubility of a salt is the concept of the solubility product for poorly soluble substances. The experimental consequences of this phenomenon are that if the concentration of a common ion is high, then the other ion becomes low in a saturated solution of the substance; that is, precipitation occurs. Conversely, the effect of foreign ions on the solubility of sparingly soluble salts is just the opposite, and the solubility increases. This is called the salt effect.

4.4.3.3 Temperature

As dissolution is usually an endothermic process, an increase in the solubility of solids with a rise in temperature is the general rule. Therefore, most graphs of solubility plotted against temperature show a continuous rise, but there are exceptions; for example, the solubility of sodium chloride is almost invariant, while that for calcium hydroxide falls slightly from a solubility of 0.185 g/mL at 0°C to 0.077 g/mL at 100°C.

4.5 Measurement Strategies

The understanding of the factors that affect the values of pK_a or $\log P$ obtained, as discussed previously, is essential in making the best use of the multitude of techniques available to measure these parameters and then interpret them to the drug discovery group. The limitations faced by the preformulation group at this stage include the following:

- *Solubility of the compound.* There must be some solubility. The pK_a of poorly soluble compounds must be measured in aqueous methanol solution. If several titrations are carried out with different ratios of methanol:water, the Yesuda–Shedlovsky equation can reveal the theoretical pK_a in purely aqueous solution. Similarly, for poorly soluble compounds, provided the log P is high enough, the compound may be determined by titration, by the addition of the sample to the octanol first. The compound will then back partition into the aqueous layer. If this fails, spectroscopic methods have to be employed, as more dilute solutions may be used.
- *Stability of the compound.* The compound must be able to withstand the rigors of testing, such as not breaking down during the time it takes to establish equilibrium between the two phases.
- *Purity of the compound.* Substances submitted for pK_a and log P studies need to be pure, of accurately known composition, and be submitted as free bases or inorganic acid salts. In general, no reliable measurements can be made on organic acid salts.
- *Single compound.* It is preferred to prepare a series of compounds to validate methods of testing, to validate a trend, and to obviate many experimental problems.

Table 4.5 summarizes the advantages and disadvantages of the most commonly used methods to measure pK_a and log P. These are presented together, because in many instances, both parameters can be obtained from unified experimental runs, a strategy that is very useful when the quantity of the substance available is limited, as is the case in most instances.

Most companies would do well by studying the available equipment from Sirius (6). Table 4.6 lists the available equipment and their applications.

4.5.1 Ion Pair Log *P*

Ion pair log Ps might be determined by at least two or preferably three titrations in different ratios of octanol to water. The apparent pK_a in the presence of octanol, the poK_a, can be used to determine the presence of ion pair partitioning according to the equations:

$$P_{XH} = \frac{\begin{array}{c} r_2(10^{P_aK_a(2)-pK_a} - r_1 10^{P_aK_a(1)-pK_a} - (r_2 - r_1)) \\ \times 10^{P_aK_a(1)+pK_a+P_aK_a(2)-2pK} \end{array}}{r_1 r_2(10^{P_aK_a(1)-pK_a} - 10^{P_aK_a(2)-pK_a})} \tag{4.64}$$

$$P_X = \frac{r_1(10^{P_aK_a(2)-pK_a} - r_2 10^{P_aK_a(1)-pK_a} - r_2 - r_1}{r_1 r_2(10^{P_aK_a(1)-pK_a} - 10^{P_aK_a(2)-pK_a})} \tag{4.65}$$

where r is the octanol:water ratio.

TABLE 4.5

Advantages and Disadvantages of pK_a and Log P Measurement Techniques

Method	Measures	Advantage	Disadvantage	Concentration Required	Sample Size
Sirius Potentiometric pKa/log P	pKa, log P, log P app	Rapid, convenient	Insoluble or neutral samples cannot be measured	0.0001 M (0.1 mM)	1–5 mg
Sirius Yesuda-Shedlovsky	pKa	pKa for insoluble samples	Takes three or more titrations	0.0005 M (0.5 mM)	5 mg
Sirius ion-pair log P	log P, log P (ip)	Predict log D more accurately	Takes three or more titrations	0.0001 M (0.1 mM)	3–15 mg
Manual potentiometric pKa	pKa	Simple, rapid	Not for low or overlapping pKas; precipitation when titrated to neutral species; multiple experiments required	>0.0025 M (2.5 mM)	50 mg
pKa by UV	pKa	pKa for poorly soluble or scarce compounds	Slow	0.000025 M (25 μM)	6 mg
pKa by solubility	pKa	pKa for highly insoluble compounds	Slow, low accuracy	Below 0.0005 M (0.5 mM)	10 mg
Log P by filter probe	Log P	Log P for poorly soluble compounds, reliable > log P of 0.2	Messy, slow to set up, requires care. Inaccurate below log P of 0.2	0.000025 M (25 μM)	6 mg
Log D by filter probe	pKa, log P, log D	Can determine log Papp at any pH	Only possible with compounds possessing isobestic point	0.000025 M (25 μM)	6 mg
Log P by shake flask	Log P, log D at chosen pH	Low log P values. Can investigate surface effects	Slow, tedious, messy	0.000025 M (25 μM)	6 mg
Log P by HPLC	Log D at pH 7	Many compounds can be measured at once. Small sample size	Inaccurate, generally only carried out at pH 7	~2.5 mM	0.5 mg

^a A wavelength, wavenumber, or frequency at which the total absorbance of a sample does not change during a chemical reaction, or a physical change of the sample, such as when one molecular entity is converted into another, which has the same molar absorption coefficient at a given wavelength.

Abbreviations: HPLC, high-performance liquid chromatography; UV, ultraviolet.

TABLE 4.6

Equipment Available for Sirius for pK_a, Log P, and Solubility Measurement and Data Handling

Instrument	Features
GLpK_a: simultaneous pK_a, log P, and solubility determination	• pH range of 1.8–12.2 (for standard titrations) • Up to 30 samples in 24°hour • Automated operation • Measurements below 10–4°M • Built-in traceability and reminders • Supports D-PAS for spectrophotometric pK_a
D-PAS: spectrophotometric pK_a	• Concentrations as low as 10–6°M • Sample weight down to 50°μg • Single- or multiprotic molecules • Macro- and microconstants easily fitted to Sirius GLpK_a or PCA200
PCA200: entry-level pK_a, log P, and solubility	• Measures pK_a, log P, and intrinsic solubility • Ideal for smaller workloads or academic research • Uses the pH-metric technique and RefinementPro2 software • Automated addition of acid and base titrants • Supports D-PAS (UV method)
ProfilerSGA: rapid pK_a measurement	• Fully automated physicochemical profiling • Measures pK_a in just 2°min • Multiwavelength spectrophotometric technique • Open access option • Automated data handling and processing • Full computer control • Microplate format • Measures below 10–5°M concentration • 300 assays in 24 hours • MDM mixed solvent system
ProfilerLDA: log D/P octanol/water partitioning	• Fully automated log D determination • Multiwavelength spectrophotometric technique • Open access (administrator and user profiles) • Automated data handling and processing • Full computer control • Microplate format (96- and 384-well) • Remote network monitoring • Performance monitoring
ProfilerLDA: log D/P octanol/water partitioning	• Fully automated log d determination • Multiwavelength spectrophotometric technique • Open access (administrator and user profiles) • Automated data handling and processing • Full computer control • Microplate format (96- and 384-well) • Remote network monitoring • Performance monitoring

(*Continued*)

TABLE 4.6 (*Continued*)

Equipment Available for Sirius for pK_a, Log *P*, and Solubility Measurement and Data Handling

Instrument	Features
GLpH: automated pH measurement	• High degree of accuracy
	• Easy to use
	• Automatic calibration and reminders
	• Available in single-sample or autosampler versions
	• One-button operation for most measurements
	• built-in GLP
	• "Normal" and "supervisor" access modes
RefinementPro2: automatic clipping of data	• Automatic selection of reference ranges for D-PAS assay
	• Dataset quality marker
	• Improved "Approx" function with Auto-Bjerrum analysis
	• GLpK_a /D-PAS to be used with a laptop
	• Turbidity sensing with D-PAS probe (optional)
	• Assay planner (optional)
	• Autorefinement of pH-metric and D-PAS data
CheqSol: solubility on GLpK_a, with results in less than 1 hour	• Equilibrium and kinetic result
	• Sample does not require chromophore
	• Result confirmed within same experiment
	• Most samples measured without cosolvent
	• No filtration or separation required
	• No need to speculate whether sample is at equilibrium
	• Wide measurement range
Fast D-PAS: pK_a values in just 4 minutes	• Fast D-PAS is a new way to measure pK_a values
	• It combines the power of UV spectroscopy with the flexibility of pH-metric titration
	• Gains speed by titrating in the presence of a unique linear buffer solution
	• Fast D-PAS assays take about 4 minutes, including the time required to fill
	• Dispensers, move probes, titrate, read spectra, and clean up after assay

Source: From http://www.sirius-ai.com/index.htm.

Note: Aqueous titrations using Sirius instruments is the easiest method for pK_a and log *P* measurements and provides detailed information on the partitioning characteristics of a sample at all pH values. The PCA200 and GLpK_a and pK_a/log *P* analyzers are based on a potentiometric titration method. The basic principle of operation is to determine the pK_a by titration followed by a back titration to determine the apparent pK_a in the presence of octanol. Any partitioning by the compound will shift the equilibrium and cause a change in the apparent pK_a. From this shift, the log *P* may be calculated. Sophisticated software allows detailed iterative calculations to be made and values to be carefully refined. If a sample is soluble, then it is possible to determine all its pK_a values, its log *P*, and the apparent log *P* at every pH. In addition, log *P* values of ionized species where they occur may also be calculated. The technique can be performed on samples at a concentration of 0.0001 M or above, the ideal concentration being 0.0005 M. Using the PCA200 for a suitable molecule, the analysis time would be a few hours, including calculation time. The GLpK_a has an autosampler and can also do multiple titrations on each sample. If the sample is highly insoluble, then the log *P* cannot be measured. The pK_a can be measured by either partial titration or by a Yesuda–Shedlovsky experiment where three titrations in aqueous methanol are performed, each with a different proportion of methanol. From the results, a corrected extrapolation gives the theoretical aqueous value; the technique can be performed on samples at a concentration of 0.0005 M (6).

Abbreviations: CheqSol, chasing equilibrium solubility; UV, ultraviolet.

Both the log P and the log D values may be severely affected if one or more of the charged species is partitioned. Ion-pairing effects may be fully determined with the Sirius instruments, even in the cases of polyprotic compounds, where any of the charged or neutral species may partition.

4.5.1.1 Manual Titration

While manual titration has mostly been replaced by automated techniques described previously, the principle remains the same, wherein a pH electrode and a volumetric pipette are used. The technique may be carried out on compounds with reasonable aqueous solubilities (>0.0025 M) and that are available in amounts greater than 30 mg. This method is rapid, simple, and accurate; however, very low pK_as ($pK_a < 3$) and overlapping pK_as cannot be determined. A computer program or spreadsheet to calculate pK_a values from the experimental data can be written to speed up the calculations. Analysis time is a few hours. The reader may refer to *Excel for Chemists* by E. Joseph Billo, John Wiley & Sons, New York (2001), for help on setting up the spreadsheets.

4.5.1.2 Spectroscopy

Where the compounds are poorly soluble or where the quantity of compound available is small, pK_a values are calculated from ultraviolet (UV) spectrophotometric measurements. The method simply relies on the change in UV spectra at different pH values. An adaptation of the filter probe method (described next) is used. Sample concentrations down to 4 mg/400 mL may be determined (approximately 0.000025 M). Sirius Analytical Instruments supplies the D-PAS probe, which enables spectrophotometric determinations by using the GLpK_a instrument (Table 4.6).

The UV spectroscopy often proves to be a very useful tool if the new compound contains a chromophore (e.g., a group containing a double bond or other electron-rich zones; most suitable for compounds with an ionizing group close to or within an aromatic ring, as in such instances, the shift is large on ionization). A simple plot of UV absorption as a function of change in pH gives instant results (provided the compound has sufficient solubility to yield a stable UV absorption reading). If the compound contains an UV chromophore that changes with the extent of ionization, then a method involving UV spectroscopy can be used. This method involves measuring the UV spectrum of the compound as a function of pH. Mathematical analysis of the spectral shifts can then be used to determine the pK_a or pK_as of the compound. The pK_a of a compound may be estimated using the ACDpKa software, which also contains a large database of the measured pK_a data. The computer program SPARC (scalable processor architecture) is also used for estimating the pK_a of pharmaceuticals (8).

Generally, the quantity of substance required when the spectroscopy method is used is about 1 mg (traditional titrimetry requires about 3 mg). To maximize the utility of the small quantities available, the preformulation scientist would perform a multipurpose experiment; the compound is partitioned between a mixture of water and octanol (or a buffer), separating the two layers, centrifuged to separate any emulsification. Both layers are analyzed by HPLC method and then by using the aqueous layer to titrate or by using UV spectroscopy to determine the pH shift at pK_a. These microscale techniques form the strong basis of preformulation studies. With newer techniques of quantitation such as time of flight (TOF) mass spectroscopy (MS) and liquid chromatography-tandem mass spectroscopy (LC-MS/MS), becoming available, the burden to produce significant amounts of the lead compound is substantially reduced. This has also broadened the involvement of preformulation scientists at the earliest stages of drug discovery.

4.5.2 Solubility Method

Where the compounds have extremely low solubility, pK_a values may be measured by the solubility method. An aqueous solution of a substance is titrated in the direction of its neutral species until the free base or free acid is precipitated. pK_a can then be calculated from the solubility product. This method is not very accurate but may be used for very dilute solutions.

4.5.3 Filter Probe Method

The log P determination using the filter probe method is essentially a variation of the shake-flask method, except that it is rapid and relies on continuous sampling. An aqueous solution of the sample under test is placed in a reaction vessel and circulated through a spectrophotometric flow cell. The absorbance of the aqueous solution is measured before and after the addition of octanol. A solvent inlet filter prevents any octanol from passing through to the detector. The method is rapid and reliable for log P values from around 0.2 upward, but low log P values are difficult to measure owing to the resulting insignificant change in absorbance. The reason for this is that below a phase volume ratio of 40 (400 mL water/10 mL octanol), the octanol tends to break through the filter. In cases of low log P, the shake-flask method must be adopted. Sample concentrations down to 4 mg/400 mL may be determined (approximately 0.000025 M).

Log D profiles may be obtained by performing the filter probe experiment over a range of pH values. The critical part of the experiment is to discover whether the compound of interest has an isosbestic point in its UV spectrum. If it does not, the experiment cannot be performed; if it does, both log P and pK_a values may be determined. This method is similar to the potentiometric method described earlier, except that the amount of unpartitioned substance is determined by spectroscopy rather than by potentiometry. The advantage of this method is that only one experiment needs to be performed to yield log P, log $P_{app,}$ and pK_as, but not all compounds have an isosbestic point. Sample concentrations down to 4 mg/400 mL may be determined (approximately 0.000025 M).

4.5.4 Shake-Flask Method

The most common method for determining the partition and distribution coefficients is the shake-flask method. In this technique, the candidate drug is shaken between octanol (previously shaken together or presaturate each phase with the other) and water layers, from which an aliquot is taken and analyzed using UV absorption, HPLC, or titration. The shake-flask method is the oldest and the most tedious way of measuring log *P* values. The UV absorbance of an aqueous solution is measured before and after being shaken with a known volume of octanol. Despite its disadvantages, this remains the only method that can be used in cases of very low log *P* values. One advantage of this method is that the appearance of the compound in the octanol may be checked against the disappearance from the aqueous phase to see if any surface effects have occurred. Some molecules may form effective surfactants. It is very important to presaturate the solvents in prolonged shake-flask experiments. The experiment must be performed over 3 days or more to ensure that the equilibrium is reached; however, the actual time taken for the experiment is a few hours.

4.5.5 High-Pressure Liquid Chromatography

This chromatography may be used to estimate log *P* values. Compounds with known log *P*s are injected onto a C18 reverse-phase HPLC column, and their capacity factors are used to create a calibration curve. Unknown compounds are then injected, and their capacity factors are used to predict log *P*. Strictly, this technique is valid only for neutral molecules. Charged molecules have more complex retention behavior than simple partition. Some liquid–liquid experiments have been reported using an octanol saturated column and an aqueous mobile phase; however, the method is messy and requires frequent regeneration of the column.

The chromatographic methods suffer the disadvantage that the retention time is linearly related to the partition coefficient; that is, for a doubling of the log *P*, there is a 10-fold increase in the retention. This often requires columns of different lengths to be used—short ones for high log *P* values and long ones for low log *P* values. In addition, where strong charged molecules are involved, the data become less reliable. However, reasonable correlation is seen with neutral compounds or with those that are uncharged at pH 7.4. In cases where the molecule is charged and the pK_a is known, a correction factor may be added to correct the log *D* measurement to log *P*.

The discrepancies with the HPLC method are probably because of the imperfect nature of the C18-silica columns. Some of the new-generation reverse-phase materials, such as C18-alumina, polymeric C18, ultra-high carbon-loaded C18, and porous graphitic carbon, may overcome these problems. A recent development is an immobilized artificial membrane (IAM) column, which should more closely model the biological membranes.

The main advantage of the HPLC method is that a range of compounds may be determined at the same time. A new rapid technique has been reported in which all compounds and standards are simultaneously injected, and the identity of each peak is determined by mass spectroscopy. A refinement of this technique is the determination of log k_0'. This is achieved by measuring log k' in several different concentrations of aqueous methanol mobile phases and extrapolating back to 0% methanol. The resultant log k_0' values have been correlated to log *P* values more successfully. The concerns about polar interactions and the charge present on the analytes still remain.

4.5.6 Capillary Zone Electrophoresis

Capillary electrophoresis (CE) has emerged as a method of choice for determining compound pK_a values, as it possesses many favorable qualities, as outlined in the following:

- Potential impurities and degradants can be separated from the target compound.
- Knowledge of sample concentration is not required for analysis.
- Sparingly soluble compounds with a suitable UV chromophore can be analyzed.
- No changes in spectral properties are required for the detection of a pK_a value.
- Minimal sample amounts are required for analysis (<1 mg).

Single CE–UV systems possess a throughput of approximately one compound per hour when analyzing 12 pH points per compound. Using the 96-capillary cePRO 9600™ system (9), it is possible to analyze 12 compounds per hour over 24 pH points. This breakthrough results in a significant increase in sample throughput, in combination with an extended pH range and improved data quality.

High-performance liquid chromatography techniques have also been used in the determination of log P values. A potential problem with the use of HPLC retention data is that it is not a direct method and thus requires calibration. Furthermore, there may be problems with performing experiments at pH greater than 8.

4.5.7 Plate Method for Solubility Testing

The MultiScreen Solubility filter plate method is a screening method that provides a fast, convenient, automation-compatible, and high-throughput means to estimate the aqueous solubility of hundreds of compounds per day. It correlates well with standard shake-flask methodology and can be implemented readily for this method in the typical drug discovery laboratory. Using a single-point calibration, the screening ratio is derived simply and quickly, and compound solubility is approximated easily. Multiple samples, each requiring approximately 200 nmol (~100 μg) per result, can be run in parallel. This method allows for the analysis of approximately 45 compounds (duplicate determinations) per plate, with the capability of completing four or more plates in a standard 8-hour day. The assay is inherently compatible with the method by which most compound libraries are produced (e.g., as stock solutions in dimethylsulfoxide [DMSO]) and is integrated easily into the existing chemical profiling and early absorption, distribution, metabolism, and excretion (ADME) workflows. The method's resultant filtrate quickly provides a particulate-free and known soluble compound that can be used with confidence for other downstream ADME analysis.

Using this method, entire libraries can be screened for solubility. This narrows the number of candidates to only those that can meet solubility levels consistent with predicted oral bioavailability levels (especially when combined with permeability results) necessary to proceed down the pipeline.

High-throughput screening (HTS) assays are a routine for preformulation group. Where the solubility is low, highly unreliable data are often seen, particularly if there are molecules that skew the correlation significantly. Though compound aggregation has been determined as the cause of many false-positives, compound solubility is often not addressed until late in the ADME process. Screening compounds earlier (pharmacologic profiling) in the drug discovery process can minimize these issues, saving time and unnecessary expense. The shake-flask method, the standard method for solubility testing, has significant drawbacks, especially as an early screening tool. Long incubation times, tedious analysis requirements, and the need for large quantities of solid compounds preclude its usefulness in screening high numbers of candidates. An HTS method using a 96-well filter plate (Figure 4.12) (MultiScreen® Solubility Filter Plate, Millipore, Billerica, Massachusetts, U.S.; Ref. 10) is a suitable substitute for the classical flask method. Studies report good correlation between this method and the classical flask method. An additional benefit is that the resultant filtrate can be used for downstream ADME analysis, because it contains both a known concentration and known soluble compounds. The 96-well plate method can be easily introduced into the drug discovery workflow, because the new entities are typically stored in DMSO, a condition that is readily integrated with this methodology. This eliminates the need for the large quantities of solid compounds required in the shake-flask method. The 96-well filter plate design meets new American National Standard Institute/Society for Biomolecular Screening (ANSI/SBS) 2004 standards and is compatible with all standard laboratory robotics and analytical equipment. Incubation time for this assay is less than 2 hours, and hundreds of compounds can be evaluated on a given day.

This automatable assay can provide aqueous solubility data (in triplicate) for up to 120 drug compounds per (8 hours) day. pK_a data on compounds with ionizing groups

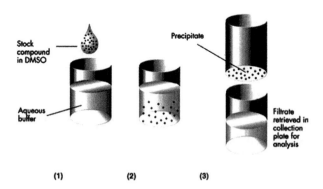

FIGURE 4.12 Filter plate method for solubility testing. (**1**) Add compound dissolved in organic solvent to aqueous buffer. (**2**) Shake for 90 minutes to allow insoluble compound to precipitate. (**3**) Apply vacuum to filter solution into collection plate. Precipitates remain on membrane. Analyze filtrate in collection plate to quantify the amount of the compound still in the solution. (Courtesy of Millipore Corporation, Billerica, MA.)

can also be obtained when solubility is determined, versus pH. There are, however, some important limitations to this method. Compounds must remain soluble, especially standards, over the duration of the assay, in whatever solvent system is used. Certain compounds, if not soluble in 20% aqueous acetonitrile (ACN), may produce visible precipitate and cloudiness, which can interfere with the UV spectroscopic analysis. If the precipitate is found, other analytical methods, such as HPLC and LC/MS/MS, may be used. Some compounds, on visual inspection, may contain color-producing chromophores, so the spectral range should be increased beyond 500 nm. The fact that the sample is made up in a 5% (v/v) DMSO solution may result in an overestimation of the compound's solubility in a purely aqueous solution. Lowering the amount of DMSO (e.g., 0.5%) may improve the correlation between the aqueous solubility method and the shake-flask method. If the compound is less than 95% pure, the UV spectroscopy method may not be suitable. A complex mixture would require some sort of chromatographic separation prior to analysis. It is essential that the compounds being investigated have sufficient UV spectroscopic molar absorptivities (extinction coefficients) to provide the requisite analytical sensitivity.

With these limitations in mind, the assay is still well suited as a high-throughput tool for a number of compound-screening applications, including the determination of structure–solubility relationships and establishing appropriate dosing concentration ranges for subsequent in vitro testing programs.

This method also allows the use of multiple-wavelength measurement and estimation of solubility. By analyzing the compound using spectroscopy at six wavelengths, the relative solubility, in the form of a screening ratio, can be calculated using the ratio of the pre- and postfiltered test samples. The calculated screening ratio provides a fast method for identifying compounds that are highly, moderately, or marginally soluble in aqueous solutions. As the screening ratio approaches unity, the sample approaches the upper limit of solubility—500 μM— as measured by the assay. If the screening ratio has a value less than 1 but greater than 0.5, the solubility of the compound is known to be between 100 and 500 μM. A screening ratio of less than 0.5 indicates that the compound's solubility is likely to be less than 100 μM.

$$\text{If: } \frac{(\sum \text{AU at 280, 300, 320, 340, 360 nm}) - (\text{AU at 800 nm}) \text{Filtrate}}{(\sum \text{AU at 280, 300, 320, 340, 360 nm}) - (\text{AU at 800 nm}) \text{Standard}} \approx 1.00 \quad (4.66)$$

$$\text{If: } \frac{(\sum \text{AU at 280, 300, 320, 340, 360 nm}) - (\text{AU at 800 nm}) \text{Filtrate}}{(\sum \text{AU at 280, 300, 320, 340, 360 nm}) - (\text{AU at 800 nm}) \text{Standard}} \leq 0.5 \quad (4.67)$$

Then: Aqueous solubility ≤ 100 μM

$$\text{If: } \frac{(\sum \text{AU at 280, 300, 320, 340, 360 nm}) - (\text{AU at 800 nm}) \text{Filtrate}}{(\sum \text{AU at 280, 300, 320, 340, 360 nm}) - (\text{AU at 800 nm}) \text{Standard}} < 1.00 \text{ and} > 0.5$$

Then: 100 μM < Aqueous solubility ≤ 500 μM

$$(4.68)$$

WEB REFERENCES

1. http://www.iupac.org/index_to.html
2. http://www.nist.gov
3. http://www.cqsar.com/medchem/chem/qsar-db/
4. http://www.biobyte.com
5. http://www.pion-inc.com/pSOL.htm
6. http://www.sirius-ai.com/index.htm
7. http://ibmlc2.chem.uga.edu/sparc/
8. http://www.combisep.com/pka.html
9. http://www.millipore.com/userguides.nsf/docs/p36523

BIBLIOGRAPHY

Avdeef A. pH-metric log *P*. II: Refinement of partition coefficients and ionization constants of multiprotic substances. *J Pharm Sci*. 1993;82(2):183–190.

RECOMMENDED READING

Acid Dissociation Constant

Ahlfors, C. E. (2016). "The bilirubin binding panel: A Henderson–Hasselbalch approach to neonatal hyperbilirubinemia." *Pediatrics* 138(4):e20154378.

Poor plasma bilirubin binding increases the risk of bilirubin neurotoxicity in newborns with hyperbilirubinemia. New laboratory tests may soon make it possible to obtain a complete bilirubin binding panel when evaluating these babies. The 3 measured components of the panel are the plasma total bilirubin concentration (BTotal), which is currently used to guide clinical care; the bilirubin binding capacity (BBC); and the concentration of nonalbumin bound or free bilirubin (BFree). The fourth component is the bilirubin-albumin equilibrium dissociation constant, KD, which is calculated from BTotal, BBC, and BFree. The bilirubin binding panel is comparable to the panel of components used in the Henderson–Hasselbalch approach to acid–base assessment. Bilirubin binding population parameters (not prospective studies to determine whether the new bilirubin binding panel components are better predictors of bilirubin neurotoxicity than BTotal) are needed to expedite the clinical use of bilirubin binding. At any BTotal, the BFree and the relative risk of bilirubin neurotoxicity increase as the KD/BBC ratio increases (i.e., bilirubin binding worsens). Comparing the KD/BBC ratio of newborns with BTotal of concern with that typical for the population helps determine whether the risk of bilirubin neurotoxicity varies significantly from the inherent risk at that BTotal Furthermore, the bilirubin binding panel individualizes care because it helps to determine how aggressive intervention should be at any BTotal, irrespective of whether it is above or below established BTotal guidelines. The bilirubin binding panel may reduce anxiety, costs, unnecessary treatment, and the likelihood of undetected bilirubin neurotoxicity.

Anderson, K. S. (2010). "A transient kinetic approach to investigate nucleoside inhibitors of mitochondrial DNA polymerase gamma." *Methods* 51(4):392–398.

Nucleoside analogs play an essential role in treating human immunodeficiency virus (HIV) infection since the beginning of the AIDS epidemic and work by inhibition of HIV-1 reverse transcriptase (RT), a viral polymerase essential for DNA replication. Today, over 90% of all regimens for HIV treatment contain at least one nucleoside. Long-term use of nucleoside analogs has been associated with adverse effects including mitochondrial toxicity due to inhibition of the mitochondrial polymerase, DNA polymerase gamma (mtDNA pol gamma). In this review, we describe our efforts to delineate the molecular mechanism of nucleoside inhibition of HIV-1 RT and mtDNA pol gamma based upon a transient kinetic approach using rapid chemical quench methodology. Using transient kinetic methods, the maximum rate of polymerization (k(pol)), the dissociation constant for the ground state binding (K(d)), and the incorporation efficiency (k(pol)/K(d)) can be determined for the nucleoside analogs and their natural substrates. This analysis allowed us to develop an understanding of the structure–activity relationships that allow correlation between the structural and stereochemical features of the nucleoside analog drugs with their mechanistic behavior toward the viral polymerase, RT, and the host cell polymerase, mtDNA pol gamma. An in-depth understanding of the mechanisms of inhibition of these enzymes is imperative in overcoming problems associated with toxicity.

Locatelli, M. et al. (2012). "Recent application of analytical methods to phase I and phase II drugs development: A review." *Biomed Chromatogr* 26(3):283–300.

Drug development is a time-consuming and costly process. It is usually divided into four phases, although it is not always possible to draw a sharp line between the various stages. In phase I and II there are many molecules investigate and it is necessary to analyze all of them in a short period of time, with lower costs, and with high-throughput assay. During phase I relevant chemical–physical parameters like the acid dissociation constant, lipophilicity, solubility and stability must be analyzed. Classic techniques such as "shake-flask" can be used, but instrumental analytical methods such as HPLC may be helpful to improve and enhance the productivity and reproducibility of the results. During phase II the activity of a drug and factors that may have an influence on it, like metabolic profile and transformations, impurities and plasma binding proteins, must be considered. In this field, recent hyphenated analytical methods, such as LC-MS/MS, GC-MS/MS or more complex couplings, can provide more complete information. The aim of this review is to report the processes required for the validation of drug efficacy with reference to the description of "classic" and modern techniques used.

Nowak, P. et al. (2015). "Application of capillary electrophoresis in determination of acid dissociation constant values." *J Chromatogr A* 1377:1–12.

The chemical groups undergoing protonation or deprotonation in solution are described by the acid dissociation constant value, the key parameter for physicochemical characterization of biologically and pharmacologically important compounds. Capillary electrophoresis (CE) proved to be suitable technique for its determination: it enables automated and accurate measurements even for minute amount of sample, does not require the information about concentration, and handle both the impure and complex samples. In this review, a number of contributions reporting on the application of CE in pKa prediction has been summarized and critically discussed. The reader will find herein the brief introduction of theory, summary of all works published in the last decade, considerations on the most important innovations and achievements, and the discussion of pKa-related issues as e.g. the role of pKa shifts in the chiral separation mechanism or the elucidation of migration order reversals observed during CE-mediated separations.

Shan, L. (2004). *Hyperpolarized (13)C-labeled bicarbonate (H(13)CO3(−)) for in vivo pH measurement with (13)C magnetic resonance spectroscopy. Molecular Imaging and Contrast Agent Database (MICAD).* Bethesda, MD: National Center for Biotechnology Information (US).

Magnetic resonance spectroscopy (MRS) is a technique that allows the noninvasive detection of multiple small metabolites within cells or extracellular spaces in vivo (1–4). Although MRS is theoretically applicable to any nucleus possessing spin, the more frequently investigated applications are in proton ((1)H) and carbon-13 ((13)C) (5–7). (13)C MRS is superior to (1)H MRS in many respects (3,7–9). (13)C MRS can provide specific information about the identity and structure of biologically important compounds. The chemical shift range for carbon (~250 ppm) is much larger than that for proton (~15 ppm), allowing for improved resolution of metabolites. However, (13)C MRS is limited by the low natural abundance of (13)C (1.1%) and its very low nuclear spin polarization ($2.5 \times 10(−6)$ polarization at 3 T and 37 masculineC) (2,3). Several techniques have been used to overcome these limitations, including dynamic nuclear polarization (DNP), which introduces one or more (13)C molecules into a metabolic substrate (2,3,9). Because the T1 relaxation time of (13)C in small molecules is much longer than that of (1)H (0.1–2.0 seconds in a magnetic field of 0.1–3.0 T), hyperpolarized (13)C-labeled tracers can be generated outside the subject and the magnetic resonance scanner (7). Nearly 100% nuclear polarization for (1)H and 50% for (13)C can be achieved in various organic molecules when DNP is performed in a strong magnetic field and at cryogenic temperatures. Replacing the (12)C isotope (98.9% natural abundance) with the (13)C isotope at a specific carbon or carbons in a metabolic substrate does not affect the substrate's biochemistry. Hyperpolarized (13)C-labeled substrates can provide >10,000-fold enhancement of the (13)C MRS signals from the substrate and its subsequent metabolic products, allowing the assessment of changes in metabolic fluxes in vivo and the imaging of blood vessels and tissue perfusion without background signal from surrounding tissues (1,3,4,10–14). (13)C MRS with DNP technique has also been investigated for measuring tissue pH in vivo (4,15). HCO3(−) is the primary extracellular buffer, and it resists changes in pH through interconversion with CO2 in the reaction catalyzed by carbonic anhydrase. In principal, tissue pH can be determined from (13)C MRS measurements of endogenous H(13)CO3(−) and (13)CO2 because their concentration ratio can be used to calculate pH from the Henderson–Hasselbalch equation with an acid dissociation constant (pKa) of 6.17 in vivo. On the basis of this principal, Schroeder et al. measured the pH in diseased and healthy cardiac myocytes with simultaneous detection of hyperpolarized [1–(13)C]pyruvate-derived H(13)CO3(−) and (13)CO2 (15). Their results suggest that hyperpolarized [1–(13)C]pyruvate with MRS detection of its derived H(13)CO3(−) and (13)CO2 can be used to measure the intracellular pH (pHi) of cardiomyocytes in vivo. Similarly, Gallagher et al. generated a nontoxic, pH-probe, hyperpolarized H(13)CO3(−) and exploited the pH in tumors with measurement of the H(13)CO3(−) and (13)CO2 concentration ratio after administration of hyperpolarized H(13)CO3(−) (4). The tumor microenvironment is characterized by low extracellular pH (pHe) and neutral-to-alkaline pHi (16,17). The average pHe could be as low as 6.0. A pH gradient (pHi > pHe) exists across the cell membrane in tumors. This gradient is contrary to that found in normal tissues, in which pHi (7.2–7.4) is lower than pHe. In addition, diffusion of the H(+) ions along concentration gradients from tumors into adjacent normal tissues creates a peritumoral acid gradient. Accurate measurement of the pH in tissues is of diagnostic and therapeutic value. Imaging with small-molecule agents has been tested for measuring tumor pH. However, agents based on (1)H, (31)P, or (19)F MRS are limited by the inherent low sensitivity of spectroscopy and small pH-dependent chemical shift of these agents (18,19). The approach with gadolinium (Gd(3+)) chelate relaxation agents, which show a pH-dependent hydrogen exchange to the Gd(3+)-bound water, requires an accurate determination of the agent concentration, which in practice is difficult to achieve in vivo (20). Although positron emission tomography and optical imaging are sensitive, they appear have difficulty obtaining a pH map at high resolution (21–23). Furthermore, most of the published probes predominantly measure the pH within cells, which is more resistant to pH changes than the extracellular space. The data obtained by Gallagher et al. from hyperpolarized H(13)CO3(–) indicated that hyperpolarized H(13)CO3(–) provided a means to measure the pHe rather than the pHi (4). Given the range of pathological conditions in which the acid–base balance is altered, this technique may prove to be of diagnostic value not only in oncology but also in the imaging of ischemia and inflammation (4).

Shumyantseva, V. V. et al. (2015). "Electrochemical methods for biomedical investigations." *Biomed Khim* 61(2):188–202.

In the review, authors discussed recently published experimental data concerning highly sensitive electrochemical methods and technologies for biomedical investigations in the postgenomic era. Developments in electrochemical biosensors systems for the analysis of various bio objects are also considered: cytochrome P450s, cardiac markers, bacterial cells, the analysis of proteins based on electro oxidized amino acids as a tool for analysis of conformational events. The electroanalysis of catalytic activity of cytochromes P450 allowed developing system for screening of potential substrates, inhibitors or modulators of catalytic functions of this class of hemoproteins. The highly sensitive quartz crystal microbalance (QCM) immunosensor has been developed for analysis of bio affinity interactions of antibodies with troponin I in plasma. The QCM technique allowed real-time monitoring of the kinetic differences in specific interactions and nonspecific sorption, without multiple labeling procedures and separation steps. The affinity binding process was characterized by the association (ka) and the dissociation (kd) kinetic constants and the equilibrium association (K) constant, calculated using experimental data. Based on the electroactivity of bacterial cells, the electrochemical system for determination of sensitivity of the microbial cells to antibiotics cefepime, ampicillin, amikacin, and erythromycin was proposed. It was shown that the minimally detectable cell number corresponds to 106 CFU per electrode. The electrochemical method allows estimating the degree of *E. coli* JM109 cells resistance to antibiotics within 2–5°h. Electrosynthesis of polymeric analogs of antibodies for myoglobin (molecularly imprinted polymer, MIP) on the surface of graphite screen-printed electrodes as sensor elements with o-phenylenediamine as the functional monomer was developed. Molecularly imprinted polymers demonstrate selective complementary binding of a template protein molecule (myoglobin) by the "key-lock" principle.

Siligardi, G. et al. (2014). "Ligand- and drug-binding studies of membrane proteins revealed through circular dichroism spectroscopy." *Biochim Biophys Acta* 1838(1 Pt A):34–42.

A great number of membrane proteins have proven difficult to crystallize for use in X-ray crystallographic structural determination or too complex for NMR structural studies. Circular dichroism (CD) is a fast and relatively easy spectroscopic technique to study protein conformational behavior. In this review examples of the applications of CD and synchrotron radiation CD (SRCD) to membrane protein ligand binding interaction studies are discussed. The availability of SRCD has been an important advancement in recent progress, most particularly because it can be used to extend the spectral region in the far-UV region (important for increasing the accuracy of secondary structure estimations) and for working with membrane proteins available in only small quantities for which SRCD has facilitated molecular recognition studies. Such studies have been accomplished by probing in the near-UV region the local tertiary structure of aromatic amino acid residues upon addition of chiral or nonchiral ligands using long pathlength cells of small volume capacity. In particular, this review describes the most recent use of the technique in the following areas: to obtain quantitative data on ligand binding (exemplified by the FsrC membrane sensor kinase receptor); to distinguish between functionally similar drugs that exhibit different mechanisms of action towards membrane proteins (exemplified by secretory phospholipase A2); and to identify suitable detergent conditions to observe membrane protein–ligand interactions using stabilized proteins (exemplified by the antiseptic transporter SugE). Finally, the importance of characterizing in solution the conformational behavior and ligand binding properties of proteins in both far- and near-UV regions is discussed. This article is part of a Special Issue entitled: Structural and biophysical characterization of membrane protein–ligand binding.

Xiao, Z. and A. G. Wedd (2010). "The challenges of determining metal-protein affinities." *Nat Prod Rep* 27(5):768–789.

A key property of metalloproteins and -enzymes is the affinity of metal ion M for protein ligand P as defined by the dissociation constant $KD = [M][P]/[MP]$. Its accurate determination is essential for a quantitative understanding of metal selection and speciation. However, the surfaces of proteins are defined by the sidechains of amino acids and so abound in good metal ligands (e.g., imidazole of histidine, thiol of cysteine, carboxylate of aspartic and glutamic acids, etc.). Consequently, adventitious binding of metal ions to protein surfaces is common with KD values $>$ or $= 10(-6)$ M. On the other hand, transport proteins responsible for 'chaperoning' essential metals to their cellular destinations appear to bind the metal ions selectively ($KD < 10(-7)$ M), both for speciation and to minimize the toxic effects of 'free' metal ions. These ions are normally bound with still higher affinities at their ultimate destinations (the active sites of metalloproteins and -enzymes). This review surveys possible approaches to estimation of these dissociation constants and pinpoints the various problems associated with each approach.

Solubility

Allen, L. V., Jr. (2008). "Dosage form design and development." *Clin Ther* 30(11):2102–2111.

BACKGROUND: Drugs must be properly formulated for administration to patients, regardless of age. Pediatric patients provide some additional challenges to the formulator in terms of compliance and therapeutic efficacy. Due to the lack of sufficient drug products for the pediatric population, the pharmaceutical industry and compounding pharmacies must develop and provide appropriate medications designed for children. OBJECTIVE: The purpose of this article was to review the physical, chemical, and biological characteristics of drug substances and pharmaceutical ingredients to be used in preparing a drug product. In addition, stability, appearance, palatability, flavoring, sweetening, coloring, preservation, packaging, and storage are discussed. METHODS: Information for the current article was gathered from a literature review; from presentations at professional and technical meetings; and from lectures, books, and publications of the author, as well as from his professional experience. Professional society meetings and standards-setting bodies were also used as a resource. RESULTS: The proper design and formulation of a dosage form requires consideration of the physical, chemical, and biological characteristics of all of the drug substances and pharmaceutical ingredients (excipients) to be used in fabricating the product. The drug and pharmaceutical materials utilized must be compatible and produce a drug product that is stable, efficacious, palatable, easy to administer, and well tolerated. Preformulation factors include physical properties such as particle size, crystalline structure, melting point, solubility, partition coefficient, dissolution, membrane permeability, dissociation constants, and drug stability. CONCLUSIONS: Successful development of a formulation includes multiple considerations involving the drug, excipients, compliance, storage, packaging, and stability, as well as patient considerations of taste, appearance, and palatability.

Baghel, S. et al. (2016). "Polymeric amorphous solid dispersions: A review of amorphization, crystallization, stabilization, solid-state characterization, and aqueous solubilization of biopharmaceutical classification system class II Drugs." *J Pharm Sci* 105(9):2527–2544.

Poor water solubility of many drugs has emerged as one of the major challenges in the pharmaceutical world. Polymer-based amorphous solid dispersions have been considered as the major advancement in overcoming limited aqueous solubility and oral absorption issues. The principle drawback of this approach is that they can lack necessary stability and revert to the crystalline form on storage. Significant upfront development is, therefore, required to generate stable amorphous formulations. A thorough understanding of the processes occurring at a molecular level is imperative for the rational design of amorphous solid dispersion products. This review attempts to address the critical molecular and thermodynamic aspects governing the physicochemical properties of such systems. A brief introduction to Biopharmaceutical Classification System, solid dispersions, glass transition, and solubility advantage of amorphous drugs is provided. The objective of this review is to weigh the current understanding of solid dispersion chemistry and to critically review the theoretical, technical, and molecular aspects of solid dispersions (amorphization and crystallization) and potential advantage of polymers (stabilization and solubilization) as inert, hydrophilic, pharmaceutical carrier matrices. In addition, different preformulation tools for the rational selection of polymers, state-of-the-art techniques for preparation and characterization of polymeric amorphous solid dispersions, and drug supersaturation in gastric media are also discussed.

Bergstrom, C. A. et al. (2014). "Early pharmaceutical profiling to predict oral drug absorption: Current status and unmet needs." *Eur J Pharm Sci* 57:173–199.

Preformulation measurements are used to estimate the fraction absorbed in vivo for orally administered compounds and thereby allow an early evaluation of the need for enabling formulations. As part of the Oral Biopharmaceutical Tools (OrBiTo) project, this review provides a summary of the pharmaceutical profiling methods available, with focus on in silico and in vitro models typically used to forecast active pharmaceutical ingredient's (APIs) in vivo performance after oral administration. An overview of the composition of human, animal and simulated gastrointestinal (GI) fluids is provided and state-of-the art methodologies to study API properties impacting on oral absorption are reviewed. Assays performed during early development, i.e. physicochemical characterization, dissolution profiles under physiological conditions, permeability assays and the impact of excipients on these properties are discussed in detail and future demands on pharmaceutical profiling are identified. It is expected that innovative computational and experimental methods that better describe molecular processes involved in vivo during dissolution and absorption of APIs will be developed in the OrBiTo. These methods will provide early insights into successful pathways (medicinal chemistry or formulation strategy) and are anticipated to increase the number of new APIs with good oral absorption being discovered.

Gajdziok, J. and B. Vranikova (2015). "Enhancing of drug bioavailability using liquisolid system formulation." *Ceska Slov Farm* 64(3):55–66.

One of the modern technologies of how to ensure sufficient bioavailability of drugs with limited water solubility is represented by the preparation of liquisolid systems. The functional principle of these formulations is the sorption of a drug in a liquid phase to a porous carrier (aluminometasilicates, microcrystalline cellulose, etc.). After addition of further excipients, in particular a coating material (colloidal silica), a powder is formed with the properties suitable for conversion to conventional solid unit dosage forms for oral administration (tablets, capsules). The drug is subsequently administered to the GIT already in a dissolved state, and moreover, the high surface area of the excipients and their surface hydrophilization by the solvent used, facilitates its contact with and release to the dissolution medium and GI fluids. This technology, due to its ease of preparation, represents an interesting alternative to the currently used methods of bioavailability improvement. The article follows up, by describing the specific aspects influencing the preparation of liquid systems, on the already published papers about the bioavailability of drugs and the possibilities of its technological improvement. Key words: liquisolid systems bioavailability porous carrier coating material preformulation studies.

Hofmann, M. and H. Gieseler (2018). "Predictive screening tools used in high-concentration protein formulation development." *J Pharm Sci* 107(3):772–777.

This review examines the use of predictive screening approaches in high-concentration protein formulation development. In addition to the normal challenges associated with protein formulation development, for high-concentration formulations, solubility, viscosity, and physical protein degradation play major roles. To overcome these challenges, multiple formulation conditions need to be evaluated such that it is desirable to have predictive but also low-volume and high-throughput methods in order to identify optimal formulation conditions very early in development without time- and material-consuming setups. Many screening techniques have been reported for use in high-concentration formulation development, but not all fulfill the requirements mentioned previously. This review summarizes the advantages and disadvantages of different screening approaches currently used in formulation development and the correlation of predictive data to protein solubility, viscosity, and stability at high protein concentrations.

Kawakami, K. (2012). "Modification of physicochemical characteristics of active pharma-
    ceutical ingredients and application of supersaturatable dosage forms for improving
    bioavailability of poorly absorbed drugs." *Adv Drug Deliv Rev* 64(6):480–495.

New chemical entities are required to possess physicochemical characteristics that
result in acceptable oral absorption. However, many promising candidates need physicochemical modification or application of special formulation technology. This review
discusses strategies for overcoming physicochemical problems during the development
at the preformulation and formulation stages with emphasis on overcoming the most
typical problem, low solubility. Solubility of active pharmaceutical ingredients can be
improved by employing metastable states, salt forms, or cocrystals. Since the usefulness of salt forms is well recognized, it is the normal strategy to select the most suitable
salt form through extensive screening in the current developmental study. Promising
formulation technologies used to overcome the low solubility problem include liquid-
filled capsules, self-emulsifying formulations, solid dispersions, and nanosuspensions.
Current knowledge for each formulation is discussed from both theoretical and practical viewpoints, and their advantages and disadvantages are presented.

Kerns, E. H. et al. (2008). "In vitro solubility assays in drug discovery." *Curr Drug Metab*
    9(9):879–885.

The solubility of a compound depends on its structure and solution conditions. Structure
determines the lipophilicity, hydrogen bonding, molecular volume, crystal energy and
ionizability, which determine solubility. Solution conditions are affected by pH, cosolvents, additives, ionic strength, time and temperature. Many drug discovery experiments
are conducted under "kinetic" solubility conditions. In drug discovery, solubility has a
major impact on bioassays, formulation for in vivo dosing, and intestinal absorption.
A good goal for the solubility of drug discovery compounds is >60 µg/mL. Equilibrium
solubility assays can be conducted in moderate throughput, by incubating excess solid
with buffer and agitating for several days, prior to filtration and HPLC quantitation.
Kinetic solubility assays are performed in high throughput with shorter incubation
times and high throughput analyses using plate readers. The most frequently used of
these are the nephelometric assay and direct UV assay, which begin by adding a small
volume of DMSO stock solution of each test compound to buffer. In nephelometry,
this solution is serially diluted across a microtiter plate and undissolved particles are
detected via light scattering. In direct UV, undissolved particles are separated by filtration, after which the dissolved material is quantitated using UV absorption. Equilibrium
solubility is useful for preformulation. Kinetic solubility is useful for rapid compound
assessment, guiding optimization via structure modification, and diagnosing bioassays. It is often useful to customize solubility experiments using conditions that answer
specific research questions of drug discovery teams, such as compound selection and
vehicle development for pharmacology and PK studies.

Narayan, P. (2011). "Overview of drug product development." *Curr Protoc Pharmacol*
    Chapter 7: Unit 7(3): 1–29.

The process for developing drug delivery systems has evolved over the past two
decades with more scientific rigor, involving a collaboration of various fields, i.e.,
biology, chemistry, engineering, and pharmaceutics. Drug products, also commonly
known in the pharmaceutical industry as formulations or "dosage forms," are used for

administering the active pharmaceutical ingredient (API) for purposes of assessing safety in preclinical models, early- to late-phase human clinical trials, and for routine clinical/commercial use. This overview discusses approaches for creating small-molecule API dosage forms, from preformulation to commercial manufacturing.

Yalkowsky, S. H. and D. Alantary (2018). "Estimation of melting points of organics." *J Pharm Sci* 107(5):1211–1227.

Unified physicochemical property estimation relationship is a system of empirical and theoretical relationships that relate 20 physicochemical properties of organic molecules to each other and to chemical structure. Melting point is a key parameter in the unified physicochemical property estimation relationships scheme because it is a determinant of several other properties including vapor pressure, and solubility. This review describes the first-principals calculation of the melting points of organic compounds from structure. The calculation is based on the fact that the melting point, Tm, is equal to the ratio of the heat of melting, DeltaHm, to the entropy of melting, DeltaSm. The heat of melting is shown to be an additive constitutive property. However, the entropy of melting is not entirely group additive. It is primarily dependent on molecular geometry, including parameters which reflect the degree of restriction of molecular motion in the crystal to that of the liquid. Symmetry, eccentricity, chirality, flexibility, and hydrogen bonding, each affect molecular freedom in different ways and thus make different contributions to the total entropy of fusion. The relationships of these entropy determining parameters to chemical structure are used to develop a reasonably accurate means of predicting the melting points over 2000 compounds.

Partitioning

Al-Badr, A. A. and G. A. Mostafa (2014). "Pravastatin sodium." *Profiles Drug Subst Excip Relat Methodol* 39:433–513.

Pravastatin sodium is an [HMG-CoA] reductase inhibitor and is a lipid-regulating drug. This monograph includes the description of the drug: nomenclature, formulae, elemental composition, solubility, appearance, and partition coefficient. The uses and the methods that have been reported for the synthesis of this drug are described. The physical methods that were used to characterize the drug are the X-ray powder diffraction pattern, thermal methods, melting point, and differential scanning calorimetry. This chapter also contains the following spectra of the drug: the UV spectrum, the vibrational spectrum, the nuclear magnetic resonance spectra, and the mass spectrum. The compendial methods of analysis include the British Pharmacopoeia and the United States Pharmacopoeia methods. Other methods of analysis that are included in this profile are spectrophotometric, electrochemical, polarographic, voltammetric and chromatographic, and immunoassay methods. The chapter also contains the pharmacokinetics, metabolism, stability, and articles that reviewed pravastatin sodium manufacturing, characterization, and analysis. One hundred and sixty-two references are listed at the end of this comprehensive profile.

Andres, A. et al. (2015). "Setup and validation of shake-flask procedures for the determination of partition coefficients (logD) from low drug amounts." *Eur J Pharm Sci* 76:181–191.

Several procedures based on the shake-flask method and designed to require a minimum amount of drug for octanol–water partition coefficient determination have been established and developed. The procedures have been validated by a 28-substance set with a lipophilicity range from −2.0 to 4.5 (logD 7.4). The experimental partition is carried out using aqueous phases buffered with phosphate (pH 7.4) and n-octanol saturated with buffered water and the analysis is performed by liquid chromatography. In order to have accurate results, four procedures and eight different ratios between phase volumes are proposed. Each procedure has been designed and optimized (for partition ratios) for a specific range of drug lipophilicity (low, regular and high lipophilicity) and solubility (high and low aqueous solubility). The procedures have been developed to minimize the measurement in the octanolic phase. Experimental logD 7.4 values obtained from different procedures and partition ratios show a standard deviation lower than 0.3 and there is a nice agreement when these values are compared with the reference literature ones.

Bittermann, K. et al. (2016). "Comparison of different models predicting the phospholipid-membrane water partition coefficients of charged compounds." *Chemosphere* 144:382–391.

A large fraction of commercially used chemicals is ionizable. This results in the need for mechanistic models to describe the physicochemical properties of ions, like the membrane–water partition coefficient (K(mw)), which is related to toxicity and bio-accumulation. In this work we compare 3 different and already existing modeling approaches to describe the liposome–water partition coefficient (K(lipw)) of organic ions, including 36 cations, 56 anions, 2 divalent cations and 2 zwitterions (plus 207 neutral compounds for ensuring model consistency). 1) The empirical correlation with the octanol–water partition coefficient of the corresponding neutral species yielded better results for the prediction of anions (RMSE = 0.79) than for cations (RMSE = 1.14). Though describing most anions reasonably well, the lack of mechanistic basis and the poor performance for cations constrain the usage of this model. 2) The polyparameter linear free energy relationship (pp-LFER) model performs worse (RMSE = 1.26/1.12 for anions/cations). The different physicochemical environments, due to different sorption depths into the membrane of the different species, cannot be described with a single pp-LFER model. 3) COSMOmic is based on quantum chemistry and fluid phase thermodynamics and has the widest applicability domain. It was the only model applicable for multiply charged ions and gave the best results for anions (RMSE = 0.66) and cations (RMSE = 0.71). We expect COSMOmic to contribute to a better estimation of the environmental risk of ionizable emerging pollutants.

Brown, T. N. et al. (2016). "Dermal permeation data and models for the prioritization and screening-level exposure assessment of organic chemicals." *Environ Int* 94:424–435.

High-throughput screening (HTS) models are being developed and applied to prioritize chemicals for more comprehensive exposure and risk assessment. Dermal pathways are possible exposure routes to humans for thousands of chemicals found in personal care products and the indoor environment. HTS exposure models rely on skin permeability coefficient (KP; cm/h) models for exposure predictions. An initial database of approximately 1000 entries for empirically based KP data was compiled from the literature and a subset of 480 data points for 245 organic chemicals derived from testing with human skin only and using only water as a vehicle was selected. The selected dataset includes chemicals with log octanol–water partition coefficients (KOW) ranging from −6.8 to 7.6 (median=1.8; 95% of the data range from −2.5 to 4.6) and molecular weight (MW) ranging from 18 to 765 g/mol (median=180); only 3% >500 g/mol. Approximately 53% of the chemicals in the database have functional groups which are ionizable in the pH range of 6 to 7.4, with 31% being appreciably ionized. The compiled log KP values ranged from −5.8 to 0.1 cm/h (median= −2.6). The selected subset of the KP data was then used to evaluate eight representative KP models that can be readily applied for HTS assessments, i.e., parameterized with KOW and MW. The analysis indicates that a version of the SKINPERM model performs the best against the selected dataset. Comparisons of representative KP models against model input parameter property ranges (sensitivity analysis) and against chemical datasets requiring human health assessment were conducted to identify regions of chemical properties that should be tested to address uncertainty in KP models and HTS exposure assessments.

Caron, G. et al. (2018). "Log *P* as a tool in intramolecular hydrogen bond considerations." *Drug Discov Today Technol* 27:65–70.

Intramolecular hydrogen bonding (IMHB) considerations are gaining relevance in drug discovery and a molecular descriptor which can predict very early the capacity of a compound to form IMHB is needed to speed up the optimization process of drug candidates. Although log *P*oct is largely used for optimization purposes, in this paper we firstly use the Block Relevance (BR) analysis to theoretically show how log *P*oct is not a convenient choice to assess IMHB properties of candidates. Then, we discuss the limits of log *P*oct and introduce Deltalog *P*oct-tol, i.e., the difference between log *P*oct and log *P*tol (the logarithm of the partition coefficient in the toluene/water system). Finally, we provided some examples also, including bRo5 protease inhibitors, to clarify how to interpret Deltalog *P*oct-tol values.

Cordero, C. et al. (2015). "Comprehensive two-dimensional gas chromatography and food sensory properties: Potential and challenges." *Anal Bioanal Chem* 407(1):169–191.

Modern omics disciplines dealing with food flavor focus the analytical efforts on the elucidation of sensory-active compounds, including all possible stimuli of multimodal perception (aroma, taste, texture, etc.) by means of a comprehensive, integrated treatment of sample constituents, such as physicochemical properties, concentration in the matrix, and sensory properties (odor/taste quality, perception threshold). Such analyses require detailed profiling of known bioactive components as well as advanced fingerprinting techniques to catalog sample constituents comprehensively, quantitatively, and comparably across samples. Multidimensional analytical platforms support comprehensive investigations required for flavor analysis by combining information on analytes' identities, physicochemical behaviors (volatility, polarity, partition coefficient, and solubility), concentration, and odor quality. Unlike other omics, flavor metabolomics and sensomics include the final output of the biological phenomenon (i.e., sensory perceptions) as an additional analytical dimension, which is specifically and exclusively triggered by the chemicals analyzed. However, advanced omics platforms, which are multidimensional by definition, pose challenging issues not only in terms of coupling with detection systems and sample preparation, but also in terms of data elaboration and processing. The large number of variables collected during each analytical run provides a high level of information but requires appropriate strategies to exploit fully this potential. This review focuses on advances in comprehensive two-dimensional gas chromatography and analytical platforms combining two-dimensional gas chromatography with olfactometry, chemometrics, and quantitative assays for food sensory analysis to assess the quality of a given product. We review instrumental advances and couplings, automation in sample preparation, data elaboration, and a selection of applications.

Dahan, A. et al. (2016). "The solubility-permeability interplay and oral drug formulation design: Two heads are better than one." *Adv Drug Deliv Rev* 101:99–107.

Poor aqueous solubility is a major challenge in today's biopharmaceutics. While solubility-enabling formulations can significantly increase the apparent solubility of the drug, the concomitant effect on the drug's apparent permeability has been largely overlooked. The mathematical equation to describe the membrane permeability of a drug comprises the membrane/aqueous partition coefficient, which in turn is dependent on the drug's apparent solubility in the GI milieu, suggesting that the solubility and the permeability are closely related, exhibit a certain interplay between them, and treating the one irrespectively of the other may be insufficient. In this article, an overview of this solubility–permeability interplay is provided, and the available data is analyzed in the context of the effort to maximize the overall drug exposure. Overall, depending on the type of solubility–permeability interplay, the permeability may decrease, remain unchanged, and even increase, in a way that may critically affect the formulation capability to improve the overall absorption. Therefore, an intelligent design of solubility-enabling formulation needs to consider both the solubility afforded by the formulation and the permeability in the new luminal environment resulting from the formulation.

Dapson, R. W. (2013). "Alternative methods for estimating common descriptors for QSAR studies of dyes and fluorescent probes using molecular modeling software: 1. Concepts and procedures." *Biotech Histochem* 88(8):477–488.

Quantitative structure–activity relation (QSAR) models were developed to predict uptake and intracellular localization of probes or dyes in living cells. Many of the QSAR parameters used in such models are determined manually. Unfortunately, this requires a depth of chemical knowledge that biologists who wish to use these predictive tools do not necessarily possess. Moreover, some of the parameters are not easily obtained for all dyes and probes, which further restricts widespread use of QSAR methodology. Alternatives to some of these QSAR descriptors are defined and explained here. Estimation of these novel parameters using molecular modeling software, widely available and readily usable on personal computers in a variety of forms and brands, is described here. QSAR researchers need only draw the molecular structure and, with the proper commands, obtain either the parameters directly or the information to calculate them. I also demonstrate how the same software can generate some of the standard QSAR parameters, e.g., MW, Z, CBN, more reliably and conveniently than the manual procedures. A particularly problematic descriptor is log P, the logarithm of the octanol/water partition coefficient of a probe. This is discussed in detail and a novel alternative measure, the hydrophilic/lipophilic index (HLI), is introduced together with preliminary validation.

DiDomenico, C. D. and L. J. Bonassar (2018). "How can 50 years of solute transport data in articular cartilage inform the design of arthritis therapeutics?" *Osteoarthritis Cartilage*.

OBJECTIVE: For the last half century, transport of nutrients and therapeutics in articular cartilage has been studied with various in vitro systems that attempt to model in vivo conditions. However, experimental technique, tissue species, and tissue storage condition (fresh/frozen) vary widely and there is debate on the most appropriate model system. Additionally, there is still no clear overarching framework with which to predict solute transport properties based on molecular characteristics. This review aims to develop such a framework, and to assess whether experimental procedure affects trends in transport data. METHODS: Solute data from 31 published papers that investigated transport in healthy articular cartilage were obtained and analyzed for trends. RESULTS: Here, we show that diffusivity of spherical and globular solutes in cartilage can be predicted by molecular weight (MW) and hydrodynamic radius via a power–law relationship. This relationship is robust for many solutes, spanning 5 orders of magnitude in MW and was not affected by variations in cartilage species, age, condition (fresh/frozen), and experimental technique. Traditional models of transport in porous media exhibited mixed effectiveness at predicting diffusivity in cartilage but were good in predicting solute partition coefficient. CONCLUSION: Ultimately, these robust relationships can be used to accurately predict and improve transport of solutes in adult human cartilage and enable the development of better optimized arthritis therapeutics.

DiDomenico, C. D. et al. (2018). "Molecular transport in articular cartilage—what have we learned from the past 50 years?" *Nat Rev Rheumatol* 14(7):393–403.

Developing therapeutic molecules that target chondrocytes and locally produced inflammatory factors within arthritic cartilage is an active area of investigation. The extensive studies that have been conducted over the past 50 years have enabled the accurate prediction and reliable optimization of the transport of a wide variety of molecules into cartilage. In this Review, the factors that can be used to tune the transport kinetics of therapeutics are summarized. Overall, the most crucial factor when designing new therapeutic molecules is solute size. The diffusivity and partition coefficient of a solute both decrease with increasing solute size as indicated by molecular mass or by hydrodynamic radius. Surprisingly, despite having an effective pore size of ~6 nm, molecules of ~16 nm radius can diffuse through the cartilage matrix. Alteration of the shape or charge of a solute and the application of physiological loading to cartilage can be used to predictably improve solute transport kinetics, and this knowledge can be used to improve the development of therapeutic agents for osteoarthritis that target the cartilage.

Enache, M. et al. (2016). "Mitoxantrone-surfactant interactions: A physicochemical overview." *Molecules* 21(10):1356.

Mitoxantrone is a synthetic anticancer drug used clinically in the treatment of different types of cancer. It was developed as a doxorubicin analogue in a program to find drugs with improved antitumor activity and decreased cardiotoxicity compared with the anthracyclines. As the cell membrane is the first barrier encountered by anticancer drugs before reaching the DNA sites inside the cells and as surfactant micelles are known as simple model systems for biological membranes, the drugs–surfactant interaction has been the subject of great research interest. Further, quantitative understanding of the interactions of drugs with biomimicking structures like surfactant micelles may provide helpful information for the control of physicochemical properties and bioactivities of encapsulated drugs in order to design better delivery systems with possible biomedical applications. The present review describes the physicochemical aspects of the interactions between the anticancer drug mitoxantrone and different surfactants. Mitoxantrone-micelle binding constants, partitions coefficient of the drug between aqueous and micellar phases and the corresponding Gibbs free energy for the above processes, and the probable location of drug molecules in the micelles are discussed.

Gala, U. and H. Chauhan (2015). "Principles and applications of Raman spectroscopy in pharmaceutical drug discovery and development." *Expert Opin Drug Discov* 10(2):187–206.

INTRODUCTION: In recent years, Raman spectroscopy has become increasingly important as an analytical technique in various scientific areas of research and development. This is partly due to the technological advancements in Raman instrumentation and partly due to detailed fingerprinting that can be derived from Raman spectra. Its versatility of applications, rapidness of collection and easy analysis have made Raman spectroscopy an attractive analytical tool. AREAS COVERED: The following review describes Raman spectroscopy and its application within the pharmaceutical industry. The authors explain the theory of Raman scattering and its variations in Raman spectroscopy. The authors also highlight how Raman spectra are interpreted, providing examples. EXPERT OPINION: Raman spectroscopy has a number of potential applications within drug discovery and development. It can be used to estimate the molecular activity of drugs and to establish a drug's physicochemical properties such as its partition coefficient. It can also be used in compatibility studies during the drug formulation process. Raman spectroscopy's immense potential should be further investigated in future.

Gurram, A. K. et al. (2015). "Role of components in the formation of self-microemulsifying drug delivery systems." *Indian J Pharm Sci* 77(3):249–257.

Pharmaceutical research is focused in designing novel drug delivery systems to improve the bioavailability of poorly water-soluble drugs. Self-microemulsifying drug delivery systems, one among the lipid-based dosage forms were proven to be promising in improving the oral bioavailability of such drugs by enhancing solubility, permeability and avoiding first-pass metabolism via enhanced lymphatic transport. Further, they have been successful in avoiding both inter and intra individual variations as well as the dose disproportionality. Aqueous insoluble drugs, in general, show greater solubility in lipid-based excipients, and hence they are formulated as lipid-based drug delivery systems. The extent of solubility of a hydrophobic drug in lipid excipients, i.e., oil, surfactant and cosurfactant (components of self-microemulsifying drug delivery systems) greatly affects the drug loading and in producing stable self-microemulsifying drug delivery systems. The present review highlighted the influence of physicochemical factors and structural features of the hydrophobic drug on its solubility in lipid excipients and an attempt was made to explore the role of each component of self-microemulsifying drug delivery systems in the formation of stable microemulsion upon dilution.

Heger, M. et al. (2014). "The molecular basis for the pharmacokinetics and pharmacodynamics of curcumin and its metabolites in relation to cancer." *Pharmacol Rev* 66(1):222–307.

This review addresses the oncopharmacological properties of curcumin at the molecular level. First, the interactions between curcumin and its molecular targets are addressed on the basis of curcumin's distinct chemical properties, which include H-bond donating and accepting capacity of the beta-dicarbonyl moiety and the phenylic hydroxyl groups, H-bond accepting capacity of the methoxy ethers, multivalent metal and nonmetal cation binding properties, high partition coefficient, rotamerization around multiple C–C bonds, and the ability to act as a Michael acceptor. Next, the in vitro chemical stability of curcumin is elaborated in the context of its susceptibility to photochemical and chemical modification and degradation (e.g., alkaline hydrolysis). Specific modification and degradatory pathways are provided, which mainly entail radical-based intermediates, and the in vitro catabolites are identified. The implications of curcumin's (photo)chemical instability are addressed in light of pharmaceutical curcumin preparations, the use of curcumin analogues, and implementation of nanoparticulate drug delivery systems. Furthermore, the pharmacokinetics of curcumin and its most important degradation products are detailed in light of curcumin's poor bioavailability. Particular emphasis is placed on xenobiotic phase I and II metabolism as well as excretion of curcumin in the intestines (first pass), the liver (second pass), and other organs in addition to the pharmacokinetics of curcumin metabolites and their systemic clearance. Lastly, a summary is provided of the clinical pharmacodynamics of curcumin followed by a detailed account of curcumin's direct molecular targets, whereby the phenotypical/biological changes induced in cancer cells upon completion of the curcumin-triggered signaling cascade(s) are addressed in the framework of the hallmarks of cancer. The direct molecular targets include the ErbB family of receptors, protein kinase C, enzymes involved in prostaglandin synthesis, vitamin D receptor, and DNA.

Heilig, A. et al. (2016). "Determination of aroma compound partition coefficients in aqueous, polysaccharide, and dairy matrices using the phase ratio variation method: A review and modeling approach." *J Agric Food Chem* 64(22):4450–4470.

The partition of aroma compounds between a matrix and a gas phase describes an individual compound's specific affinity toward the matrix constituents affecting orthonasal sensory perception. The static headspace phase ratio variation (PRV) method has been increasingly applied by various authors to determine the equilibrium partition coefficient K in aqueous, polysaccharide, and dairy matrices. However, reported partition coefficients are difficult to relate and compare due to different experimental conditions, e.g., aroma compound selection, matrix composition, equilibration temperature. Due to its specific advantages, the PRV method is supposed to find more frequent application in the future, this Review aims to summarize, evaluate, compare, and relate the currently available data on PRV-determined partition coefficients. This process was designed to specify the potentials and the limitations as well as the consistency of the PRV method, and to identify open fields of research in aroma compound partitioning in food-related, especially dairy matrices.

Hendrickx, J. et al. (2016). "Inhaled anaesthetics and nitrous oxide: Complexities overlooked: Things may not be what they seem." *Eur J Anaesthesiol* 33(9):611–619.

This review re-examines existing pharmacokinetic and pharmacodynamic concepts of inhaled anesthetics. After showing where uptake is hidden in the classic FA/FI curve, it is argued that target-controlled delivery of inhaled agents warrants a different interpretation of the factors affecting this curve (cardiac output, ventilation and blood/gas partition coefficient). Blood/gas partition coefficients of modern agents may be less important clinically than generally assumed. The partial pressure cascade from delivered to inspired to end-expired is re-examined to better understand the effect of rebreathing during low-flow anesthesia, including the possibility of developing a hypoxic inspired mixture despite existing machine standards. Inhaled agents are easy to administer because they are transferred according to partial pressure gradients. In addition, the narrow dose–response curves for the three end points of general anesthesia (loss of response to verbal command, immobility and autonomic reflex control) allow the clinical use of MACawake, MAC and MACBAR to determine depth of anesthesia. Opioids differentially affect these clinical effects of inhaled agents. The effect of ventilation–perfusion relationships on gas uptake is discussed, and it is shown how moving beyond Riley's useful but simplistic model allows us to better understand both the concept and the magnitude of the second gas effect of nitrous oxide. It is argued that nitrous oxide remains a clinically useful drug. We hope to bring old (but ignored) and new (but potentially overlooked) information into the educational and clinical arenas to stimulate discussion among clinicians and researchers. We should not let technology pass by our all too engrained older concepts.

Hussein, Y. H. A. and M. Youssry (2018). "Polymeric micelles of biodegradable diblock copolymers: Enhanced encapsulation of hydrophobic drugs." *Materials* (Basel) 11(5):668.

Polymeric micelles are potentially efficient in encapsulating and performing the controlled release of various hydrophobic drug molecules. Understanding the fundamental physicochemical properties behind drug(-)polymer systems in terms of interaction strength and compatibility, drug partition coefficient (preferential solubilization), micelle size, morphology, etc., encourages the formulation of polymeric nanocarriers with enhanced drug encapsulating capacity, prolonged circulation time, and stability in the human body. In this review, we systematically address some open issues which are considered to be obstacles inhibiting the commercial availability of polymer-based therapeutics, such as the enhancement of encapsulation capacity by finding better drug(-)polymer compatibility, the drug-release kinetics and mechanisms under chemical and mechanical conditions simulating to physiological conditions, and the role of preparation methods and solvents on the overall performance of micelles.

Ita, K. B. (2016). "Prodrugs for transdermal drug delivery—trends and challenges." *J Drug Target* 24(8):671–678.

Prodrugs continue to attract significant interest in the transdermal drug delivery field. These moieties can confer favorable physicochemical properties on transdermal drug delivery candidates. Alkyl chain lengthening, pegylation are some of the strategies used for prodrug synthesis. It is usually important to optimize partition coefficient, water and oil solubilities of drugs. In this review, progress made in the field of prodrugs for percutaneous penetration is highlighted and the challenges discussed.

Kadam, A. A. et al. (2015). "Techniques to measure sorption and migration between small molecules and packaging. A critical review." *J Sci Food Agric* 95(7):1395–1407.

The mass transfer parameters diffusion and sorption in food and packaging or between them are the key parameters for assessing a food product's shelf-life in reference to consumer safety. This has become of paramount importance owing to the legislations set by the regulated markets. The technical capabilities that can be exploited for analyzing product–package interactions have been growing rapidly. Different techniques categorized according to the state of the diffusant (gas or liquid) in contact with the packaging material are emphasized in this review. Depending on the diffusant and on the analytical question under review, the different ways to study sorption and/or migration are presented and compared. Some examples have been suggested to reach the best possible choice, consisting of a single technique or a combination of different approaches.

Keyte, I. J. et al. (2013). "Chemical reactivity and long-range transport potential of polycyclic aromatic hydrocarbons—a review." *Chem Soc Rev* 42(24):9333–9391.

Polycyclic aromatic hydrocarbons (PAHs) are of considerable concern due to their well-recognized toxicity and especially due to the carcinogenic hazard which they present. PAHs are semi-volatile and therefore partition between vapor and condensed phases in the atmosphere and both the vapor and particulate forms undergo chemical reactions. This article briefly reviews the current understanding of vapor-particle partitioning of PAHs and the PAH deposition processes, and in greater detail, their chemical reactions. PAHs are reactive towards a number of atmospheric oxidants, most notably the hydroxyl radical, ozone, the nitrate radical (NO_3) and nitrogen dioxide. Rate coefficient data are reviewed for reactions of lower-molecular-weight PAH vapor with these species as well as for heterogeneous reactions of higher-molecular-weight compounds. Whereas the data for reactions of the 2–3-ring PAH vapor are quite extensive and generally consistent, such data are mostly lacking for the 4-ring PAHs and the heterogeneous rate data (5 and more rings), which are dependent on the substrate type and reaction conditions, are less comprehensive. The atmospheric reactions of PAH lead to the formation of oxy and nitro derivatives, reviewed here, too. Finally, the capacity of PAHs for long range transport and the results of numerical model studies are described. Research needs are identified.

Khan, N. R. et al. (2015). "Nanocarriers and their actions to improve skin permeability and transdermal drug delivery." *Curr Pharm Des* 21(20):2848–2866.

Transdermal drug delivery is impeded by the natural barrier of epidermis namely stratum corneum. This limits the route to transport of drugs with a log octanol–water partition coefficient of 1–3, molecular weight of less than 500 Da and melting point of less than 200°C. Nanotechnology has received widespread investigation as nanocarriers are deemed to be able to fluidize the stratum corneum as a function of size, shape, surface charges, and hydrophilicity–hydrophobicity balance, while delivering drugs across the skin barrier. This review provides an overview and update on the latest designs of liposomes, ethosomes, transfersomes, niosomes, magnetosomes, oilin–water nanoemulsions, water-in-oil nanoemulsions, bicontinuous nanoemulsions, covalently crosslinked polysaccharide nanoparticles, ionically crosslinked polysaccharide nanoparticles, polyelectrolyte coacervated nanoparticles, and hydrophobically modified polysaccharide nanoparticles with respect to their ability to fuse or fluidize lipid/protein/tight junction regimes of skin, and effect changes in skin permeability and drug flux. Universal relationships of nanocarrier size, zeta potential and chemical composition on transdermal permeation characteristics of drugs will be developed and discussed.

Kiang, T. K. et al. (2014). "A comprehensive review on the pharmacokinetics of antibiotics in interstitial fluid spaces in humans: Implications on dosing and clinical pharmacokinetic monitoring." *Clin Pharmacokinet* 53(8):695–730.

The objective of the current review was to provide an updated and comprehensive summary on pharmacokinetic data describing the distribution of antimicrobials into interstitial fluid (ISF) by comparing drug concentration versus time profiles between ISF and blood/plasma in healthy individuals and/or diseased populations. An extensive literature search identified 55 studies detailing 87 individual comparisons. For each antibiotic (antibacterial) (or antibiotic class), we comment on dosing implications based on tissue ISF distribution characteristics and determine the suitability of conducting clinical pharmacokinetic monitoring (CPM) using a previously published scoring algorithm. Using piperacillin as an example, there is evidence supporting different degrees of drug penetration into the ISF of different tissues. A higher dose of piperacillin may be required to achieve an adequate ISF concentration in soft tissue infections. To achieve these higher doses, alternative administration regimens such as intravenous infusions may be utilized. Data also suggest that piperacillin can be categorized as a 'likely suitable' agent for CPM in ISF. Regression analyses of data from the published studies, including protein binding, molecular weight, and predicted partition coefficient (using Xlog $P3$) as dependent variables, indicated that protein binding was the only significant predictor for the extent of drug distribution as determined by ratios of the area under the concentration–time curve between muscle ISF/total plasma (R (2) = 0.65, $p < 0.001$) and adipose ISF/total plasma (R (2) = 0.48, $p < 0.004$). Although recurrent limitations (i.e., small sample size, lack of statistical comparisons, lack of steady-state conditions, high individual variability) were identified in many studies, these data are still valuable and allowed us to generate general dosing guidelines and assess the suitability of using ISF for CPM.

Kiem, S. and J. J. Schentag (2014). "Interpretation of epithelial lining fluid concentrations of antibiotics against methicillin resistant staphylococcus aureus." *Infect Chemother* 46(4):219–225.

Although antibiotics whose epithelial lining fluid (ELF) concentrations are reported high tend to be preferred in treatment of pneumonia, measurement of ELF concentrations of antibiotics could be misled by contamination from lysis of ELF cells and technical errors of bronchoalveolar lavage (BAL). In this review, ELF concentrations of antimethicillin-resistant *Staphylococcus aureus* (MRSA) antibiotics were interpreted considering above confounding factors. An equation used to explain antibiotic diffusion into CSF (cerebrospinal fluid) was adopted: ELF/free serum concentration ratio = $0.96 + 0.091 \times$ ln (partition coefficient/molecular weight (1/2)). Seven anti-MRSA antibiotics with reported ELF concentrations were fitted to this equation to see if their ELF concentrations were explainable by the penetration capacity only. Then, outliers were modeled under the assumption of varying contamination from lysed ELF cells (test range 0%–10% of ELF volume). ELF concentrations of oritavancin, telavancin, tigecycline, and vancomycin were well described by the diffusion equation, with or without additional impact from cell lysis. For modestly high ELF/free serum concentration ratio of linezolid, technical errors of BAL should be excluded. Although teicoplanin and iclaprim showed high ELF/free serum ratios also, their protein binding levels need to be cleared for proper interpretation. At the moment, it appears very premature to use ELF concentrations of anti-MRSA antibiotics as a relevant guide for treatment of lung infections by MRSA.

Kollipara, S. and R. K. Gandhi (2014). "Pharmacokinetic aspects and in vitro–in vivo correlation potential for lipid-based formulations." *Acta Pharm Sin B* 4(5):333–349.

Lipid-based formulations have been an attractive choice among novel drug delivery systems for enhancing the solubility and bioavailability of poorly soluble drugs due to their ability to keep the drug in solubilized state in the gastrointestinal tract. These formulations offer multiple advantages such as reduction in food effect and interindividual variability, ease of preparation, and the possibility of manufacturing using common excipients available in the market. Despite these advantages, very few products are available in the present market, perhaps due to limited knowledge in the in vitro tests (for prediction of in vivo fate) and lack of understanding of the mechanisms behind pharmacokinetic and biopharmaceutical aspects of lipid formulations after oral administration. The current review aims to provide a detailed understanding of the in vivo processing steps involved after oral administration of lipid formulations, their pharmacokinetic aspects and in vitro in vivo correlation (IVIVC) perspectives. Various pharmacokinetic and biopharmaceutical aspects such as formulation dispersion and lipid digestion, bioavailability enhancement mechanisms, impact of excipients on efflux transporters, and lymphatic transport are discussed with examples. In addition, various IVIVC approaches towards predicting in vivo data from in vitro dispersion/precipitation, in vitro lipolysis and ex vivo permeation studies are also discussed in detail with help of case studies.

Lydy, M. J. et al. (2014). "Passive sampling methods for contaminated sediments: State of the science for organic contaminants." *Integr Environ Assess Manag* 10(2):167–178.

This manuscript surveys the literature on passive sampler methods (PSMs) used in contaminated sediments to assess the chemical activity of organic contaminants. The chemical activity in turn dictates the reactivity and bioavailability of contaminants in sediment. Approaches to measure specific binding of compounds to sediment components, for example, amorphous carbon or specific types of reduced carbon, and the associated partition coefficients are difficult to determine, particularly for native sediment. Thus, the development of PSMs that represent the chemical activity of complex compound–sediment interactions, expressed as the freely dissolved contaminant concentration in porewater (Cfree), offer a better proxy for endpoints of concern, such as reactivity, bioaccumulation, and toxicity. Passive sampling methods have estimated Cfree using both kinetic and equilibrium operating modes and used various polymers as the sorbing phase, for example, polydimethylsiloxane, polyethylene, and polyoxymethylene in various configurations, such as sheets, coated fibers, or vials containing thin films. These PSMs have been applied in laboratory exposures and field deployments covering a variety of spatial and temporal scales. A wide range of calibration conditions exist in the literature to estimate Cfree, but consensus values have not been established. The most critical criteria are the partition coefficient between water and the polymer phase and the equilibrium status of the sampler. In addition, the PSM must not appreciably deplete Cfree in the porewater. Some of the future challenges include establishing a standard approach for PSM measurements, correcting for nonequilibrium conditions, establishing guidance for selection and implementation of PSMs, and translating and applying data collected by PSMs.

Mackay, D. et al. (2014). "QSARs for aquatic toxicity: Celebrating, extending and display-
	ing the pioneering contributions of Ferguson, Konemann and Veith." *SAR QSAR
	Environ Res* 25(5):343–355.

Significant advances were made in the development of QSARs relating molecular structure to aquatic toxicity by three studies over 30 years ago by Ferguson in 1939, Konemann
in 1981, and Veith and colleagues in 1983. We revisit the original concepts and data from
these studies and review these contributions from the bases of current perspectives on the
hypothesized mechanism of baseline narcotic toxicity and the underlying thermodynamic
and kinetic aspects. The relationships between LC50, octanol–water partition coefficient,
aqueous solubility, chemical activity and chemical volume fraction in lipid phases are
outlined including kinetic influences on measured toxicities. These relationships provide
a compelling and plausible explanation of the success of these and other QSARs for
aquatic toxicity. Suggestions are made for further advances in these QSARs to improve
assessments of toxicity by baseline narcotic toxicity and selective modes of action, especially using emerging quantum chemical computational capabilities.

Manaargadoo-Catin, M. et al. (2016). "Hemolysis by surfactants—A review." *Adv Colloid
	Interface Sci* 228:1–16.

An overview of the use of surfactants for erythrocyte lysis and their cell membrane
action mechanisms is given. Erythrocyte membrane characteristics and its association with the cell cytoskeleton are presented in order to complete understanding of the
erythrocyte membrane distortion. Cell homeostasis disturbances caused by surfactants might induce changes starting from shape modification to cell lysis. Two main
mechanisms are hypothesized in literature which are osmotic lysis and lysis by solubilization even if the boundary between them is not clearly defined. Another specific
mechanism based on the formation of membrane pores is suggested in the particular
case of saponins. The lytic potency of a surfactant is related to its affinity for the
membrane and the modification of the lipid membrane curvature. This is to be related
to the surfactant shape defined by its hydrophobic and hydrophilic moieties but also
by experimental conditions. As a consequence, prediction of the hemolytic potency of
a given surfactant is challenging. Several studies are focused on the relation between
surfactant erythrolytic potency and their physicochemical parameters such as the critical micellar concentration (CMC), the hydrophile–lipophile balance (HLB), the surfactant membrane/water partition coefficient (K) or the packing parameter (P). The
CMC is one of the most important factors considered even if a lytic activity cut-off
effect points out that the only consideration of CMC not enough predictive. The relation K.CMC must be considered in addition to the CMC to predict the surfactant lytic
capacity within the same family of nonionic surfactant. Those surfactant structure/
lytic activity studies demonstrate the requirement to take into account a combination
of physicochemical parameters to understand and foresee surfactant lytic potency.

Mansour, F. R. and N. D. Danielson (2017). "Solidification of floating organic droplet
	in dispersive liquid–liquid microextraction as a green analytical tool." *Talanta*
	170:22–35.

Dispersive liquid–liquid microextraction (DLLME) is a special type of microextraction in which a mixture of two solvents (an extracting solvent and a disperser) is
injected into the sample. The extraction solvent is then dispersed as fine droplets
in the cloudy sample through manual or mechanical agitation. Hence, the sample

is centrifuged to break the formed emulsion and the extracting solvent is manually separated. The organic solvents commonly used in DLLME are halogenated hydrocarbons that are highly toxic. These solvents are heavier than water, so they sink to the bottom of the centrifugation tube which makes the separation step difficult. By using solvents of low density, the organic extractant floats on the sample surface. If the selected solvent such as undecanol has a freezing point in the range 10–25°C, the floating droplet can be solidified using a simple ice-bath, and then transferred out of the sample matrix; this step is known as solidification of floating organic droplet (SFOD). Coupling DLLME to SFOD combines the advantages of both approaches together. The DLLME-SFOD process is controlled by the same variables of conventional liquid–liquid extraction. The organic solvents used as extractants in DLLME-SFOD must be immiscible with water, of lower density, low volatility, high partition coefficient and low melting and freezing points. The extraction efficiency of DLLME-SFOD is affected by types and volumes of organic extractant and disperser, salt addition, pH, temperature, stirring rate and extraction time. This review discusses the principle, optimization variables, advantages and disadvantages and some selected applications of DLLME-SFOD in water, food and biomedical analysis.

Mazak, K. and B. Noszal (2014). "Drug delivery: A process governed by species-specific lipophilicities." *Eur J Pharm Sci* 62:96–104.

Drug delivery is a cascade of molecular migration processes, in which the active principle dissolves in and partitions between several biological media of various hydrophilic and lipophilic character. Membrane penetration and other partitions are controlled by a number of physicochemical parameters, the eminent ones are species-specific basicity and lipophilicity. Latter is a molecular property of immense importance in pharmacy, bio-, and medicinal chemistry, expressing the affinity of the molecule for a lipophilic environment. This review gives an overview of the types and definitions of the partition coefficient, the most widespread lipophilicity parameter, focusing on the species-specific (microscopic) partition coefficients. We survey the pertinent literature and summarize our recent works that enabled the determination of previously inaccessible species-specific partition coefficients for coexisting, inseparable protonation isomers too. This thorough insight provides explanation why some drugs unexpectedly get into the CNS and sheds some light on the submolecular mechanism of pharmacokinetic processes. The contribution of the various ionic forms to the overall partition can now be quantitated. As a result, there is clear-cut evidence that passive diffusion into lipophilic media is not necessarily predominated by the noncharged species, contrary to the widespread misbelief.

Mazak, K. and B. Noszal (2016). "Advances in microspeciation of drugs and biomolecules: Species-specific concentrations, acid–base properties and related parameters." *J Pharm Biomed Anal* 130:390–403.

The pharmacokinetic and pharmacodynamic behavior of drugs and the interacting biomolecules are highly influenced by their species-specific physicochemical properties. The first of such biorelevant, structure-dependent properties were the species-specific acid–base constants and the codependent concentrations, but the past decade brought significant advances to previously uncharted territories, including the experimental determination of species-specific partition coefficients, solubilities and redox equilibrium constants. This review gives an overview of the types and definitions of species-specific physicochemical and analytical properties. We survey the pertinent literature, the fundamental relationships, and summarize some of our recent work that enabled the determination of species-specific partition coefficients for coexisting, inseparable protonation isomers and pH-independent, microscopic redox equilibrium constants. The thorough insight provided by these species-specific properties improves our understanding of the submolecular mechanism of pharmacokinetic processes. As a result, there are some pieces of clear-cut evidence of practical significance. A few of them are as follows: passive diffusion into lipophilic media is not necessarily predominated by the noncharged species, contrary to the widespread misbelief. The reactive microspecies in structure-controlled, highly specific biochemical reactions is not necessarily the major one—a preventive defense system against oxidative stress can be based upon thiol-disulfide equilibria of custom-tailored redox potentials.

Moller, M. N. and A. Denicola (2018). "Diffusion of nitric oxide and oxygen in lipoproteins and membranes studied by pyrene fluorescence quenching." *Free Radic Biol Med* 128:137–143.

Oxygen and nitric oxide are small hydrophobic molecules that usually need to diffuse a considerable distance to accomplish their biological functions and necessarily need to traverse several lipid membranes. Different methods have been used to study the diffusion of these molecules in membranes and herein we focus in the quenching of fluorescence of pyrenes inserted in the membrane. The pyrene derivatives have long fluorescence lifetimes (around 200 ns) that make them very sensitive to fluorescence quenching by nitric oxide, oxygen and other paramagnetic species. Results show that the apparent diffusion coefficients in membranes are similar to those in water, indicating that diffusion of these molecules in membranes is not considerably limited by the lipids. This high apparent diffusion in membranes is a consequence of both a favorable partition of these molecules in the hydrophobic interior of membranes and a high diffusion coefficient. Altering the composition of the membrane results in slight changes in diffusion, indicating that in most cases the lipid membranes will not hinder the passage of oxygen or nitric oxide. The diffusion of nitric oxide in the lipid core of low-density lipoprotein is also very high, supporting its role as an antioxidant. In contrast to the high permeability of membranes to nitric oxide and oxygen, the permeability to other reactive species such as hydrogen peroxide and peroxynitrous acid is nearly five orders of magnitude lower.

Pascolutti, M. and R. J. Quinn (2014). "Natural products as lead structures: Chemical transformations to create lead-like libraries." *Drug Discov Today* 19(3):215–221.

In this review, we analyze and illustrate the variation of the two main lead-like descriptors (molecular weight [MW] and the partition coefficient [log *P*]) in the generation of libraries in which a natural product (NP) is used as the guiding structure. Despite the different approaches used to create NP-like libraries, controlling these descriptors during the synthetic process is important to generate lead-like libraries. From this analysis, we present a schematic approach to the generation of lead-like libraries that can be applied to any starting NP.

Pearl, D. L. (2014). "Making the most of clustered data in laboratory animal research using multi-level models." *Ilar J* 55(3):486–492.

In the following review article, I address the fitting of multilevel models for the analysis of hierarchical data in laboratory animal medicine. Using an example of paternal dietary effects on the weight of offspring in a mouse model, this review outlines the reasons and benefits of using a multilevel modeling approach. To start, the concept of clustered/autocorrelated data is introduced, and the implications of ignoring the effects of clustered data on measures of association/model coefficients and their statistical significance are discussed. The limitations of other methods compared with multilevel modeling for analyzing clustered data are addressed in terms of statistical power, control of potential confounding effects associated with group membership, proper estimation of associations and their statistical significance, and adjusting for multiple levels of clustering. In addition, the benefits of being able to estimate variance partition coefficients and intraclass correlation coefficients from multilevel models is described, and the concepts of more complex correlation structures and various methods for fitting multilevel models are introduced. The current state of learning materials including textbooks, websites, and software for the nonstatistician is outlined to describe the accessibility of multilevel modeling approaches for laboratory animal researchers.

Raffy, G. et al. (2018). "Oral bioaccessibility of semi-volatile organic compounds (SVOCs) in settled dust: A review of measurement methods, data and influencing factors." *J Hazard Mater* 352:215–227.

Many semivolatile organic compounds (SVOCs), suspected of reprotoxic, neurotoxic or carcinogenic effects, were measured in indoor settled dust. Dust ingestion is a nonnegligible pathway of exposure to some of these SVOCs, and an accurate knowledge of the real exposure is necessary for a better evaluation of health risks. To this end, the bioaccessibility of SVOCs in dust needs to be considered. In the present work, bioaccessibility measurement methods, SVOCs' oral bioaccessibility data and influencing factors were reviewed. SVOC bioaccessibilities (%) ranged from 11 to 94, 8 to 100, 3 to 92, 1 to 81, 6 to 52, and 2 to 17, for brominated flame retardants, organophosphorus flame retardants, polychlorobiphenyls, phthalates, pesticides and polycyclic aromatic hydrocarbons, respectively. Measurements method produced varying results depending on the inclusion of food and/or sink in the model. Characteristics of dust, e.g., organic matter content and particle size, also influenced bioaccessibility data. Last, results were influenced by SVOC properties, such as octanol/water partition coefficient and migration pathway into dust. Factors related to dust and SVOCs could be used in prediction models. To this end, more bioaccessibility studies covering more substances should be performed, using methods that are harmonized and validated by comparison to in vivo studies.

Rao, G. and E. P. Vejerano (2018). "Partitioning of volatile organic compounds to aerosols: A review." *Chemosphere* 212:282–296.

Although volatile organic compounds (VOCs) exist mainly in the gas phase rather than in aerosols, the concentrations of VOCs measured from aerosols are comparable to those of semivolatile organic compounds, which preferentially partition into aerosols. VOCs that partition into aerosols may raise health effects that are generally not exerted by aerosols or by VOCs alone. So far, only scant reports on VOC/aerosol partitioning are available in the extant literature. In this review, we discuss findings presented in recent studies on the partition mechanism, factors affecting the partition process, existing knowledge gaps, and recommendations to help address these gaps for future research. Also, we have surveyed the different models that can be applied to predict partition coefficients and the inherent advantage and shortcoming of the assumptions in these models. A better understanding of the partition mechanism and partition coefficient of VOCs into aerosols can improve prediction of the global fate and transport of VOCs in the environment and enhance assessment of the health effects from exposure to VOCs.

Sahoo, S. et al. (2016). "A short review of the generation of molecular descriptors and their applications in quantitative structure–property/activity relationships." *Curr Comput Aided Drug Des* 12(3):181–205.

BACKGROUND: Synthesis of organic compounds with specific biological activity or physicochemical characteristics needs a thorough analysis of the enumerable data set obtained from literature. Quantitative structure–property(QSP)/activity relationships (ARs) have made it simple by predicting the structure of the compound with any optimized activity. For that there is a paramount data set of molecular descriptors (MD). This review is a survey on the generation of the molecular descriptors and its probable applications in QSP/AR. METHODS: Literatures have been collected from a wide class of research journals, citable web reports, seminar proceedings and books. The MDs were classified according to their generation. The applications of the MDs on the QSP/AR have also been reported in this review. RESULTS: The MDs can be classified into experimental and theoretical types, having a sub classification of the later into structural and quantum chemical descriptors. The structural parameters are derived from molecular graphs or topology of the molecules. Even the pixel of the molecular image can be used as molecular descriptor. In QSPR studies the physicochemical properties include boiling point, heat capacity, density, refractive index, molar volume, surface tension, heat of formation, octanol–water partition coefficient, solubility, chromatographic retention indices etc. Among biological activities toxicity, antimalarial activity, sensory irritant, potencies of local anesthetic, tadpole narcosis, antifungal activity, enzyme inhibiting activity are some important parameters in the QSAR studies. CONCLUSION: The classification of the MDs is mostly generic in nature. The application of the MDs in QSP/AR also has a generic link. Experimental MDs are more suitable in correlation analysis than the theoretical ones but are more expensive for generation. In advent of sophisticated computational tools and experimental design proliferation of MDs is inevitable, but for a highly optimized MD, studies on generation of MD is an unending process.

Selvaraj, S. et al. (2015). "Influence of membrane lipid composition on flavonoid–membrane interactions: Implications on their biological activity." *Prog Lipid Res* 58:1–13.

The membrane interactions and localization of flavonoids play a vital role in altering membrane-mediated cell signaling cascades as well as influence the pharmacological activities such as antitumor, antimicrobial and antioxidant properties of flavonoids. Various techniques have been used to investigate the membrane interaction of flavonoids. These include partition coefficient, fluorescence anisotropy, differential scanning calorimetry, NMR spectroscopy, electrophysiological methods and molecular dynamics simulations. Each technique will provide specific information about either alteration of membrane fluidity or localization of flavonoids within the lipid bilayer. Apart from the diverse techniques employed, the concentrations of flavonoids and lipid membrane composition employed in various studies reported in literature also are different and together these variables contribute to diverse findings that sometimes contradict each other. This review highlights different techniques employed to investigate the membrane interaction of flavonoids with special emphasis on erythrocyte model membrane systems and their significance in understanding the nature and extent of flavonoid–membrane interactions. We also attempt to correlate the membrane localization and alteration in membrane fluidity with the biological activities of flavonoids such as antioxidant, anticancer and antimicrobial properties.

Swami, R. and A. Shahiwala (2013). "Impact of physiochemical properties on pharmacokinetics of protein therapeutics." *Eur J Drug Metab Pharmacokinet* 38(4):231–239.

Physicochemical properties, such as molecular weight, size, partition coefficient, acid dissociation constant and solubility have a great impact on pharmacokinetics of traditional small molecule drugs and substantially used in development of small drugs. However, predicting pharmacokinetic fate (absorption, distribution, metabolism, and elimination) of protein therapeutics from their physicochemical parameters is extremely difficult due to the macromolecular nature of therapeutic proteins and peptides. Their structural complexity and immunogenicity are other contributing factors that determine their biological fate. Therefore, to develop generalized strategies concerning development of therapeutic proteins and peptides are highly challenging. However, reviewing the literature, authors found that physiochemical properties, such as molecular weight, charge and structural modification are having great impact on pharmacokinetics of protein therapeutics and an attempt is made to provide the major findings in this manuscript. This manuscript will serve to provide some bases for developing protein therapeutics with desired pharmacokinetic profile.

Todo, H. (2017). "Transdermal permeation of drugs in various animal species." *Pharmaceutics* 9(3):33.

Excised human skin is utilized for in vitro permeation experiments to evaluate the safety and effect of topically applied drugs by measuring its skin permeation and concentration. However, ethical considerations are the major problem for using human skin to evaluate percutaneous absorption. Moreover, large variations have been found among human skin specimens as a result of differences in age, race, and anatomical donor site. Animal skins are used to predict the in vivo human penetration/permeation of topically applied chemicals. In the present review, skin characteristics, such as thickness of skin, lipid content, hair follicle density, and enzyme activity in each model are compared to human skin. In addition, intra- and interindividual variation in animal models, permeation parameter correlation between animal models and human skin, and utilization of cultured human skin models are also descried. Pig, guinea pig, and hairless rat are generally selected for this purpose. Each animal model has advantages and weaknesses for utilization in in vitro skin permeation experiments. Understanding of skin permeation characteristics such as permeability coefficient (P), diffusivity (D), and partition coefficient (K) for each skin model would be necessary to obtain better correlations for animal models to human skin permeation.

Toprak, M. (2016). "Fluorescence study on the interaction of human serum albumin with Butein in liposomes." *Spectrochim Acta A Mol Biomol Spectrosc* 154:108–113.

The interaction of Butein with human serum albumin in L-egg lecithin phosphatidylcholine (PC) liposome has been investigated by fluorescence and absorption spectroscopy. The results of the fluorescence measurement indicated that Butein effectively quenched the intrinsic fluorescence of HSA via static quenching. The Stern-Volmer plots in all the liposome solutions showed a positive deviation from the linearity. According to the thermodynamic parameters, the hydrophobic interactions appeared be the major interaction forces between Butein and HSA. The effect of Butein on the conformation of HSA was also investigated by the synchronous fluorescence under the same experimental conditions. In addition, the partition coefficient of the Butein in the PC liposomes was also determined by using the fluorescence quenching process. The obtained results can be of biological significance in pharmacology and clinical medicine.

Treu, G. et al. (2015). "The dessau workshop on bioaccumulation: State of the art, challenges and regulatory implications." *Environ Sci Eur* 27(1):34.

Bioaccumulation plays a vital role in understanding the fate of a substance in the environment and is key to the regulation of chemicals in several jurisdictions. The current assessment approaches commonly use the octanol–water partition coefficient (log KOW) as an indicator for bioaccumulation and the bioconcentration factor (BCF) as a standard criterion to identify bioaccumulative substances show limitations. The log KOW does not take into account active transport phenomena or special structural properties (e.g., amphiphilic substances or dissociating substances) and therefore additional screening criteria are required. Regulatory BCF studies are so far restricted to fish and uptake through the gills. Studies on (terrestrial) air-breathing organisms are missing. Though there are alternative tests such as the dietary exposure bioaccumulation fish test described in the recently revised OECD test guideline 305, it still remains unclear how to deal with results of alternative tests in regulatory decision-making processes. A substantial number of bioaccumulation fish tests are required in regulation. The development of improved test systems following the 3R principles, namely, to replace, reduce and refine animal testing, is thus required. All these aspects stress the importance to further develop the assessment of bioaccumulation. The Dessau Workshop on Bioaccumulation which was held from June 26 to June 27, 2014, in Dessau, Germany, provided a comprehensive overview of the state of the art of bioaccumulation assessment, provided insights into the problems and challenges addressed by the regulatory authorities and described new research concepts and their regulatory implications. The event was organized by UBA (Dessau, Germany) and Fraunhofer IME (Schmallenberg, Germany). About 50 participants from industry, regulatory bodies and academia listened to 14 lectures on selected topics and joined the plenary discussions.

Tsopelas, F. et al. (2017). "Lipophilicity and biomimetic properties to support drug discovery." *Expert Opin Drug Discov* 12(9):885–896.

INTRODUCTION: Lipophilicity, expressed as the octanol–water partition coefficient, constitutes the most important property in drug action, influencing both pharmacokinetic and pharmacodynamics processes as well as drug toxicity. On the other hand, biomimetic properties defined as the retention outcome on HPLC columns containing a biological relevant agent, provide a considerable advance for rapid experimental–based estimation of ADME properties in early drug discovery stages. Areas covered: This review highlights the paramount importance of lipophilicity in almost all aspects of drug action and safety. It outlines problems brought about by high lipophilicity and provides an overview of the drug-like metrics which incorporate lower limits or ranges of log *P*. The fundamental factors governing lipophilicity are compared to those involved in phospholipophilicity, assessed by immobilized artificial membrane chromatography (IAM). Finally, the contribution of biomimetic properties to assess plasma protein binding is evaluated. Expert opinion: Lipophilicity and biomimetic properties have important distinct and overlapping roles in supporting the drug discovery process. Lipophilicity is unique in early drug design for library screening and for the identification of the most promising compounds to start with, while biomimetic properties are useful for the experimentally-based evaluation of ADME properties for the synthesized novel compounds, supporting the prioritization of drug candidates and guiding further synthesis.

Wei, W. et al. (2018). "Influence of indoor environmental factors on mass transfer parameters and concentrations of semi-volatile organic compounds." *Chemosphere* 195:223–235.

Semivolatile organic compounds (SVOCs) in indoor environments can partition among the gas phase, airborne particles, settled dust, and available surfaces. The mass transfer parameters of SVOCs, such as the mass transfer coefficient and the partition coefficient, are influenced by indoor environmental factors. Subsequently, indoor SVOC concentrations and thus occupant exposure can vary depending on environmental factors. In this review, the influence of six environmental factors, i.e., indoor temperature, humidity, ventilation, airborne particle concentration, source loading factor, and reactive chemistry, on the mass transfer parameters and indoor concentrations of SVOCs was analyzed and tentatively quantified. The results show that all mass transfer parameters vary depending on environmental factors. These variations are mostly characterized by empirical equations, particularly for humidity. Theoretical calculations of these parameters based on mass transfer mechanisms are available only for the emission of SVOCs from source surfaces when airborne particles are not present. All mass transfer parameters depend on the temperature. Humidity influences the partition of SVOCs among different phases and is associated with phthalate hydrolysis. Ventilation has a combined effect with the airborne particle concentration on SVOC emission and their mass transfer among different phases. Indoor chemical reactions can produce or eliminate SVOCs slowly. To better model the dynamic SVOC concentration indoors, the present review suggests studying the combined effect of environmental factors in real indoor environments. Moreover, interactions between indoor environmental factors and human activities and their influence on SVOC mass transfer processes should be considered.

Wong, T. W. (2014). "Electrical, magnetic, photomechanical and cavitational waves to overcome skin barrier for transdermal drug delivery." *J Control Release* 193:257–269.

Transdermal drug delivery is hindered by the barrier property of the stratum corneum. It limits the route to transport of drugs with a log octanol–water partition coefficient of 1–3, molecular weight of less than 500 Da and melting point of less than 200 degrees C. Active methods such as iontophoresis, electroporation, sonophoresis, magnetophoresis and laser techniques have been investigated for the past decades on their ability, mechanisms and limitations in modifying the skin microenvironment to promote drug diffusion and partition. Microwave, an electromagnetic wave characterized by frequencies range between 300 MHz and 300 GHz, has recently been reported as the potential skin permeation enhancer. Microwave has received a widespread application in food, engineering and medical sectors. Its potential use to facilitate transdermal drug transport is still in its infancy stage of evaluation. This review provides an overview and update on active methods utilizing electrical, magnetic, photomechanical and cavitational waves to overcome the skin barrier for transdermal drug administration with insights into mechanisms and future perspectives of the latest microwave technique described.

Xu, S. et al. (2014). "Critical review and interpretation of environmental data for volatile methylsiloxanes: Partition properties." *Environ Sci Technol* 48(20):11748–11759.

Volatile methylsiloxanes (VMS) enter the environment through industrial activities and the use of various consumer products. Reliable measurements of environmental partition properties for these compounds are critical for accurate prediction of their environmental fate, distribution, transport, exposure and potential effects. In this study, the measured partition properties including air/water (K(AW)), octanol/water (K(OW)), and octanol/air partitioning coefficients (K(OA)), soil organic carbon/water distribution coefficient (K(OC)), and biological medium/fluid partition coefficients, and their temperature dependence were critically reviewed. Based on these results, organosilicon compounds such as methylsiloxanes are expected to behave differently in the environment compared to conventional hydrophobic environmental contaminants, as a result of their inherent characteristics related to molecular size and capacity for different types of molecular interactions that control partitioning. The differences are critical and need to be taken into consideration in environmental exposure and risk analyses of these compounds.

Yang, Y. J. and J. S. Ding (2016). "Progress in study of nitroimidazole as hypoxia imaging agents in tumor." *Yao Xue Xue Bao* 51(8):1227–1232.

Radionuclide hypoxia imaging has become an indispensable core of tumor diagnosis. Nitroimidazole derivatives have been extensively used as the hypoxia imaging agents in preclinical and clinical research. It is the key to design the ideal structure for promising agents. The type and quantity of nitroimidazole, the linker structure and chiral may have an impact on the imaging results. The characteristics of the imaging agents including single electron reduction potential (SERP), oil–water partition coefficient (log *P*) and pharmacokinetics are also the key factors. In this review, we highlight the factors for hypoxia imaging, providing clues for the structure design of new agents.

5

Release, Dissolution, and Permeation

Meditation is the dissolution of thoughts in Eternal awareness or Pure consciousness without objectification, knowing without thinking, merging finitude in infinity.

Voltaire

5.1 Introduction

Newly discovered lead compounds that are ultimately formulated into drug delivery systems should be capable of existing either in a molecular dispersion, such as solutions, or in an aggregate state, such as tablets, capsules, and suspensions, so that are readily rendered into finer state of dispersion and dissolution. Regardless of the stage of aggregation in the final formulation, the active pharmaceutical ingredient (API) must be released from the drug delivery system and, as the first step, should be dissolved in an aqueous environment; this will then be followed possibly by one or more transfers across nonaqueous barriers. The scope of preformulation studies has changed significantly over the past couple of decades with the availability of techniques to study the release and permeation characteristics of lead compounds. Although the design of drug delivery systems can alter release characteristics to some extent, the basic permeation characteristics remain an innate property based on the physicochemical nature of the drug.

In the recent years, several new approaches to study permeation that can be of great use in assessing the lead compound potential have been developed. The need to study the release and permeation patterns has become a pivotal part of preformulation studies, since the U.S. Food and Drug Administration (U.S. FDA) adopted a system of classification of drugs: the Biopharmaceutics Classification System (BCS), which was suggested by Gordon Amidon and his group in 1995, allows prediction of in vivo pharmacokinetic performance of drug products from measurements of permeability (determined as the extent of oral absorption) and solubility and thus forms the scientific basis to allow waiver of in vivo bioavailability and bioequivalence testing of immediate-release solid dosage forms for high-permeability drugs that also exhibit rapid dissolution (1). Later in the chapter, a detailed discussion will be presented regarding this classification system.

5.2 Release

Drug absorption depends on the release of the drug substance from the drug product (dissolution), the solubility, and the permeability across the gastrointestinal (GI) tract. The release characteristics of a drug delivery system are often determined by the manufacture of the product and highly affected by drug solubility, which also affects dissolution rates. The release step is followed by dissolution of the active ingredient. Dissolution of a pure substance follows the classic Noyes–Whitney equation:

$$dc/dt = kS(Cs - Ct) \qquad (5.1)$$

where dc/dt is the rate of dissolution, k is the dissolution rate constant, S is the surface area of the dissolving solid, Cs is the saturation concentration of drug in the diffusion layer, and Ct is the concentration of drug in dissolution media (or the bulk).

This equation is of great value in the formulation studies, wherein increase in the surface area of aggregates is the most powerful tool to optimize dissolution. The innate property in the equation that is subject to much of preformulation work refers to the solubility of the compound. In dissolution theory, it is assumed that an aqueous diffusion layer or stagnant liquid film of thickness h exists at the surface of a solid undergoing dissolution, as observed in Figure 5.1. This thickness h represents a stationary layer of solvent in which the solute molecules exist in concentrations from Cs to C. Beyond the static diffusion layer, at x greater than h, mixing occurs in the solution, and the drug is found at a uniform concentration, C, throughout the bulk phase (Figure 5.1).

The diffusion layer model of dissolution assumes that the dissolution of drug at the solid–liquid interface into a concentrated layer surrounding the solid particle is more rapid than the diffusion of dissolved drug from that layer into the bulk solution. This diffusion is therefore rate-limiting in observed dissolution. As diffusion involves kinetic energy, it is highly dependent on the temperature. For an ideal solution, no heat is absorbed or given off on dissolution; however, for a real solution, the heat of the solution (ΔH) can be either negative (heat is given off) or positive (heat is absorbed). The mathematical relationship of solubility (Cs) to temperature is:

$$\log Cs = (-\Delta H/2.303\, RT) + \text{constant} \qquad (5.2)$$

where R is the gas constant and T is the absolute temperature. A plot of log Cs versus $1/T$ gives the value of the constant. A heat effect depends on whether the material

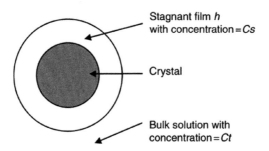

Stagnant film h
with concentration $= Cs$

Crystal

Bulk solution with
concentration $= Ct$

FIGURE 5.1 Diffusion layer model of dissolution.

absorbs heat (an endothermic process) or gives off heat (an exothermic process) when it dissolves. Most materials absorb heat as they dissolve. According to the Le Chatelier's principle, a system at equilibrium will adjust in such a manner as to reduce external stress. Therefore, if a substance absorbs heat when it dissolves and heat is added to the system, equilibrium can be restored, that is, the external stress can be reduced, by the absorption of heat. This can only be done in such a system by the dissolution of more substance, that is, an increase in solubility at the higher temperature, until the equilibrium is restored.

The thermodynamic driving force for dissolution is therefore the heat of solution of the substance. For a crystalline solid, this represents the difference between the heat of sublimation of the compound and the heat of hydration of the ions. The heat of sublimation is the heat required to bring ions from the solid state to the gaseous state and is a measure of the energy required to pull apart the crystalline lattice. The heat of hydration is the heat given off by the hydration of those ions. For dissolution to be an endothermic process, the heat of sublimation is greater than the heat of hydration, and ΔH is positive, that is, the heat is absorbed upon dissolution; therefore, solubility increases with an increase in temperature. If heat of sublimation is equal to the heat of hydration, solubility is independent of temperature.

As discussed in the previous chapter, the solubility of ionizable compounds is pH-dependent. For weak acids, as pH decreases, the solubility decreases. At equilibrium:

$$[HA] \text{ solid} \leftrightarrow [HA] \text{ solution} \tag{5.3}$$

while the molar solubility (So) remains unchanged as a function of pH. The equilibrium dissociation constant is:

$$K_a = [H_3O^+] * [A^-]/[HA] \tag{5.4}$$

or

$$[A^-] = K_a * [HA]/[H_3O^+] = K_a * So/[H_3O^+] \tag{5.5}$$

The total solubility (*S*) is expressed as:

$$S = [A^-] + [HA] \tag{5.6}$$

or

$$S = K_a * So/[H_3O^+] + So \tag{5.7}$$

or

$$S - So = K_a * So/[H_3O^+] \tag{5.8}$$

$$\log(S - So) = \log K_a + \log So - \log[H_3O^+] \tag{5.9}$$

$$\log[(S - So)/So] = -pK_a + pH \tag{5.10}$$

Plotting $\log[(S-So)/S]$ versus pH (Figure 5.2) allows experimental determination of *S* and So.

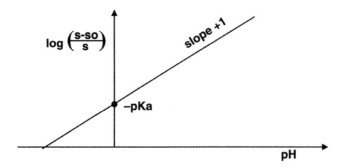

FIGURE 5.2   Calculation of solubility as a function of pH.

Therefore, because So is assumed to remain constant and pK_a is a constant, if pH decreases, the value of S must also decrease. In a similar manner, the solubility of a weak base decreases as pH increases.

There are several new ways emerging to measure the solubility of ionizable drugs, such as using the method called CheqSol® (chasing equilibrium solubility). Not only does CheqSol measure equilibrium and kinetic solubility rapidly and accurately, but it also provides insights into compound behavior that will be of value for the better understanding of drug bioavailability, for modeling of precipitation processes, and for investigating changes of crystalline form in suspensions.

The solubility of drug is an important physicochemical property, because it affects the bioavailability of the drug, the rate of drug release into the dissolution medium, and, consequently, the therapeutic efficacy of the pharmaceutical product. The solubility of a molecule in various solvents is determined as a first step. This information is valuable in developing a formulation. Solubility is usually determined in a variety of commonly used solvents and some oils if the molecule is lipophilic.

The solubility of a material is usually determined by the equilibrium solubility method, which employs a saturated solution of the material, obtained by stirring an excess of the material in the solvent for a prolonged period, until equilibrium is achieved. Common solvents used for solubility determination are as follows:

- Water
- Polyethylene glycols
- Propylene glycol
- Glycerin
- Sorbitol
- Ethyl alcohol
- Methanol
- Benzyl alcohol
- Isopropyl alcohol
- Tweens
- Polysorbates
- Castor oil

- Peanut oil
- Sesame oil
- Buffers at various pHs

5.2.1 Solubility Modulation

Poorly soluble compounds represent an estimated 60% of compounds in development and many major marketed drugs. It is important to measure and predict solubility and permeability accurately at an early stage and interpret these data to help assess the potential for the development of the candidates. This requires the development of an effective strategy to select the most appropriate tools to examine and improve the solubility in each phase of development and the optimization of solid-state approaches to enhance solubility, including the use of polymorphs, cocrystals, and amorphous solids. All of these would affect the dissolution rates and bioavailability that can be studied with nanocrystal technology.

With this trend of increasingly insoluble drugs stretching resources, many companies are now reevaluating their strategy. They know that there are many available technologies to measure and predict and finally improve solubility, and several new techniques are emerging. Studies that encompass this scope would include how membrane permeation of drugs can be enhanced by means of solubilizing agents, how the solid state is characterized and modified to improve solubility and drug performance, how salt screening and selection can impact the dissolution rate and oral absorption, the application of nanocrystal technology to increase dissolution rate, and the analysis of the use of pharmaceutical co-crystals in enhancing drug properties.

Many different approaches have been developed to overcome the solubility problem of poorly soluble drugs, for example, solubilization, inclusion compounds, and complexation. A basic disadvantage in these formulation approaches is that these can be applied only to a certain number of drugs exhibiting special features required for implementing the formulation principle (e.g., molecule fits into the cavity of the cyclodextrin ring). The use of solvent mixtures is also very limited owing to toxicological considerations. In addition, more and more newly developed drugs are poorly soluble in aqueous media and simultaneously in organic media, thus excluding the use of solvent mixtures. Ideally, the formulation principle should be able to be applied to all or at least most of the poorly soluble drugs.

Solubilizers (e.g., organic solvents, detergents, and Pluronics) are often used to solubilize drugs in aqueous solution without considering their effects on biological systems, such as lipid membranes and multidrug-resistance (MDR) efflux transporters (e.g., P-glycoprotein and MDR1). Liposomal solubilization is an effective approach for the delivery of potent, insoluble drug candidates. An alternative to other methods developed is the production of drug nanoparticles by high-pressure homogenization, either as pearl milling or as the continuous high-pressure homogenization. Of importance is the consideration of metallic contamination during fast speed milling processes to keep it less than 1 ppm. Drug nanoparticles are produced by the dispersion of drug powder in an aqueous surfactant solution; the obtained presuspension is passed through a high-pressure piston-gap homogenizer, for example, 5–20 homogenization cycles at typically 1000–1500 bars, and works on the principle that cavitation occurs in the aqueous phase. The particle suspension has a very high flow velocity when passing the tiny gap of the homogenizer; the static pressure on the water decreases below the vapor pressure of water; the water starts boiling at room temperature, leading to the formation of gas bubbles; and at the exit of the gap, the gas bubbles implode. The implosion shock waves disintegrate the drug particles to drug nanoparticles. Further improvement on nanoparticle production includes homogenization in the nonaqueous phases or with reduced water content to produce more pronounced cavitation at higher temperatures. The chemical stability of the drugs is less impaired when homogenizing in nonaqueous or water-reduced media at low temperatures. The drug powder is dispersed in a nonaqueous medium (e.g., polyethylene glycol [PEG] 600 and Miglyol 812) or in a water-reduced mixture (e.g., water-ethanol), and the presuspension is homogenized in a piston-gap homogenizer. A suitable machine for lab scale is the Micron Lab 40 (APV Deutschland GmbH, Lübeck, Germany). Ostwald ripening occurs because of different saturation solubilities in the vicinity of very small and large particles. The particles produced are relatively homogeneous. The differences in the size, in combination with the generally poor solubility of the drug nanoparticles, are sufficiently low to avoid Ostwald ripening. Aqueous drug nanoparticle suspensions generally prove to be physically stable for several years.

The application of micronization and nanonization increases the surface area, leading to an increased dissolution rate, according to the Noyes–Whitney equation. However, this is only one aspect. The dissolution pressure is a function of the curvature of the surface that is much stronger for a curved surface of nanoparticles. For a size less than approximately 1–2 μm, the dissolution pressure increases distinctly, leading to an increase in saturation solubility. In addition, the diffusional distance h on the surface of drug nanoparticles is decreased, thus leading to an increased concentration gradient $(Cs-Cx)/h$. The increase in surface area and concentration gradient leads to a greater increase in the dissolution velocity compared with a micronized product. In addition, the saturation solubility is also increased, even though it is a thermodynamic parameter; the increase in solubility occurs as the supersaturation stage is reached. Saturation solubility and dissolution velocity are important parameters affecting the bioavailability of orally administered drugs. From this, nanoparticles have the potential to overcome these limiting steps.

Nanoparticle-based products are likely to have some unique characteristics: general adhesiveness of nanoparticles to the gut wall; adhesion to the gut wall being a reproducible process, thus minimizing variation in drug absorption, increase in dissolution velocity overcoming this rate-limiting step; and an additional increase in the saturation solubility, leading to an increased concentration gradient between the gut and blood. Orally administered drug nanoparticles can increase the bioavailability and can be the only tool available to achieve sufficient bioavailability with poorly soluble drugs. However, the possibility of faster absorption may have drawbacks, both from pharmacology and stability in the gut. For intravenous administration, the drug nanoparticles should possess a bulk population in the nanometer range by simultaneously having a low microparticle content, that is, especially particles larger than 5 μm, which can cause capillary blockade. The homogenization process yields a product with a minimized content of particles larger than 1 μm. Intravenous administration of drug nanoparticles allows the achievement of sufficient blood levels and finds good application in the evaluation of new compounds. In addition, toxicologically critical excipients, such as Cremophor EL used in Taxol formulations can be avoided when stabilizing the drug nanoparticles with accepted emulsifiers, for example, lecithin and

Tween 80. It is interesting to note that when Taxol is administered with Cremophor EL, the pharmacokinetics of the drug turns out to be nonlinear. For intravenous administration, a small particle size of less than 150 nm is desirable only in cases where one wants to pass fenestrated endothelia (e.g., treatment of tumors); however, this is a very limited case. More realistic and short-term achievable goal is passive targeting of drugs to treat mononuclear phagocytic system (MPS) infections (i.e., targeting the macrophages, e.g., treatment of *Mycobacterium tuberculosis* and *Mycobacterium avium* infections, especially in human immunodeficiency virus [HIV]-infected patients). Here, it is more desirable to have larger particles to ensure fast and efficient removal from the bloodstreams by the macrophages. Another therapeutic goal is the creation of stealth drug nanoparticles circulating in the blood, minimizing free-drug concentration, and simultaneously prolonging the drug release by slow dissolution. For this purpose, very small particles are not suitable, because they will dissolve too fast. Another therapeutic goal is targeting the non-MPS targets, for example, the brain and the bone marrow.

The particle size should be customized depending on the therapeutic requirements and purpose. The nanoparticle suspensions are physically stable for a long period of time if they are stabilized by emulsifiers or polymers in optimized composition. However, aqueous suspensions might not be the most convenient dosage form for the patient. The nanoparticle suspension can be used as granulation fluid for tablet production or as wetting liquid for pellet production. The dispersions can also be spray-dried to be filled into hard gelatin capsules or sachets. Drug nanoparticles produced in PEG 600 or Miglyol can directly be filled into soft gelatin capsules. Lyophilization of drug nanoparticles produced in a water-reduced media can be used to produce fast-dissolving delivery systems. For parenteral application, nanoparticles can be lyophilized and reconstituted with isotonic media prior to injection (e.g., water with glycerol). There are also other areas of application, for example, ocular delivery (prolonged retention time) and topical application (increased saturation solubility, leading to increased diffusion pressure into the skin).

5.3 Assay Systems

As the U.S. FDA has begun accepting recommendations for waiver of bioequivalence requirement, protocols proving extremely expensive in the drug development cycle, there is a greater need to develop surrogate models that might prove useful sometime in securing waivers for all classes of drugs. Generally, the methods available currently show that the complexity of assay is directly proportional to its correlation with the absorption of drugs in humans (Figure 5.3). Studies that correlated log P with human absorption profile and the suitability or lead candidates are elaborated in Chapter 4. In this chapter, we will examine more complex assay systems.

Drug transport across epithelial cell barriers, especially the human small intestine, is difficult to predict. The intestinal epithelial cell barrier is a sophisticated organ that has evolved over hundreds of millions of years to become a "smart," effective, and selective xenobiotic screen. Nevertheless, there is large interindividual variability in the intestinal transport of drugs. Genetic variability in key proteins is believed to be causal. There is a pressing need to better understand the key processes and how the system components interact at the molecular, cellular, and tissue levels to control drug transport and determine drug absorption in small intestines.

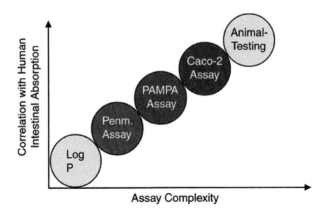

FIGURE 5.3 Assay complexity versus correlation with human absorption. Data from both complex biological and artificial permeation assays can provide valuable information regarding the absorption of a drug. (Courtesy of Millipore Corporation, Billerica, MA.)

Is it feasible to construct an in silico framework to represent the drug absorption in small intestines at the cellular level, with internal dynamic property, and concert with the update molecular biochemical mechanism? This new generation of models and computational tools might integrate the available and emerging information at different levels to better account for and predict the observed experimental results. Predicting aqueous solubility is possible using in silico tools. It is, however, difficult to measure accurately, especially for poorly soluble compounds, and thus, numerous in silico models have been developed for its prediction. Some in silico models can predict aqueous solubility of simple, uncharged organic chemicals reasonably well; however, solubility prediction for charged species and drug-like chemicals is not very accurate. However, extrapolating solubility data to intestinal absorption from pharmacokinetic and physicochemical data and elucidating crucial parameters for absorption and the potential for improvement of bioavailability are important at the preformulation stages.

The poor oral bioavailability of drugs is generally assumed to be due to physiochemical problems, which result in poor solubility in the GI tract or difficulty in diffusion through small intestine epithelial membrane. Furthermore, the biochemical process also contributes to oral bioavailability. The in vitro cell culture models of the intestinal epithelial cell barrier have evolved to become widely used experimental devices.

In the previous chapter, the log *P* factor was discussed in detail; in this chapter, we will examine other methods of testing transport across membranes.

5.3.1 Permeability Assays

The permeability assay uses an artificial membrane composed of hexadecane.

The automated systems comprise of multiwell systems is shown in Figure 5.4.

The protocol for permeability assay is outlined as follows:

1. Into each well, add 15 µL of a 5% solution of hexadecane in hexane.
2. Dry for 45 minutes–1 hour to ensure complete evaporation of hexane.

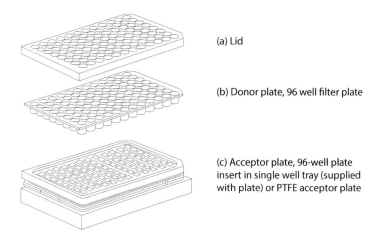

(a) Lid

(b) Donor plate, 96 well filter plate

(c) Acceptor plate, 96-well plate insert in single well tray (supplied with plate) or PTFE acceptor plate

FIGURE 5.4 The 96-well permeability testing method. The support membrane is a 3-μm track etched polycarbonate of 10°μm thick; the artificial membrane is hexadecane, and the recommended incubation time is 4–6 hours. (Courtesy of Millipore Corporation, Billerica, MA.)

3. Add 300 μL of buffer with 5% dimethylsulfoxide (DMSO) at the desired pH to the acceptor plate.
4. Place donor plate into the acceptor plate, making sure that the underside of the membrane is in contact with the buffer.
5. Dissolve drugs of interest to the desired concentration. Add 150 μL of the drug at the desired concentration in 5% DMSO/phosphate buffer saline (PBS) at the desired pH to each well in the donor plate.
6. Cover and incubate at room temperature for 4–6 hours.
7. Transfer 100 μL/well from the donor plate and 250 μL/well from the acceptor plate to separate ultraviolet (UV)/visible (Vis) compatible plates, and measure the UV/Vis absorption from 250 to 500 nm (SPECTRAmax® plate reader, Molecular Devices) for both plates.
8. Prepare drug solutions at the theoretical equilibrium (i.e., the resulting concentration if the donor and acceptor solutions were simply combined), and measure UV/Vis absorption from 250 to 500 nm for 250 μL/well of each.
9. Calculate log P_e and membrane retention using Eq. 5.11:

$$\log P_e = \log\left\{C* - \ln\left\{1 - \frac{[\text{drug}]_{\text{acceptor}}}{[\text{drug}]_{\text{equlibrium}}}\right\}\right\} \text{where}$$

(5.11)

$$C = \left\{\frac{V_D * V_A}{(V_D + V_A)\,\text{area}*\text{time}}\right\}$$

5.3.2 Parallel Artificial Membrane Permeability Analysis

Early drug discovery ADME (absorption and distribution in the body, metabolism and elimination from the body) assays, such as fast Caco-2 screens, can help in rejecting test compounds that lack good pharmaceutical profiles. The parallel artificial membrane permeability analysis (PAMPA), a cost-effective, high-throughput method that uses a phospholipid artificial membrane that models the passive transport of epithelial cells, is becoming increasingly popular. The PAMPA assay utilizes a range of lipid components that model a variety of different plasma membranes. The support membrane is 0.45 μm hydrophobic polyvinylidene fluoride, with a thickness of 130 μm, and the artificial membrane is lecithin in dodecane; recommended incubation time is 16–24 hours. The protocol is as follows:

1. Dissolve drugs of interest to the desired concentration.
2. Add 300 μL of the buffer with 5% DMSO at the desired pH to the acceptor plate.
3. Into each well, add 5 μL of lipids in organic solvent (e.g., 2% lecithin in dodecane).
4. Add 150 μL of the drug at the desired pH and concentration in 5% DMSO/PBS to each well in the donor plate.
5. Place donor plate into the acceptor plate, making sure that the underside of the membrane is in contact with the buffer. Steps 3–5 should be completed quickly, within 10 minutes.
6. Cover and incubate at room temperature for 16–24 hours.
7. Transfer 100 μL/well from the donor plate and 250 μL/well from the acceptor plate to separate UV/Vis compatible plates, and measure the UV/Vis absorption from 250 to 500 nm (SPECTRAmax plate reader, Molecular Devices) for both plates.
8. Prepare drug solutions at the theoretical equilibrium (i.e., the resulting concentration if the donor and acceptor solutions were simply combined), and measure UV/Vis absorption from 250 to 500 nm for 250 μL/well of each.
9. Calculate log P_e and membrane retention using Eq. 5.11, described earlier.

The permeability and PAMPA assays, as described, are robust and reproducible assays for determining passive, transcellular compound permeability. Permeability and PAMPA are automation compatible, relatively fast (4–16 hours), inexpensive, and straightforward, and their results correlate with human drug absorption values from published methods. The PAMPA assay provides the benefits of a more biologically relevant system. It is also possible to tailor the lipophilic constituents, so that they mimic specific membranes, such as the blood–brain barrier (BBB). Optimization of incubation time, lipid mixture, and lipid concentration will also enhance the assay's ability to predict compound permeability.

Modifications of the permeability and PAMPA systems have been reported, for example, using the pION PAMPA Evolution 96 System with double-sink and gut-box (2) as a new surrogate assay that predicts the GI tract absorption of candidate drug molecules at different pH conditions. Using Beckman Coulter's Biomek FX Single-Bridge Laboratory Automation Workstation PAMPA Assay System that features a

30-minute incubation time and an on-deck integrated gut-box and a SpectraMax microplate spectrophotometer, the permeability coefficients of drug standards with diverse physiochemical properties can be compared from both the PAMPA and Caco-2 assays. It is automated using the Biomek FX Workstation.

These automated assays can be used for high-throughput ADME screening in early drug discovery. The double-sink PAMPA permeability assay mimics in vivo conditions, using a chemical sink in the acceptor wells and pH gradient in the donor wells. The use of the pION gut-box integrated on the deck has shortened the PAMPA assay incubation time to 30 minutes. The permeability coefficient and rank order correlate well with the data obtained using the in vitro Caco-2 assay and in vivo permeability properties measured in rat intestinal perfusions.

5.3.3 Caco-2 Drug Transport Assays

Drug absorption generally occurs through passive transcellular or paracellular diffusion, active carrier transport, or active efflux mechanisms. Several methods have been developed to aid in the understanding of the absorption of new lead compounds. The most common ones use an immortalized cell line (e.g., Caco-2, Madin-Darby canine kidney, and the like) to mimic the intestinal epithelium. These in vitro models provide more predictive permeability information than the artificial membrane systems (i.e., PAMPA and permeability assays, described previously), based on the cells' ability to promote (active transport) or resist (efflux) transport. Various in vitro methods are listed in the U.S. FDA guidelines. These are acceptable to evaluate the permeability of a drug substance and include a monolayer of suitable epithelial cells, and one such epithelial cell line that has been widely used as a model system of intestinal permeability is the Caco-2 cell line.

The kinetics of intestinal drug absorption, permeation enhancement, chemical moiety structure–permeability relationships, dissolution testing, in vitro–in vivo correlation, bioequivalence, and the development of novel polymeric materials are closely associated with the concept of Caco-2. As most drugs are known to absorb via intestines without using cellular pumps, passive permeability models came into the limelight. In a typical Caco-2 experiment, a monolayer of cells is grown on a filter separating two stacked micro-well plates. The permeability of drugs through the cells is determined after the introduction of a drug on one side of the filter. The entire process is automated, and when used in conjunction with chromatography and/or mass spectroscopy (MS) detection, it enables any drug's permeability to be determined. The method requires careful sample analysis to calculate permeability correctly. Limitations of Caco-2 experiments are 21 days for preparing a stable monolayer and stringent storage conditions; however, tight-junction formation prior to use is a better choice. The villus in the small intestine contains more than one cell type; the Caco-2 cell line does not produce the mucus, as observed in the small intestine, and no P-450 metabolizing enzyme activity has been found in the Caco-2 cell line. Test compound solubility may pose a problem in Caco-2 assays because of the assay conditions. Finally, Caco-2 cells also contain endogenous transporter and efflux systems, the latter of which works against the permeability process and can complicate data interpretation for some drugs.

The Caco-2 cell line is heterogeneous and was derived from a human colorectal adenocarcinoma. Caco-2 cells are used as in vitro permeability models to predict human intestinal absorption, because they exhibit many features of absorptive intestinal cells. This includes their ability to spontaneously differentiate into polarized enterocytes that express high levels of brush border hydrolases and form well-developed junctional complexes. Consequently, it becomes possible to determine whether passage is transcellular or paracellular, based on a compound's transport rate. Caco-2 cells also express a variety of transport systems, including dipeptide transporters and P-glycoproteins (Pgp). Owing to these features, drug permeability in Caco-2 cells correlates well with human oral absorption, making Caco-2 an ideal in vitro permeability model. Additional information can be gained on metabolism and potential drug–drug interactions as the drug undergoes transcellular diffusion through the Caco-2 transport model.

Although accurate and well researched, the Caco-2 cell model requires a high investment of time and resources. Depending on a number of factors, including initial seeding density, culturing conditions, and passage number, Caco-2 cells can take as much as 20 days to reach confluence and achieve full differentiation. During this 20-day period, they require manual or automated exchange of media as frequently as every other day. The transport assays consume valuable drug compounds and normally require expensive, post-transport sample analyses (e.g., liquid chromatography [LC]/MS). Therefore, the use of the Caco-2 transport model in a high-throughput laboratory setting is possible only if the platform is robust, automation compatible, and reproducible and provides high-quality data that correlate well with established methodologies.

The Millipore MultiScreen Caco-2 assay system is a reliable 96-well platform for predicting human oral absorption of drug compounds (using Caco-2 cells or other cell lines whose drug transport properties have been well characterized). The MultiScreen system format is automation compatible and is designed to offer more cost-effective and high-throughput screening (HTS) of drugs than a 24-well system. The MultiScreen Caco-2 assay system exhibits good uniformity of cell growth and drug permeability across all 96 wells and low variability between production lots.

The plate design supports the use of lower volumes of expensive media and reduced amounts of test compounds. Using the MultiScreen Caco-2 assay system, standard drug compounds are successfully categorized as either "high" or "low" permeable, as defined by the FDA, and the permeability data correlate well with the established human absorption values. The components of the Caco-2 assay system are shown in Figure 5.5.

The apparent permeability (P_{app}), in units of centimeters per second, can be calculated for Caco-2 drug transport assays by using the following equation:

$$P_{app} = \left(\frac{V_A}{area * time} \right) * \left(\frac{[drug]_{acceptor}}{[drug]_{initial,donor}} \right) \tag{5.12}$$

where V_A is the volume (in mL) in the acceptor well, area is the surface area of the membrane (0.11 cm^2 for MultiScreen Caco-2 plate and 0.3 cm^2 for the 24-well plate), and time is the total transport time in seconds. For radio-labeled drug transport experiments, the counters per minute units obtained from the Trilux Multiwell

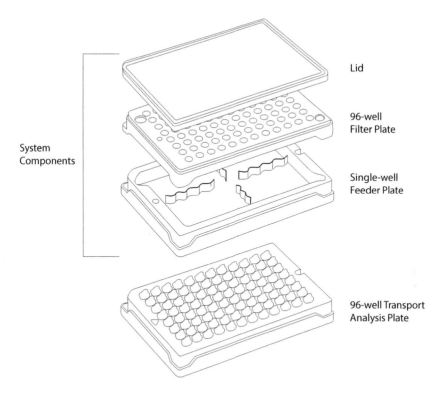

FIGURE 5.5 MultiScreen Caco-2 assay system. Components with single-well feeder plate and 96-well transport analysis plate. (Courtesy of Millipore Corporation, Billerica, MA.)

Plate Scintillation Counter are used directly for the drug acceptor and the initial concentrations such that the formula becomes:

$$P_{app} = \left(\frac{V_A}{area * time} \right) * \left(\frac{CPM_{acceptor}}{CPM_{initial,donor}} \right) \tag{5.13}$$

Historically, it has been shown that a sigmoidal relationship exists between drug absorption rates, as measured with the in vitro Caco-2 model and human absorption:

$$\% \text{ human absorption} = 100 \times \exp(a + b \times P_{app}) / \tag{5.14}$$
$$[1 + \exp(a + b \times P_{app})]$$

Caco-2 cells are heterogeneous, and their properties in final culture may differ based on the selection pressures of a particular laboratory. A direct comparison of compound permeability rates between laboratories is not possible unless the same Caco-2 cells and conditions are used. Therefore, transport rates and permeability classification ranges of specific drugs are expected to vary between reported studies. Most important is the ability to successfully classify compounds as low-, medium-, or high-permeable drugs and to produce transport results that correlate to established human absorption values.

Several modifications of Caco-2 cell model have been tested; for example, CYP3A4-transfected Caco-2 cells are also used to define the biochemical absorption barriers. Oral bioavailability and intestinal drug absorption can be significantly limited by metabolizing enzymes and efflux transporters in the gut. The most prevalent oxidative drug-metabolizing enzyme present in the intestine is cytochrome P4503A4 (CYP3A4). Currently, more than 50% of the drugs in the market metabolized by P450 enzymes are metabolized by CYP3A4. Oral absorption of CYP3A4 substrates can also be limited by the MDR transporter Pgp, as there is extensive substrate overlap between these two proteins. Pgp is an ATP-dependent transporter on the apical plasma membrane of enterocytes that functions to limit the entry of drugs into the cell. There is a significant interaction between CYP3A4 and Pgp in the intestine. Although Caco-2 cells express a variety of uptake and efflux transporters found in the human intestine, a major drawback to the use of Caco-2 cells is that they lack CYP3A4. As such, no data regarding the importance of intestinal metabolism on limiting drug absorption can be obtained from normal Caco-2 cells. Caco-2 cells pretreated with 1,25-dihydroxyvitamin-D3 (vitamin D3) express higher levels of CYP3A4 compared with Caco-2 but still underestimate the amount of CYP3A4 in the human intestine. In the CYP3A4-transfected Caco-2 cells, Pgp can enhance the metabolism of orally dosed drugs by repeated cycling of the drug at the apical membrane.

5.3.4 Animal Model Testing

The quantity of substance available at the preformulation stages is generally small; however, in some instances, early animal testing for absorption potential is needed, particularly if the solid form of the new drug offers many options, such as amorphous forms, solvates, and so on. The absorption models used in animals are well described and will not be discussed here. Establishing good in vitro–in vivo correlation (IVIVC) at this stage proves useful because of a limited access to sufficient compounds to run the entire absorption profiles. The IVIVC analysis can be made extensive, or general conclusions can be drawn from limited studies; the choice depends on the amount of compound available and the nature or robustness of correlation observed.

5.3.5 In Vitro–In Vivo Correlation

The selection of a drug candidate marks the most crucial stage in the life cycle of drug development. Such selection is primarily based on the drug "developability" criteria, which include physicochemical properties of the drug and the results obtained from preliminary studies involving several in vitro systems and in vivo animal models, which address the efficacy and toxicity issues. During this stage, exploring the relationship between in vitro and in vivo properties of the drug in animal models provides an idea about the feasibility of the drug delivery system for a given drug. In such correlations, study designs, including study of more than one formulation of the modified-release dosage forms and a rank order of release (fast/slow) of the formulations, should be incorporated. Even though the formulations and methods used at this stage are not optimal, they prompt better design and development efforts in the future.

There are four levels of IVIVC that have been described in the FDA guidance, which include levels A, B, C, and multiple C.

- *Level A correlation*: This correlation represents a point-to-point relationship between in vitro dissolution and in vivo dissolution (input/absorption rate). Level A IVIVC is also viewed as a predictive model for the relationship between the entire in vitro release time course and the entire in vivo response time course. In general, correlations are linear at this level. Although a concern of acceptable nonlinear correlation has been addressed, no formal guidance on the nonlinear IVIVC has been established. Level A correlation is the most informative and very useful from a regulatory perspective.

- *Level B correlation*: In Level B correlation, the mean in vivo dissolution or the mean residence time is compared with the mean in vitro dissolution time by using statistical moment analytical methods. This type of correlation uses all in vitro and in vivo data; thus, it is not considered as a point-to-point correlation. This is of limited interest and use because more than one kind of plasma curve produces similar mean residence time.

- *Level C correlation*: This correlation describes a relationship between the amount of drug dissolved (e.g., percent dissolved in 1 hour) at one time point and one pharmacokinetic parameter (e.g., either area under the curve [AUC] or C_{max}). Level C correlation is considered the lowest correlation level, as it does not reflect the complete shape of the plasma concentration time curve. Similarly, a multiple Level C correlation relates one or more pharmacokinetic parameters to the percent drug dissolved at several time points of the dissolution profile and thus may be more useful. Levels B and C correlations can be useful in early formulation development, including the selection of the appropriate excipients and the optimization of manufacturing processes, for quality control purposes, and in the characterization of the release patterns of newly formulated immediate-release and modified-release products relative to the reference.

The most basic IVIVC models are expressed as a simple linear equation between the in vivo drug absorption and in vitro drug dissolved (released):

$$Y \text{ (in vivo absorbed)} = mX \text{ (in vitro drug dissolved)} + C \qquad (5.15)$$

In this equation, m is the slope of the relationship and C is the intercept. Ideally, $m = 1$ and C = 0, indicating a linear relationship. However, depending on the nature of the modified-release system, some data are better fitted by using nonlinear models, such as Sigmoid, Weibull, Higuchi, and Hixson–Crowell.

In vivo release rate (X'_{vivo}) can also be expressed as a function of in vitro release rate ($X'_{rel,vitro}$), with parameters (a, b), which may be empirically selected and refined by using appropriate mathematical processes:

$$X'_{vivo}(t) = X'_{rel, vitro}(a + bt) \qquad (5.16)$$

An iterative process may be used to compute the time-scaling and time-shifting parameters. Model validation is integral to the model development exercise, and it can be accomplished by using data from the formulations used to build the model (internal validation) or by using data obtained from a different (new) formulation (external validation). While internal validation serves the purpose of providing a basis for the acceptability of the model, external validation is superior and affords greater "confidence" in the model.

Generally, a plot of the fraction of drug absorbed (F_a) against the fraction drug dissolved (F_d) is made, wherein the fraction absorbed is obtained by deconvoluting the plasma profile. Often the goal is to develop a profile that need not a priori be a linear or even a predefined function. For example,

$$F_a = \frac{1}{f_a}\left(1 - \frac{\alpha}{\alpha - 1}(1 - F_d) + \frac{1}{\alpha - 1}(1 - F_d)^\alpha\right) \tag{5.17}$$

where F_a is the fraction of the total amount of drug absorbed at time t, f_a is the fraction of the dose absorbed at $t = \#$, α is the ratio of the apparent first-order permeation rate constant (k_{paap}) to the first-order dissolution rate constant (k_d), and F_d is the fraction of the drug dose dissolved at time t.

5.3.5.1 Internal Validation

Using the IVIVC model, for each formulation, the relevant exposure parameters (C_{max} and AUC) are predicted and compared with the actual (observed) values. The prediction errors are calculated using:

$$\text{Prediction error (\% PE)} = [(C_{max,observed} - C_{max,predicted})/ \tag{5.18}$$
$$C_{max,observed}] \times 100$$

The C_{max} can be replaced with corresponding AUC. The criteria set in the FDA guidance on IVIVC are as follows: for C_{max} and AUC, the mean absolute percent prediction error (% PE) should not exceed 10%, and the PE for individual formulations should not exceed 15%.

For establishing external predictability, the exposure parameters for a new formulation are predicted using its in vitro dissolution profile and the IVIVC model, and the predicted parameters are compared with the observed parameters. The PEs are computed as for the internal validation. For C_{max} and AUC, the PE for the external validation formulation should not exceed 10%. A PE of 10–20% indicates inconclusive predictability and illustrates the need for further study, using additional data sets. For drugs with a narrow therapeutic index, external validation is required despite acceptable internal validation, whereas internal validation is usually sufficient with nonnarrow therapeutic index drugs.

Several commercial software programs are available to study IVIVC; for example, PDx-IVIVC (3), which is a comprehensive IVIVC software program that performs deconvolution, calculating the fraction or percentage of drug absorbed and correlating it with in vitro fraction or percent of dissolved data. It also allows Level C correlations (single or multiple), wherein a single-point relationship between a dissolution parameter, for example, percent dissolved in 4 hours and a pharmacokinetic parameter (e.g., AUC, C_{max}, and T_{max}), is determined. A successful IVIVC model can be developed if in vitro dissolution is the rate-limiting step in the sequence of events, leading to the appearance of the drug in the systemic circulation following oral or other routes of administration. Thus, the dissolution test can be utilized as a surrogate for bioequivalence studies (involving human subjects) if the developed IVIVC is predictive of in vivo performance of the product.

5.4 Waiver of In Vivo Bioavailability and Bioequivalence Studies for Immediate-Release Solid Oral Dosage Forms Based on a Biopharmaceutics Classification System: Guidance for Industry[1]

[This section maintains the original FDA document released in December 2017 to allow easy reference; the footnotes refer to the marked footnotes]

Introduction

This guidance provides recommendations for sponsors of investigational new drug applications (INDs), and applicants who submit new drug applications (NDAs), abbreviated new drug applications (ANDAs), and supplements to these applications for immediate-release (IR) solid oral dosage forms, and who wish to request a waiver of an in vivo bioavailability (BA) and/or bioequivalence (BE) study requirement. These recommendations are intended to apply to waivers requested during the IND period and the NDA stage or for ANDAs, i.e., (1) subsequent in vivo BA or BE studies of formulations after the initial establishment of the in vivo BA of IR solid oral dosage forms during the IND period, and (2) in vivo BE studies of IR solid oral dosage forms in NDAs, ANDAs, and supplements to these applications.

Regulations at 21 CFR 320 address the requirements for BA and BE data for approval of NDAs, ANDAs, and supplemental applications. Provision for waivers of in vivo BA/BE studies (biowaivers) under certain conditions is provided at 21 CFR 320.22.[2] This guidance finalizes the guidance for industry on *Waiver of In Vivo Bioavailability and Bioequivalence Studies for Immediate-Release Solid Oral Dosage Forms Based on a Biopharmaceutics Classification System*,[3] published in May 2015, and explains when biowaivers can be requested for IR solid oral dosage forms based on an approach

---

[1] This guidance has been prepared by the Office of Pharmaceutical Quality and the Office of Translational Sciences in the Center for Drug Evaluation and Research (CDER) at the Food and Drug Administration.

[2] In addition to waiver of an in vivo BE requirement under 21 CFR 320.22, there are certain circumstances in which BE can be evaluated using in vitro approaches under 21 CFR 320.24(b)(6). The scientific principles described in this guidance regarding waiver of an in vivo requirement also apply to consideration of in vitro data under that regulation. In such circumstances, an in vivo data requirement is not waived, but rather, FDA has determined that in vitro data is the most accurate, sensitive, and reproducible for a product, as required under 21 CFR 320.24(a).

Nonetheless, for ease of the reader, in this guidance we will refer to either the decision to waive an in vivo BE requirement under 21 CFR 320.22 or the decision to accept in vitro BE data in accordance with 21 CFR 320.24(a) as a "biowaiver."

[3] We update guidances periodically. To make sure you have the most recent version of a guidance, check the FDA Drugs guidance web page at http://www.fda.gov/Drugs/GuidanceComplianceRegulatory Information/Guidances/default.htm.

termed the Biopharmaceutics Classification System (BCS).[4] This guidance includes biowaiver extension to BCS class 3 drug products, and additional modifications, such as criteria for high permeability and high solubility.

In general, FDA's guidance documents do not establish legally enforceable responsibilities. Instead, guidances describe the Agency's current thinking on a topic and should be viewed only as recommendations, unless specific regulatory or statutory requirements are cited. The use of the word *should* in Agency guidances means that something is suggested or recommended, but not required.

The Biopharmaceutics Classification System

[Note: This section uses a different numbering system]

The BCS is a scientific framework for classifying drug substances based on their aqueous solubility and intestinal permeability. When combined with the dissolution of the drug product, the BCS takes into account three major factors that govern the rate and extent of drug absorption from IR solid oral dosage forms: (1) dissolution, (2) solubility, and (3) intestinal permeability.[5]

According to the BCS, drug substances are classified as follows:

Class 1: High Solubility—High Permeability
Class 2: Low Solubility—High Permeability
Class 3: High Solubility—Low Permeability
Class 4: Low Solubility—Low Permeability

In addition, some IR solid oral dosage forms are categorized as having rapid or very rapid[6] dissolution. Within this framework, when certain criteria are met, the BCS can be used as a drug development tool to help sponsors/applicants justify requests for biowaivers.

Observed in vivo differences in the rate and extent of absorption of a drug from two pharmaceutically equivalent solid oral products may be due to differences in drug dissolution in vivo.[4] However, when the in vivo dissolution of an IR solid oral dosage form is rapid or very rapid in relation to gastric emptying and the drug has high solubility, the rate and extent of drug absorption is unlikely to be dependent on drug dissolution and/or GI transit time. Under such circumstances, demonstration of in vivo BA or BE may not be necessary for drug products containing class 1 and class 3 drug substances, as long as the inactive ingredients used in the dosage form do not significantly affect absorption of the active ingredients.

---

[4] See *The Biopharmaceutics Classification System (BCS) Guidance* at: http://www.fda.gov/aboutfda/centersoffices/officeofmedicalproductsandtobacco/cder/ucm128219.htm.
[5] Amidon GL, Lennernäs H, Shah VP, and Crison JR, 1995, A Theoretical Basis for a Biopharmaceutics Drug Classification: The Correlation of In Vitro Drug Product Dissolution and In Vivo Bioavailability, Pharm Res, 12: 413–420.
[6] Yu LX, Amidon GL, Polli JE, Zhao H, Mehta MU, Conner DP et al, 2002, Biopharmaceutics classification system: The scientific basis for biowaiver extensions, Pharm Res, 19(7):921–5.

The BCS approach outlined in this guidance can be used to justify biowaivers for highly soluble and highly permeable drug substances (i.e., class 1) as well as highly soluble and low permeable drug substances (i.e., class 3) in IR solid oral dosage forms that exhibit rapid or very rapid in vitro dissolution using the recommended test methods. The recommended methods for determining solubility, permeability, and in vitro dissolution are discussed below.

Solubility

The solubility class boundary is based on the highest strength of an IR product that is the subject of a biowaiver request. A drug substance is considered *highly soluble* when the highest strength is soluble in 250 mL or less of aqueous media within the pH range of 1–6.8 at 37°C $\pm$ 1°C. The volume estimate of 250 mL is derived from typical BE study protocols that prescribe administration of a drug product to fasting human volunteers with an 8-fluid ounce glass of water.

Permeability

The permeability class boundary is based indirectly on the extent of absorption (fraction of dose absorbed, not systemic BA) of a drug substance in humans, and directly on measurements of the rate of mass transfer across human intestinal membrane. Alternatively, other systems capable of predicting the extent of drug absorption in humans can be used (e.g., in situ animal, in vitro epithelial cell culture methods). A drug substance is considered to be *highly permeable* when the systemic BA or the extent of absorption in humans is determined to be 85% or more of an administered dose based on a mass balance determination (along with evidence showing stability of the drug in the GI tract) or in comparison to an intravenous reference dose.

Dissolution[7]

An IR drug product is considered *rapidly dissolving* when a mean of 85% or more of the labeled amount of the drug substance dissolves within 30 minutes, using *United States Pharmacopeia* (USP) Apparatus 1 at 100 rpm or Apparatus 2 at 50 rpm (or at 75 rpm when appropriately justified (see section III.C.) in a volume of 500 mL or less (or 900 mL when appropriately justified) in each of the following media: (1) 0.1 N HCl or Simulated Gastric Fluid USP without enzymes; (2) a pH 4.5 buffer; and (3) a pH 6.8 buffer or Simulated Intestinal Fluid USP without enzymes.

An IR product is considered *very rapidly dissolving* when a mean of 85% or more of the labeled amount of the drug substance dissolves within 15 minutes, using the above-mentioned conditions.

---

[7] See also the draft guidance for industry *Dissolution Testing of Immediate Release Solid Oral Dosage Forms*. When final, this guidance will represent the FDA's current thinking on this topic.

Recommended Methodology for Classifying a Drug Substance and for Determining the Dissolution Characteristics of a Drug Product

The following approaches are recommended for classifying a drug substance and determining the dissolution characteristics of an IR drug product according to the BCS.

Determining Drug Substance Solubility Class

An objective of the BCS approach is to determine the equilibrium solubility of a drug substance under physiological pH conditions. The pH-solubility profile of the test drug substance should be determined at 37°C ± 1°C in aqueous media with a pH in the range of 1–6.8. A sufficient number of pH conditions should be evaluated to accurately define the pH-solubility profile within the pH range of 1–6.8. The number of pH conditions for a solubility determination can be based on the ionization characteristics of the test drug substance to include pH = pKa, pH = pKa + 1, pH = pKa − 1, and at pH = 1 and 6.8. A sufficient number of pH conditions should be determined for both ionizable and non-ionizable compounds. A minimum of three replicate determinations of solubility in each pH condition is recommended. Depending on study variability, additional replicates may be necessary to provide a reliable estimate of solubility.

Standard buffer solutions described in the USP are considered appropriate for use in solubility studies. If these buffers are not suitable for physical or chemical reasons, other buffer solutions can be used with justification. Solution pH should be verified (measured and adjusted to the target pH if required) after addition of the drug substance to a buffer. Solution pH should also be measured at the end of the equilibrium solubility study.

Methods other than the traditional shake-flask method, such as acid or base titration methods, can also be used with justification supporting the ability of such methods to predict equilibrium solubility of the test drug substance. The concentration of the drug substance in selected buffers (or pH conditions) should be determined using a validated stability-indicating assay that can distinguish the drug substance from its degradation products.[8] If degradation of the drug substance is observed as a function of buffer composition and/or pH, it should be reported. The solubility class should be determined by calculating the volume of an aqueous medium sufficient to dissolve the highest strength in the pH range of 1–6.8. A drug substance should be classified as highly soluble when the highest strength is soluble in ≤250 mL of aqueous media over the pH range of 1–6.8. In other words, the highest strength divided by 250 should be less than or equal to the lowest solubility observed over the entire pH range of 1–6.8.

For drug products where the highest single dose administered is higher than the highest strength, additional information may be necessary. If the solubility classification is likely to change with the highest single dose as criterion, additional PK dose proportionality information in a wide dose range covering the therapeutic dose range will be necessary.

---

[8] Refer to the guidance for industry *Submitting Documentation for the Stability of Human Drugs and Biologics*.

Determining Drug Substance Permeability Class

The permeability class of a drug substance can be determined via human pharmacokinetic studies (mass balance, or absolute BA) which are preferred methods, or through in vivo intestinal perfusion in human subjects. Alternatively, methods not involving human subjects, which include in vivo or in situ intestinal perfusion in a suitable animal model (e.g., rats), and in vitro permeability methods using excised intestinal tissues, or monolayers of suitable epithelial cells, may also be used.

A single method may be sufficient: (i) when the absolute BA is 85% or more, or (ii) when 85% or more of the administered drug is excreted unchanged in urine, or (iii) when 85% or more of the administered drug is recovered in urine as parent and metabolites with evidence indicating stability in the GI tract. When a single method fails to conclusively demonstrate a permeability classification, two different methods may be advisable. In case of conflicting information from different types of studies, it is important to note that human data supersede in vitro or animal data.

Pharmacokinetic Studies in Humans

Mass Balance Studies   Pharmacokinetic (PK) mass balance studies using unlabeled, stable isotopes or a radiolabeled drug substance can be used to document the extent of absorption of a drug. A sufficient number of subjects should be enrolled to provide a reliable estimate of extent of absorption.

When mass balance studies are used to demonstrate high permeability, additional data to document the drug's stability in the GI tract is required, unless 85% or more of the drug is excreted unchanged in urine. Please see method details in section III.B.3.

Absolute Bioavailability Studies   Oral BA determination using intravenous administration as a reference can be used. Depending on the variability of the studies, a sufficient number of subjects should be enrolled in a study to provide a reliable estimate of the extent of absorption. When the absolute BA of a drug is shown to be 85% or more, additional data to document drug stability in the GI fluid is not necessary.

Intestinal Permeability Methods

The following methods can be used to determine the permeability of a drug substance from the GI tract: (1) in vivo intestinal perfusion studies in humans; (2) in vivo or in situ intestinal perfusion studies using suitable animal models; (3) in vitro permeation studies using excised human or animal intestinal tissues; or (4) in vitro permeation studies across a monolayer of cultured epithelial cells.

In vivo or in situ animal models and in vitro methods, such as those using cultured monolayers of animal or human epithelial cells, are considered appropriate for passively transported drugs. The observed low permeability of some drug substances in humans could be caused by efflux of drugs via membrane efflux transporters such as P-glycoprotein (P-gp), breast cancer resistance protein (BCRP) and/or multidrug resistance associated protein 2 (MRP2). When the efflux transporters are absent in these models, or their degree of expression is low compared to that in humans, there may be a greater likelihood of misclassification of permeability class for a drug subject to efflux compared to a drug transported passively. Expression of known transporters in selected study systems should be characterized. Functional expression of efflux systems (e.g., P-gp, BCRP, MRP2) can be demonstrated with techniques such as bidirectional transport studies, demonstrating a higher rate of transport in the basolateral-to-apical direction as compared to apical-to-basolateral direction (efflux ratio >2)[9,10] using selected model drugs or chemicals at concentrations that do not saturate the efflux system (e.g., digoxin, vinblastine, rhodamine 123, and methotrexate). The use of animal or in vitro permeability test methods is recommended only for drug substances that are transported by passive mechanisms (efflux ratio of the test drug should be <2). PK studies on dose linearity or proportionality may provide useful information for evaluating the relevance of observed in vitro efflux of a drug. For example, there may be fewer concerns associated with the use of in vitro methods for a drug that has a higher rate of transport in the basolateral-to-apical direction at low drug concentrations but exhibits linear PK in humans.

For BCS-based permeability determination, an apparent passive transport mechanism can be assumed when one of the following conditions is satisfied:

A proportional relationship between the dose (e.g., relevant clinical dose range) and measures of BA (area under the concentration-time curve) or linear PK of a drug is demonstrated in humans.

Lack of dependence of the measured in vivo or in situ permeability is demonstrated in an animal model on initial drug concentration (e.g., 0.01, 0.1, and 1 times the highest strength dissolved in 250 mL) in the perfusion fluid.

Lack of dependence of the measured in vitro permeability on initial drug concentration (e.g., 0.01, 0.1, and 1 times the highest strength dissolved in 250 mL) is demonstrated, or lack of dependence on transport direction (i.e., efflux ratio 0.5–2) using a suitable in vitro cell culture method that has been shown to express known efflux transporters (e.g., Pgp, BCRP, and MRP2).

METHOD SUITABILITY: One of the critical steps in using in vivo or in situ perfusion, or in vitro permeability methods for permeability classification is to demonstrate the suitability of the method. To demonstrate suitability of a permeability method intended for BCS-based permeability determination, a rank-order relationship between experimental permeability values and the extent of drug absorption data in human subjects should be established using a sufficient number of model drugs. For in vivo intestinal perfusion studies in humans, six model drugs are recommended. For in vivo or in situ intestinal perfusion studies in animals, and for in vitro tissue or cell monolayer methods, twenty model drugs are recommended. Depending on study variability, a sufficient number of subjects, animals, excised tissue samples, or cell monolayers should be used in a study to provide a reliable estimate of drug permeability (e.g., a minimum of three per group). This relationship should allow accurate differentiation between drug substances of low and high intestinal permeability attributes.

To demonstrate the suitability of a method, model drugs should represent a range of zero, low (e.g., <50%), moderate (e.g., 50%–84%), and high (≥85%) absorption.

---

[9] KM Giacomini, SM Huang, DJ Tweedie, LZ Benet, KLR Brouwer, X Chu, A Dahlin, R Evers, V Fischer et al. March 2010, The International Transporter Consortium, Membrane transporters in drug development, *Nature Reviews Drug Discovery*, 9:215–236.

[10] See the guidance for industry *Drug Interaction Studies—Study Design, Data Analysis, Implications for Dosing, and Labeling Recommendations*. When final, this guidance will represent the FDA's current thinking on this topic.

Sponsors/applicants may select compounds from the list of drugs and/or chemicals provided in Attachment A, or they may select other drugs for which there is information available on mechanism of absorption and reliable estimates of the extent of drug absorption in humans.

For a given test method with set conditions, selection of a high permeability internal standard with permeability in close proximity to the low/high permeability class boundary may be used to facilitate classification of a test drug substance. For instance, a test drug substance may be determined to be highly permeable when its permeability value is equal to or greater than that of the selected internal standard with high permeability.

After demonstrating suitability of a method and maintaining the same study protocol, it is not necessary to retest all selected model drugs for subsequent studies intended to classify a drug substance. Instead, a low and a high permeability model drug should be used as internal standards (i.e., included in the perfusion fluid or donor fluid along with the test drug substance). These two internal standards are in addition to the fluid volume marker (or a zero-permeability compound such as PEG 4000) that is included in certain types of perfusion techniques (e.g., closed loop techniques). The choice of internal standards should be based on compatibility with the test drug substance (i.e., they should not exhibit any significant physical, chemical, or permeation interactions). When it is not feasible to follow this protocol, the permeability of internal standards should be determined in the same subjects, animals, tissues, or monolayers, following (or, if appropriate, in parallel to) evaluation of the test drug substance. The permeability values of the two internal standards should not differ substantially between experiments conducted to demonstrate the assay's method suitability and those for the test drug. For example, the laboratory may set acceptance criteria for the permeability values of its high, low, and zero permeability standard compounds.

At the end of an in vitro test, the amount of drug in the tissue or cell monolayer, apical and basolateral chambers should be determined to assist in calculation of mass balance. If recovery from the apical and basolateral chambers is >80%, there is no need to measure drug in the tissue or cell monolayers.

When intestinal permeability methods are used to demonstrate high permeability, additional data to document the drug's stability in the GI tract is required. Please see method details in section III.B.3.

Instability in the Gastrointestinal Tract

Determining the extent of absorption in humans based on mass balance studies using total radioactivity in urine does not take into consideration the extent of degradation of a drug in the GI fluid prior to intestinal membrane permeation. In addition, some methods for determining permeability could be based on loss or clearance of a drug from fluids perfused into the human and/or animal GI tract either in vivo or in situ. Documenting the fact that drug loss from the GI tract arises from intestinal membrane permeation, rather than a degradation process, will help establish permeability. Stability in the GI tract may be documented using simulated gastric and intestinal fluids. Obtaining GI fluids from human subjects requires intubation and may be difficult. Stability in the GI tract may therefore be documented using simulated gastric and intestinal fluids such as Gastric and Intestinal Fluids USP or, with suitable justification, other biorelevant media.

Drug solutions in these fluids should be incubated at 37°C for a period that is representative of in vivo drug contact with these fluids, for example, one hour in gastric fluid and three hours in intestinal fluid. Drug concentrations should then be determined using a validated stability- indicating assay method. Significant degradation (>5%) of a drug in this study could suggest potential instability.

Determining Drug Product Dissolution Characteristics and Dissolution Profile Similarity[7]

Dissolution testing should be carried out in USP Apparatus 1 (typically at 100 rpm) or USP Apparatus 2 (typically at 50 rpm, or at 75 rpm when appropriately justified) using 500 mL (or 900 mL with appropriate justification) of the following dissolution media: (1) 0.1 N HCl or Simulated Gastric Fluid USP without enzymes; (2) a pH 4.5 buffer; and (3) a pH 6.8 buffer or Simulated Intestinal Fluid USP without enzymes. For gelatin capsules and tablets with gelatin coating, Simulated Gastric and Intestinal Fluids USP (with enzymes) can be used.

The dissolution testing apparatus used in this evaluation should conform to the requirements in USP (<711> Dissolution) and FDA's guidance on Mechanical Calibration of Dissolution Apparatus 1 and 2.[11] Selection of the dissolution testing apparatus (USP Apparatus 1 or 2) during drug development should be based on a comparison of in vitro dissolution and in vivo PK data available for the product. The USP Apparatus 1 (*basket method*) is generally preferred for capsules and products that tend to float, and USP Apparatus 2 (*paddle method*) is generally preferred for tablets. For some tablet dosage forms, in vitro (but not in vivo) dissolution may be slow due to the manner in which the disintegrated product settles at the bottom of a dissolution vessel. In such situations, USP Apparatus 1 may be preferred over Apparatus 2, or alternatively, rotation speed for Apparatus 2 may be modified with justification. If the testing conditions need to be modified to better reflect rapid in vivo dissolution (e.g., use of a different rotating speed), such modifications can be justified by comparing in vitro dissolution with in vivo absorption data (e.g., a relative BA study using a simple aqueous solution as the reference product).

A minimum of 12 dosage units of the test and reference drug product for each strength should be evaluated to support a biowaiver request. Samples should be collected at a sufficient number of intervals to characterize the entire dissolution profile of the drug product (e.g., 5, 10, 15, 20, and 30 minutes).

When comparing the test and reference products, dissolution profiles should be compared using a similarity factor (f2).

$$f2 = 50 \bullet \log \{[1 + (1/n)\Sigma t \; n \; (Rt - Tt)2] - 0.5 \bullet 100\}$$

The similarity factor is a logarithmic reciprocal square root transformation of the sum of squared error and is a measurement of the similarity in the percent of dissolution between the two curves; where n is the number of time points, Rt is the dissolution value of the reference batch at time t, and Tt is the dissolution value of the test batch at time t.

---

[11] See the guidance for industry *The Use of Mechanical Calibration of Dissolution Apparatus 1 and 2—Current Good Manufacturing Practice (CGMP)*.

Two dissolution profiles are considered similar when the f2 value is ≥50. To allow the use of mean data, the coefficient of variation should not be more than 20% at the earlier time points (e.g., 15 minutes), and should not be more than 10% at other time points. Only one measurement should be considered after 85% dissolution of both products. In addition, when both test and reference products dissolve 85% or more of the label amount of the drug in 15 minutes using all three dissolution media recommended above, the profile comparison with an f2 test is unnecessary.

Biowaivers Based on BCS

This guidance is applicable for BA/BE waivers (biowaivers) based on BCS, for BCS class 1 and class 3 IR solid oral dosage forms.

For BCS class 1 drug products, the following should be demonstrated:

The drug substance is highly soluble

The drug substance is highly permeable

The drug product (test and reference) is rapidly dissolving, and

The product does not contain any excipients that will affect the rate or extent of absorption of the drug

For BCS class 3 drug products, the following should be demonstrated:

The drug substance is highly soluble

The drug product (test and reference) is very rapidly dissolving, and

The test product formulation is qualitatively the same and quantitatively very similar

Additional Considerations for Requesting a Biowaiver

When requesting a BCS-based biowaiver for in vivo BA/BE studies for IR solid oral dosage forms, sponsors/applicants should note that the following factors can affect their request or the documentation of their request.

Excipients

BCS class 1 drug products: Excipients can sometimes affect the rate and extent of drug absorption. In general, using excipients that are currently in FDA-approved IR solid oral dosage forms will not affect the rate or extent of absorption of a highly soluble and highly permeable drug substance that is formulated in a rapidly dissolving IR product. To support a biowaiver request, the quantity of excipients in the IR drug product should be consistent with the intended function (e.g., lubricant). When new excipients or atypically large amounts of commonly used excipients are included in an IR solid dosage form, additional information documenting the absence of an impact on BA of the drug may be requested by the Agency. Such information can be provided with a relative BA study using a simple aqueous solution as the reference product. Excessive quantities of certain excipients, such as surfactants (e.g., polysorbate 80) and sweeteners (e.g., mannitol or sorbitol) may be problematic, and sponsors/applicants are encouraged to contact the review division[12] when this is a factor.

BCS class 3 drug products: Unlike for BCS class 1 products, for a bio-waiver to be scientifically justified, BCS class 3 test drug product must contain the same excipients as the reference product. This is due to the concern that excipients can have a greater impact on absorption of low permeability drugs. The composition of the test product must be quali-tatively the same (except for a different color, flavor, or preservative that could not affect the BA) and should be quantitatively very similar to the reference product. Quantitatively very similar includes the following allowable differences:

Changes in the Technical Grade of an Excipient

Changes in excipients, expressed as percent (w/w) of the total formulation less than or equal to the following percent ranges:

Filler ($\pm 10\%$)

Disintegrant, Starch ($\pm 6\%$); Disintegrant, Other ($\pm 2\%$); Binder ($\pm 1\%$)

Lubricant, Calcium or Magnesium Stearate ($\pm 0.5\%$)

Lubricant, Other ($\pm 2\%$)

Glidant, Talc ($\pm 2\%$)

Glidant, Other ($\pm 0.2\%$)

Film Coat ($\pm 2\%$)

The total additive effect of all excipient changes should not be more than 10%.

Prodrugs

Permeability of prodrugs will generally depend on the mechanism and (anatomical) site of conversion to the drug substance. When the prodrug-to-drug (i.e., active moiety) conversion is shown to occur predominantly after intestinal membrane permeation, the permeability of the prodrug should be measured. When this conversion occurs prior to intestinal permeation, the permeability of the drug should be determined. Dissolution and pH-solubility data on both prodrug and drug can be relevant. Sponsors may wish to consult with appropriate review staff[12] before applying the BCS approach to IR products containing prodrugs.

---

[12] When the submission is for an NDA, contact the specific drug product's review division with questions. When the submission is for an ANDA, submit a Controlled Correspondence via email to GenericDrugs@fda.hhs.gov.

Fixed Dose Combinations Containing BCS Class 1, or Class 3, or a Combination of Class 1 and 3 Drugs

If all active components belong to BCS class 1: BCS-based biowaivers are applicable for IR fixed dose combination products if all the drugs in the combination belong to BCS class 1, provided there is no PK interaction[13] between the components, and the excipients fulfill the considerations (i). If there is a PK interaction, the excipients should fulfill the considerations (ii). Otherwise, in vivo bioequivalence testing is required.

If all components of the combination belong to BCS class 3 or a combination of class 1 and 3: BCS-based biowaivers are applicable for IR fixed dose combination products in this situation provided the excipients fulfill the considerations (ii). Otherwise, in vivo bioequivalence testing is required.

For fixed drug combination products where BCS classes 1 or 3 are combined with any other BCS class drugs, this biowaiver approach is not applicable.

Exceptions

BCS-based biowaivers are not applicable for the following:

Narrow Therapeutic Index Drugs[14]

This guidance does not apply to narrow therapeutic index (NTI) drug products because of the critical relationship between the bioavailable dose and clinical performance. Sponsors should contact the appropriate review division[15] to determine whether a drug should be considered to have a narrow therapeutic index.

Products Designed to be Absorbed in the Oral Cavity

A request for a waiver of in vivo BA/BE studies based on the BCS is not appropriate for dosage forms intended for absorption in the oral cavity (e.g., sublingual or buccal tablets). Similarly, a biowaiver based on BCS for an orally disintegrating tablet can be considered only if the absorption from the oral cavity can be ruled out. The sponsor/applicant can discuss the information required to rule out absorption from oral cavity with the Agency.[16]

Regulatory Applications of the BCS–Based Biowaivers

INDs/NDAs

Evidence demonstrating in vivo BA or information to permit FDA to waive this evidence must be included in NDAs (21 CFR 320.21(a)). A specific objective of such BA information is to establish in vivo performance of the dosage form used in the clinical studies that provided primary evidence of efficacy and safety. Sponsors/applicants may

---

[13] See the guidance for industry *Drug Interaction Studies —Study Design, Data Analysis, Implications for Dosing, and Labeling Recommendations*. When final, this guidance will represent the FDA's current thinking on this topic.

[14] This guidance uses the term *narrow therapeutic range* instead of *narrow therapeutic index*, although the latter is more commonly used.

[15] See footnote 12.

[16] Ibid.

wish to determine the relative BA of an IR solid oral dosage form by comparison with an oral solution, suspension, or intravenous injection (21 CFR 320.25(d)(2) and 320.25(d)(3)). The BA of the clinical trial dosage form should be optimized during the IND period.

Once the in vivo BA of a formulation is established during the IND period, waivers of subsequent in vivo BE studies, following changes in components, composition, and/or method of manufacture may be possible using the BCS-based waiver approach. BCS-based biowaivers are applicable to the to-be-marketed formulation when changes in components, composition, and/or method of manufacture occur to the clinical trial formulation, as long as the dosage forms exhibit either rapid or very rapid dissolution (as appropriate), have similar in vitro dissolution profiles (see sections II and III), and for a BCS class 3 IR drug product, it meets the criteria for allowable differences in composition described previously (see section V). This approach is useful only when the drug substance belongs to BCS class 1 or 3, and the formulations pre- and post-change are pharmaceutical equivalents (under the definition at 21 CFR 320.1(c)). BCS-based biowaivers are intended only for subsequent in vivo BA or BE studies. They do not apply to food effect BA studies or other PK studies. BCS-based biowaivers may be applicable for pharmaceutical alternatives including other oral dosage forms (e.g., powders), if appropriately justified. The sponsor should contact the appropriate review division in such situations.

ANDAs

BCS-based biowaivers are appropriate for IR generic drug products that meet the criteria for BCS class 1 or 3 as discussed in section II and III. The proposed drug product (i.e., test product) should exhibit similar dissolution profiles to the reference listed drug product (see sections II and III). The choice of dissolution apparatus (USP Apparatus 1 or 2) should be the same as that established for the reference listed drug product.

Supplemental NDAs/ANDAs (Postapproval Changes)

BCS-based biowaivers are appropriate for postapproval changes in components, composition and manufacturing process for an IR solid oral drug product that meets the criteria for BCS class 1 or 3 as discussed above, and both pre- and post-change products exhibit similar dissolution profiles (see sections II and III). This approach is useful only when the drug products pre- and post- change are pharmaceutical equivalents.

Data to Support a Biowaiver Request

As described above, the drug product for which a biowaiver is being requested should include a drug substance that is highly soluble (BCS class 1 and BCS class 3) and highly permeable (BCS class 1), and the drug product should be rapidly dissolving (BCS class 1) or very rapidly dissolving (BCS class 3). Sponsors/applicants requesting biowaivers based on the BCS should submit the following information to the Agency for review.

Data Supporting High Solubility

Data supporting high solubility of the test drug substance should be developed (see section III.A). The following information should be included in the application:

A description of test methods, including information on analytical method(s) and composition of the buffer solutions.

Information on chemical structure, molecular weight, nature of the drug substance (acid, base, amphoteric, or neutral), and dissociation constants (pKa(s)).

Test results (mean, standard deviation, and coefficient of variation) summarized in a table under solution pH, drug solubility (e.g., mg/mL), and volume of media required to dissolve the highest strength.

A graphic representation of mean pH-solubility profile.

Data Supporting High Permeability

Data supporting high permeability of the test drug substance should be developed (Refer to section III.B. of this guidance: Determining Drug Substance Permeability Class). The following information and data should be included in the application:

A description of test methods, including information on analytical method(s) and composition of the buffer solutions.

A rationale for the dose or drug concentrations used in studies.

For human PK studies, information on study design and methods used along with the PK data.

For direct permeability methods, information supporting the suitability of a selected method that encompasses a description of the study method, criteria for selection of human subjects, animals, or epithelial cell line, drug concentrations in the donor fluid, description of the analytical method, method used to calculate extent of absorption or permeability, and where appropriate, information on efflux potential (e.g., bidirectional transport data).

A list of selected model drugs along with data on extent of absorption in humans (mean, standard deviation, coefficient of variation) used to establish suitability of a method, permeability values for each model drug (mean, standard deviation, coefficient of variation), permeability class of each model drug, and a plot of the extent of absorption as a function of permeability (mean ± standard deviation or 95% confidence interval) with identification of the low/high permeability class boundary and selected internal standard. Information to support high permeability of a test drug substance (mean, standard deviation, coefficient of variation) should include permeability data on the test drug substance, the internal standards, GI stability information, data supporting passive transport mechanism where appropriate, and methods used to establish high permeability of the test drug substance.

Data Supporting Rapid, Very Rapid, and Similar Dissolution

For submission of a biowaiver request, an IR product should be rapidly dissolving (BCS class 1) or very rapidly dissolving (BCS class 3). Data supporting rapid dissolution attributes of the test and reference products should be developed (see section III.C). The following information should be included in the application:

A description of test methods, including information on analytical method(s) and composition of the buffer solutions.

A brief description of the IR products used for dissolution testing, including information on batch or lot number, expiry date, dimensions, strength, and weight.

Dissolution data obtained with 12 individual units of the test and reference products using recommended test methods in section III.C for each of the proposed strengths. The percentage of labeled claim dissolved at each specified testing interval should be reported for each individual dosage unit. The mean percent dissolved, range (highest and lowest) of dissolution, and coefficient of variation (relative standard deviation), should be tabulated. A graphic representation of the mean dissolution profiles for the test and reference products in the three media should also be included.

Data supporting similarity in dissolution profiles between the test and reference products in each of the three media (see section III.C.).

Dissolution data supporting rapid or very rapid dissolution should be demonstrated for each strength to be marketed.

Additional Information

The manufacturing process used to make the test product should be described briefly to provide information on the method of manufacture (e.g., wet granulation versus direct compression).

A list of excipients used, and their intended functions should be provided for both the test and reference products. Ideally, excipients used in the test product should have been used previously in FDA-approved IR solid oral dosage forms. In addition, it is important to provide a quantitative comparison of excipients between the test and reference product for BCS class 3 drug products.

Attachment A

This attachment includes model drugs suggested for use in establishing suitability of a permeability method as described in section III. Zero permeability markers and efflux substrates are also identified.

Group	Drug
High Permeability (fa ≥ 85%)	Antipyrine, Caffeine, Ketoprofen, Naproxen, Theophylline, Metoprolol, Propranolol, Carbamazepine, Phenytoin, Disopyramide, Minoxidil
Moderate Permeability (fa = 50%–84%)	Chlorpheniramine, Creatinine, Terbutaline, Hydrochlorothiazide, Enalapril, Furosemide, Metformin, Amiloride Atenolol, Ranitidine
Low Permeability (fa < 50%)	Famotidine, Nadolol, Sulpiride, Lisinopril, Acyclovir, Foscarnet, Mannitol, Chlorothiazide Polyethylene glycol, 400 Enalaprilat
Zero Permeability	FITC-Dextran (MW ≥ 3000) Polyethylene glycol, 4000 Lucifer yellow Inulin Lactulose
Efflux Substrates	Digoxin, Paclitaxel, Quinidine, Vinblastine

5.5 Using BDCS in Preformulation

The testing methodology must be based on the physiological and physical–chemical properties controlling drug absorption. Generally, no IVIVC may be expected for rapidly dissolving (85% dissolved in less than 15 minutes) low-permeability drugs; where permeability is not a problem, even a simple one-point dissolution test is all that is needed to insure bioavailability. For slowly dissolving drugs, a dissolution profile is required with multiple time points in systems, which would include low pH, physiological pH, and surfactants, and the in vitro conditions should mimic the conditions of the in vivo processes (Table 5.1).

The biopharmaceutics drug classification system (BDCS) should serve the needs of the earliest stages of discovery research, where it can be useful in predicting routes of elimination, effects of efflux, and absorptive transporters on oral absorption, when transporter–enzyme interplay will yield clinically significant effects, such as low bioavailability and drug–drug interactions, the direction and importance of food effects, and transportor effects on postabsorption systemic levels following oral and intravenous doses.

Leads obtained through HTS tend to have higher molecular weights (MWs) and greater lipophilicity than leads in the pre-HTS era. Poor absorption or permeation is more likely when there are more than five H-bond donors, 10 H-bond acceptors, the MW is greater than 500, and the calculated log P is greater than five. This is also often referred to as Rule 5 of Lipinski. However, Lipinski specifically states that the Rule 5 only hold for compounds that are *not* substrates for active transporters. As almost all drugs are substrates for some transporter or the other, much remains to be studied about the Lipinski's rule. In addition, unless a drug molecule can passively gain intracellular access, it is possible to simply investigate whether the molecule is a substrate for efflux transporters.

Several generalizations can be made about the interplay of transporters and the BDCS classification:

1. *Transporter effects are minimal for class 1 compounds.* The high permeability or high solubility of such compounds allows high concentrations in the gut to saturate any transporter, both efflux and absorptive. Class 1 compounds may be substrates for both uptake and efflux transporters in vitro in cellular systems under the right conditions (e.g., midazolam and nifedipine are substrates for Pgp), but transporter effects will not be important clinically. It is therefore possible that some compounds that should be considered class 1 in terms of drug absorption and disposition are not class 1 in BDCS, owing to the requirement of good solubility and rapid dissolution at low-pH values. Such pH effects would not be limiting in vivo, where absorption takes place from the intestine. Examples of this include the nonsteroidal anti-inflammatory drugs (NSAIDs) diclofenac, diflunisal, flurbiprofen, indomethacin, naproxen, and piroxicam; warfarin is almost completely bioavailable. In contrast, ofloxacin is listed as class 2 because of its low solubility at pH 7.5.

2. *Efflux transporter effects will predominate for class 2 compounds.* The high permeability of these compounds will allow ready access into the gut membranes, and uptake transporters will have no effect on absorption, but the low solubility will limit the concentrations coming into the enterocytes,

TABLE 5.1

The Biopharmaceutics Drug Classification System, as Defined by the Food and Drug Administration and Modified by Recent Findings

High solubility (e.g., when the highest dose strength is soluble in 250 mL or less of aqueous media over a pH range of 1–7.5 at 37°C	Low solubility
High permeability (e.g., absorption >90% compared with intravenous dose) (drug + metabolite)	Class 1 (generally about 8% of new leads): • High solubility • High permeability • Rapid dissolution for biowaiver • Route of elimination: metabolism, extensive • Transporter effects: minimal *Examples:* Abacavir; Acetaminophen; *Acyclovir; Amiloride*[S,I]; *Amitriptyline*[S,I]; antipyrine; *Atropine;* **Buspirone;** Caffeine; *Captopril;* Chloroquine[S,I]; **Chlorpheniramine;** Cyclophosphamide; Desipramine; **Diazepam; Diltiazem**[S,I]; **dihenhydramine;** Disopyramide; **Doxepin;** oxycycline; Enalapril; Ephedrine; Ergonovine; Ethambutol; Ethinyl estradiol; Fluoxetine[I]; Glucose; Imipramine[I]; Ketoprofen; **Ketorolac;** Labetolol; Levodopa[S]; Levofloxacin[S]; **Lidocaine**[I]; Lomefloxacin: **Meperidine;** Metoprolol; Metronidazole; **Midazolam**[S,I]; **Minocycline; Misoprostol; Nifedipine**[S]; Phenobarbital; Phenylalanine; Prednisolone; **Primaquine**[S]; Promazine; Propranolol[I]; **Quinidine**[S,I]; **Rosiglitazone;** Salicylic acid; Theophylline; Valproic acid; **Verapamil**[I]; Zidovudine	Class 2: • Low solubility • High permeability • Route of elimination: metabolism, extensive • Transporter: efflux transporter effects predominant *Examples:* **Amiodarone**[I]; **Atorvastatin**[S,I]; **Azithromycin**[S,I]; **Carbamazepine**[S,I]; **Carvedilol;** Chlorpromazine[I]; Ciprofloxacin[S]; **Cisapride**[S]; **Cyclosporine**[S,I]; **Danazol; Dapsone;** Diclofenac; Diflunisal; Digoxin[S]; *Erythromycin*[S,I]; Flurbiprofen; **Glipizide;** Glyburide[S,I]; Griseofulvin; Ibuprofen; **Indinavir**[S]; **Indomethacin; Itraconazole**[S,I]; **Ketoconazole**[I]; **Lansoprazole**[I]; **Lovastatin**[S,I]; *Mebendazole;* Naproxen; Nelfinavir[S,I]; Ofloxacin; Oxaprozin; Phenazopyridine; Phenytoin[S]; Piroxicam; Raloxifene[S]; **Ritonavir**[S,I]; **Saquinavir**[S,I]; **Sirolimus**[S]; Sirolimus[S]; Spironolactone[I]; Spironolactone[I]; **Tacrolimus**[S,I]; Tacrolimus[S,I]; Talinolol[S]; Talinolol[S]; **Tamoxifen**[I]; Tamoxifen[I]; **Terfenadine**[I]; Terfenadine[I]; Warfarin

(Continued)

TABLE 5.1 (*Continued*)

The Biopharmaceutics Drug Classification System, as Defined by the Food and Drug Administration and Modified by Recent Findings

Low permeability

Class 3:
- High solubility
- Low permeability
- Route of elimination: renal and/or biliary elimination of unchanged drugs; metabolism is poor
- Transporter: absorptive effects predominant

Examples: Acyclovir, Amiloride[S,I], Amoxicillin[S,I], Atenolol; Atropine; Bidisomide; Bisphosphonates; *Captopril; Cefazolin;* Cetirizine; Cimetidine[S]; *Ciprofloxacin[S];* Cloxacillin; Dicloxacillin[S]; *Erythromycin[S,I];* Famotidine; Fexofenadine[S]; Folinic acid: *Furosemide;* Ganciclovir; *Hydrochlorothiazide;* Lisinopril; Metformin: *Methotrexate;* Nadolol: Penicillins; Pravastatin[S]; Ranitidine[S]; Tetracycline; Trimethoprim[S]; Valsartan; Zalcitabine

Class 4:
- Low solubility
- Low permeability
- Route of elimination: renal and/or biliary elimination of unchanged drug; metabolism is poor
- Transporter: absorptive and efflux transporters can be predominant

Examples: Amphotericin B; Chlorothiazide; Chlorthalidone; *Ciprofloxacin;* Colistin; *Furosemide; Hydrochlorothiazide; Mebendazole; Methotrexate;* Neomycin

Notes: The compounds listed in *italic* are those that fall in more than one category according to different authors, which could be a result of the definition of the experimental conditions. The compounds listed in **bold** are primarily cytochrome P450 (CYP3A) substrates, where metabolism accounts for more than 70% of the elimination; superscript I and/or S indicate P-glycoprotein inhibitors and/or substrates, respectively. Classes 1 and 2 compounds are eliminated primarily via metabolism, whereas Classes 3 and 4 compounds are primarily eliminated unchanged into the urine and bile.

thereby preventing the saturation of the efflux transporters. Consequently, efflux transporters will affect the extent of oral bioavailability and the rate of absorption of class 2 compounds.

3. *Transporter-enzyme interplay in the intestines will be important, primarily for class 2 compounds that are substrates for CYP3A and phase 2 conjugation enzymes.* For such compounds, intestinal uptake transporters will generally be unimportant, owing to the rapid permeation of the drug molecule into the enterocytes as a function of their high lipid solubility. That is, the absorption of class 2 compounds is primarily passive and a function of lipophilicity. However, owing to the low solubility of these compounds, there will be little opportunity to saturate apical efflux transporters and intestinal enzymes, such as CYP3A4 and UDPglucuronosyltransferases (UGTs). Thus, changes in transporter expression and inhibition or induction of efflux transporters will cause changes in the intestinal metabolism of drugs that are substrates for the intestinal metabolic enzymes. Note the large number of class 2 compounds in Table 5.1 that are primarily substrates for CYP3A (compounds listed in bold), as well as substrates or inhibitors of the efflux transporter Pgp (indicated by superscripts S and I, respectively). Work in our laboratory has characterized this interplay in the absorptive process for the investigational cysteine protease inhibitor K77 and sirolimus, substrates for CYP3A and Pgp, and more recently for raloxifene, a substrate for UGTs and Pgp.

4. *Absorptive transporter effects will predominate for class 3 compounds.* For class 3 compounds, sufficient drug will be available in the gut lumen owing to good solubility, but an absorptive transporter will be necessary to overcome the poor permeability characteristics of these compounds. However, intestinal apical efflux transporters may also be important for the absorption of such compounds when sufficient enterocyte penetration is achieved via an uptake transporter.

RECOMMENDED READING

Dissolution

Batchelor, H. K. et al. (2014). "Paediatric oral biopharmaceutics: Key considerations and current challenges." *Adv Drug Deliv Rev* 73:102–126.

The complex process of oral drug absorption is influenced by a host of drug and formulation properties as well as their interaction with the GI environment in terms of drug solubility, dissolution, permeability, and presystemic metabolism. For adult dosage forms the use of biopharmaceutical tools to aid in the design and development of medicinal products is well documented. This review considers current literature evidence to guide development of bespoke pediatric biopharmaceutics tools and reviews current understanding surrounding extrapolation of adult methodology into a pediatric population. Clinical testing and the use of in silico models were also reviewed. The results demonstrate that further work is required to adequately characterize the pediatric GI tract to ensure that biopharmaceutics tools are appropriate to predict performance within this population. The most vulnerable group was found to be neonates and infants up to 6 months where differences from adults were greatest.

Censi, R. et al. (2018). "Hot melt extrusion: Highlighting physicochemical factors to be investigated while designing and optimizing a hot melt extrusion process." *Pharmaceutics* 10(3):89.

Hot-melt extrusion (HME) is a well-accepted and extensively studied method for preparing numerous types of drug delivery systems and dosage forms. It offers several advantages: no solvents are required, it is easy to scale up and employ on the industrial level, and, in particular, it offers the possibility of improving drug bioavailability. HME involves the mixing of a drug with one or more excipients, in general polymers and even plasticizers, which can melt, often forming a solid dispersion of the drug in the polymer. The molten mass is extruded and cooled, giving rise to a solid material with designed properties. This process, which can be realized using different kinds of special equipment, may involve modifications in the drug physicochemical properties, such as chemical, thermal, and mechanical characteristics, thus affecting the drug physicochemical stability and bioavailability. During process optimization, the evaluation of the drug solid state and stability is thus of paramount importance to guarantee stable drug properties for the duration of the drug product shelf life. This manuscript reviews the most important physicochemical factors that should be investigated while designing and optimizing a hot melt extrusion process, and by extension, during the different preformulation, formulation and process, and postformulation phases. It offers a comprehensive evaluation of the chemical and thermal stability of extrudates, the solid physical state of extrudates, possible drug-polymer interactions, the miscibility/solubility of the drug-polymer system, the rheological properties of extrudates, the physicomechanical properties of films produced by hot melt extrusion, and drug particle dissolution from extrudates. It draws upon the last ten years of research, extending inquiry as broadly as possible.

Davis, M. and G. Walker (2018). "Recent strategies in spray drying for the enhanced bioavailability of poorly water-soluble drugs." *J Control Release* 269:110–127.

Poorly water-soluble drugs are a significant and ongoing issue for the pharmaceutical industry. An overview of recent developments for the preparation of spray-dried delivery systems is presented. Examples include amorphous solid dispersions, spray dried dispersions, microparticles, nanoparticles, surfactant systems, and self-emulsifying drug delivery systems. Several aspects of formulation are considered, such as prescreening, choosing excipient(s), the effect of polymer structure on performance, formulation optimization, ternary dispersions, fixed-dose combinations, solvent selection, and component miscibility. Process optimization techniques including nozzle selection are discussed. Comparisons are drawn with other preparation techniques such as hot melt extrusion, freeze drying, milling, electro spinning, and film casting. Novel analytical and dissolution techniques for the characterization of amorphous solid dispersions are included. Progress in understanding of amorphous supersaturation or recrystallisation from solution gathered from mechanistic studies is discussed. Aspects of powder flow and compression are considered in a section on downstream processing. Overall, spray drying has a bright future due to its versatility, efficiency, and the driving force of poorly soluble drugs.

Ghadi, R. and N. Dand (2017). "BCS class IV drugs: Highly notorious candidates for formulation development." *J Control Release* 248:71–95.

BCS class IV drugs (e.g., amphotericin B, furosemide, acetazolamide, ritonavir, paclitaxel) exhibit many characteristics that are problematic for effective oral and per oral delivery. Some of the problems associated include low aqueous solubility, poor permeability, erratic and poor absorption, inter- and intrasubject variability, and significant positive food effect, which leads to low and variable bioavailability. Also, most of the class IV drugs are substrate for P-glycoprotein (low permeability) and substrate for CYP3A4 (extensive presystemic metabolism) which further potentiates the problem of poor therapeutic potential of these drugs. A decade back, extreme examples of class IV compounds were an exception rather than the rule, yet today many drug candidates under development pipeline fall into this category. Formulation and development of an efficacious delivery system for BCS class IV drugs are herculean tasks for any formulator. The inherent hurdles posed by these drugs hamper their translation to actual market. The importance of the formulation composition and design to successful drug development is especially illustrated by the BCS class IV case. To be clinically effective these drugs require the development of a proper delivery system for both oral and per oral delivery. Ideal oral dosage forms should produce both a reasonably high bioavailability and low inter- and intrasubject variability in absorption. Also, ideal systems for BCS class IV should produce a therapeutic concentration of the drug at reasonable dose volumes for intravenous administration. This article highlights the various techniques and upcoming strategies, which can be employed for the development of highly notorious BCS class IV drugs. Some of the techniques employed are lipid-based delivery systems, polymer based nanocarriers, crystal engineering (nanocrystals and cocrystals), liquisolid technology, self-emulsifying solid dispersions and miscellaneous techniques addressing the Pgp efflux problem. The review also focuses on the roadblocks in the clinical development of the aforementioned strategies such as problems in scale up, manufacturing under cGMP guidelines, appropriate quality control tests, validation of various processes, variable therein, etc. It also brings to forefront the current lack of regulatory guidelines which poses difficulties during preclinical and clinical testing for submission of NDA and subsequent marketing. Today, the pharmaceutical industry has as its disposal a series of reliable and scalable formulation strategies for BCS Class IV drugs. However, due to lack of understanding of the basic physical chemistry behind these strategies' formulation development is still driven by trial and error.

He, Y. and C. Ho (2015). "Amorphous solid dispersions: Utilization and challenges in drug discovery and development." *J Pharm Sci* 104(10):3237–3258.

Amorphous solid dispersion (ASD) can accelerate a project by improving dissolution rate and solubility, offering dose escalation flexibility and excipient acceptance for toxicology studies, as well as providing adequate preclinical and clinical exposure. The prerequisite physicochemical properties for a compound to form a stable ASD are glass-forming ability and low-crystallization tendency, which can be assessed using computational tools and experimental methods. Polymer excipient screening by in silico miscibility prediction and experimental screening techniques is discussed. Improved technologies for polymer screening with minimal quantity of drug substance and the scalability of ASD from bench to commercial are reviewed. Considerations of in vitro evaluations, preclinical animal selection, and the translation of the preclinical results to clinical studies are also discussed. Better understanding of how polymers improve the stability of the amorphous phase in the solid state and how ASD improves bioavailability have facilitated the applications of ASD ranging from discovery research to preclinical development and further to commercialization. With the understanding of how ASDs are currently used in the pharmaceutical industry and what challenges remain to be solved, ASD can be applied to solve drug formulation problems at given research and development stages.

Jambhekar, S. S. and P. J. Breen (2013). "Drug dissolution: Significance of physicochemical properties and physiological conditions." *Drug Discov Today* 18(23–24):1173–1184.

Oral bioavailability of a drug is determined by a number of properties, including drug dissolution rate, solubility, intestinal permeability, and presystemic metabolism. Frequently, the rate limiting step in drug absorption from the GI tract is drug release and drug dissolution from the dosage form. Therapeutic agents with aqueous solubilities less than 100 µg/mL often present dissolution limitations to absorption. Physicochemical, formulation-related and physiological factors can all influence drug dissolution. In this review, the authors will discuss the important physicochemical properties of a drug and physiological conditions in the GI tract that play an important part in drug dissolution and absorption processes and, consequently, the bioavailability of a drug.

Parrott, N. et al. (2009). "Predicting pharmacokinetics of drugs using physiologically based modeling—application to food effects." *AAPS J* 11(1):45–53.

Our knowledge of the major mechanisms underlying the effect of food on drug absorption allows reliable qualitative prediction based on biopharmaceutical properties, which can be assessed during the preclinical phase of drug discovery. Furthermore, several recent examples have shown that physiologically based absorption models incorporating biorelevant drug solubility measurements can provide quite accurate quantitative prediction of food effect. However, many molecules currently in development have distinctly suboptimal biopharmaceutical properties, making the quantitative prediction of food effect for different formulations from in vitro data very challenging. If such drugs reach clinical development and show undesirable variability when dosed with food, improved formulation can help to reduce the food effect and carefully designed in vivo studies in dogs can be a useful guide to clinical formulation development. Even so, such in vivo studies provide limited throughput for screening, and food effects seen in dog cannot always be directly translated to human. This paper describes how physiologically based absorption modeling can play a role in the prediction of food effect by integrating the data generated during preclinical and clinical research and development. Such data include physicochemical and in vitro drug properties, biorelevant solubility and dissolution, and in vivo preclinical and clinical pharmacokinetic data. Some background to current physiological absorption models of human and dog is given, and refinements to models of in vivo drug solubility and dissolution are described. These are illustrated with examples using GastroPlus to simulate the food effect in dog and human for different formulations of two marketed drugs.

Stuurman, F. E. et al. (2013). "Oral anticancer drugs: Mechanisms of low bioavailability and strategies for improvement." *Clin Pharmacokinet* 52(6):399–414.

The use of oral anticancer drugs has increased during the last decade, because of patient preference, lower costs, proven efficacy, lack of infusion-related inconveniences, and the opportunity to develop chronic treatment regimens. Oral administration of anticancer drugs is, however, often hampered by limited bioavailability of the drug, which is associated with a wide variability. Since most anticancer drugs have a narrow therapeutic window and are dosed at or close to the maximum tolerated dose, a wide variability in the bioavailability can have a negative impact on treatment outcome. This review discusses mechanisms of low bioavailability of oral anticancer drugs and strategies for improvement. The extent of oral bioavailability depends on many factors, including release of the drug from the pharmaceutical dosage form, a drug's stability in the GI tract, factors affecting dissolution, the rate of passage through the gut wall, and the presystemic metabolism in the gut wall and liver. These factors are divided into pharmaceutical limitations, physiological endogenous limitations, and patient-specific limitations. There are several strategies to reduce or overcome these limitations. First, pharmaceutical adjustment of the formulation or the physicochemical characteristics of the drug can improve the dissolution rate and absorption. Second, pharmacological interventions by combining the drug with inhibitors of transporter proteins and/or presystemic metabolizing enzymes can overcome the physiological endogenous limitations. Third, chemical modification of a drug by synthesis of a derivative, salt form, or prodrug could enhance the bioavailability by improving the absorption and bypassing physiological endogenous limitations. Although the bioavailability can be enhanced by various strategies, the development of novel oral products with low solubility or cell membrane permeability remains cumbersome and is often unsuccessful. The main reasons are unacceptable variation in the bioavailability and high investment costs. Furthermore, novel oral anticancer drugs are frequently associated with toxic effects including unacceptable GI adverse effects. Therefore, compliance is often suboptimal, which may negatively influence treatment outcome.

Release

Agashe, H. et al. (2012). "Formulation and delivery of microbicides." *Curr HIV Res* 10(1):88–96.

The development of preexposure prophylactics or microbicide products for the reduction or elimination of the sexual transmission of HIV has numerous challenges or barriers to success. Historically traditional dosage forms such as gels have been developed in the field but more recently controlled release dosage forms such as vaginal rings and novel dosage forms such as polymeric thin films have been studied. Studies have begun to incorporate scientific strategies into the formulation design of microbicide products in order to develop safer and more effective products. In addition, advanced drug delivery strategies to overcome barriers to delivery and specific drug targeting methods are being employed. In the present review, a comprehensive discussion of formulation efforts and novel delivery strategies in the field of microbicide product development is presented.

Aggarwal, A. et al. (2016). "Aripiprazole lauroxil long-acting injectable: The latest addition to second-generation long-acting agents." *Clin Schizophr Relat Psychoses* 10(1):58–63.

Antipsychotics have long been the mainstay for the treatment of schizophrenia and other psychotic disorders. Long-acting injectables (LAI) of antipsychotics-provided once every two weeks to once every three months-promise to reduce the incidence of nonadherence. ARISTADA (aripiprazole lauroxil; ALLAI) extended-release inject-able suspension was approved by the U.S. FDA in October 2015 for the treatment of schizophrenia and is the newest entrant in the LAI market. ALLAI is available as a single-use, prefilled syringe, can be started in three different dosages, and also has the option of every six-week dosing. Treatment with oral aripiprazole is recommended for the first twenty-one days after the first ALLAI injection, which is a potential disadvantage. Adverse effects include sensitivity to extrapyramidal symptoms, espe-cially akathisia, which is well documented in other aripiprazole preparations. There is no available data comparing ALLAI to other antipsychotics, and more head-to-head trials comparing different LAI formulations are needed. Based on the available data, ALLAI is an effective and safe option for treatment of schizophrenia. Further studies and postmarketing data will provide better understanding of this formulation.

Amsden, B. G. (2011). "Delivery approaches for angiogenic growth factors in the treatment of ischemic conditions." *Expert Opin Drug Deliv* 8(7):873–890.

INTRODUCTION: Despite current medical treatments, cardiovascular disease resulting in local ischemia remains a significant clinical problem. Therapeutic angio-genesis, that is, the growth and remodeling of new blood vessels from preexisting blood vessels to the ischemic area, is a promising solution to this problem. AREAS COVERED: Therapeutic angiogenesis can be generated in vivo through the local release of various proangiogenic factors. This review describes the various formula-tion approaches that have been devised for this purpose, highlighting the advantages and disadvantages of each. EXPERT OPINION: Formulations that release single proangiogenic growth factors have not yet been demonstrated to achieve functional therapeutic angiogenesis. Formulations capable of multiple growth factor delivery are needed; however, the complexity of the physiologic process requires the examination of appropriate growth factor doses, as well as release sequence, to guide effectively new formulation design. Furthermore, new formulation approaches need to be tested in vivo in appropriate animal models over extended time periods to assess clearly the potential of the delivery approach.

Burness, C. B. et al. (2014). "Lanreotide autogel®: A review of its use in the treatment of patients with acromegaly." *Drugs* 74(14):1673–1691.

Lanreotide Autogel® (ATG) [Somatuline® Autogel®, Somatuline® Depot®] is a prolonged-release, supersaturated aqueous gel formulation of the somatostatin ana-logue lanreotide acetate that acts via somatostatin receptors to reduce both growth hormone and insulin-like growth factor-I levels. It is indicated for the treatment of patients with acromegaly who have had an inadequate response to or cannot be treated with surgery and/or radiotherapy. This article reviews the clinical efficacy and tolerability of lanreotide ATG in the treatment of acromegaly, as well as sum-marizing its pharmacological properties. Results of clinical trials and extension studies of up to 4 years duration showed that deep subcutaneous lanreotide ATG was a generally effective treatment in treatment-naive and treatment-experienced adults with acromegaly. Lanreotide ATG provided hormonal control and improved both health-related quality of life and acromegaly symptoms in most patients; it also reduced tumor volume to a clinically significant extent in studies of primary therapy. Moreover, lanreotide ATG was generally no less effective than intramuscular lanreotide long-acting microparticles and was as effective as intramuscular octreotide long-acting release in switching or crossover studies, including those with standard or extended dosing intervals. Lanreotide ATG is generally well tolerated; the most frequently reported adverse events were mild or moderate transient GI symptoms. Lanreotide ATG also has the advantage of being available in a convenient prefilled syringe and is given subcutaneously rather than intramuscularly. Thus, lanreotide ATG continues to be a valuable option in the treatment of acromegaly, with potential advantages being ease of administration and longer dosing intervals in patients who have an adequate response to initial therapy.

Chen, D. et al. (2017). "Plasma protein adsorption and biological identity of systemically administered nanoparticles." *Nanomedicine* (Lond) 12(17):2113–2135.

Although a variety of nanoparticles (NPs) have been used for drug delivery applications, their surfaces are immediately covered by plasma protein corona upon systemic administration. As a result, the adsorbed proteins create a unique biological identity of the NPs that lead to unpredictable performance. The protein corona on NPs could also impede active targeting, induce off-target effects, trigger particle clearance, and even provoke toxicity. This article reviews the fundamentals of NP-plasma protein interaction, the consequences of the interactions, and provides insights into the correlations of protein corona with biodistribution and cellular delivery. We hope that this review will trigger additional questions and possible solutions that lead to more favorable developments in NP-based targeted delivery systems.

Chowdhury, P. et al. (2017). "Magnetic nanoformulations for prostate cancer." *Drug Discov Today* 22(8):1233–1241.

Magnetic nanoparticles (MNPs) play a vital role for improved imaging applications. Recently, a number of studies demonstrate MNPs can be applied for targeted delivery, sustained release of therapeutics, and hyperthermia. Based on stable particle size and shape, biocompatibility, and inherent contrast enhancement characteristics, MNPs have been encouraged for preclinical studies and human use. As a theranostic platform development, MNPs need to balance both delivery and imaging aspects. Thus, this review provides significant insight and advances in the theranostic role of MNPs through the documentation of unique magnetic nanoparticles used in prostate cancer, their interaction with prostate cancer cells, in vivo fate, targeting, and biodistribution. Specific and custom-made applications of various novel nanoformulations in prostate cancer are discussed.

Coghill, D. et al. (2013). "Long-acting methylphenidate formulations in the treatment of attention-deficit/hyperactivity disorder: A systematic review of head-to-head studies." *BMC Psychiatry* 13:237.

BACKGROUND: The stimulant methylphenidate (MPH) has been a mainstay of treatment for attention-deficit/hyperactivity disorder (ADHD) for many years. Owing to the short half-life and the issues associated with multiple daily dosing of immediate-release MPH formulations, a new generation of long-acting MPH formulations has emerged. Direct head-to-head studies of these long-acting MPH formulations are important to facilitate an evaluation of their comparative pharmacokinetics and efficacy; however, to date, relatively few head-to-head studies have been performed. The objective of this systematic review was to compare the evidence available from head-to-head studies of long-acting MPH formulations and provide information that can guide treatment selection. METHODS: A systematic literature search was conducted in MEDLINE and PsycINFO in March 2012 using the MeSH terms: attention deficit disorder with hyperactivity/drug therapy; methylphenidate/therapeutic use and All Fields: Concerta; Ritalin LA; OROS and ADHD; Medikinet; Equasym XL and ADHD; long-acting methylphenidate; Diffucaps and ADHD; SODAS and methylphenidate. No filters were applied, and no language, publication date, or publication status limitations were imposed. Articles were selected if the title indicated a comparison of two or more long-acting MPH preparations in human subjects of any age; nonsystematic review articles and unpublished data were not included. RESULTS: Of 15,295 references returned in the literature search and screened by title, 34 articles were identified for inclusion: nine articles from pharmacokinetic studies (nine studies); nine articles from laboratory school studies (six studies); two articles from randomized controlled trials (two studies); three articles from switching studies (two studies) and three articles from one observational study. CONCLUSIONS: Emerging head-to-head studies provide important data on the comparative efficacy of the formulations available. At a group level, efficacy across the day generally follows the pharmacokinetic profile of the MPH formulation. No formulation is clearly superior to another; careful consideration of patient needs and subtle differences between formulations is required to optimize treatment. For patients achieving suboptimal symptom control, switching long-acting MPH formulations may be beneficial. When switching formulations, it is usually appropriate to titrate the immediate-release component of the formulation; a limitation of current studies is a focus on total daily dose rather than equivalent immediate-release components. Further studies are necessary to provide guidance in clinical practice, particularly in the treatment of adults and preschool children and the impact of comorbidities and symptom severity on treatment response.

Daminet, S. et al. (2014). "Best practice for the pharmacological management of hyperthyroid cats with antithyroid drugs." *J Small Anim Pract* 55(1):4–13.

Pharmacological management of feline hyperthyroidism offers a practical treatment option for many hyperthyroid cats. Two drugs have been licensed for cats in the last decade: methimazole and its prodrug carbimazole. On the basis of current evidence and available tablet sizes, starting doses of 2.5 mg methimazole twice a day and 10–15 mg once a day for the sustained release formulation of carbimazole are recommended. These doses should then be titrated to effect in order to obtain circulating total thyroxine (TT4) concentrations in the lower half of the reference interval. Treated cases should be monitored for side effects, especially during the first months of treatment. Some side effects may require discontinuation of treatment. At each monitoring visit, clinical condition and quality of life should also be evaluated, with special attention to possible development of azotemia, hypertension, and iatrogenic hypothyroidism. When euthyroidism has been achieved, monitoring visits are recommended after 1 month, 3 months, and biannually thereafter. Cats with preexisting azotemia have shorter survival times. However, development of mild azotemia during the initial course of treatment, unless associated with hypothyroidism, does not appear to decrease survival time. The long-term effects of chronic medical management require further study.

Davis, M. and G. Walker (2018). "Recent strategies in spray drying for the enhanced bioavailability of poorly water-soluble drugs." *J Control Release* 269:110–127.

Poorly water-soluble drugs are a significant and ongoing issue for the pharmaceutical industry. An overview of recent developments for the preparation of spray-dried delivery systems is presented. Examples include amorphous solid dispersions, spray-dried dispersions, microparticles, nanoparticles, surfactant systems, and self-emulsifying drug delivery systems. Several aspects of formulation are considered, such as prescreening, choosing excipient(s), the effect of polymer structure on performance, formulation optimization, ternary dispersions, fixed-dose combinations, solvent selection, and component miscibility. Process optimization techniques including nozzle selection are discussed. Comparisons are drawn with other preparation techniques such as hot melt extrusion, freeze drying, milling, electro spinning, and film casting. Novel analytical and dissolution techniques for the characterization of amorphous solid dispersions are included. Progress in understanding of amorphous supersaturation or recrystallisation from solution gathered from mechanistic studies is discussed. Aspects of powder flow and compression are considered in a section on downstream processing. Overall, spray drying has a bright future due to its versatility, efficiency, and the driving force of poorly soluble drugs.

Deng, C. et al. (2010). "The role of histaminergic H1 and H3 receptors in food intake: A mechanism for atypical antipsychotic-induced weight gain?" *Prog Neuropsychopharmacol Biol Psychiatry* 34(1):1–4.

Atypical antipsychotics such as olanzapine and clozapine are effective at treating the multiple domains of schizophrenia, with a low risk of extra-pyramidal side effects. However, a major downfall to their use is metabolic side effects particularly weight gain/obesity, which occurs by unknown mechanisms. The present paper explores the potential candidature of histaminergic neurotransmission in the mechanisms of atypical antipsychotic-induced weight gain, with a focus on the histaminergic H1 and H3 receptors. Olanzapine and clozapine have a high affinity for the H1 receptor, and meta-analyses show a strong correlation between risk of weight gain and H1 receptor affinity. In addition, olanzapine treatment decreases H1 receptor binding and mRNA expression in the rat hypothalamus. Furthermore, a complex role is emerging for the histamine H3 receptor in the control of hunger. The H3 receptor is a presynaptic autoreceptor that inhibits the synthesis and release of histamine, and a heteroreceptor that inhibits other neurotransmitters such as serotonin (5-HT), noradrenaline (NA), and acetylcholine (ACh), which are also implicated in the regulation of food intake. Thus, the H3 receptor is in a prime position to regulate food intake, both through its control of histamine and its influence on other feeding pathways. We proposed that a mechanism for atypical antipsychotic-induced weight gain may be partly through the H3 receptor, as a drug-induced decrease in H1 receptor activity may decrease histamine tone through the H3 autoreceptors, compounding the weight gain problem. In addition, atypical antipsychotics may affect food intake by influencing 5-HT, NA, and ACh release via interactions with the H3 heteroreceptor.

Desai, K. G. et al. (2018). "Japan-specific key regulatory aspects for development of new biopharmaceutical drug products." *J Pharm Sci* 107(7):1773–1786.

Japan represents the third largest pharmaceutical market in the world. Developing a new biopharmaceutical drug product for the Japanese market is a top business priority for global pharmaceutical companies while aligning with ethical drivers to treat more patients in need. Understanding Japan-specific key regulatory requirements is essential to achieve successful approvals. Understanding the full context of Japan-specific regulatory requirements/expectations is challenging to global pharmaceutical companies due to differences in language and culture. This article summarizes key Japan-specific regulatory aspects/requirements/expectations applicable to new drug development, approval, and postapproval phases. Formulation excipients should meet Japan compendial requirements with respect to the type of excipient, excipient grade, and excipient concentration. Preclinical safety assessments needed to support clinical phases I, II, and III development are summarized. Japanese regulatory authorities have taken appropriate steps to consider foreign clinical data, thereby enabling accelerated drug development and approval in Japan. Other important topics summarized in this article include: Japan new drug application-specific bracketing strategies for critical and noncritical aspects of the manufacturing process, regulatory requirements related to stability studies, release specifications and testing methods, standard processes involved in pre- and postapproval inspections, management of postapproval changes, and Japan regulatory authority's consultation services available to global pharmaceutical companies.

Fernandes, E. et al. (2015). "New trends in guided nanotherapies for digestive cancers: A systematic review." *J Control Release* 209:288–307.

Digestive tract tumors are among the most common and deadliest malignancies worldwide, mainly due to late diagnosis and lack of efficient therapeutics. Current treatments essentially rely on surgery associated with (neo)adjuvant chemotherapy agents. Despite an upfront response, conventional drugs often fail to eliminate highly aggressive clones endowed with chemoresistant properties, which are responsible for tumor recurrence and disease dissemination. Synthetic drugs also present severe adverse systemic effects, hampering the administration of biologically effective dosages. Nanoencapsulation of chemotherapeutic agents within biocompatible polymeric or lipid matrices holds great potential to improve the pharmacokinetics and efficacy of conventional chemotherapy while reducing systemic toxicity. Tagging nanoparticle surfaces with specific ligands for cancer cells, namely monoclonal antibodies or antibody fragments, has provided means to target more aggressive clones, further improving the selectivity and efficacy of nanodelivery vehicles. In fact, over the past twenty years, significant research has translated into a wide array of guided nanoparticles, providing the molecular background for a new generation of intelligent and more effective anticancer agents. Attempting to bring awareness among the medical community to emerging targeted nanopharmaceuticals and foster advances in the field, we have conducted a systematic review about this matter. Emphasis was set on ongoing preclinical and clinical trials for liver, colorectal, gastric, and pancreatic cancers. To the best of our knowledge this is the first systematic and integrated overview on this field. Using a specific query, 433 abstracts were gathered and narrowed to 47 manuscripts when matched against inclusion/exclusion criteria. All studies showed that active targeting improves the effectiveness of the nanodrugs alone, while lowering its side effects. The main focus has been on hepatocarcinomas, mainly by exploring glycans as homing molecules. Other ligands such as peptides/small proteins and antibodies/antibody fragments, with affinity to either tumor vasculature or tumor cells, have also been widely and successfully applied to guide nanodrugs to GI carcinomas. Conversely, few solutions have been presented for pancreatic tumors. To this date only three nanocomplexes have progressed beyond preclinical stages: (i) PK2, a galactosamine-functionalized polymeric-DOX formulation for hepatocarcinomas; (ii) MCC-465, an anti-(myosin heavy chain a) immunoliposome for advanced stage metastatic solid tumors; and (iii) MBP-426, a transferrin-liposome-oxaliplatin conjugate, also for advanced stage tumors. Still, none has been approved for clinical use. However, based on the high amount of preclinical studies showing enthusiastic results, the number of clinical trials is expected to increase in the near future. A more profound understanding about the molecular nature of chemoresistant clones and cancer stem cell biology will also contribute to boost the field of guided nanopharmacology towards more effective solutions.

Figueroa, C. et al. (2009). "Pharmacokinetic profiles of extended release quetiapine fumarate compared with quetiapine immediate release." *Prog Neuropsychopharmacol Biol Psychiatry* 33(2):199–204.

This 10-day, single-center, open-label, randomized, crossover study compared pharmacokinetic profiles, and tolerability of extended release quetiapine fumarate (quetiapine XR) with quetiapine immediate release (quetiapine IR) in patients with schizophrenia, schizoaffective disorder or bipolar disorder. After a 2-day lead-in period during which patients received quetiapine XR 300 mg once daily, patients were randomized to quetiapine IR 150 mg twice daily followed by quetiapine XR 300 mg once daily, or quetiapine XR 300 mg once daily followed by quetiapine IR 150 mg twice daily. Pharmacokinetic parameters were evaluated at the end of each 4-day treatment period at steady state. Vital signs, laboratory values, and adverse events (AEs) were recorded throughout the study. The least squares mean (90% confidence interval) of the ratio of the area under the plasma concentration–time curve over a 24 hours dosing interval (AUC ([0–24 hours])) for quetiapine XR/IR was 1.04 (0.92–1.19) and within the predefined range set for equivalence (0.80–1.25). Maximum plasma concentration at steady state (C(max)) was approximately 13% lower for quetiapine XR than for quetiapine IR (495.3 vs. 568.1 ng/mL), time to reach C(max) (t(max)) was 5 hours versus 2 hours and mean concentration at the end of 24 hours dosing interval (C(min)) was 95.3 versus 96.5 ng/mL, respectively. No patients withdrew from the study owing to AEs and there were no serious AEs or deaths related to study medication. No unexpected AEs, changes in vital signs or laboratory values were observed. These findings suggest that modifying the formulation does not change the overall absorption or elimination of quetiapine, and support emerging clinical evidence for the use of quetiapine XR as a once daily treatment in patients initiating therapy or those established on quetiapine IR.

Fitzgerald, K. A. et al. (2015). "Life in 3D is never flat: 3D models to optimize drug delivery." *J Control Release* 215:39–54.

The development of safe, effective and patient-acceptable drug products is an expensive and lengthy process and the risk of failure at different stages of the development life cycle is high. Improved biopharmaceutical tools which are robust, easy to use, and accurately predict the in vivo response are urgently required to help address these issues. In this review, the advantages and challenges of in vitro 3D versus 2D cell culture models will be discussed in terms of evaluating new drug products at the preclinical development stage. Examples of models with a 3D architecture including scaffolds, cell-derived matrices, multicellular spheroids, and biochips will be described. The ability to simulate the microenvironment of tumors and vital organs including the liver, kidney, heart, and intestine, which have major impact on drug absorption, distribution, metabolism, and toxicity will be evaluated. Examples of the application of 3D models including a role in formulation development, pharmacokinetic profiling, and toxicity testing will be critically assessed. Although utilization of 3D cell culture models in the field of drug delivery is still in its infancy, the area is attracting high levels of interest and is likely to become a significant in vitro tool to assist in drug product development thus reducing the requirement for unnecessary animal studies.

Ghadi, R. and N. Dand (2017). "BCS class IV drugs: Highly notorious candidates for formulation development." *J Control Release* 248:71–95.

BCS class IV drugs (e.g., amphotericin B, furosemide, acetazolamide, ritonavir, and paclitaxel) exhibit many characteristics that are problematic for effective oral and per oral delivery. Some of the problems associated include low aqueous solubility, poor permeability, erratic and poor absorption, inter- and intrasubject variability, and significant positive food effect, which leads to low and variable bioavailability. Also, most of the class IV drugs are substrate for P-glycoprotein (low permeability) and substrate for CYP3A4 (extensive presystemic metabolism), which further potentiates the problem of poor therapeutic potential of these drugs. A decade back, extreme examples of class IV compounds were an exception rather than the rule, yet today many drug candidates under development pipeline fall into this category. Formulation and development of an efficacious delivery system for BCS class IV drugs are herculean tasks for any formulator. The inherent hurdles posed by these drugs hamper their translation to actual market. The importance of the formulation composition and design to successful drug development is especially illustrated by the BCS class IV case. To be clinically effective these drugs require the development of a proper delivery system for both oral and per oral delivery. Ideal oral dosage forms should produce both a reasonably high bioavailability and low inter- and intrasubject variability in absorption. Also, ideal systems for BCS class IV should produce a therapeutic concentration of the drug at reasonable dose volumes for intravenous administration. This article highlights the various techniques and upcoming strategies which can be employed for the development of highly notorious BCS class IV drugs. Some of the techniques employed are lipid-based delivery systems, polymer based nanocarriers, crystal engineering (nanocrystals and cocrystals), liquisolid technology, self-emulsifying solid dispersions, and miscellaneous techniques addressing the Pgp efflux problem. The review also focuses on the roadblocks in the clinical development of the aforementioned strategies such as problems in scale up, manufacturing under cGMP guidelines, appropriate quality control tests, validation of various processes, and variable therein. It also brings to forefront the current lack of regulatory guidelines which poses difficulties during preclinical and clinical testing for submission of NDA and subsequent marketing. Today, the pharmaceutical industry has as its disposal a series of reliable and scalable formulation strategies for BCS Class IV drugs. However, due to lack of understanding of the basic physical chemistry behind these strategies' formulation development is still driven by trial and error.

Horky, K. (2010). "Direct renin inhibitor aliskiren in the treatment of cardiovascular and renal diseases." *Vnitr Lek* 56(2):120–126.

The role of renin-angiotensin-aldosterone system (RAAS) in regulating the volume and composition of extracellular fluid, blood pressure (BP), as well as onset and progression of cardiovascular and renal diseases has been studied for more than 150 years. The compounds that block the vital stages of the RAAS cascade, such as ACE-inhibitors (ACEI), AT1-receptor blockers (ARB), and aldosterone receptor antagonists, importantly extended our treatment options. However, the positive therapeutic effects of these compounds also have certain negative consequences. Administration of ACEIs and ARBs interrupts physiological feedback for renal renin release and leads to reactive elevation of circulating active renin and greater production of angiotensin I and angiotensin II with subsequent return of aldosterone secretion to the pretreatment levels ("escape" phenomenon). These possible adverse effects of the intermediary products of incomplete RAAS blockade leading to organ complications have facilitated the efforts to develop compounds blocking the initial stages of renin-angiotensin cascade—i.e., direct renin blockers. After several years of unsuccessful attempts, the recent years have seen development of the first nonpeptide, orally long-term effective renin inhibitor, aliskiren fumarate. In monotherapy or in combination with other antihypertensives (hydrochlorothiazide, ARB, ACEI), aliskiren reduces BP in a dose-dependent manner (75–600 mg/den). Aliskiren reduces plasma renin activity (PRA) and neutralizes hydrochlorothiazide-induced RAAS activation. Once daily administration of the drug leads to longer than 24-hour activity, and its prolonged blocking effects on the kidneys are the basis for its renoprotectivity. In addition to the significant antihypertensive effect, clinical studies also showed a range of organoprotective properties in patients with left ventricle hypertrophy (ALLAY study), heart failure (ALOFT study) and diabetic nephropathy (AVOID study). Similar to other AT1-blockers, aliskiren has a minimum of adverse side effects. Aliskiren for hypertension therapy was launched in clinical practice in USA in 2007 (Tekturna and combination formulation Tekturna HCl, respectively) and shortly after that in European Union as Rasilez. In the Czech Republic, aliskiren (Rasilez) was released for clinical use by diabetologists and nephrologists in patients with hypertension and concomitant diabetes, nephropathy, and proteinuria in doses of 150–300 mg per day on August 1, 2009. It is recommended as monotherapy or in combination with other antihypertensives to treat conditions with elevated PRA, including PRA elevation following diuretic, ACEI or ARB administration. Aliskiren might be used in patients who do not tolerate ACEIs as well as in patients in whom angiotensin II participates in the pathogenesis of their diseases. Renoprotective properties leading to a reduction in proteinuria and delaying renal failure progression were observed in patients with diabetic as well as nondiabetic nephropathy. The drug is the subject to similar precautions and contraindications as ACEIs and ARBs, i.e., pregnancy and bilateral renal artery stenosis. To make meaningful conclusions about the so far positive contribution of this new treatment class and its broad applicability for the therapy of hypertension and other cardiovascular diseases, it will be imperative to assess its long-term effects on morbidity and mortality as well as to compare these agents with other RAAS blockers in long-term clinical studies; this represents a research effort for another 7–8 years.

Jambhekar, S. S. and P. J. Breen (2013). "Drug dissolution: Significance of physicochemical properties and physiological conditions." *Drug Discov Today* 18(23–24):1173–1184.

Oral bioavailability of a drug is determined by a number of properties, including drug dissolution rate, solubility, intestinal permeability, and presystemic metabolism. Frequently, the rate limiting step in drug absorption from the GI tract is drug release and drug dissolution from the dosage form. Therapeutic agents with aqueous solubilities less than 100 μg/mL often present dissolution limitations to absorption. Physicochemical, formulation-related, and physiological factors can all influence drug dissolution. In this review, the authors will discuss the important physicochemical properties of a drug and physiological conditions in the GI tract that play an important part in drug dissolution and absorption processes and, consequently, the bioavailability of a drug.

Jost, W. H. and L. Bergmann (2010). "Clinical data of the prolonged-release formulation of ropinirole." *Fortschr Neurol Psychiatr* 78 Suppl 1:S20–S24.

Ropinirole is a nonergoline dopamine agonist with medium elimination half time, which has been licensed for the therapy of idiopathic Parkinson syndrome in mono- and add-on therapy for more than 10 years. Since 2008 a prolonged-release formulation has been available in Germany, which can be taken once daily. This formulation results in less plasma level fluctuations compared to the thrice-daily immediate-release formulation enabling smoother dopaminergic therapy with symptomatic efficacy day and night. Ropinirole PR has shown good efficacy and tolerability in controlled trials in monotherapy in early patients as well as in add-on studies in advanced patients. In a head-to-head comparison of both formulations as add-on therapy in advanced patients, higher doses were achieved with ropinirole PR accompanied by a higher mean decrease of L-Dopa dose. Under these conditions significantly higher efficacy was observed. The titration regime of ropinirole PR is faster with significant efficacy versus placebo as early as in week 2. Especially in patients with preexisting Parkinson-related poor sleep quality positive effects on sleep and nocturnal symptoms were shown.

Koudelka, S. et al. (2015). "Liposomal delivery systems for anti-cancer analogues of vitamin E." *J Control Release* 207:59–69.

Proapoptotic analogues of vitamin E (VE) exert selective anticancer effect on various animal cancer models. Neither suitable formulation of alpha-tocopheryl succinate (alpha-TOS), representative semi-synthetic VE analogue ester, nor suitable formulations of the other VE analogues for clinical application have been reported yet. The major factor limiting the use of VE analogues is their low solubility in aqueous solvents. Due to the hydrophobic character of VE analogues, liposomes are predetermined as suitable delivery system. Liposomal formulation prevents undesirable side effects of the drug, enhances the drug biocompatibility, and improves the drug therapeutic index. Liposomal formulations of VE analogues, especially of alpha-TOS and alpha-tocopheryl ether-linked acetic acid (alpha-TEA), have been developed. The anti-cancer effect of these liposomal VE analogues has been successfully demonstrated in preclinical models in vivo. Present achievements in: (i) preparation of liposomal formulations of VE analogues, (ii) physicochemical characterization of these developed systems, and (iii) testing of their biological activity such as induction of apoptosis and evaluation of anti-cancer effect are discussed in this review.

Lammers, T. et al. (2011). "Theranostic nanomedicine." *Acc Chem Res* 44(10):1029–1038.

Nanomedicine formulations aim to improve the biodistribution and the target site accumulation of systemically administered (chemo)therapeutic agents. Many different types of nanomedicines have been evaluated over the years, including, for instance, liposomes, polymers, micelles, and antibodies, and a significant amount of evidence has been obtained showing that these submicrometer-sized carrier materials are able to improve the balance between the efficacy and the toxicity of therapeutic interventions. Besides for therapeutic purposes, nanomedicine formulations have in recent years also been increasingly employed for imaging applications. Moreover, paralleled by advances in chemistry, biology, pharmacy, nanotechnology, medicine, and imaging, several different systems have been developed in the last decade in which disease diagnosis and therapy are combined. These so-called (nano) theranostics contain both a drug and an imaging agent within a single formulation, and they can be used for various different purposes. In this Account, we summarize several exemplary efforts in this regard, and we show that theranostic nanomedicines are highly suitable systems for monitoring drug delivery, drug release, and drug efficacy. The (pre)clinically most relevant applications of theranostic nanomedicines relate to their use for validating and optimizing the properties of drug delivery systems, and to their ability to be used for prescreening patients and enabling personalized medicine. Regarding the former, the combination of diagnostic and therapeutic agents within a single formulation provides real-time feedback on the pharmacokinetics, the target site localization and the (off-target) healthy organ accumulation of nanomedicines. Various examples of this will be highlighted in this Account, illustrating that by non-invasively visualizing how well carrier materials are able to deliver pharmacologically active agents to the pathological site, and how well they are able to prevent them from accumulating in potentially endangered healthy tissues, important information can be obtained for optimizing the basic properties of drug delivery systems, as well as for improving the balance between the efficacy and the toxicity of targeted therapeutic interventions. Regarding personalized medicine, it can be reasoned that only in patients which show high levels of target site accumulation, and which respond well to the first couple of treatment cycles, targeted therapy should be continued, and that in those in which this is not the case, other therapeutic options should be considered. Based on these insights, we expect that ever more efforts will be invested in developing theranostic nanomedicines, and that these systems and strategies will contribute substantially to realizing the potential of personalized medicine.

Lammers, T. et al. (2012). "Drug targeting to tumors: Principles, pitfalls and (pre-) clinical progress." *J Control Release* 161(2):175–187.

Many different systems and strategies have been evaluated for drug targeting to tumors over the years. Routinely used systems include liposomes, polymers, micelles, nanoparticles, and antibodies, and examples of strategies are passive drug targeting, active drug targeting to cancer cells, active drug targeting to endothelial cells, and triggered drug delivery. Significant progress has been made in this area of research both at the preclinical and at the clinical level, and a number of (primarily passively tumor-targeted) nanomedicine formulations have been approved for clinical use. Significant progress has also been made with regard to better understanding the (patho-) physiological principles of drug targeting to tumors. This has led to the identification of several important pitfalls in tumor-targeted drug delivery, including (I) overinterpretation of the EPR effect; (II) poor tumor and tissue penetration of nanomedicines; (III) misunderstanding of the potential usefulness of active drug targeting; (IV) irrational formulation design, based on materials which are too complex and not broadly applicable; (V) insufficient incorporation of nanomedicine formulations in clinically relevant combination regimens; (VI) negligence of the notion that the highest medical need relates to metastasis, and not to solid tumor treatment; (VII) insufficient integration of noninvasive imaging techniques and theranostics, which could be used to personalize nanomedicine-based therapeutic interventions; and (VIII) lack of (efficacy analyses in) proper animal models, which are physiologically more relevant and more predictive for the clinical situation. These insights strongly suggest that besides making ever more nanomedicine formulations, future efforts should also address some of the conceptual drawbacks of drug targeting to tumors, and that strategies should be developed to overcome these shortcomings.

Malik, T. et al. (2017). "'Fusion and binding inhibition' key target for HIV-1 treatment and pre-exposure prophylaxis: Targets, drug delivery and nanotechnology approaches." *Drug Deliv* 24(1):608–621.

More than 35 million people are living with HIV worldwide with approximately 2.3 million new infections per year. Cascade of events (cell entry, virus replication, assembly, and release of newly formed virions) is involved in the HIV-1 transmission process. Every single step offers a potential therapeutic strategy to halt this progression and HIV fusion into the human host cell is one such stage. Controlling the initial event of HIV-1 transmission is the best way to control its dissemination especially when prophylaxis is concerned. Action is required either on the HIV's or host's cell surface which is logically more rational when compared with other intracellular acting moieties. Aim of this manuscript is to detail the significance and current strategies to halt this initial step, thus blocking the entry of HIV-1 for further infection. Both HIV-1 and the possible host cell's receptors/coreceptors are under focus while specifying the targets available for inhibiting this fusion. Current and under-investigation moieties are categorized based on their versatile mechanisms. Advanced drug delivery and nanotechnology approaches present a key tool to exploit the therapeutic potential in a boosted way. Current drug delivery and the impact of nanotechnology in potentiating this strategy are detailed.

Mohamed-Ahmed, A. H. et al. (2016). "Non-human tools for the evaluation of bitter taste in the design and development of medicines: A systematic review." *Drug Discov Today* 21(7):1170–1180.

Taste evaluation is a crucial factor for determining acceptance of medicines by patients. The human taste panel test is the main method used to establish the overall palatability and acceptability of a drug product to a patient towards the end of development. Nonhuman in vitro and in vivo taste-evaluation tools are very useful for preformulation, quality control, and screening of formulations. These nonhuman taste assessment tools can be used to evaluate all aspects of taste quality. The focus of this review is bitterness because it is a key aspect of taste in association with the development of medicines. In this review, recent in vitro (analytical) and in vivo (non-human) tools are described for the assessment of the bitter taste of medicines. Their correlations with human taste data are critically discussed. The potential for their use in early screening of the taste of active pharmaceutical ingredients (APIs) to expedite pediatric formulation development is also considered.

Farrell, N. P. (2011). "Platinum formulations as anticancer drugs clinical and pre-clinical studies." *Curr Top Med Chem* 11(21):2623–2631.

This review summarizes clinical and preclinical results on platinum anticancer drug formulations. A concise summary of the use of oxidation state to modulate cancer pharmacology is given for Pt(IV) complexes, distinct from the clinically used Pt(II) drugs. The chemistry of platinum drug formulation combines aspects of kinetics of active moiety release from nominally weak-binding ligands (bond cleavage from platinum-carboxylate and platinum-phosphate) in polymers and nanoparticles with pharmacological considerations of plasma distribution and cellular accumulation. The action of any molecular entity as a drug is influenced by its ADME profile—absorption, distribution, metabolism, and excretion. The purpose of drug formulation is to alter any or all of these parameters with the ultimate goal of improving the efficacy and reducing side effects with the possibility to target drugs directly to the tumor site. The diverse array of approaches includes liposomes, polymers (not limited to peptides, dendrimers, biodegradable polymers, polysaccharides, and metallic nanoparticles). Functionalization of the surfaces of nanoparticles with antibodies or cellular surface recognition motifs may further target specific cancers.

Nunes, R. et al. (2014). "Formulation and delivery of anti-HIV rectal microbicides: Advances and challenges." *J Control Release* 194:278–294.

Men and women engaged in unprotected receptive anal intercourse (RAI) are at higher risk of acquiring HIV from infected partners. The implementation of preventive strategies is urgent and rectal microbicides may be a useful tool in reducing the sexual transmission of HIV. However, preclinical and first clinical trials have been able to identify limitations of candidate products, mostly related with safety issues, which can in turn enhance viral infection. Indeed, the development of suitable formulations for the rectal delivery of promising antiretroviral drugs is not an easy task and has been mostly based on products specifically intended for vaginal delivery, but these have been shown to provide suboptimal outcomes when administered rectally. Research and development in the rectal microbicide field are now charting their own path and important information is now available. In particular, specific formulation requirements of rectal microbicide products that need to be met have just recently been acknowledged despite additional work being still required. Desirable rectal microbicide product features regarding characteristics such as pH, osmolality, excipients, dosage forms, volume to be administered, and the need for applicator use have been studied and defined in recent years, and specific guidance is now possible. This review provides a synopsis of the field of rectal microbicides, namely past and ongoing clinical studies, and details on formulation and drug delivery issues regarding the specific development of rectal microbicide products. Also, future work, as required for the advancement of the field, is discussed.

Peltonen, L. (2018). "Practical guidelines for the characterization and quality control of pure drug nanoparticles and nano-cocrystals in the pharmaceutical industry." *Adv Drug Deliv Rev* 131:101–115.

The number of poorly soluble drug candidates is increasing, and this is also seen in the research interest towards drug nanoparticles and (nano-)cocrystals; improved solubility is the most important application of these nanosystems. In order to confirm the functionality of these nanoparticles throughout their lifecycle, repeatability of the formulation processes, functional performance of the formed systems in predetermined way and system stability, a thorough physicochemical understanding with the aid of necessary analytical techniques is needed. Even very minor deviations in for example particle size or size deviation in nanoscale can alter the product bioavailability, and the effect is even more dramatic with the smallest particle size fractions. Also, small particle size sets special requirements for the analytical techniques. In this review, most important physicochemical properties of drug nanocrystals and nano-cocrystals are presented, suitable analytical techniques, their pros and cons, are described with the extra input on practical point of view.

Pires, P. C. and A. O. Santos (2018). "Nanosystems in nose-to-brain drug delivery: A review of non-clinical brain targeting studies." *J Control Release* 270:89–100.

The treatment of neurodegenerative and psychiatric disorders remains a challenge in medical research. Several strategies have been developed over the years, either to overcome the blood–brain barrier or to achieve a safer or faster brain delivery, one of them being intranasal (IN) administration. The possibility of direct nose-to-brain transport offers enhanced targeting and reduced systemic side effects. Nevertheless, labile, low soluble, low permeant, and/or less potent drugs might need a formulation other than the common solutions or suspensions. For that, the formulation of nanosystems is considered to be a promising approach, since it can protect drugs from chemical and/or metabolic degradation, enhance their solubility, or offer transport through biological membranes. However, the understanding of the factors promoting efficient brain targeting when using nanosystems through the nasal route is currently patchy and incomplete. The main purpose of the present review was to evaluate the association between brain delivery efficacy (in terms of brain targeting, brain bioavailability, and time to reach the brain) and nanosystem type. For that, we performed a systematic bibliographic search and analysis. Furthermore, study designs, nanosystem properties, and reporting quality were also analyzed and discussed. It was found a high heterogeneity in how preclinical brain targeting studies have been conducted, analyzed, and reported in scientific literature, which surely originates a significant degree of bias and data dispersion. This review attempts to provide some systematization recommendations, which may be useful for researchers entering the field, and assist in increasing the uniformity of future reports. The analysis of literature data confirmed that there is evidence of the advantage of the IN route (when compared to the intravenous route) and in using carrier nanosystems (when compared to IN solutions) for brain delivery of a large set of drugs. Among the most represented nanosystem classes, microemulsions had some of the lowest pharmacokinetic ratio values, while polymeric micelles had some of the best. Nevertheless, brain targeting efficacy comparisons between nanosystem groups had little statistical significance, and the superiority of the polymeric micelles group disappeared when nanosystems were compared to the respective IN drug solutions. In fact, some drugs reached the brain so efficiently, even as drug solutions, that further benefit from formulating them into nanosystems became less evident.

Rodriguez, P. C. et al. (2010). "Clinical development and perspectives of CIMAvax EGF, Cuban vaccine for non–small-cell lung cancer therapy." *MEDICC Rev* 12(1):17–23.

INTRODUCTION: CIMAvax EGF is a therapeutic anticancer vaccine developed entirely in Cuba and licensed in Cuba for use in adult patients with stage IIIB/IV non–small-cell lung cancer (NSCLC). The vaccine is based on active immunotherapy by which an individual's immune response is manipulated to release its own effector antibodies (Abs) against the epidermal growth factor (EGF). OBJECTIVE: Review preclinical and clinical research conducted during development of CIMAvax EGF, primarily studies published by Cuban investigators in international peer-reviewed scientific journals. METHODS: An automated search for "vaccine" and "EGF" was conducted in PubMed, resulting in 17 articles published by Cuban authors between January 1, 1994, and September 30, 2009. Main findings were described and discussed, along with unpublished preliminary findings of an initial ongoing phase III clinical trial. RESULTS: Articles reviewed describe five phase I/II and one phase II clinical trials conducted in Cuba in 1995–2005. A noncontrolled 1995–1996 study resulted in the earliest published scientific evidence of the feasibility of inducing an immune response against autologous EGF in patients with different advanced stage tumors. Subsequent controlled, randomized trials included patients with advanced stage (IIIB/IV) NSCLC. The 2nd and 3rd phase I/II trials differentiated immunized patients as poor antibody responders (PAR) and good antibody responders (GAR), according to their anti-EGF antibody response, and confirmed greater immunogenicity with Montanide ISA 51 adjuvant in the vaccine formulation, as well as the benefits of low-dose cyclophosphamide treatment 72 hours before the first immunization. The 4th phase I/II trial found increased immunogenicity with an increased dose divided in 2 anatomical sites and also established correlation between Ab titers, serum EGF concentration and length of survival. In the first 4 phase I/II trials and the phase II trial, vaccine was administered after chemotherapy (ChTVV schedule). In the 5th phase I/III trial, longer survival and increased immunogenicity were achieved using a VChTV schedule and dividing the vaccine dose in 4 anatomical sites. The phase II clinical trial confirmed results of earlier studies as well as the mild-to-moderate adverse event profile associated with CIMAvax EGF Longer survival was observed in all vaccinated patients compared to controls, and the difference was significant ($p < 0.05$) in the group aged <60 years. CONCLUSIONS: CIMAvax EGF's benefits in earlier NSCLC stages and in other tumor locations, as well as in patients unfit for chemotherapy, need to be evaluated. Evidence of the vaccine's safety for chronic use also needs to be systemized.

Shadrack, D. M. et al. (2018). "Polyamidoamine dendrimers for enhanced solubility of small molecules and other desirable properties for site specific delivery: Insights from experimental and computational studies." *Molecules* 23(6):1419.

Clinical applications of many small molecules are limited due to poor solubility and lack of controlled release besides lack of other desirable properties. Experimental and computational studies have reported on the therapeutic potential of polyamidoamine (PAMAM) dendrimers as solubility enhancers in preclinical and clinical settings.

Besides formulation strategies, factors such as pH, PAMAM dendrimer generation, PAMAM dendrimer concentration, nature of the PAMAM core, special ligand and surface modifications of PAMAM dendrimer have an influence on drug solubility, and other recommendable pharmacological properties. This review, therefore, compiles the recently reported applications of PAMAM dendrimers in preclinical and clinical uses as enhancers of solubility and other desirable properties such as sustained and controlled release, bioavailability, biodistribution, toxicity reduction or enhancement, and targeted delivery of small molecules with emphasis on cancer treatment.

Shakya, P. et al. (2011). "Palatal mucosa as a route for systemic drug delivery: A review." *J Control Release* 151(1):2–9.

Rapid developments in the field of molecular biology and gene technology resulted in generation of many macromolecular drugs including peptides, proteins, polysaccharides, and nucleic acids in great number possessing superior pharmacological efficacy with site specificity and devoid of untoward and toxic effects. However, the main impediment for the oral delivery of these drugs as potential therapeutic agents is their extensive presystemic metabolism, instability in acidic environment resulting into inadequate and erratic oral absorption. Parenteral route of administration is the only established route that overcomes all these drawbacks associated with these orally less/inefficient drugs. But, these formulations are costly, have least patient compliance, require repeated administration, in addition to the other hazardous effects associated with this route. Over the last few decades pharmaceutical scientists throughout the world are trying to explore transdermal and transmucosal routes as an alternative to injections. Historically, oral transmucosal drug delivery has received intensive interest since ancient times for the most widely utilized route of administration for the systemic delivery of drugs. In more recent years, better systemic bioavailability of many drugs has been achieved by oromucosal route. Among the various transmucosal sites available, soft-palatal mucosa was also found to be the most convenient and easily accessible novel site for the delivery of therapeutic agents for systemic delivery as retentive dosage forms, because it has abundant vascularization and rapid cellular recovery time after exposure to stress. Smooth surface of the soft palate and its good flexibility are prerequisites to prevent mechanical irritation and local discomfort. The objective of this review is to provide an update on the most promising advances in novel noninvasive soft-palatal route and the conceptual and technical approaches to the design and formulation of soft-palatal drug delivery systems. In this area, the development of mucoadhesive delivery systems appears to be the most promising strategy.

Staatz, C. E. and S. E. Tett (2015). "Clinical pharmacokinetics of once-daily tacrolimus in solid-organ transplant patients." *Clin Pharmacokinet* 54(10):993–1025.

Tacrolimus is a pivotal immunosuppressant agent used in solid-organ transplantation. It was originally formulated for oral administration as Prograf®, a twice-daily immediate-release capsule. In an attempt to improve patient adherence, retain manufacturer market share and/or reduce health care costs, newer once-daily prolonged-release formulations of tacrolimus (Advagraf® and Envarsus® XR) and various generic versions of Prograf® are becoming available. Tacrolimus has a narrow therapeutic index. Small variations in drug exposure due to formulation differences can have a significant impact on patient outcomes. The aim of this review is to critically analyze the published data on the clinical pharmacokinetics of once-daily tacrolimus in solid-organ transplant patients. Forty-three traditional (noncompartmental) and five population pharmacokinetic studies were identified and evaluated. On the basis of the stricter criteria for narrow-therapeutic-index drugs, Prograf®, Advagraf® and Envarsus® XR are not bioequivalent [in terms of the area under the concentration–time curve from 0 to 24 hours (AUC0-24) or the minimum concentration (C min)]. Patients may require a daily dosage increase if converted from Prograf® to Advagraf®, while a daily dosage reduction appears necessary for conversion from Prograf® to Envarsus® XR. Prograf® itself, or generic immediate-release tacrolimus, can be administered in a once-daily regimen with a lower than double daily dose being reported to give 24-hours exposure equivalent to that of a twice-daily regimen. Intense clinical and concentration monitoring is prudent in the first few months after any conversion to once-daily tacrolimus dosing; however, there is no guarantee that therapeutic drug monitoring strategies applicable to one formulation (or twice-daily dosing) will be equally applicable to another. The correlation between the tacrolimus AUC0-24 and C min is variable and not strong for all three formulations, indicating that trough measurements may not always give a good indication of overall drug exposure. Further investigation is required into whether the prolonged-release formulations have reduced within-subject pharmacokinetic variability, which would be a distinct advantage. Whether the effects of factors that influence tacrolimus absorption and presystemic metabolism (patient genotype status; GI disease and disorders) and drug interactions differ across the formulations needs to be further elucidated. Most pharmacokinetic comparison studies to date have involved relatively stable patients, and many have been sponsored by the pharmaceutical companies manufacturing the new formulations. Larger randomized, controlled trials are needed in different transplant populations to determine whether there are differences in efficacy and toxicity across the formulations and whether formulation conversion is worthwhile in the longer term. While it has been suggested that once-daily administration of tacrolimus may improve patient compliance, further studies are required to demonstrate this. Mistakenly interchanging different tacrolimus formulations can lead to serious patient harm. Once-daily tacrolimus is now available as an alternative to twice-daily tacrolimus and can be used de novo in solid-organ transplant recipients or as a different formulation for existing patients, with appropriate dosage modifications. Clinicians need to be fully aware of pharmacokinetic and possible outcome differences across the different formulations of tacrolimus.

Stuurman, F. E. et al. (2013). "Oral anticancer drugs: Mechanisms of low bioavailability and strategies for improvement." *Clin Pharmacokinet* 52(6):399–414.

The use of oral anticancer drugs has increased during the last decade, because of patient preference, lower costs, proven efficacy, lack of infusion-related inconveniences, and the opportunity to develop chronic treatment regimens. Oral administration of anticancer drugs is, however, often hampered by limited bioavailability of the drug, which is associated with a wide variability. Since most anticancer drugs have a narrow therapeutic window and are dosed at or close to the maximum tolerated dose, a wide variability in the bioavailability can have a negative impact on treatment outcome. This review discusses mechanisms of low bioavailability of oral anticancer drugs and strategies for improvement. The extent of oral bioavailability depends on many factors, including release of the drug from the pharmaceutical dosage form, a drug's stability in the GI tract, factors affecting dissolution, the rate of passage through the gut wall, and the presystemic metabolism in the gut wall and liver. These factors are divided into pharmaceutical limitations, physiological endogenous limitations, and patient-specific limitations. There are several strategies to reduce or overcome these limitations. First, pharmaceutical adjustment of the formulation or the physicochemical characteristics of the drug can improve the dissolution rate and absorption. Second, pharmacological interventions by combining the drug with inhibitors of transporter proteins and/or presystemic metabolizing enzymes can overcome the physiological endogenous limitations. Third, chemical modification of a drug by synthesis of a derivative, salt form, or prodrug could enhance the bioavailability by improving the absorption and bypassing physiological endogenous limitations. Although the bioavailability can be enhanced by various strategies, the development of novel oral products with low solubility or cell membrane permeability remains cumbersome and is often unsuccessful. The main reasons are unacceptable variation in the bioavailability and high investment costs. Furthermore, novel oral anticancer drugs are frequently associated with toxic effects including unacceptable GI adverse effects. Therefore, compliance is often suboptimal, which may negatively influence treatment outcome.

Van Peer, A. (2010). "Variability and impact on design of bioequivalence studies." *Basic Clin Pharmacol Toxicol* 106(3):146–153.

In 2008, the European Agency for the Evaluation of Medicinal Products released a draft guidance on the investigation of bioequivalence for immediate release dosage forms with systemic action to replace the former guidance of a decade ago. Revisions of the regulatory guidance are based upon many questions over the past years and sometimes continuing scientific discussions on the use of the most suitable statistical analysis methods and study designs, particularly for drugs and drug products with high within-subject variability. Although high within-subject variability is usually associated with a coefficient of variation of 30% or more, new approaches are available in the literature to allow a gradual increase and a levelling off of the bioequivalence limits to some maximum wider values (e.g., 75%–133%), dependent on the increase in the within-subject variability. The two-way, crossover single-dose study measuring parent drug is still the design of first choice. A partial replicate design with repeating the reference product and scaling the bioequivalence for the reference variability are proposed for drugs with high within-subject variability. In case of high variability, more regulatory authorities may accept a two-stage or group-sequential bioequivalence design using appropriately adjusted statistical analysis. This review also considers the mechanisms why drugs and drug products may exhibit large variability. The physiological complexity of the GI tract and the interaction with the physicochemical properties of drug substances may contribute to the variation in plasma drug concentration–time profiles of drugs and drug products and to variability between and within subjects. A review of submitted bioequivalence studies at the FDA's Office of Generic Drugs over the period 2003–2005 indicated that extensive presystemic metabolism of the drug substance was the most important explanation for consistently high variability drugs, rather than a formulation factor. These scientific efforts are expected to further lead to revisions of earlier regulatory guidance in other regions as is the current situation in Europe.

Vural, E. M. et al. (2014). "Optimal dosages for melatonin supplementation therapy in older adults: A systematic review of current literature." *Drugs Aging* 31(6):441–451.

BACKGROUND: Melatonin is a hormone that regulates circadian rhythm, and its levels decline with age. As melatonin levels decrease, older adults are prone to develop disorders related to an altered circadian rhythm. The effective dose of melatonin supplementation in these disorders remains unclear. OBJECTIVES: Our objective was to define the optimal dosage of exogenous melatonin administration in disorders related to altered melatonin levels in older adults aged 55 years and above by determining the dose–response effect of exogenous administered melatonin on endogenous levels. METHODS: We conducted a systematic review through PubMed/MEDLINE and Embase, both from 1980 until November 2013. Included articles studied the effect of exogenous melatonin administration on endogenous melatonin levels in either serum, urine, or saliva in humans aged 55 years and above. RESULTS: We included 16 articles, nine of which were randomized controlled trials (RCTs). The mean age varied from 55.3 to 77.6 years. Melatonin dosage varied from 0.1 mg to 50 mg/kg and was administered orally in all studies. Pre- and postintervention levels revealed a significant elevation of the postintervention melatonin levels in a dose-dependent fashion. The maximum concentrations measured in serum and urine were all elevated compared with placebo, and a higher elevation in older adults than in younger adults was demonstrated. Even though there were no differences between times to reach maximum concentration in serum and urine, melatonin levels with higher doses were maintained longer above a certain threshold than were lower doses. CONCLUSION: In older adults, we advise the use of the lowest possible dose of immediate-release formulation melatonin to best mimic the normal physiological circadian rhythm of melatonin and to avoid prolonged, supraphysiological blood levels.

Permeation

Aguirre, T. A. et al. (2015). "In vitro and in vivo preclinical evaluation of a minisphere emulsion-based formulation (SmPill(R)) of salmon calcitonin." *Eur J Pharm Sci* 79:102–111.

Salmon calcitonin (sCT, MW 3432Da) is a benchmark molecule for an oral peptide delivery system because it is degraded and has low intestinal epithelial permeability. Four dry emulsion minisphere prototypes (SmPill(R)) containing sCT were coformulated with permeation enhancers (PEs): sodium taurodeoxycholate (NaTDC), sodium caprate (C10) or coco-glucoside (CG), or with a pH acidifier, citric acid (CA). Minispheres protected sCT from thermal degradation and the released sCT retained high bioactivity, as determined by cyclic AMP generation in T47D cells. Preminisphere emulsions of PEs combined with sCT increased absolute bioavailability (F) compared to native sCT following rat intrajejunal (i.j.) and intracolonic (i.c.) loop instillations, an effect that was more pronounced in colon. Minispheres corresponding to ~2000 I.U. (~390 μg) sCT/kg were instilled by i.j. or i.c. instillations and hypocalcaemia resulted from all prototypes. The absolute F (i.j.) of sCT was 11.0, 4.8, and 1.4% for minispheres containing NaTDC (10 μmol/kg), CG (12 μmol/kg) or CA (32 μmol/kg) respectively. For i.c. instillations, the largest absolute F (22% in each case) was achieved for minispheres containing either C10 (284 μmol/kg) or

CG (12 μmol/kg), whilst the absolute F was 8.2% for minispheres loaded with CA (32 μmol/kg). In terms of relative F, the best data were obtained for minispheres containing NaTDC (i.j.), a 4-fold increase over sCT solution, and also for either C10 or CG (i.c.), where there was a 3-fold increase over sCT solution. Histology of instilled intestinal loops indicated that neither the minispheres nor components thereof caused major perturbation. In conclusion, selected SmPill(R) minisphere formulations may have the potential to be used as oral peptide delivery systems when delivered to jejunum or colon.

Bhalekar, M. et al. (2015). "Formulation and evaluation of Adapalene-loaded nanoparticulates for epidermal localization." *Drug Deliv Transl Res* 5(6):585–595.

Adapalene (ADP), a topically administered antiacne drug, finds limitation due to poor penetration, limited localization, and associated incompatibility of photosensitization and skin irritation. To explicate an innovative and safe method for ADP administration and alleviating the associated limitations, solid lipid nanoparticles (SLN) of ADP have been fabricated and evaluated for efficacy in the present work. The SLN were prepared using preemulsion sonication method and incorporated into convenient topical dosage form, hydrogels. In vitro permeation studies of the hydrogels through HCS indicated gel containing ADP-SLN showed 2-fold more accumulation in skin layers as compared to conventional ADP gel. Rheological studies demonstrated ADP-SLN gel to possess pseudoplastic behavior, occlusion and hydration studies revealed permeation effectiveness of ADP-SLN gel over conventional ADP gel while primary skin irritation studies established safety of the ADP-SLN gel upon topical application. Hence, it was concluded that the studied ADP-SLN formulation with skin localizing ability may be a promising carrier for topical delivery of ADP.

Bijukumar, D. et al. (2016). "Design of an inflammation-sensitive polyelectrolyte-based topical drug delivery system for arthritis." *AAPS PharmSciTech* 17(5):1075–1085.

The most successful treatment strategy for arthritis is intra-articular injections that are costly and have reduced patient compliance. The purpose of the current study was to develop an inflammation-sensitive system for topical drug administration. Multimacromolecular alginate-hyaluronic acid-chitosan (A-H-C) polyelectrolyte complex nanoparticles, loaded with indomethacin were developed employing pregel and postgel techniques in the presence of dodecyl-L-pyroglutamate (DLP). In addition to in vitro studies, in silico simulations were performed to affirm and associate the molecular interactions inherent to the formulation of core all-natural multicomponent biopolymeric architectures composed of an anionic (alginate), a cationic (chitosan), and an amphi-ionic polyelectrolytic (hyaluronic acid) macromolecule. The results demonstrated that DLP significantly influenced the size of the synthesized nanoparticles. Drug-content analysis revealed higher encapsulation efficiency (77.3%) in the presence of DLP, irrespective of the techniques used. Moreover, in vitro drug release studies showed that indomethacin release from the nanosystem was significantly improved (98%) in Fenton's reagent. Drug permeation across a cellulose membrane using a Franz diffusion cell system showed an initial surge flux (0.125 mg/cm(-2)/h), followed by sustained release of indomethacin for the postgel nanoparticles revealing its effective skin permeation efficiency. In conclusion, the study presents novel nanoparticles which could effectively encapsulate and deliver hydrophobic drugs to the target site, particularly for arthritis.

Candido, T. M. et al. (2018). "Safety and antioxidant efficacy profiles of rutin-loaded ethosomes for topical application." *AAPS PharmSciTech* 19(4):1773–1780.

Topical application of dermocosmetics containing antioxidant and/or the intake of antioxidants through diet or supplementation are remarkable tools in an attempt to slow down some of the harmful effects of free radicals. Rutin is a strong antioxidant compound used in food and pharmaceutical industries. It was established that rutin presents a low skin permeation rate, a property that could be considered an inconvenience to the satisfactory action for a dermocosmetic formulation to perform its antioxidant activity onto the skin. Therefore, it is indispensable to improve its delivery, aiming at increasing its antioxidant capacity in deeper layers of the epidermis, being a possibility to associate the rutin to liposomal vesicles, such as ethosomes. Thus, in this work, the preclinical safety of rutin-loaded ethosomes was investigated employing an in vitro method, and the clinical safety and efficacy were also assessed. Rutin-loaded ethosomes were efficaciously obtained in a nanoscale dimension with a relevant bioactive compound loading (80.2%) and provided antioxidant in vitro activity in comparison with the blank sample. Preclinical and clinical safety assays assured the innocuous profile of the rutin-loaded ethosomes. The ethosomes containing the bioactive compound accomplished a more functional delivery system profile, since in the tape stripping assay, the deeper layers presented higher rutin amounts than the active delivered in its free state. However, the ex vivo antioxidant efficacy test detected no positive antioxidant activity from the rutin-loaded ethosomes, even though the in vitro assay demonstrated an affirmative antioxidant action.

Christensen, J. M. et al. (2011). "Hydrocortisone diffusion through synthetic membrane, mouse skin, and epiderm cultured skin." *Arch Drug Inf* 4(1):10–21.

OBJECTIVES: The penetration of hydrocortisone (HC) from six topical over-the-counter products along with one prescription cream through cultured normal human-derived epidermal keratinocytes (Epiderm), mouse skin and synthetic nylon membrane was performed as well as the effect hydrating the skin by prewashing was explored using the Upright Franz Cell. METHOD AND RESULTS: Permeation of HC through EpiDerm, mouse skin, and synthetic membrane was highest with the topical HC gel formulation with prewash treatment of the membranes among seven products evaluated, $198 \pm 32 \, \mu g/cm^2$, $746.32 \pm 12.43 \, \mu g/cm^2$, and $1882 \pm 395.18 \, \mu g/cm^2$, respectively. Prewashing to hydrate the skin enhanced HC penetration through EpiDerm and mouse skin. The 24-hours HC released from topical gel with prewash treatment was $198.495 \pm 32 \, \mu g/cm^2$ and $746.32 \pm 12.43 \, \mu g/cm^2$, while without prewash, the 24-hours HC released from topical gel was $67.2 \pm 7.41 \, \mu g/cm^2$ and $653.43 \pm 85.62 \, \mu g/cm^2$ through EpiDerm and mouse skin, respectively. HC penetration through synthetic membrane was 10 times greater than through mouse skin and EpiDerm. Generally, the shape, pattern, and rank order of HC diffusion from each commercial product was similar through each membrane.

Cianetti, S. et al. (2010). "Enhancement of intestinal absorption of 2-methyl cytidine prodrugs." *Drug Deliv* 17(4):214–222.

The purpose of this study was to investigate the in vivo absorption enhancement of a nucleoside (phosphoramidate prodrug of 2′-methyl-cytidine) antiviral agent of proven efficacy by means of intestinal permeation enhancers. Natural nucleosides are hydrophilic molecules that do not rapidly penetrate cell membranes by diffusion and their absorption relies on specialized transporters. Therefore, the oral absorption of nucleoside prodrugs and the target organ concentration of the biologically active nucleotide can be limited due to poor permeation across the intestinal epithelium. In the present study, the specificity, concentration dependence, and effect of four classes of absorption promoters, i.e., fatty acids, steroidal detergents, mucoadhesive polymers, and secretory transport inhibitors, were evaluated in a rat in vivo model. Sodium caprate and alpha-tocopheryl-polyethyleneglycol-1000-succinate (TPGS) showed a significant effect in increasing liver concentration of nucleotide (5-fold). These results suggested that both excipients might be suited in a controlled release matrix for the synchronous release of the drug and absorption promoter directly to the site of absorption and highlights that the effect is strictly dependent on the absorption promoter dose. The feasibility of such a formulation approach in humans was evaluated with the aim of developing a solid dosage form for the peroral delivery of nucleosides and showed that these excipients do provide a potential valuable tool in preclinical efficacy studies to drive discovery programs forward.

Davies, L. B. et al. (2017). "Accelerating topical anaesthesia using microneedles." *Skin Pharmacol Physiol* 30(6):277–283.

BACKGROUND/AIMS: Topical anesthetics reduce pain during venous access procedures in children. However, clinical use is hindered by a significant anesthetic onset time. Restricted diffusion of the topical anesthetic through the stratum corneum barrier is the principal reason for the delayed onset. Microneedles can painlessly pierce the skin. This study evaluated microneedle pretreatment of ex vivo human skin as a means to increase the rate of tetracaine permeation, in order to accelerate the onset of anesthesia. METHODS: Franz-type diffusion cells were used to determine permeation of a commercial tetracaine formulation, Ametop gel, through human skin epidermis. Microneedle-assisted permeation was compared to untreated epidermis. Upon completion of the permeation studies, the epidermal membranes were visually characterized. RESULTS: At 30 minutes, 5.43 $\mu g/cm^2$ of tetracaine had permeated through the untreated membrane compared to 12.13 $\mu g/cm^2$ through the microneedle-treated membrane. Insertion of a hypodermic needle created a large single channel in the epidermis (approx. 4,250 μm^2), whilst the punctured surface area following microneedle treatments was estimated to be 75,000 μm^2. CONCLUSION: Pretreatment of skin with microneedles significantly enhances the permeation of tetracaine. Microneedles have the potential to more than halve the onset time for anesthesia when applying Ametop gel.

Dubey, S. and Y. N. Kalia (2014). "Understanding the poor iontophoretic transport of lysozyme across the skin: When high charge and high electrophoretic mobility are not enough." *J Control Release* 183:35–42.

The original aim of the study was to investigate the transdermal iontophoretic delivery of lysozyme and to gain further insight into the factors controlling protein electrotransport. Initial experiments were done using porcine skin. Lysozyme transport was quantified by using an activity assay based on the lysis of Micrococcus lysodeikticus and was corrected for the release of endogenous enzyme from the skin during current application. Cumulative iontophoretic permeation of lysozyme during 8 hours at 0.5 mA/cm^2 (0.7 mM; pH 6) was surprisingly low (5.37 $\pm$ 3.46 $\mu g/cm^2$ in 8 hours) as compared to electrotransport of cytochrome c (Cyt c) and ribonuclease A (RNase A) under similar conditions (923.0 $\pm$ 496.1 and 170.71 $\pm$ 92.13 μg/cm^2, respectively)—despite its having a higher electrophoretic mobility. The focus of the study then became to understand and explain the causes of its poor iontophoretic transport. Lowering formulation pH to 5 increased histidine protonation in the protein and decreased the ionization of fixed negative charges in the skin (pI ~4.5) and resulted in a small but statistically significant increase in permeation. Co-iontophoresis of acetaminophen revealed a significant inhibition of electroosmosis; inhibition factors of 12–16 were indicative of strong lysozyme binding to skin. Intriguingly, lidocaine electrotransport, which is due almost exclusively to electromigration, was also decreased (approximately 2.7-fold) following skin pretreatment by lysozyme iontophoresis (cf. iontophoresis of buffer solution)—suggesting that lysozyme was also able to influence subsequent cation electromigration. In order to elucidate the site of skin binding, different porcine skin models were tested (dermatomed skin with thicknesses of 250 and 750 μm, tape-stripped skin and heat-separated dermis). Although no difference was seen between permeation across 250 and 750 μm dermatomed skin (13.57 $\pm$ 12.20 and 5.37 $\pm$ 3.46 μg/cm^2, respectively), there was a statistically significant increase across tape-stripped skin and heat-separated dermis (36.86 $\pm$ 7.48 and 43.42 $\pm$ 13.11 μg/cm^2, respectively)—although transport was still much less than that seen across intact skin for Cyt c or RNase A. Furthermore, electroosmotic inhibition factors fell to 2.2 and 1.0 for tape-stripped skin and heat-separated dermis—indicating that lysozyme affected convective solvent flow through interactions with the epidermis and predominantly the stratum corneum. Finally, cation exchange and hydrophobic interaction chromatography confirmed that although lysozyme had greater positive charge than Cyt c or RNase A under the conditions used for iontophoresis, it also possessed the highest surface hydrophobicity, which may have facilitated the interactions with the transport pathways and encouraged aggregation in the skin microenvironment. Thus, high charge and electrophoretic mobility seem to be inadequate descriptors to predict the transdermal iontophoretic transport of proteins whose complex three-dimensional structures can facilitate interactions with cutaneous transport pathways.

Feturi, F. G. et al. (2018). "Mycophenolic acid for topical immunosuppression in vascularized composite allotransplantation: Optimizing formulation and preliminary evaluation of bioavailability and pharmacokinetics." *Front Surg* 5:20.

Mycophenolic acid (MPA), is the active form of the ester prodrug mycophenolate mofetil (MMF). MMF is an FDA approved immunosuppressive drug that has been successfully used in systemic therapy in combination with other agents for the prevention of acute rejection (AR) following solid organ transplantation (SOT) as well as in vascularized composite allotransplantation (VCA). Systemic use of MMF is associated with GI adverse effects. Topical delivery of the prodrug could thus provide graft-targeted immunosuppression while minimizing systemic drug exposure. Our goal was to develop a topical formulation of MPA with optimal in vitro/in vivo characteristics such as release, permeation, and tissue bioavailability to enable safety and efficacy evaluation in clinical VCA. Permeation studies were performed with a solution of MPA (10 mg/mL). In vitro release and permeation studies were performed for different semisolid formulations (Aladerm, Lipoderm, emollient, and VersaBase) of MPA (1% w/w) using a Franz Diffusion Cell System (FDCS). In vivo pharmacokinetic characterization of MPA release from Lipoderm was performed in rats.

MPA in solution exhibited a steady state flux (3.8 ± 0.1 µg/cm^2/h) and permeability ($1.1 \times 10(-7) \pm 3.2 \times 10(-9)$ cm/s). MPA in Lipoderm exhibited a steady state flux of 1.12 ± 0.24 µg/cm^2/h, and permeability of $6.2 \times 10(-09) \pm 1.3 \times 10(-9)$ cm/s across the biomimetic membrane. The cumulative release of MPA from Lipoderm, showed a linear single-phase profile with a R(2) of 0.969. In vivo studies with MPA in Lipoderm showed markedly higher local tissue MPA levels and lower systemic MPA exposure as compared to values obtained after intravenous delivery of the same dose of drug ($p < 0.05$). We successfully developed for the first time, a topical formulation of MPA in Lipoderm with optimal in vitro/in vivo permeability characteristics and no undesirable local or systemic adverse effects in vivo. Our study provides key preliminary groundwork for translational efficacy studies of topical MPA in preclinical large animal VCA models and for effectiveness evaluation in patients receiving VCA.

Fiala, S. et al. (2010). "A fundamental investigation into the effects of eutectic formation on transmembrane transport." *Int J Pharm* 393(1–2):68–73.

Eutectic systems enhance the permeation of therapeutic agents across biological barriers, but the mechanism by which this occurs has not previously been elucidated. Using human skin, it has proven difficult to isolate the fundamental effects of eutectic formation on molecule diffusion and partition from those that arise as a consequence of the simultaneous application of two agents. The aim of this work was to employ a model hydrophobic membrane to understand the fundamental permeation characteristics of two agents when applied as a eutectic mixture. Lidocaine and prilocaine were selected as model agents and infinite-dose permeation studies were carried out using precalibrated Franz diffusion cells with two thicknesses of silicone membrane. Membrane solubility was determined by HCl solution extraction and the membrane diffusion coefficients were calculated from the permeation lag times. The maximum permeation enhancement was achieved using a eutectic mixture at a 0.7:0.3 prilocaine/lidocaine ratio. A higher solubility of both agents in silicone membrane, enhanced diffusivity of prilocaine and superior release of both drugs, all contributed to produce enhanced permeation from the eutectic mixtures. Deconvolution of the transmembrane transport process suggests that the eutectic enhancement phenomena is a consequence of more favorable permeation characteristics of the two molecules in the absence of a formulation vehicle which competes in the transport process.

Folzer, E. et al. (2014). "Comparison of skin permeability for three diclofenac topical formulations: An in vitro study." *Pharmazie* 69(1):27–31.

Diclofenac is a hydrophilic nonsteroidal anti-inflammatory drug (NSAID) widely used in humans and animals. There are limited published studies evaluating diclofenac's skin permeation following topical administration. The aim of our study was to evaluate and compare the in vitro permeation of three different diclofenac-containing formulations (patch, gel, solution) over 24 hours. These formulations were applied ($n = 6$ per formulation) to pig skin sandwiched between the two chambers in a static Franz diffusion cell and aliquots from the receptor medium were sampled at predefined time points. An HPLC method with UV detection was developed and validated with the aim of characterizing the transepidermal penetration in the in vitro system. Using this assay to determine the permeation parameters, results at 24 hours showed that the Flector patch released the highest drug amount (54.6%), whereas a lower drug amount was delivered with the Voltaren Emulgel (38.2%) and the solution (34.4%). The commercial gel showed the highest flux (39.9 ± 0.9 μg/cm²/h) and the shortest lag time (1.97 ± 0.02 hours). Based on these in vitro results using pig skin, the transdermal patch resulted in a long-lasting controlled release of diclofenac, while the gel had the shortest lag time.

Ghadi, R. and N. Dand (2017). "BCS class IV drugs: Highly notorious candidates for formulation development." *J Control Release* 248:71–95.

BCS class IV drugs (e.g., amphotericin B, furosemide, acetazolamide, ritonavir, paclitaxel) exhibit many characteristics that are problematic for effective oral and per oral delivery. Some of the problems associated include low aqueous solubility, poor permeability, erratic and poor absorption, inter and intra subject variability and significant positive food effect which leads to low and variable bioavailability. Also, most of the class IV drugs are substrate for P-glycoprotein (low permeability) and substrate for CYP3A4 (extensive presystemic metabolism) which further potentiates the problem of poor therapeutic potential of these drugs. A decade back, extreme examples of class IV compounds were an exception rather than the rule, yet today many drug candidates under development pipeline fall into this category. Formulation and development of an efficacious delivery system for BCS class IV drugs are herculean tasks for any formulator. The inherent hurdles posed by these drugs hamper their translation to actual market. The importance of the formulation composition and design to successful drug development is especially illustrated by the BCS class IV case. To be clinically effective these drugs require the development of a proper delivery system for both oral and per oral delivery. Ideal oral dosage forms should produce both a reasonably high bioavailability and low inter and intra subject variability in absorption. Also, ideal systems for BCS class IV should produce a therapeutic concentration of the drug at reasonable dose volumes for intravenous administration. This article highlights the various techniques and upcoming strategies which can be employed for the development of highly notorious BCS class IV drugs. Some of the techniques employed are lipid-based delivery systems, polymer based nanocarriers, crystal engineering (nanocrystals and cocrystals), liquisolid technology, self-emulsifying solid dispersions, and miscellaneous techniques addressing the Pgp efflux problem. The review also focuses on the roadblocks in the clinical development of the aforementioned strategies such as problems in scale up, manufacturing under cGMP guidelines, appropriate quality control tests, validation of various processes and variable therein etc. It also brings to forefront the current lack of regulatory guidelines which poses difficulties during preclinical and clinical testing for submission of NDA and subsequent marketing. Today, the pharmaceutical industry has as its disposal a series of reliable and scalable formulation strategies for BCS Class IV drugs. However, due to lack of understanding of the basic physical chemistry behind these strategies' formulation development is still driven by trial and error.

Giannos, S. A. et al. (2018). "Formulation stabilization and disaggregation of bevacizumab, ranibizumab and aflibercept in dilute solutions." *Pharm Res* 35(4):78.

PURPOSE: Studies were conducted to investigate dilute solutions of the monoclonal antibody (mAb) bevacizumab, mAb fragment ranibizumab and fusion protein aflibercept, develop common procedures for formulation of low concentration mAbs and identify a stabilizing formulation for anti-VEGF mAbs for use in vitro permeation studies. METHODS: Excipient substitutions were screened. The most stabilizing formulation was chosen. Standard dilutions of bevacizumab, ranibizumab and aflibercept were prepared in PBS, manufacturer's formulation, and the new formulation. Analysis was by SE-HPLC and ELISA. Stability, disaggregation and preexposure tests were studied. RESULTS: When Avastin, Lucentis and Eylea are diluted in PBS or manufacturer's formulation, there is a 40%–50% loss of monomer concentration and drug activity. A formulation containing 0.3% NaCl, 7.5% trehalose, 10 mM arginine and 0.04% Tween 80 at a pH of 6.78 stabilized the mAbs and minimized the drug loss. The formulation also disaggregates mAb aggregation while preserving the activity. Degassing the formulation increases recovery. CONCLUSIONS: We developed a novel formulation that significantly stabilizes mAbs under unfavorable conditions such as low concentration or body temperature. The formulation allows for tissue permeation experimentation. The formulation also exhibits a disaggregating effect on mAbs, which can be applied to the manufacture/packaging of mAbs and bioassay reagents.

Grammen, C. et al. (2014). "Development and in vitro evaluation of a vaginal microbicide gel formulation for UAMC01398, a novel diaryltriazine NNRTI against HIV-1." *Antiviral Res* 101:113–121.

Diaryltriazines (DATAs) constitute a class of nonnucleoside reverse transcriptase inhibitors (NNRTIs) that are being investigated for use as anti-HIV microbicides. The aim of the present study was (1) to assess the biopharmaceutical properties of the DATA series, (2) to select the lead candidate as vaginal microbicide and (3) to develop and evaluate gel formulations of the lead candidate. First, the vaginal tissue permeation potential of the different DATAs was screened by performing permeability and solubility measurements. To obtain a suitable formulation of the lead microbicide candidate, several hydroxyethylcellulose-based gels were assessed for their cellular toxicity, stability and ability to enable UAMC01398 epithelial permeation. Also, attention was given to appropriate preservative selection. Because of its favourable in vitro activity, safety and biopharmaceutical profile, UAMC01398 was chosen as the lead microbicide candidate among the DATA series. Formulating UAMC01398 as a vaginal gel did not affect its anti-HIV activity. Safe and chemically stable gel formulations of UAMC01398 (0.02%) included a nonsolubilizing gel and a gel containing sulfobutyl ether-beta-cyclodextrin (SBE-betaCD, 5%) as solubilizing excipient. Inclusion of SBE-betaCD in the gel formulation resulted in enhanced microbicide flux across HEC-1A epithelial cell layers, to an extent that could not be achieved by simply increasing the dose of UAMC01398. The applied rational (pre)formulation approach resulted in the development of aqueous-based gel formulations that are appropriate for further in vivo investigation of the anti-HIV microbicide potential of the novel NNRTI UAMC01398.

Gupta, V. et al. (2011). "Reduction in cisplatin genotoxicity (micronucleus formation) in non target cells of mice by protransfersome gel formulation used for management of cutaneous squamous cell carcinoma." *Acta Pharm* 61(1):63–71.

Cisplatin-loaded protransfersome system was prepared and characterized for in vitro drug permeation, drug deposition and antitumor effect. A histopathological study and a genotoxicity study were also done. The skin permeation data of cisplatin from protransfersome gel formulation revealed 494.33 ± 11.87 µg/cm^2, which was significantly higher than that from the control plain drug solution in 0.9% NaCl ($p < 0.001$). Untreated group of animals showed invasive moderately differentiated keratinizing squamous cell carcinoma (malignant stage). However, with cisplatin loaded protransfersome gel system simple epithelial hyperplasia (precancerous stage) with no cancerous growth was observed. Also, a significant induction in micronucleus formation was found in the group that was treated with injectable intraperitoneal cis-platin preparation in 0.9 % saline as compared to the group treated with topical pro-transfersome gel formulation. The findings of this research work appear to support improved, site-specific and localized drug action in the skin, thus providing a better option for dealing with skin related problems like squamous cell carcinoma.

Han, S. M. et al. (2017). "Emulsion-based intradermal delivery of melittin in rats." *Molecules* 22(5):836.

Bee venom (BV) has long been used as a traditional medicine. The aim of the present study was to formulate a BV emulsion with good rheological properties for dermal application and investigate the effect of formulation on the permeation of melittin through dermatomed rat skin. A formulated emulsion containing 1% (w/v) BV was prepared. The emulsion was compared with distilled water (DW) and 25% (w/v) N-methyl-2-pyrrolidone (NMP) in DW. Permeation of melittin from aqueous solution through the dermatomed murine skin was evaluated using the Franz diffusion cells. Samples of receptor cells withdrawn at predetermined time intervals were measured for melittin amount. After the permeation study, the same skin was used for melittin extraction. In addition, a known amount of melittin (5 µg/mL) was added to stratum corneum, epidermis, and dermis of the rat skin, and the amount of melittin was mea-sured at predetermined time points. The measurement of melittin from all samples was done with HPLC-MS/MS. No melittin was detected in the receptor phase at all time points in emulsion, DW, or NMP groups. When the amount of melittin was fur-ther analyzed in stratum corneum, epidermis, and dermis from the permeation study, melittin was still not detected. In an additional experiment, the amount of melittin added to all skin matrices was corrected against the amount of melittin recovered. While the total amount of melittin was retained in the stratum corneum, less than 10% of melittin remained in epidermis and dermis within 15 and 30 minutes, respectively. Skin microporation with BV emulsion facilitates the penetration of melittin across the stratum corneum into epidermis and dermis, where emulsified melittin could have been metabolized by locally occurring enzymes.

Hoeller, S. et al. (2009). "Lecithin based nanoemulsions: A comparative study of the influence of non-ionic surfactants and the cationic phytosphingosine on physicochemical behaviour and skin permeation." *Int J Pharm* 370(1–2):181–186.

Charged drug delivery systems are interesting candidates for the delivery of drugs through skin. In the present study, it was possible to create negatively and positively charged oil/water nanoemulsions by using sucrose laureate and polysorbate 80 as nonionic surfactants. The positively charged nanoemulsions were generated by add-ing cationic phytosphingosine (PS). The relationship between the physicochemical properties of the nanoemulsions was shown by particle size and zeta potential mea-surements. These properties were dependent on the type of nonionic surfactant and the concentration of PS. Furthermore the cationic PS had a positive impact on the skin permeation rates (flux) of the incorporated model drugs fludrocortisone acetate and flumethasone pivalate. An enhancement factor between 1.1 and 1.5 was obtained in relation to the control. The interaction of preimpregnated porcine skin with positively and negatively charged nanoemulsions was confirmed by DSC analysis. The generated DSC-curves showed a slight difference in the phase transition temperature assigned to the characteristic lipid transition. However, it was not possible to assign the effect to one of the ingredients in the multicomponent system.

Hussain, I. et al. (2016). "Fabrication of anti-vitiligo ointment containing Psoralea corylifolia: In vitro and in vivo characterization." *Drug Des Devel Ther* 10:3805–3816.

BACKGROUND: Vitiligo is a repugnant and odious dermatological malady of the time. It has an detrimental impact on the pigmentation of the human skin as a result of the destruction of cutaneous melanocytes. It affects 1%–2% of the population worldwide. Different therapeutic regimens have been deployed to treat vitiligo, but none of them could stand alone to be stated as a perfect cure. Recently, a change has been observed through novel experimental-designed optimization leading to the development of an antivitiligo ointment containing Psoralea corylifolia (PC) seed powder. AIM: The aim of this study was to explore the clinical outcomes of ointment containing powdered seeds of PC. MATERIALS AND METHODS: Guided by the protocol Response Surface Methodology, 13 formulations of concentration variance of permeation enhancers were prepared. The formulation fulfilling the required criteria (pH; temperature stability tests at $8°C \pm 0.1°C$, $25°C \pm 0.1°C$, and $40°C \pm 0.1°C$; and the physical properties such as color, bleeding and rheology) was selected for clinical trials. Fourier transform infrared spectroscopy studies of seed powder of PC and selected formulation of the seed powder were performed. After obtaining informed consents and with prior approval of university and hospital ethical review boards, 20 patients (age range 25–65 years) were included in the present study. Formulations were applied on the affected body parts of patients, and some affected portion of the same patient was taken as control (self-control study design). The pigmentation of white spots of vitiligo was photographically evaluated before, during and after 12 weeks of treatment. Analysis of the measured values was performed using GraphPad Prism version 5 statistical software. A paired sample t-test was performed to observe variation between repigmented patches and white patches of self-control. RESULTS: Hydrophilic ointment (10% w/w) prepared with seed powder of PC was fabricated. The ointment was found effective for small circular white lesions of vitiligo as compared to self-control. Pre and posttreatment differences in the levels of pigmentation were statistically significant ($P \leq 0.05$). CONCLUSION: Ointment containing seed powder of PC could be an effective monotherapy for small circular white lesions of vitiligo.

Iyire, A. et al. (2016). "Pre-formulation and systematic evaluation of amino acid assisted permeability of insulin across in vitro buccal cell layers." *Sci Rep* 6:32498.

The aim of this work was to investigate alternative safe and effective permeation enhancers for buccal peptide delivery. Basic amino acids improved insulin solubility in water while 200 and 400 µg/mL lysine significantly increased insulin solubility in HBSS. Permeability data showed a significant improvement in insulin permeation especially for 10 µg/mL of lysine ($p < 0.05$) and 10 µg/mL histidine ($p < 0.001$), 100 µg/mL of glutamic acid ($p < 0.05$) and 200 µg/mL of glutamic acid and aspartic acid ($p < 0.001$) without affecting cell integrity; in contrast to sodium deoxycholate which enhanced insulin permeability but was toxic to the cells. It was hypothesized that both amino acids and insulin were ionized at buccal cavity pH and able to form stable ion pairs which penetrated the cells as one entity; while possibly triggering amino acid nutrient transporters on cell surfaces. Evidence of these transport mechanisms was seen with reduction of insulin transport at suboptimal temperatures as well as with basal-to-apical vectoral transport, and confocal imaging of transcellular insulin transport. These results obtained for insulin are the first indication of a possible amino acid mediated transport of insulin via formation of insulin-amino acid neutral complexes by the ion pairing mechanism.

Kesarla, R. et al. (2016). "Preparation and evaluation of nanoparticles loaded ophthalmic in situ gel." *Drug Deliv* 23(7):2363–2370.

CONTEXT: Conventional ophthalmic solutions often eliminate rapidly after administration and cannot provide and maintain an adequate concentration of drug in the precorneal area. OBJECTIVES: Above problem can be overcome by the use of in situ gel forming systems that are instilled as drops in to the eye and undergo a sol-gel transition in the cul-de-sac. METHODS: An ion sensitive polymer gellan gum was used as gelling agent which formed immediate gel and remained for extended time period. Nanoparticles of moxifloxacin, prepared by solvent evaporation, were separated by freeze drying. The rheological properties and in vitro drug release test of in situ gel loaded with nanoparticles were evaluated and compared with marketed preparation. In vitro release study demonstrated diffusion-controlled release for moxifloxacin from formulations over a period of 12 hours. RESULTS: The developed formulation was stable and showed enhanced contact time minimizing the frequency of administration. Confocal microscopy showed clear permeation of drug loaded nanoparticles across L/S of cornea. CONCLUSION: The formulation of moxifloxacin was found liquid at the formulated pH and formed gel in the presence of mono or divalent cations. The gel formed in situ showed sustained drug release over a period of 10–12 hours. The formulations were less viscous before instillation and formed strong gel after instilling it into cul-de-sac. It is thus concluded that by adopting a systematic formulation approach, an optimum point can be reached in the shortest time with minimum efforts to achieve desirable rheological and in vitro release property for in situ gel forming system.

Khalil, S. K. et al. (2012). "Preparation and evaluation of warfarin-beta-cyclodextrin loaded chitosan nanoparticles for transdermal delivery." *Carbohydr Polym* 90(3):1244–1253.

The main objective of the present work was to prepare warfarin-beta-cyclodextrin (WAF-beta-CD) loaded chitosan (CS) nanoparticles for transdermal delivery. CS is a hydrophilic carrier therefore, to overcome the hydrophobic nature of WAF and allow its incorporation into CS nanoparticles, WAF was first complexed with beta-cyclodextrin (beta-CD). CS nanoparticles were prepared by ionotropic pregelation using tripolyphosphate (TPP). Morphology, size and structure characterization of nanoparticles were carried out using SEM, TEM and FTIR, respectively. Nanoparticles prepared with 3:1 CS:TPP weight ratio and 2 mg/mL final CS concentration were found optimum. They possessed spherical particles (35 ± 12 nm diameter) with narrow size distribution (PDI = 0.364) and 94% entrapment efficiency. The in vitro release as well as the ex vivo permeation profiles of WAF-beta-CD from the selected nanoparticle formulation were studied at different time intervals up to 8 hours. In vitro release of WAF-beta-CD from CS nanoparticles followed a Higuchi release profile whereas its ex vivo permeation (at pH 7.4) followed a zero-order permeation profile. Results suggested that the developed WAF-beta-CD loaded CS carrier could offer a controlled and constant delivery of WAF transdermally.

Liu, R. et al. (2016). "Liquid crystalline nanoparticles as an ophthalmic delivery system for tetrandrine: Development, characterization, and in vitro and in vivo evaluation." *Nanoscale Res Lett* 11(1):254.

The purpose of this study was to develop novel liquid crystalline nanoparticles (LCNPs) that display improved preocular residence time and ocular bioavailability and that can be used as an ophthalmic delivery system for tetrandrine (TET). The delivery system consisted of three primary components, including glyceryl monoolein, poloxamer 407, and water, and two secondary components, including Gelucire 44/14 and amphipathic octadecyl-quaternized carboxymethyl chitosan. The amount of TET, the amount of glyceryl monoolein, and the ratio of poloxamer 407 to glyceryl monoolein were selected as the factors that were used to optimize the dependent variables, which included encapsulation efficiency and drug loading. A three-factor, five-level central composite design was constructed to optimize the formulation. TET-loaded LCNPs (TET-LCNPs) were characterized to determine their particle size, zeta potential, entrapment efficiency, drug loading capacity, particle morphology, inner crystalline structure, and in vitro drug release profile. Corneal permeation in excised rabbit corneas was evaluated. Preocular retention was determined using a noninvasive fluorescence imaging system. Finally, pharmacokinetic study in the aqueous humor was performed by microdialysis technique. The optimal formulation had a mean particle size of 170.0 ± 13.34 nm, a homogeneous distribution with polydispersity index of 0.166 ± 0.02, a positive surface charge with a zeta potential of 29.3 ± 1.25 mV, a high entrapment efficiency of $95.46\% \pm 4.13\%$, and a drug loading rate of $1.63\% \pm 0.07\%$. Transmission electron microscopy showed spherical particles that had smooth surfaces. Small-angle X-ray scattering profiles revealed an inverted hexagonal phase. The in vitro release assays showed a sustained drug release profile. A corneal permeation study showed that the apparent permeability coefficient of the optimal formulation was 2.03-fold higher than that of the TET solution. Preocular retention capacity study indicated that the retention of LCNPs was significantly longer than that of the solution ($p < 0.01$). In addition, a pharmacokinetic study of rabbit aqueous humors demonstrated that the TET-LCNPs showed 2.65-fold higher ocular bioavailability than that of TET solution. In conclusion, a LCNP system could be a promising method for increasing the ocular bioavailability of TET by enhancing its retention time and permeation into the cornea.

Mah, C. S. et al. (2013). "A miniaturized flow-through cell to evaluate skin permeation of endoxifen." *Int J Pharm* 441(1–2):433–440.

Endoxifen, an anti-estrogenic agent, has been recently implicated in the use of breast cancer. Its physicochemical properties make it a good candidate for transdermal delivery. However, as an investigative drug, its limited supply makes it difficult to conduct extensive preformulation studies. To address this issue, a miniaturized flow-through diffusion cell has been fabricated that utilized minimal amounts of the drug for in vitro skin permeation studies. The novel flow-through cells have been validated against horizontal diffusion cells and shown to cause no noticeable damage to the applied skin, as observed by histological sectioning. The cells were also demonstrated to be useful in search of suitable enhancers for endoxifen. Endoxifen permeation using permeation enhancers was tested by using this new device and limonene was found to achieve highest flux, attaining the requirement for clinical applications. The fabricated cells can thus be useful in carrying out preformulation studies for expensive, new drug entities, both in industrial as well as academic research.

Maher, S. et al. (2016). "Intestinal permeation enhancers for oral peptide delivery." *Adv Drug Deliv Rev* 106(Pt B):277–319.

Intestinal permeation enhancers (PEs) are one of the most widely tested strategies to improve oral delivery of therapeutic peptides. This article assesses the intestinal permeation enhancement action of over 250 PEs that have been tested in intestinal delivery models. In depth analysis of preclinical data is presented for PEs as components of proprietary delivery systems that have progressed to clinical trials. Given the importance of copresentation of sufficiently high concentrations of PE and peptide at the small intestinal epithelium, there is an emphasis on studies where PEs have been formulated with poorly permeable molecules in solid dosage forms and lipoidal dispersions.

Martin, C. J. et al. (2017). "Development and Evaluation of Topical Gabapentin Formulations." *Pharmaceutics* 9(3):31.

Topical delivery of gabapentin is desirable to treat peripheral neuropathic pain conditions whilst avoiding systemic side effects. To date, reports of topical gabapentin delivery in vitro have been variable and dependent on the skin model employed, primarily involving rodent and porcine models. In this study a variety of topical gabapentin formulations were investigated, including Carbopol® hydrogels containing various permeation enhancers, and a range of proprietary bases including a compounded Lipoderm® formulation; furthermore, microneedle facilitated delivery was used as a positive control. Critically, permeation of gabapentin across a human epidermal membrane in vitro was assessed using Franz-type diffusion cells. Subsequently this data was contextualized within the wider scope of the literature. Although reports of topical gabapentin delivery have been shown to vary, largely dependent upon the skin model used, this study demonstrated that 6% (w/w) gabapentin 0.75% (w/w) Carbopol® hydrogels containing 5% (w/w) DMSO or 70% (w/w) ethanol and a compounded 10% (w/w) gabapentin Lipoderm® formulation were able to facilitate permeation of the molecule across human skin. Further preclinical and clinical studies are required to investigate the topical delivery performance and pharmacodynamic actions of prospective formulations.

Montaseri, H. et al. (2013). "Enhanced oral bioavailability of paclitaxel by concomitant use of absorption enhancers and P-glycoprotein inhibitors in rats." *J Chemother* 25(6): 355–361.

Paclitaxel (PCT) is a cytotoxic agent with a broad antineoplastic activity. IV formulation of PCT causes hypersensitivity reactions in some patients and oral administration is an alternative to decrease the side effects. PCT is not orally available because of low solubility, lack of intestinal permeability, and efflux by pumps in intestinal wall. PCT solution in cremophor EL: ethanol (100 mg/kg) was administered orally to rats after pretreatment by mefenamic acid, ibuprofen, verapamil, cyclosporine, and verapamil + ibuprofen in individual groups. Ibuprofen presented positive effect on intestinal permeation of PCT. C(max) and area under the serum concentration versus time curve (AUC) after pretreatment by ibuprofen was decreased when the oral dose of PCT was decreased to 50 and 25 mg/kg, while dose-blood concentration relationship was nonlinear. Rise in oral bioavailability of PCT after pretreatment by cyclosporine was lower than ibuprofen. It seems that by using ibuprofen in concomitant with potent Pgp inhibitors before PCT solution, oral delivery of PCT could be promising.

Monti, D. et al. (2014). "Ciclopirox vs amorolfine: In vitro penetration into and permeation through human healthy nails of commercial nail lacquers." *J Drugs Dermatol* 13(2):143–147.

One of the prerequisite for a successful topical antifungal drug indicated for onychomycosis is its bioavailability into the nail unit for achieving fungal eradication and clinical benefit. The aim of this study was to compare in vitro permeation/penetration through and into human nails of amorolfine (MRF) from a 5% anhydrous commercial formulation (Loceryl® and ciclopirox (CPX) from the 8% aqueous formulation in hydroxypropyl chitosan (HPCH) technology (Onytec®. The ability of the active ingredient to reach efficacious concentrations to inhibit nail pathogens was also evaluated. The amounts of drug permeated and retained in human healthy nails were determined using a suitably modified diffusion apparatus. HPLC analysis of the samples was performed. The HPCH-based CPX formulation demonstrated an efficient penetration into and permeation through the nail plates. Conversely, Loceryl(R) produced an amount of MRF permeated through and penetrated into the human toenails significantly lower than CPX. The evaluation of the efficacy index showed a higher potential efficacy of Onytec(R) with respect to Loceryl(R) on nail pathogens. The present work not only reinforced the previous results on different experimental substrates, but pointed out the superiority of HPCH-based Onytec(R) formulation containing CPX with respect to Loceryl(R) commercial product with MRF, both in terms of higher permeation through and penetration into the human nail, and for the efficacy towards the most common ungual pathogens.

Nayak, A. et al. (2016). "Lidocaine carboxymethylcellulose with gelatine co-polymer hydrogel delivery by combined microneedle and ultrasound." *Drug Deliv* 23(2):658–669.

A study that combines microneedles (MNs) and sonophoresis pretreatment was explored to determine their combined effects on percutaneous delivery of lidocaine from a polymeric hydrogel formulation. Varying ratios of carboxymethylcellulose and gelatine (NaCMC/gel ranges 1:1.60–1:2.66) loaded with lidocaine were prepared and characterized for zeta potential and particle size. Additionally, variations in the formulation drying techniques were explored during the formulation stage. Ex vivo permeation studies using Franz diffusion cells measured lidocaine permeation through porcine skin after pretreatment with stainless steel MNs and 20 kHz sonophoresis for 5- and 10-minutes durations. A stable formulation was related to a lower gelatine mass ratio because of smaller mean particle sizes and high zeta potential. Lidocaine permeability in skin revealed some increases in permeability from combined MN and ultrasound pretreatment studies. Furthermore, up to 4.8-fold increase in the combined application was observed compared with separate pretreatments after 30 minutes. Sonophoresis pretreatment alone showed insignificant enhancement in lidocaine permeation during the initial 2 hours period. MN application increased permeability at a time of 0.5 hours for up to approximately 17-fold with an average up to 4-fold. The time required to reach therapeutic levels of lidocaine was decreased to less than 7 minutes. Overall, the attempted approach promises to be a viable alternative to conventional lidocaine delivery methods involving painful injections by hypodermic needles. The mass transfer effects were fairly enhanced and the lowest amount of lidocaine in skin was 99.7% of the delivered amount at a time of 3 hours for lidocaine NaCMC/GEL 1:2.66 after low-frequency sonophoresis and MN treatment.

Rai, V. et al. (2011). "Effect of surfactants and pH on naltrexone (NTX) permeation across buccal mucosa." *Int J Pharm* 411(1–2):92–97.

The objective of this preformulation study was to systematically investigate the effects of two surfactants (Brij 58® and Tween 80® and change in solution pH on in vitro permeation of naltrexone HCl (NTX-HCl) across tissue engineered human buccal mucosa. For the study, 10 mg/mL solutions of Tween 80® (0.1 and 1%, w/v) and Brij 58® (1%, w/v) were prepared in standard artificial saliva buffer solution (pH 6.8). For studying pH effects, solution pH was adjusted to either 7.5 or 8.2. As controls, three concentrations of NTX-HCl (2.5, 10, and 25 mg/mL) were prepared. Using NTX standard solution (10 mg/mL; pH 6.8), the permeation was observed between in vitro human and ex vivo porcine mucosa. It was observed that Brij 58® increased the permeation rates of NTX significantly. The flux of 10 mg/mL solution (pH 6.8) increased from 1.9 ± 0.6 ($\times 10(2)$) to 13.9 ± 2.2 ($\times 10(2)$) µg/(cm^{2}h) (approximately 6-fold) in presence of 1% Brij 58®. Increasing pH of NTX-HCl solution was found to increase the drug flux from 1.9 ± 0.6 ($\times 10(2)$) (pH 6.8) to 3.0 ± 0.6 ($\times 10(2)$) (pH 7.4) and 8.0 ± 3.5 ($\times 10(2)$) (pH 8.2) µg/(cm^{2}h), respectively. Histological analyses exhibited no tissue damage due to exposure of buccal tissue to Brij 58®. The mean permeability coefficients (K(p)) for 2.5, 10 and 25 mg/mL solutions of NTX-HCl (pH 6.8) were 5.0 ($\times 10(-2)$), 1.8 ($\times 10(-2)$) and 3.2 ($\times 10(-2)$) cm/h, respectively, consistent with data from published literature sources. Increase of NTX flux observed with 1% Brij 58® solution may be due to the effects of ATP. Increase in flux and the shortening of lag time observed by increasing in solution pH confirmed earlier finding that distribution coefficient (logD) of NTX is significantly affected by small increments in pH value and therefore plays an important role in NTX permeation by allowing faster diffusion across tissue engineered human buccal tissue.

Rajesh, S. Y. et al. (2018). "Impact of various solid carriers and spray drying on pre/post compression properties of solid SNEDDS loaded with glimepiride: In vitro–ex vivo evaluation and cytotoxicity assessment." *Drug Dev Ind Pharm* 44(7):1056–1069.

Development of self-nanoemulsifying drug delivery systems (SNEDDS) of glimepiride is reported with the aim to achieve its oral delivery. Lauroglycol FCC, Tween-80, and ethanol were used as oil, surfactant, and cosurfactant, respectively, as independent variables. The optimized composition of SNEDDS formulation (F1) was 10% v/v Lauroglycol FCC, 45% v/v Tween 80, 45% v/v ethanol, and 0.005% w/v glimepiride. Further, the optimized liquid SNEDDS were solidified through spray drying using various hydrophilic and hydrophobic carriers. Among the various carriers, Aerosil 200 was found to provide desirable flow, compression, dissolution, and diffusion. Both, liquid and solid-SNEDDS have shown release of more than 90% within 10 minutes. Results of permeation studies performed on Caco-2 cell showed that optimized

SNEDDS exhibited 1.54 times higher drug permeation amount and 0.57 times lower drug excretion amount than that of market tablets at 4 hours ($p < 0.01$). Further, the cytotoxicity study performed on Caco-2 cell revealed that the cell viability was lower in SNEDDS (92.22% $\pm$ 4.18%) compared with the market tablets (95.54% $\pm$ 3.22%; $p > 0.05$, i.e., 0.74). The formulation was found stable with temperature variation and freeze thaw cycles in terms of droplet size, zeta potential, drug precipitation and phase separation. Crystalline glimepiride was observed in amorphous state in solid SNEDDS when characterized through DSC, PXRD, and FT-IR studies. The study revealed successful formulation of SNEDDS for glimepiride.

Rodriguez-Luna, A. et al. (2017). "Topical application of glycolipids from isochrysis galbana prevents epidermal hyperplasia in mice." *Mar Drugs* 16(1):2.

Chronic inflammatory skin diseases such as psoriasis have a significant impact on society. Currently, the major topical treatments have many side effects, making their continued use in patients difficult. Microalgae have emerged as a source of bioactive molecules such as glycolipids with potent anti-inflammatory properties. We aimed to investigate the effects of a glycolipid (MGMG-A) and a glycolipid fraction (MGDG) obtained from the microalga Isochrysis galbana on a TPA-induced epidermal hyperplasia murine model. In a first set of experiments, we examined the preventive effects of MGMG-A and MGDG dissolved in acetone on TPA-induced hyperplasia model in mice. In a second step, we performed an in vivo permeability study by using rhodamine-containing cream, ointment, or gel to determinate the formulation that preserves the skin architecture and reaches deeper. The selected formulation was assayed to ensure the stability and enhanced permeation properties of the samples in an ex vivo experiment. Finally, MGDG-containing cream was assessed in the hyperplasia murine model. The results showed that pretreatment with acetone-dissolved glycolipids reduced skin edema, epidermal thickness, and pro-inflammatory cytokine production (TNF-alpha, IL-1beta, IL-6, and IL-17) in epidermal tissue. The in vivo and ex vivo permeation studies showed that the cream formulation had the best permeability profile. In the same way, MGDG-cream formulation showed better permeation than acetone-dissolved preparation. MGDG-cream application attenuated TPA-induced skin edema, improved histopathological features, and showed a reduction of the inflammatory cell infiltrate. In addition, this formulation inhibited epidermal expression of COX-2 in a similar way to dexamethasone. Our results suggest that an MGDG-containing cream could be an emerging therapeutic strategy for the treatment of inflammatory skin pathologies such as psoriasis.

Sala, M. et al. (2017). "Diclofenac loaded lipid nanovesicles prepared by double solvent displacement for skin drug delivery." *Pharm Res* 34(9):1908–1924.

PURPOSE: Herein, we detail a promising strategy of nanovesicle preparation based on control of phospholipid self-assembly: the Double Solvent Displacement. A systematic study was conducted and diclofenac as drug model encapsulated. In vitro skin studies were carried out to identify better formulation for dermal/transdermal delivery. METHODS: This method consists in two solvent displacements. The first one, made in a free water environment, has allowed triggering a phospholipid preorganization. The second one, based on the diffusion into an aqueous phase has led to liposome formation. RESULTS: Homogeneous liposomes were obtained with a size close to 100 nm and a negative zeta potential around −40 mV. After incorporation of acid diclofenac, we obtained nanoliposomes with a size between 101 ± 45 and 133 ± 66 nm, a zeta potential between 34 ± 2 and 49 ± 3 mV, and the encapsulation efficiency (EE%) was between 58 ± 3 and 87% ± 5%. In vitro permeation studies showed that formulation with higher EE% displayed the higher transdermal passage (18,4% of the applied dose) especially targeting dermis and beyond. CONCLUSIONS: Our results suggest that our diclofenac loaded lipid vesicles have significant potential as transdermal skin drug delivery system. Here, we produced cost effective lipid nanovesicles in a merely manner according to a process easily transposable to industrial scale. Graphical Abstract.

Salamanca, C. H. et al. (2018). "Franz diffusion cell approach for pre-formulation Characterisation of ketoprofen semi-solid dosage forms." *Pharmaceutics* 10(3):148.

This study aimed to evaluate and compare, using the methodology of Franz diffusion cells, the ketoprofen (KTP) releasing profiles of two formulations: A gel and a conventional suspension. The second aim was to show that this methodology might be easily applied for the development of semi-solid prototypes and claim proof in preformulation stages. Drug release analysis was carried out under physiological conditions (pH: 5.6–7.4; ionic strength 0.15 M; at 37°C) for 24 hours. Three independent vertical Franz cells were used with a nominal volume of the acceptor compartment of 125 mL and a diffusion area of 2.5 cm². Additionally, two different membranes were evaluated: A generic type (regenerated cellulose) and a transdermal simulation type (Strat-M®). The KTP permeation profiles demonstrated that depending on the membrane type and the vehicle used, the permeation is strongly affected. High permeation efficiencies were obtained for the gel formulation, and the opposite effect was observed for the suspension formulation. Moreover, the permeation studies using Strat-M membranes represent a reproducible methodology, which is easy to implement for preformulation stage or performance evaluation of semi-solid pharmaceutical products for topical or transdermal administration.

Sharma, V. and K. Pathak (2016). "Effect of hydrogen bond formation/replacement on solubility characteristics, gastric permeation and pharmacokinetics of curcumin by application of powder solution technology." *Acta Pharm Sin B* 6(6):600–613.

The present research aimed to improve the dissolution rate and bioavailability of curcumin using the potential of liquisolid technology. Twelve drug-loaded liquisolid systems (LS-1 to LS-12) were prepared using different vehicles (PEG 200, PEG 400 and Tween 80) and curcumin concentrations in vehicle (40%, 50%, 60% and 70%, w/w). The carrier [microcrystalline cellulose (MCC) PH102] to coat (Aerosil®) ratio was 20 in all formulations. The systems were screened for precompression properties before being compressed to liquisolid tablets (LT-1 to LT-12). Post compression tests and in vitro dissolution of LTs were conducted and the results compared with those obtained for a directly compressed tablet (DCT) made of curcumin, MCC PH102 and Aerosil®. LTs exhibited higher cumulative drug release (CDR) than the DCT and the optimum formulation, LT-9 (made using Tween 80), was studied by powder XRD, DSC, SEM and FTIR. Ex-vivo permeation of curcumin from LT-9 through goat GI mucosa was significantly (P < 0.05) enhanced and its oral bioavailability was increased 18.6-fold in New Zealand rabbits. In vitro cytotoxicity (IC50) of LT-9 towards NCL 87 cancer cells was 40.2 μmol/L substantiating its anticancer efficacy. Accelerated stability studies revealed insignificant effects of temperature and humidity on LT-9. In summary, solubility enhancement of curcumin in LTs produced significant improvements in its permeation and bioavailability.

Sierra, A. F. et al. (2013). "In vivo and in vitro evaluation of the use of a newly developed melatonin loaded emulsion combined with UV filters as a protective agent against skin irradiation." *J Dermatol Sci* 69(3):202–214.

BACKGROUND: Melatonin has attracted attention because of their high antioxidant and anticarcinogenic activity. Otherwise, the use of sunscreens is recommended for patients after chemotherapy and radiotherapy treatments or to prevent UV radiation-induced skin damages that may result in precancerous and cancerous skin lesions. OBJECTIVE: To evaluate the beneficial influence of melatonin in topical sunscreen emulsions combined with three common ultraviolet filters. METHODS: After the formulation characterization in terms of rheology, stability studies were performed. Release studies let us to evaluate its mechanism of delivery and ex vivo permeation study through human skin, the amount of melatonin retained. The antioxidant activity assay was also carried out, and finally the in vivo photoprotective effect in rats was tested as transepidermal water loss and erythema formation. RESULTS: The rheological behaviour of formulations was pseudoplastic fluid, all emulsions had good physical stability. Release studies showed a trend of enhancement in melatonin release from emulsions incorporating UV filters and followed a Weibull model. Melatonin permeation was higher from the emulsion containing melatonin combined with a mixture of three ultraviolet filters (MMIX) formulation. Equally this formulation exhibited the highest radical scavenging activity. Finally, the photoprotective assay showed that only skin areas treated with this formulation were statistically equivalent to the unirradiated control area. CONCLUSION: MMIX formulation would be a promising formulation for preventing the undesirable adverse effects of UV skin irradiation because melatonin not only acts as a potent antioxidant itself, but also is capable of activating an endogenous enzymatic protective system against oxidative stress.

Thatai, P. et al. (2016). "Progressive development in experimental models of transungual drug delivery of anti-fungal agents." *Int J Cosmet Sci* 38(1):1–12.

Preclinical development comprises of different procedures that relate drug discovery in the laboratory for commencement of human clinical trials. Preclinical studies can be designed to recognize a lead candidate from a list to develop the procedure for scale-up, to choose the unsurpassed formulation, to determine the frequency, and duration of exposure; and eventually make the foundation of the anticipated clinical trial design. The foremost aim in the pharmaceutical research and industry is the claim of drug product quality throughout a drug's life cycle. The particulars of the preclinical development process for different candidates may vary; however, all have some common features. Typically, in vitro, in vivo, or ex vivo studies are elements of preclinical studies. Human pharmacokinetic in vivo studies are often supposed to serve as the 'gold standard' to assess product performance. On the other hand, when this general assumption is revisited, it appears that in vitro studies are occasionally better than in vivo studies in assessing dosage forms.

The present review is compendious of different such models or approaches that can be used for designing and evaluation of formulations for nail delivery with special reference to antifungal agents.

Zhao, Y. et al. (2010). "The effects of particle properties on nanoparticle drug retention and release in dynamic minoxidil foams." *Int J Pharm* 383(1–2):277–284.

Nanocarriers may act as useful tools to deliver therapeutic agents to the skin. However, balancing the drug–particle interactions; to ensure adequate drug loading, with the drug–vehicle interactions; to allow efficient drug release, presents a significant challenge using traditional semi-solid vehicles. The aim of this study was to determine how the physicochemical properties of nanoparticles influenced minoxidil release pre and post dose application when formulated as a simple aqueous suspension compared to dynamic hydrofluoroalkane (HFA) foams. Minoxidil loaded lipid nanoparticles (LN, 1.4 mg/mL, 50 nm) and polymeric nanoparticles with a lipid core (PN, 0.6 mg/mL, 260 nm) were produced and suspended in water to produce the aqueous suspensions. These aqueous suspensions were emulsified with HFA using pluronic surfactant to generate the foams. Approximately 60% of the minoxidil loaded into the PN and 80% of the minoxidil loaded into the LN was released into the external aqueous phase 24 hours after production. Drug permeation was superior from the PN, i.e., it was the particle that retained the most drugs, irrespective of the formulation method. Premature drug release, i.e., during storage, resulted in the performance of the topical formulation being dictated by the thermodynamic activity of the solubilized drug not the particle properties.

Zhou, Y. et al. (2014). "Application of a continuous intrinsic dissolution–permeation system for relative bioavailability estimation of polymorphic drugs." *Int J Pharm* 473(1–2):250–258.

A new continuous dissolution–permeation system, consisting of an intrinsic dissolution apparatus and an Ussing chamber, was developed for screening and identification of high-bioavailability polymorphisms at preformulation stages. Three different solid forms of two model drugs (agomelatine and carbamazepine) were used to confirm the system's predictive ability. Ranks for cumulative permeation of the three solids were: Form III > Form I > Form II for agomelatine, and Form III > Form I > the dihydrate form for carbamazepine. Regression analysis of these parameters and published pharmacokinetics confirmed linear IVIVCs (most correlation coefficients > 0.9). To confirm dissolution–absorption relationships, permeability coefficients were calculated. Relatively constant values among various polymorphisms for each drug supported a linear dependency between polymorphism-increased dissolution and polymorphism-enhanced permeation. A combined analysis of intrinsic dissolution rates and permeability coefficients revealed that both drugs are of the BCS II class and have dissolution-limited absorption. In conclusion, our new system was valuable not only for high-bioavailability polymorphism screening, but also for drug classification within the BCS system.

6

Solid-State Properties

Humility is the solid foundation of all virtues.

Confucius

6.1 Introduction

Solid-state characterization is one of the most important functions of the preformulation group, which is assigned the responsibility of making recommendations for further formulation work on a lead compound. Physical properties have a direct bearing on both physical and chemical stabilities of the lead compound. Much of the later work on formulation will depend on how well the solid state is characterized from the decisions to compress the drug into tablets to the selection of appropriate salt forms. The studies reported in this section, of course, apply to those drugs that are available in solid form, crystalline or amorphous, pure or amalgamated.

Physical properties affected by the solid-state properties can influence both the choice of the delivery system and the activity of the drug, as determined by the rate of delivery. Chemical stability, as affected by the physical properties, can be significant. Although it is always desirable to enhance chemical stability (a pursuit of the synthetic chemist), modulation of physical properties, such as reducing the hygroscopicity by increasing the hydrophobicity of an acid or by moving to carboxylic rather than sulfonic or mineral acid or using an acid of higher pK_a to raise the pH of a solution, often provides more stable compounds. Stability is also improved by decreasing the solubility and increasing the crystallinity by increasing the melting. It is important to realize that factors that improve the chemical stability often impact the physical properties adversely. Therefore, a fine balance must be achieved when selecting between the physical properties of a chemical property modulation.

The stability of the salt could also be an important issue, and depending on the pK_a, many properties, including indirectly related physical characteristics, such as volatility (e.g., hydrochloride salts are often more volatile than sulfate salts), can change. Discoloration of the salt form of drugs is also prominent for some specific forms, as the oxidation reactions (often accompanied by hydrolysis) are a result of factors such as affinity for moisture, surface hydrophobicity, and so on. Hydrolysis of a salt back to the free base may also take place if the pK_a of the base is sufficiently weak.

6.2 Crystal Morphology

A crystalline species is defined as a solid composed of atoms, ions, or molecules arranged in a periodic, three-dimensional (3D) pattern. A 3D array is called a lattice, as shown in Figure 6.1. The requirement of a lattice is that each volume, which is called a unit cell, is surrounded by identical objects. Three vectors, a, b, and c, are defined in a right-handed sense for a unit cell. However, as three vectors are quite arbitrary, a unit cell is described by six scalars, a, b, c, α, β, and γ without directions (Figure 6.2). Several kinds of unit cells are possible, for example, if $a = b = c$ and $\alpha = \beta = \gamma = 90°$, the unit cell is cubic. It turns out that only seven different kinds of unit cells are necessary to include all the possible lattices. These correspond to the seven crystal systems, as shown in Table 6.1.

The seven different point lattices can be obtained simply by putting points at the corners of the unit cells of the seven crystal systems. However, there are more possible arrangements of points, which do not violate the requirements of a lattice.

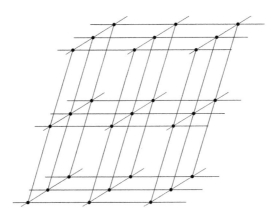

FIGURE 6.1   Crystal lattice.

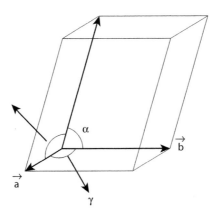

FIGURE 6.2   Scalars of lattice structure.

TABLE 6.1

Seven Crystal Systems

Crystal System	Axial Lengths and Angles
Cubic	$a = b = c$
	$\alpha = \beta = \gamma = 90°$
Tetragonal	$a = b \neq c$
	$\alpha = \beta = \gamma = 90°$
Orthorhombic	$a \neq b \neq c$
	$\alpha = \beta = \gamma = 90°$
Rhombohedral	$a = b = c$
Trigonal	$\alpha = \beta = \gamma \neq 90°$
Hexagonal	$a = b \neq c$
	$\alpha = \beta = 90°\ \gamma = 120°$
Monoclinic	$a \neq b \neq c$
	$\alpha = \gamma = 90° \neq \beta$
Triclinic	$a \neq b \neq c$
	$\alpha \neq \beta \neq \gamma \neq 90°$

The French crystallographer Bravais proposed 14 possible point lattices, as shown in Figures 6.3 and 6.4, as a result of combining the seven crystal systems and centered points.

Symmetry operations are divided into macroscopic and microscopic operations. Macroscopic operations can be deduced from the arrangement of well-developed crystal faces, without any knowledge of the atomic arrangement inside the crystals, whereas the microscopic operations depend on the atomic arrangement (Table 6.2) that cannot be inferred from the external growth of the crystal. Reflection, rotation, inversion, and rotation–inversion are included in macroscopic operations, whereas glide planes and screw axes belong to microscopic operations. The combination of macroscopic operations with the seven crystal systems leads to 32 possible groups, and they are called 32 point groups. The microscopic symmetry operations describe the way in which the atoms or molecules in crystals are combined to 32 point groups with 14 Bravais lattices, resulting in 230 combinations, called 230 space groups.

A crystalline particle is characterized by definite external and internal structures. Habit describes the external shape of a crystal, whereas polymorphic state refers to the definite arrangement of molecules inside the crystal lattice. Crystallization is invariably employed as the final step for the purification of a solid. The use of different solvents and processing conditions may alter the habit of recrystallized particles, besides modifying the polymorphic state of the solid. Subtle changes in crystal habit at this stage can lead to significant variation in raw-material characteristics. Furthermore, various indices of dosage form performance, such as particle orientation, flowability, packing, compaction, suspension stability, and dissolution can be altered even in the absence of significantly altered polymorphic state. These effects are a result of the physical effect of different crystal habits. In addition, changes in crystal habit either accompanied or not by polymorphic transformation during processing or storage, can lead to serious implications of physical stability in dosage forms. Therefore, in order to minimize the variations in raw-material characteristics, to ensure the reproducibility of results during

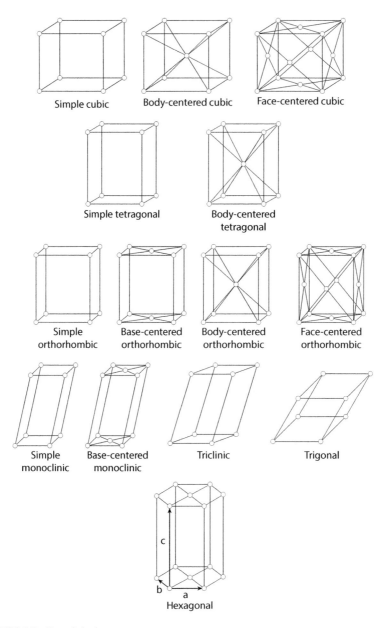

FIGURE 6.3 Bravais lattice system.

preformulation, and to correctly judge the cause of instability and poor performance of a dosage form, it is essential to recognize the importance of changes in crystal surface appearance and habit of pharmaceutical powders.

The crystal habit is also affected by impurities present in the crystallizing solution; often, these impurities provide the earliest nucleation of crystal growth and become an integral part of the crystal. In some instances, the presence of impurities inhibits

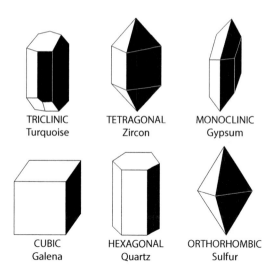

TRICLINIC
Turquoise

TETRAGONAL
Zircon

MONOCLINIC
Gypsum

CUBIC
Galena

HEXAGONAL
Quartz

ORTHORHOMBIC
Sulfur

FIGURE 6.4 Common crystal habits.

crystal growth, as shown, when certain dyes or heavy metals are mixed with solutions. If an impurity can adsorb at the growing face, it can significantly alter the course of crystal growth and geometry. The habits bound by plane faces are termed *euhedral* and those with irregularly shaped ones are called *anhedral*. The symmetry of a crystal is generally studied by using optical goniometer that allows the measurement of the angles between the crystal faces. This technique is of use only when good crystals of size greater than 0.05 mm in each direction can be obtained, which is generally not the case.

Chemical crystallography provides accurate and precise measurements of molecular dimensions in a way that no other science can begin to approach. Historically, single crystal X-ray diffraction was used to determine the structure of what was thought of as "small molecules." Twenty years ago, it was possible to solve structures with an average of only 100 nonhydrogen atoms. However, with developments in hardware and software, the upper limit has risen to about 500, and recently, even a 1000-atom structure was solved. The APEX II line of Chemical Crystallography Solutions (1) allows single-crystal structure determination. The APEX II detector is suitable for fast processing. The Brucker SHellXTL software system works well with these systems and provides a complete characterization that is suitable for publication would include the following data:

1. Data collection
   a. Source of sample and conditions of crystallization
   b. Habit, color, and dimensions of the crystal
   c. Formula and formula weight
   d. Unit cell parameters and volume with (esds). The number of data and theta range of data used to determine the cell parameters
   e. Crystal type and space group
   f. Z, density, and absorption coefficient
   g. Instrument and temperature of data collection and cell parameter determination

TABLE 6.2

Common Crystal Habits

Habit	Description	Example
Acicular	Needle-like, slender, and/or tapered	Rutile in quartz
Amygdaloidal	Almond-shaped	Heulandite
Anhedral	Poorly formed, distorted	Olivine
Bladed	Blade-like, slender, and flattened	Kyanite
Botryoidal or globular	Grape-like, hemispherical masses	Smithsonite
Columnar	Similar to fibrous: long, slender prisms often with parallel growth	Calcite
Coxcomb	Aggregated flaky or tabular crystals closely spaced	Barite
Dendritic or arborescent	Tree-like, branching in one or more direction from central point	Magnesite in opal
Dodecahedral	Dodecahedron, 12-sided	Garnet
Drusy or encrustation	Aggregate of minute crystals coating a surface	Uvarovite
Enantiomorphic	Mirror-image habit and optical characteristics; right- and left-handed crystals	Quartz
Equant, stout, stubby, or blocky	Squashed, pinnacoids dominant over prisms	Zircon
Euhedral	Well formed, undistorted	Spinel
Fibrous or columnar	Extremely slender prisms	Tremolite
Filiform or capillary	Hair-like or thread-like, extremely fine	Natrolite
Foliated or micaceous	Layered structure, parting into thin sheets	Mica
Granular	Aggregates of anhedral crystals in matrix	Scheelite
Hemimorphic	Doubly terminated crystal with two differently shaped ends	Hemimorphite
Mamillary	Breast-like: intersecting large rounded contours	Malachite
Massive or compact	Shapeless, no distinctive external crystal shape	Serpentine
Nodular or tuberose	Deposit of roughly spherical form with irregular protruberances	Geodes
Octahedral	Octahedron, eight-sided (two pyramids base to base)	Magnetite
Plumose	Fine, feather-like scales	Mottramite
Prismatic	Elongate, prism-like: all crystal faces parallel to c-axis	Tourmaline
Pseudo-hexagonal	Ostensibly hexagonal because of cyclic twinning	Aragonite
Pseudomorphous	Occurring in the shape of another mineral through pseudomorphous replacement	Tiger's eye
Radiating or divergent	Radiating outward from a central point	Pyrite suns
Reniform or colloform	Similar to mamillary: intersecting kidney-shaped masses	Hematite
Reticulated	Acicular crystals forming net-like intergrowths	Cerussite
Rosette	Platy, radiating rose-like aggregate	Gypsum
Sphenoid	Wedge-shaped	Sphene
Stalactitic	Form as stalactites or stalagmites; cylindrical or cone-shaped	Rhodochrosite
Stellate	Star-like, radiating	Pyrophyllite
Striated/striations	Surface growth lines parallel or perpendicular to c-axis	Chrysoberyl
Tabular or lamellar	Flat, tablet-shaped, prominent pinnacoid	Ruby
Wheat sheaf	Aggregates resembling hand-reaped wheat sheaves	Zeolites

2. Structure solution
    a. Number of data collected, unique [*R*(int)]
    b. Method and program used for structure solution
    c. Absorption correction details

3. Structure refinement
    a. Method and program for refinement
    b. Number of data refined, restraints, and parameters
    c. Weighting scheme
    d. *R*1 (observed data), w*R*2 (all data), and *S* values
    e. Final maximum shift/error
    f. Final maximum and minimum of difference electron density map

4. Tables and figures
    a. Positional parameters and isotropic or equivalent displacement parameters
    b. Bond distances, angles, and torsion angles
    c. Anisotropic displacement parameters
    d. Structure factor tables (often required for review but discarded by the journal)
    e. Torsion angles (optional)
    f. Least-square planes (optional)
    g. Hydrogen bond geometry (optional)
    h. A labeled figure showing the displacement ellipsoids
    i. A packing diagram showing relevant intermolecular interactions

The modeling of the habits of crystals is a subject of many sophisticated computer programs, such as CERIUS2 (2), which also provides the effect of additives. The Bravais, Friedel, Donny, and Harker (BFDH) model and the attachment energy model, in conjunction with force field methods, are used in habit prediction. The attachment energy approach gives the growth morphology of the crystal studied, but it is also possible to calculate the shape of a small particle in equilibrium with its growth environment by computing the surface energy of each relevant face.

Surface interactions between solvent molecules and growing faces can also be modeled. It is well known that the stronger the solvent binds to a particular face, the more it will inhibit the growth of that face, so as to affect the morphology. This can be simulated by the computer. The ability to predict the crystal morphology, that is, identifying the key growth faces, combined with the ability to analyze the surface chemistry of each of the faces in detail (including interactions with solvent molecules, excipients and impurities), enables rational control of morphology and crystal growth. For example, an undesirable morphology (a plate) can be transformed into a more isometrical shape.

In addition to morphological assessments of crystals, optical microscopy can be used to measure their refractive indices. To identify the crystal, it is not necessary to measure the principal refractive indices; simply measuring two that are unique and reproducible is sufficient. These are termed the key refractive indices that, according to these researches, are all that are needed to identify any particular compound.

6.3 Polymorphism

Both organic and inorganic pharmaceutical compounds can crystallize into two or more solid forms that have the same chemical composition; this is called polymorphism. Polymorphs have different relative intermolecular and/or interatomic distances and unit cells, resulting in different physical and chemical properties, such as density, solubility, dissolution rate, bioavailability, and so on. Crystal structures containing solvents (or water) are often called psudopolymorphs, with distinct physical and chemical properties. It is possible for each pseudopolymorph to have many polymorphs. In polymorphism, the crystal lattice formation can take place through two mechanisms: packing polymorphism and conformational polymorphism. Packing polymorphism represents the formation of different crystal lattices of conformationally rigid molecules that can be rearranged stably into different 3D structures through different intermolecular mechanisms. When a nonconformationally rigid molecule can be folded into alternative crystal structures, the polymorphism is categorized as conformational polymorphism.

Polymorphs and pseudopolymorphs can also be classified as monotropes or enantiotropes, depending upon whether or not one form can transform reversibly into another. In a monotropic system, Form I does transform to Form II, because the transition temperature cannot appear before the melting temperature (Figure 6.5, monotropy). In Figure 6.6 (enantiotropy), Form II is stable over a temperature range below the transition temperature, at which two solubility curves meet, and Form I is stable above the transition temperature. At the transition temperature, reversible transformation between the two forms occurs. Figure 6.7 (enantiotropy with metastable phases) shows the kinetic effects on the thermodynamic property of solubility, which shows Ostwald ripening effect.

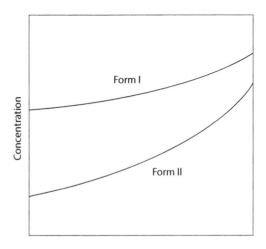

FIGURE 6.5   Monotropic system as a function of temperature (*x*-axis).

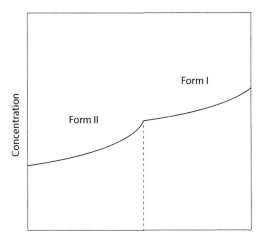

FIGURE 6.6 Enantiotropic system as a function of temperature (*x*-axis).

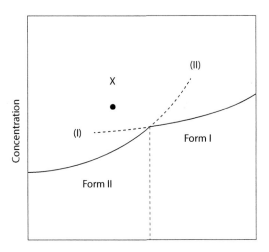

FIGURE 6.7 Enantiotropic system with metastable phases as a function of temperature (*x*-axis).

An unstable system does not necessarily transform directly into the most stable state but into one that most closely resembles its own, that is, into another transient state, whose formation from the original is accompanied by the smallest loss of free energy.

When a decision needs to be made on whether two polymorphs are enantiotropes or monotropes, it is very useful to use the thermodynamic rules developed by Burger and Ramberger, which are tabulated in Table 6.3.

The stability of polymorphs is thermodynamically related to their free energy. The more stable polymorph has the lower free energy at a given temperature. The aforementioned classification of polymorphic substances into monotropic and enantiotropic classes, from the lattice theory perspective, is not always appropriate. There is a need to explore the way in which the crystal lattice structures of polymorphs

TABLE 6.3

Thermodynamic Rules for Polymorphic Transitions

Enantiotropy	Monotropy
Transition < melting I	Transition > melting I
I stable > transition	I always stable
II stable < transition	—
Transition reversible	Transition irreversible
Solubility I higher < transition	Transition I always lower
Solubility I lower > transition	—
Transition II → I endothermic	Transition II → I exothermic
$\Delta H_f^{I} < \Delta H_f^{II}$	$\Delta H_f^{I} > \Delta H_f^{II}$
IR peak I before II	IR peak I after II
Density I < II	Density I > density II

are related. At a transition point, with the temperature and the pressure fixed, it is possible for interconversion to take place between two polymorphs only in the case where the structures of the polymorphs are related. If complete rearrangement is required by atoms or molecules during transformation, no point of contact for reversible interconversion exists. Therefore, the existence of enantiotropes or monotropes in thermodynamics and phase theory corresponds to related or unrelated lattice structures in structural theory. Transformation between polymorphs that have completely different lattice structures exhibits dramatic changes in properties. The difference in energy between polymorphs is not always considerable, as shown with diamond/graphite. In most cases, polymorphs in this category are required to break bonds and rearrange atoms or molecules, and consequently, the polymorphs have a monotropic relation.

For the study of polymorphs that are structurally related, the structural relationships between the polymorphs should be established first; second, it should be explained why a particular substance is able to arrange its structural units in two closely related lattices, and finally, there should be a description of the manner and conditions under which rearrangement of the units from one lattice type to another can happen. It is the physical form of the drugs that is responsible for its degradation in the solid state. Selection of a polymorph that is chemically more stable is a solution in many cases. Different polymorphs also lead to different morphology, tensile strength and density of powder bed, which collectively contribute to the compression characteristics of materials. Some investigation of polymorphism and crystal habit of a drug substance, as it relates to pharmaceutical processing, is desirable during its preformulation evaluation, especially when the active ingredient is expected to constitute the bulk of the tablet mass.

Various techniques are available for the investigation of the solid state. These include microscopy (including hot-stage microscopy, HSM), infrared spectrophotometry (IRS), single-crystal X-ray and X-ray powder diffraction (XRPD), thermal analysis, and dilatometry.

A preformulation study plan must challenge the crystal structure to determine if any polymorphs exist. It is possible for a new compound to show polymorphic forms only when subjected to stress—physical and chemical. Most organic compounds are capable of exhibiting polymorphism because of their complex flexible structure. The window of physicochemical stress that a drug is generally subjected to during manufacturing is at times not able to adduce the differentiation of a drug into its possible polymorphic forms. For example, enantiotropic state is the state in which one polymorph can be reversibly changed into another by varying the temperature or pressure. One way of assessing whether the solid is a metastable form of the compound is to slurry the compound in a range of solvents. In this way, a solvent-mediated phase transformation may be detected using the usual techniques. The monotropic state exists when the transformation between the two forms is irreversible. As all polymorphs are providing the lowest-energy polymorph, the most able polymorph is often needed to ensure consistency in the physicochemical properties; this is necessary for consistency in manufacturing procedures and in bioavailability. The right polymorph, at times, is not necessarily the most stable polymorph; unstable forms like amorphous forms (that are most constrained) are often used because of their higher solubility and often a better bioavailability profile.

The manufacturing factors that may be affected by the choice of a particular polymorphic form include granulation; milling and compression; stability (particularly for semisolid forms); amount of dose delivered in metered inhalers; crystallization from different solvents at different speeds and temperature, precipitation, concentration, or evaporation; crystallization from the melt, grinding, and compression; lyophilization; and spray drying. In the manufacturing processing, crystallization is a major problem, and it can be avoided by a careful study of polymorphic transition, particularly in supercritical fluids.

Polymorphism is frequently a function of the type of salt, because the presence of counter ions can make the crystals form differently, leading to widely variable physicochemical properties, as described earlier under the description of polymorphism. Generally, salts exhibiting polymorphism should be avoided.

An interesting example of polymorphic structure differentiation is that of human immunodeficiency virus (HIV) protease inhibitors. The HIV protease inhibitors pose a serious problem in their bioavailability. Invirase showed only modest market performance, and it was soon superseded by drugs, such as ritonavir (Norvir®) and indinavir sulfate (Crixivan®), that had better bioavailability. Three years after initial approval, saquinavir was reintroduced in a formulation with 6-fold higher oral bioavailability relative to the original product. Ritonavir was originally launched as a semisolid dosage form, in which the waxy matrix contained the dispersed drug, in order to achieve acceptable oral bioavailability. Two years after its introduction, ritonavir exhibited latent crystal polymorphism, which caused the semisolid capsule formulation of Norvir to be removed from the market.

The acceptance criterion for polymorphic forms in a drug substance is generally based on the considerations given in Scheme 6.1.

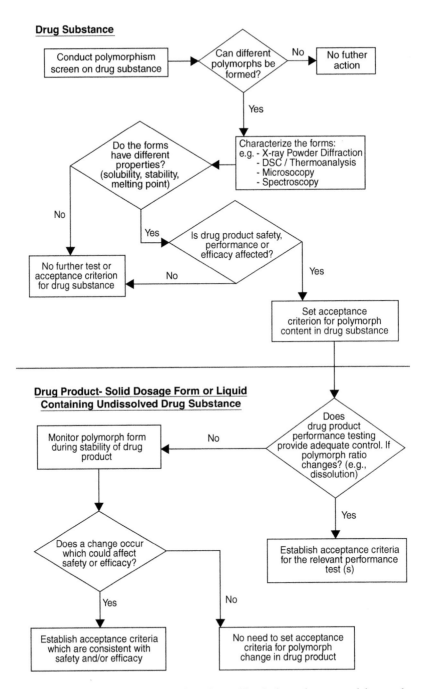

SCHEME 6.1   Some acceptance criteria for polymorphism in drug substances and drug products.
(From http://pharmquest.com.)

6.4 High-Throughput Crystal Screening

The search for crystal forms and salts of compounds emerging from discovery must rely on automation and miniaturization of crystallization trials. Currently, development chemists may experiment with 1–10 mg per trial on a total budget of tens to hundreds of milligrams. Although the material is usually recoverable at a cost in time and effort, the traditional experimentation remains linear in nature. The search for crystal forms in such a linear fashion is time consuming, and the pressure keeps mounting to test a compound in toxicology and the clinic. The technical solution provided by high-throughput (HT) crystallization is the possibility of parallel, miniaturized trials of a larger experimental space (solvents, combinations, processing parameters, and so on). In order to significantly increase the productivity of crystallization efforts, one must be able to conduct parallel experiments at the level of micrograms per trial. In this way, valuable time and material can be saved, while generating useful physicochemical information to support development decisions. For instance, if crystalline forms are found, the program can confidently move forward to assessing their utility. Even when a crystal form remains elusive, the information from crystallization trials on the compound and some of its congeners may help the medicinal chemists design the optimal compound to advance the program. High-throughput crystallization screening provides a way to address polymorphism issues much earlier and can help to avoid late discoveries of polymorphism in pharmaceutical systems; the use of such technologies as CrystalMax® (4) enables parallel, miniaturized crystallization of compounds in cycles of 1–2 weeks. With a capacity of up to 10,000 crystallization experiments per week, this technology enables the discovery and characterization of diverse solid forms of active pharmaceutical ingredients, leading to enhanced solubility and selection of salts, cocrystals, and the like. The technology allows design, execution, and analysis of thousands of crystallization trials on hundreds of micrograms of crystalline material per well in microliter volumes within a 96-well array format. The FAST® (4) HT technology from the same vendor allows the discovery of novel solution formulations of poorly soluble compounds, either for intravenous or for oral use. The technology uses a 96-well format to conduct parallel screening of thousands of combinations of semi-aqueous formulations. Other tools, such as HT crystallization tools with miniaturization, come from Symyx (5), Aventium (6), and Solvias (7).

In the recent years, sophisticated modeling tools, such as the Cerius^2 (8), have become available, where various modules allow the analysis of crystallization, crystal growth, and material form characterization. In brief, this technique uses a simulated annealing and a rigid-body Rietveld refinement procedure, whereby the calculated and measured XRPD patterns are compared; if they agree sufficiently, the structure is deemed to be solved. Other modules offered by Cerus include the following:

- C^2. HP Morphology is an advanced method for predicting crystal morphology for salts and solvates.
- C^2. Morphology predicts and analyzes the morphology of crystals from their internal crystal structure, which helps to relate morphological features to structure and understand the likely effects of solvents and growth-modifying additives.
- C^2. Polymorph predicts the polymorphs of organic crystalline materials, such as drugs, pigments, and fine chemicals, from their molecular structure.

- C^2. Polymorph is used to predict unsynthesized polymorphs or to determine structures in combination with techniques, such as Rietveld refinement. The Cereus Polymorph Predictor is based on a potential energy function program and a search program to locate potential minima of that potential function. It does have limitations; for example, by neglecting polarization effects, the results are less accurate for molecules such as salts that are common in the pharmaceutical industry. Moreover, atoms, such as fluorine and divalent sulfur, are not optimally parameterized. The molecules need to be rigid; however, a few successes for flexible molecules have been reported.

- C^2. Powder Fit provides crystal structure determination capabilities by helping to determine the parameters required to generate a simulated powder pattern by analyzing the peak positions, profiles, and background of an experimental pattern.

- C^2. Powder Indexing completes a comprehensive package of software modules for crystal structure determination from powder data. It is possible to establish unit cell and symmetry information and use this to assist Rietveld refinement or crystal structure predictions.

- C^2. Powder Solve provides crystal structure determination capabilities by sampling a vast number of trial structures, subsequently proposing a structure for which the simulated pattern most closely matches the experimental one.

- C^2. Diffraction-Amorphous simulates noncrystalline diffraction, including small-angle scattering. Comparison with experimental data helps to determine amorphous structure, polymer chain conformation, copolymer sequence structure, and orientation.

- C^2. Diffraction-Crystal simulates powder, fiber, and single-crystal diffraction from crystalline models, which helps to interpret the experimental data from molecular, inorganic, and polymeric crystalline materials.

- C^2. Diffraction-Faulted simulates powder diffraction from faulted or layered structures, which helps to characterize structures such as zeolites and clays.

- C^2. EXAFS (extended X-ray absorption fine structure) jointly developed with the CCLRC Daresbury Laboratory, U.K. (9), integrates the EXAFS analysis and refinement techniques of Daresbury's EXCURV92 software with Cerius' modeling tools, radically improving the ability to interpret the EXAFS data.

- C^2. HRTEM simulates high-resolution transmission electron microscope images from crystals, interfaces, and defect structures. One can set up and interpret electron microscope experiments that investigate technologically important materials.

- C^2. IR/Raman is a computational instrument that predicts IR/Raman spectra.

- C^2. Low electron diffraction/high electron diffraction under grazing incidence (LEED/RHEED) helps interpret low-energy electron diffraction patterns and reflection high-energy electron diffraction from surfaces.

- C^2. Rietveld performs crystal structure refinement and quantitative phase analysis, using powder diffraction data and the Rietveld method.

Combining refinement programs and advanced modeling tools allows a faster route to determining the structures of both inorganic and molecular crystals. An effective way to know the atomic structure is by means of diffraction techniques using neutrons from nuclear reactors and particle accelerators or X-rays from X-ray tubes and synchrotrons. The single-crystal diffraction technique, using relatively large crystals of the material, gives a set of separate data from which the structure can be obtained. However, the *powder* diffraction technique is used in conditions where it is not possible to grow large crystals. The drawback of this conventional *powder* method is that the data grossly overlap, thereby preventing proper determination of the structure. The "Rietveld method" creates an effective separation of these overlapping data, thereby allowing an accurate determination of the structure. An even more widely used application of the method is the determination of the components of chemical mixtures.

6.4.1 Crystalline Index of Refraction

As different polymorphs have different internal structures, they belong to different crystal systems; therefore, polymorphs can be distinguished by using polarized light and a microscope. The crystals can be either isotropic or anisotropic. In isotropic crystals, the velocity of light is the same in all directions, whereas anisotropic crystals have two or three different light velocities or refractive indices. In terms of crystal systems, only the cubic system is isotropic and the other six are anisotropic.

6.5 Solvates

In addition to polymorphs, solvates (inclusion of the solvent of crystallization) are also often formed during the crystallization process. These forms are also called pseudopolymorphs. The solvent molecules fill the spaces in the crystal lattice and generally reduce the solubility and dissolution rates. This phenomenon is thermodynamically driven. If the solvate contains an organic solvent, this would not be admitted by the regulatory authorities. According to the International Conference on Harmonization (ICH) guidelines, the class I solvents, such as benzene, carbon tetrachloride, and 1,2-dichloromethane, must be avoided, as these are carcinogenic. The class II solvents should be limited and include nongenotoxic animal carcinogens, such as cyclohexane and acetonitrile. The class III solvents, including acetic acid, alcohol, and acetone, which have low toxicity potential, are allowed as long as the daily permissible dose does not exceed 50 mg. Generally, an allowed solvate would likely be removed during the manufacturing process, but in some instances, the presence of the solvate is desired, as in the case of the beclomethasone dipropionate product of Glaxo that includes trichlorofluoromethane solvate. This solvate prevents crystal growth in sprays containing trichlorofluoromethane as a propellant. A U.S. Patent issued to Glaxo 5270305 demonstrates the use of trichlorofluoromethane.

6.5.1 Hydrates

When the solvate happens to be water, these are called hydrates, wherein water is entrapped through hydrogen bonding inside the crystal, and they strengthen the crystal structure, thereby invariably reducing the dissolution rate (Table 6.4). The water molecules can reside in the crystal either as isolate lattice, where they are not in contact with each other; as lattice channel water, where they fill space; and as metal-ion coordinated water in salts of weak acids, where the metal ion coordinates with the water molecule. Metal ion coordinates may also fill channels, such as in the case of nedocromil sodium trihydrate. Crystalline hydrates have been classified by structural aspects into three classes: isolated lattice sites, lattice channels, and

TABLE 6.4

Drug Substance Hydrate Forms, as Reported in the Pharmacopeia

Compound	Water of Hydration
Aminophylline	2
Ampicillin	3
Beclomethasone dipropionate	0 or 1
Caffeine	1
Calcium citrate	4
Calcium gluceptate	0 or variable; effloresces
Calcium gluconate	0 or 1
Dextrose	1
Diatrizoic acid	2
Dibasic sodium phosphate	0, 1, or 2
Ephedrine	½
Fluocinolone acetonide	2
Hydrocortisone hemisuccinate	1
Magnesium citrate oral solution	1
Magnesium gluconate	2
Magnesium sulfate	0, loses gradually
Monosodium sodium phosphate	0, 1, or 2
Naloxone hydrochloride	2
Nitrofurantoin	0 or 1
Potassium gluconate	0 or 1
Prednisolone	0 or 1
Saccharin sodium	1/3; effloresces
Sodium acetate	3
Sodium citrate	0 or 2
Sodium sulfate	0 or 1; effloresces
Succinyl chloride	2
Theophylline	0 or 1
Thioguanine	0 or ½
Thiothixene hydrochloride	0 or 2
Zinc sulfate	1 or 7

Source: United States Pharmacopeia (USP) 24.

metal-ion coordinated water. There are three classes that are discernible by the commonly available analytical techniques.

1. Class I includes isolated lattice sites and represents the structures with water molecules that are isolated and kept from contacting other water molecules directly in the lattice structure. Therefore, water molecules exposed to the surface of crystals may be easily lost. However, the creation of holes that were occupied by the water molecules on the surface of the crystals does not provide access for water molecules inside the crystal lattice. The thermogravimetric analysis (TGA) and differential scanning calorimetry (DSC) for the hydrates in this class show sharp endotherms. Cephradine dihydrate is an example of this class of hydrates.

2. Class II includes hydrates that have water molecules in channels. The water molecules in this class lie continuously next to the other water molecules, forming channels through the crystal. The TGA and DSC data show interesting characteristics of channel hydrate dehydration. Early-onset temperature of dehydration is expected, and broad dehydration is also characteristic of the channel hydrates. This is because the dehydration begins from the ends of channels that are open to the surface of crystals. Subsequently, dehydration keeps happening until all the water molecules are removed through the channels. Ampicillin trihydrate belongs to this class. Some hydrates have water molecules in two-dimensional (2D) space, and they are called planar hydrates.

3. Class III includes ion-associated hydrates. Hydrates contain metal-ion coordinated water and the interaction between the metal ions and water molecules is the major force in the structure of crystalline hydrates. The metal–water interactions may be quite strong relative to the other nonbonded interactions, and therefore, dehydration occurs at very high temperatures. In TGA and DSC thermograms, very sharp peaks corresponding to dehydration of water bonded with metal ions are expected at high temperatures.

Hydrates can also exist in various polymorphs, such as in the case of amiloride hydrochloride. A myriad of methods is available to study hydrates and their polymorphs, including DTA, DSC, XRPD, and moisture-uptake studies.

6.6 Amorphous Forms

Solid powders, wherein no particular order of molecules is technically noncrystalline, are called amorphous forms. The amorphous forms are formed by vapor condensation, supercooling of a melt, precipitation from solution, and milling and compaction of crystals. These are more like liquids, where the molecular interaction has weakened; in most instances, there would be some crystalline forms among the amorphous forms as well. This two-state model is described in the U.S. Pharmacopeia (USP). The amorphous forms are thermodynamically unstable, as they have high energy (that went into breaking intermolecular bonds). As a result, they might turn into a crystalline form, particularly in suspension dosage forms and even in solid dosage forms, wherein the atmospheric moisture might serve as the nucleation point.

Discovery programs frequently yield amorphous compounds as a result of time pressures, the methods used to isolate them on small scales, and the increasing complexity of newly discovered molecules. Amorphous compounds carry inherent risks because of their physicochemical nature, and as a result, very few Food and Drug Administration (FDA)-approved drugs appear in amorphous forms; examples include accupril/accuretic, intraconazole, accolate (zafirlukast), viracept (nelfinavir mesylate), and paroxetine. Other drugs that are available in amorphous forms include celecoxib, amifostine, cefuroxime axetil, cefpodoxime proxetil, and novobiocin. In addition to being a physically metastable physical form, amorphous forms are generally less stable chemically. They also tend to have very low bulk densities, making the materials difficult to isolate and handle. The irregular shape of the powder of amorphous forms creates high surface area, which attracts water molecules, making them inherently more hygroscopic.

Although all these problems can be resolved, generally, the amorphous forms are to be avoided, unless the differences in solubility make a significant impact on the bioavailability.

6.7 Hygroscopicity

Water molecules have polar ends and readily form hydrogen bonding. As a result, several compounds interact with water molecules by surface adsorption, condensation in capillaries, bulk retention, and chemical interaction and are called hygroscopic. At times, the interaction between the compounds and water is so strong that the interacting water vapors result in dissolving the compound. This process is called deliquescence, wherein a saturated layer of solution is formed around the particles. Most of these interactions are dependent on critical water vapor pressure or relative humidity (RH). Moisture also induces hydrolysis and other degradation reactions. In addition, its presence affects the physical properties, such as powder flow, dissolution, and even crystal structure. The impact of moisture on the physical or chemical properties of compounds depends on the strength of bonding between the water molecules and the surrounding space where the water molecules are contained. In a tightly bound state, the water molecules are generally not available to induce chemical reactions. Free water molecules can participate in the creation of a liquid environment around the crystal lattice, where the pH may be altered as a result of the dissolution process. Similarly, water molecules held as crystal hydrates or trapped in an amorphous form are not available to modify the milieu interior of solid powders. It is noteworthy that some hydrates on taking up moisture convert into hydrates (discussed earlier). This transition can be useful in formulation studies, and this property should be tested for hygroscopic compounds.

The classification of compounds into different hygroscopic categories is based on two types of models: (1) In the first model, the RH and temperature are kept constant, gain in the weight of compound is recorded as per the definitions of the European Pharmacopoeia, and the compound tested is stored at 25°C for 24 hours at 80% RH. A slightly hygroscopic compound would show less than 2% m/m mass gain, hygroscopic compounds show less than 15%, and very hygroscopic compounds show more than 15% m/m mass gain; the deliquescent compounds simply liquefy. The dynamic model tests hygroscopic nature at various humidities; compounds showing no mass gain at 90% are called nonhygroscopic, those that do not gain at 90% are slightly hygroscopic, and those that gain 5% over a week's period are called moderately hygroscopic. Where mass increases at 40%–50% humidity, these compounds are called very hygroscopic.

Generally, a compound that is very hygroscopic would be less desirable, but if studies show that, despite moisture uptake, the compound stays stable and workable in the formulation studies, this is an important consideration.

High hygroscopicity is undesirable for many reasons, including handling problems, requirement of special storage conditions, and problems with chemical and physical stability. It is difficult to develop acceptance criteria for the amount of moisture, and large batch-to-batch variations are inevitable. Even if it were possible to define reasonable acceptance criteria, if the compound shows changes in crystal structure as a function of moisture content, this leads to problems in solubility and dissolution profiles that may not be acceptable. Stability of salts at accelerated temperature is complicated when there is significant sorption of moisture, because the properties related to the removal of moisture will be highly dependent on the choice and amount of excipients, the manufacturing process of the final dosage form, and even the impurity profile, both in the lead compound and in the excipients. As a rule, any property, such as hygroscopicity, which makes it difficult to create acceptance criterion, should be minimized. Solid-state stability, as a result of hygroscopicity, often plays a significant role in determining the dissolution rate, for example, napsylate salts often provide a more stable physical form and thus allow better dissolution.

6.8 Solubility

Solubility is a function of hygroscopicity, polymorphism, and chemical nature or pK_a of the salt. If the pK_a is at least two units lower than the pH of the medium, complete dissolution can be achieved; the opposite holds true for basic compounds. Even though in the early phase of the study, the quantity of the compound might be limited, solubility studies need to be carried out as a function of pH, leaving sufficient quantity even after the formation of salt. The solids formed (both wet and dry) should then be studied using the usual techniques, such as DSC, TGA, and XRPD. The method of determining solubility can often provide variable results. The in situ technique often proves more useful to screen out poor-solubility compounds; the traditional methods are always preferred. Solubility increase leads to improved bioavailability and liquid formulation and can be achieved by increasing the melting point or the hydrophobicity of the conjugate anion. Reduced solubility is desired for suspension and controlled-release dosage forms and can be achieved by decreasing the pK_a and increasing the solubility of the conjugate acid.

The choice of salt is greatly determined by solubility considerations; the pH of the resultant solution is important, because the salts of the stronger acids produce liquids with a lower pH to promote the dissolution of the basic compounds. However, in places where a common-ion effect can operate, such as the use of hydrochloride in gastric fluid, the useful solubility window might be limited, and this modification might not work well. Similarly, when determining the solubility, there can often be significant differences in results obtained, depending on whether it is determined in water, saline, or buffer, as a function of the nature of salt. It is not as straightforward as in the case of hydrochloride, where a common-ion effect is clearly the most important observation. There is complex effect of pH, common-ion effect, and dielectric properties of media.

The dissolution of solid particles of salts can be inhibited if the parent acid or base precipitates at the surface of the particles undergoing dissolution. For example, stearate salts show reduced dissolution if stearic acid layer precipitates on the surface in an acidic pH environment.

The choice of salt is often determined by taste consideration, such as the use of benzathine salts of penicillin V. Low-solubility salts have lesser taste, but they also dissolve slowly and are often used for preparing depot preparations, such as benzathine salts of penicillin G and V. Similarly, the napsylate salt provides better organoleptic properties as a result of its low solubility when compared with hydrochloride forms.

The stoichiometry of the salts is established by a detailed study of the physical structure by using XRPD techniques, and it can, at times, be not what the chemical structures would generally indicate.

6.8.1 Salt Form

Combinatorial chemistry offers many advantages, including the synthesis of larger-molecular-weight drugs, which are mostly lipophilic. The bioavailability considerations require converting them into salt forms. This trend is apparent from recent regulatory approvals by the FDA, where more than 50% of the new drugs approved have been in salt forms. The common methods used for the characterization and the screening of salt forms include the following:

- XRPD analysis
- Thermal analysis (DSC, TGA, and thermomechanical analysis)
- Dynamic vapor sorption (DVS)
- Nuclear magnetic resonance (NMR)
- Dissolution (including intrinsic)
- Microscopy (light and polarized)
- Density (intrinsic and bulk)
- Particle size (optical, laser light, and light obscuration)

A process flow for the selection of the best salt form is given in Scheme 6.2.

The choice of using a cation or an anion form is always based on all the factors described earlier. There are fewer salt-forming species for weak acids than there are for weak bases, and the available information suggests that, in general, alkali metal salts exhibit greater solubility than the corresponding alkaline earth salts. Among cations, the most frequently found ion is sodium (62%), followed by potassium and calcium (10%); this is followed by zinc and meglumine (3%), lithium, magnesium diethanolamine, benzathine, ethyldiamine, aluminum, chloroprocaine, and choline (in the decreasing order of frequency). Among anions, the most frequently used counter ion is hydrochloride

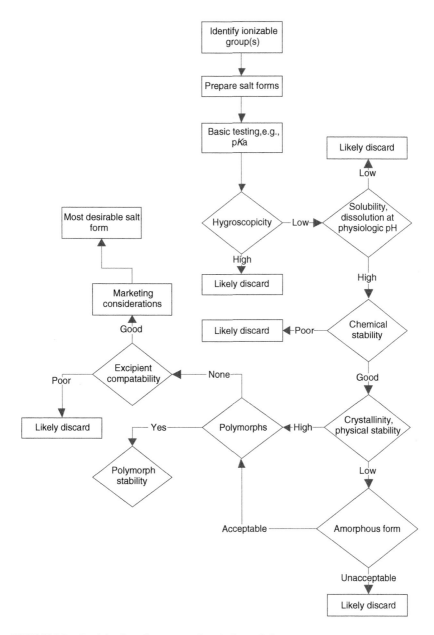

SCHEME 6.2 Decision flow diagram to select the best salt form.

(almost 50%), followed by sulfate (8%), bromide and chloride (5%), diphosphate, citrate, and maleate (3%), iodine mesylate and hydrobromide (2%), acetate and pamoate (1%), isothionate, methylsulfate, salicylate, lactate, methylbromide, nitrate, bitartrate, benzoate, dihydrochloride, gluconate, carbonate, edisylate, mandelate, methylnitrate, subacetate, succinate, benzenesulfonate, calcium edentate, camsylate, edentate, fumarate, glutamate, hydrobromine, napsylate, pantothenate, stearate, gluceptate, bicarbonate,

TABLE 6.5

The pK_a of Common Weak Acids Used in Salt Formation

Acid	pK_a
Acetate	4.76
Ascorbate	4.21
Benzoate	4.20
Besylate	2.54
Citrate	3.13
Fumarate	3.0, 4.4
Gluconate	3.60
Hydrobromide	−8.0
Hydrochloride	−6.1
Malate	3.5, 5.1
Mesylate	1.92
Napsylate	0.17
Oleate	~4.0
Phosphate	2.15, 7.20, 12.38
Succinate	4.2, 5.6
Sulfate	−3.0
Tartrate	3.0, 4.3
Tosylate	−0.51

estolate, esylate, glycollylarsinate, hexylresorcinate, lactobionate, maleate, mucate, polygalactoronate, teoclate, and triethiodide (in the decreasing order of frequency). The choice of counterions is a function of the pK_a of the weak acid involved in the formation of salt. Table 6.5 lists the pK_a values of weak acids that are most frequently used in salt formation.

To form a salt of a basic compound, the pK_a of the salt-forming acid has to be less than or equal to the pK_a of the basic center of the compound. As a result, very weak basic compounds have a pK_a value around 2. Bases with higher pK_a have a greater range of possibilities for salt formation. As most drugs are weak bases, it is not surprising that hydrochloride, sulfuric, and toluenesulfonic salts are very common.

The chances are high that a newly discovered drug substance would have polarizable groups that make the compound capable of interacting with the receptor sites. The most common polarizable ends are present in acidic or basic compounds. Neutral compounds are inert and mostly inactive; for example, perfluorodecalin is a balanced cyclohexane, wherein the ring electronegativity is neutralized by the strong fluorine molecules. This molecule is inert and is not degraded by the body. As the availability of the ionizing center leads to salt formation, the salt formation studies are one of the most important studies at the prenomination stage, because this can affect the solubility, dissolution hygroscopicity, taste, physical and chemical stability, or polymorphism properties of the newly discovered drug substance. It is most likely for these studies to be conducted after establishing the basic physicochemical properties, in order to allow the comparison with properties in various salt forms. In the order of importance, the selection process follows the following theme.

6.8.2 Melting Point

Solubility is increased when the melting point of the salt is lower or where there is improved hydrogen bonding (with water), and as a result, the hydroxyl groups in the conjugate acid improve the solubility and the hydrophobic groups reduce the solubility. Often, it is desired to prepare salts with a lower solubility to mask taste, provide slower dissolution, and increase its chemical stability. An increase in the melting point results in process problem and reduced solubility; this can be achieved by the use of more flexible aliphatic acids with aromatic bases. Move to more highly substituted acids that destroy the crystal symmetry. A decrease in the melting point generally improves the solubility and allows the formation of oil, and it can be achieved by using small counterions, for example, chloride and bromide, or aromatic conjugate anions in case of aromatic base or by using small hydroxyl acids if the drug has good hydrogen bonding potential. The melting point is generally decreased by increasing the hydroxylation of the conjugate acid and, in the cases of common ion dependence, by moving small organic acids. In the case of the sodium salt of drugs, the logarithm of aqueous solubility is often inversely related to melting point.

6.8.3 Dissolution

The factors described above affecting the solubility are important to select a salt form or a specific crystalline or polymorphic form that may affect dissolution rate, the most critical parameter. The first step in the commencement of dissolution is the wettability of solid particles—there is a direct correlation between wettability and bioavailability. As the milieu of drug administration sites is mostly aqueous in nature, low wettability makes the particles less hygroscopic.

The dissolution of the salts leads to a change in the pH of the dissolution media because of the buffering effect. A base dissolved in the acidic media increases the pH, because the acidic counterions are trapped into salt forms. Similarly, as the salts dissolve, the pH shift depends on whether it is the acid or the basic component that is weaker. The final balance is always dependent on the relative pK_a of the acidic and alkaline components. This is an important consideration, as it explains the difference in the results obtained when the studies are conducted in water or buffer. When enteric protection is desired, the dissolution rates should be determined in 0.1 N HCl, wherein many differences in the dissolution rates between water and buffer are obviated.

6.9 Study Methods

At the preformulation stage, the limitations of the quantity of the sample available determines to a great degree the type of the study to be conducted. Some physical properties are fundamental in nature, whereas others are a manifestation of these basic properties. For example, melting point determination reveals much about the internal structure of crystals and the solubility and dissolution characteristics; the latter properties are the derived properties. As a result, techniques available to study the aforementioned properties are categorized by the U.S. FDA in a decreasing order of importance (FDA, The Gold Sheet, 1985). The following is an expanded list of these methodologies available for evaluation:

- Melting point (HSM)
- IRS
- XRPD
- Thermal analytical techniques (e.g., DSC, differential thermal analysis [DTA], TGA, and the like)
- Solid-state Raman spectroscopy
- Crystalline index of refraction
- Phase solubility analysis
- Solution pH profile determination
- Solution calorimetry
- Comparative intrinsic dissolution rates
- Cross-polarization/magic angle spinning (CP/MAS) solid-state NMR
- Hygroscopicity measurement (particularly for salts)

6.9.1 Thermal Analysis

There are a number of interrelated thermal analytical techniques that can be used to characterize the salts and the polymorphs of candidate drugs. The melting point of a salt can be manipulated to produce compounds with desirable physicochemical properties for specific formulation types. Of the thermal methods available for investigating polymorphism and related phenomena, DSC, TGA, and HSM are the most widely used methods.

6.9.2 Differential Scanning Calorimetry

Differential scanning calorimetry is one of the most frequently used methods to study solid-state properties. The flux-type DSC involves heating the sample and reference samples at a constant rate by using thermocouples, to determine how much heat is flowing into each sample and thus finding the differences between the two. Examples of such DSC instrumentation are those provided by Mettler and duPont. The power compensation DSC (e.g., PerkinElmer), an exothermic or endothermic event, occurs when a sample is heated, and the power added or subtracted to one or both furnaces to compensate for the energy change occurring in the sample is measured. Thus, the system is maintained in a thermally neutral position at all times, and the amount of power required to maintain the system at equilibrium is directly proportional to the energy changes occurring in the sample. In both types of DSC measurements, only a few milligrams of the compound suffice. The sample can be heated in an open pan or in hermetically sealed chambers, where there may or may not be vents to release moisture or solvents; the compound may be subjected to pyrolysis in the testing phase.

Although the instrumentation available in the recent years has become very sophisticated, making such analysis possible with great consistency, the interpretation of the results is highly dependent on a keen understanding of the factors that affect the results. For example, such subtle factors as the type of pan, the heating rate used, the nature and mass of the compound, the particle size distribution, packing and porosity, pretreatment and dilution of the sample, and the use of the nitrogen cover can significantly alter the DSC profile obtained and should be controlled to secure consistency in the repeat results.

A well-designed and properly replicated DSC profile would yield such physical properties as melting (endothermic), solid-state transitions (endothermic), glass transitions, crystallization (endothermic), decomposition (exothermic), dehydration or desolvation (endothermic), and purity (of high purity compounds; though much less reliable than high-performance liquid chromatography, HPLC).

A heating rate of 10°C/min is a useful compromise between the speed of analysis and detecting any heating rate-dependent phenomena. If any heating rate-dependent phenomena are evident, the experiments should be repeated by varying the heating rate, in order to identify the nature of the transition that might be the result of polymorphism or particle size. It is noteworthy that milling the powder size may alter the profile significantly and can be confused with polymorphic changes. Using different heating rates often resolves this problem.

A number of parameters can be measured from the various thermal events detected by DSC. For example, for a melting endotherm, the onset, peak temperatures, and enthalpy of fusion can be derived. The onset temperature is obtained by extrapolation from the leading edge of the endotherm to the baseline. The peak temperature is the temperature corresponding to the maximum of the endotherm, and the enthalpy of fusion is derived from the area of the thermogram. It is an accepted custom that the extrapolated onset temperature is taken as the melting point; however, some users report the peak temperature in this respect. We tend to report both for completeness.

Recycling experiments can also be conducted, whereby a sample is heated and then cooled. The thermogram might show a crystallization exotherm for the sample, which might show a melting point different from the first run on subsequent reheating. In a similar way, amorphous forms can be produced by cooling the molten sample to form a glass.

The calibration of a DSC employs the use of standards; the most common ones are listed in Table 6.6. These standards must meet a certain criterion of purity. A two-point calibration is often needed, for example, using indium and lead.

TABLE 6.6

Standards for Thermal Analysis in the Order of Increasing Melting Point

Temperature (°C)	Substance
0	Water
26.87	Phenoxybenzene
114.2	Acetanilide
151.4	Adipic acid
156.6	Indium
229	Tin
232	Caffeine
327.5	Lead
419.6	Zinc

A variation of DSC is the modulated DSC (MDSC), wherein heat is applied sinusoidally, such that any thermal events are resolved into reversing and nonreversing components to allow complex and even overlapping processes to be deconvoluted. The heat flow signal in conventional DSC is a combination of "kinetic" and heat capacity responses, and Fourier transform (FT) techniques are used to separate the heat flow component from the underlying heat flow signal. The cyclic heat flow part of the signal (heat capacity, C_p × heating rate) is termed the reversing heat flow component. The nonreversing part is obtained by subtracting this value from the total heat flow curve. It is important to note that all these noises appear in the nonreversing signal. The limitations of the MDSC studies include the requirement of a sufficient number of cycles to cover thermal events. In cases where the samples do not follow the signal or where there is fluctuation in temperature during the sinusoidal ramp, these compounds may not be suitable for this study.

6.9.3 Hot-Stage Microscopy

Hot-stage microscopy is a thermal analytical technique, whereby a few milligrams of the material is spread on a microscope slide, which is then placed in the hot stage and heated at various rates and under different atmospheric environments, including very low temperatures. The events can be recorded using video systems. Hot-stage microscopy is routinely used in conjunction with other methods. Although many newer automated methods to observe the melting behavior of crystals are available, to a trained eye, this classic method remains one of the most powerful tools.

6.9.4 Thermogravimetric Analysis

Thermogravimetric analysis (TGA) is used to detect the amount of weight lost on heating a sample. It is based on a sensitive balance that records the weight of the sample (generally 5–10 mg), as it is heated under nitrogen. Thermogravimetric analysis experiments can detect the presence of water or solvent in different locations in the crystal lattice. This technique has an advantage over a Karl Fischer titration or a loss on drying experiment that can only detect the total amount of moisture present. In addition, TGA requires smaller quantities of the compounds than the other two techniques. However, the use of very little sample in TGA can yield erroneous results because of buoyancy and convection current effects. The total amount of moisture lost in TGA experiments is not affected by the heating rate; however, the temperature at which it occurs may vary. It is noteworthy that the dehydration mechanism and activation of the reaction may be dependent on the practice size and sample weight. The TGA is calibrated using magnetic standards.

6.9.5 Solution Calorimetry

Solution calorimetry involves the measurement of heat flow when a compound dissolves in a solvent. There are two types of solution calorimeters, that is, isoperibol and isothermal. In the isoperibol technique, the heat change caused by the dissolution of the solute gives rise to a change in the temperature of the solution. This results in a temperature–time plot from which the heat of the solution is calculated. In contrast, in isothermal solution calorimetry (where, by definition, the temperature is maintained constant), any heat change is compensated by an equal, but opposite, energy change, which is then the heat of solution. The latest microsolution calorimeter can be used with 3–5 mg of compound. Experimentally, the sample is introduced into the equilibrated solvent system, and the heat flow is measured using a heat conduction calorimeter.

Dissolution of a solute involves several thermal events, such as heat associated with wetting, breakage of lattice bonds, and salvation energy. The peak can be integrated directly to give an enthalpy of dissolution. The relative stability of polymorphs can be investigated in this way by the magnitude and sign (endothermic/exothermic) of the enthalpy of dissolution. A more endothermic (or less exothermic) response indicates that the energy of solvation of the solute does not compensate for the breaking of lattice bonds, and it is therefore the more stable solid (polymorphs).

Solution calorimetry can also be used to evaluate the amorphous/crystalline content in a binary mixture. The enthalpy of solution for the amorphous compound is an exothermic event, whereas that of the crystalline hydrate is endothermic. Enthalpy of a solution is a sum of several thermal events, that is, heat of wetting (incorporating sorption process, such as surface sorption and complexation), disruption of the crystal lattice, and solvation. The order of magnitude of solution enthalpy for the crystalline compound suggests that the disruption of the crystal lattice predominates over the heat of solvation. In addition, the ready solubility of the compound in aqueous media is probably governed by entropy considerations.

Solution calorimeters are calibrated using KCl in water (for endothermic processes) and Tris-HCl in 0.01 M HCl (for exothermic processes) standards. For example, the heat of solution ΔH_s of KCl at 25°C (298.15 K) is 235.86 $\pm$ 0.23 J/g. Similarly, the ΔH_s for Tris-HCl at 25°C is −29.80 kJ/mol.

6.9.6 Isothermal Microcalorimetry

Isothermal microcalorimetry can also be used to determine, among other things, the hygroscopicity of substances. In the ramp mode, this technique can be used, like DVS, to examine the milligram quantities of compound. This instrument utilizes a perfusion attachment with a precision flow switching valve. The moist gas is pumped into a reaction ampoule through two inlets, one that delivers dry nitrogen at 0% RH and the other that delivers nitrogen that has been saturated by passing it through two humidifier chambers maintained at 100% RH. The required RH is then achieved by the switching valve, which varies the proportion of dry to saturated gas. The RH can then be increased or decreased to determine the effect of moisture on the physicochemical properties of the compound.

It is probably more popular to perform microcalorimetry in the static mode. In the so-called internal hygrostat method, the compound under investigation is sealed into a vial with a sealed pipette tip containing the saturated salt solution chosen to give the required RH.

6.9.7 Infrared Spectroscopy

Infrared spectroscopy differentiates solid-state structures of compounds just as well as it differentiates and identifies the chemical structures and peculiarities. This is because the different arrangements of atoms in the solid state lead to different molecular environments, which in turn induce variability in stretching frequencies.

These differences are used to distinguish the polymorphic forms of a compound. The presence of solvent or water can be detected using this technique as a result of the "broad–OH" stretch associated with water.

The IRS is applied to studies in a number of ways: by Nujol mull, KBr disc, or the diffuse reflectance (DR) technique. In the KBr disc technique, the compound is mixed with KBr and compressed into a disc by using a press and a die. This compression can be a disadvantage if the compound undergoes a polymorphic transformation under pressure.

Nowadays, most instruments use an FT-infrared (FT-IR) system, a mathematical operation used to translate a complex curve into its component curves. In an FT-IR instrument, the complex curve is an interferogram or the sum of the constructive and destructive interferences generated by overlapping light waves, and the component curves are the IR spectrum. The standard IR spectrum is calculated from the FT interferogram, giving a spectrum in percent transmittance (%T) versus light frequency (cm^{-1}).

An interferogram is generated because of the unique optics of an FT-IR instrument. The key components are a moveable mirror and a beam splitter. The moveable mirror is responsible for the quality of the interferogram, and it is very important to move the mirror at a constant speed. For this reason, the moveable mirror is often the most expensive component of an FT-IR spectrometer. The beam splitter is just a piece of semireflective material, usually Mylar film sandwiched between two pieces of an IR-transparent material. The beam splitter splits the IR beam 50/50 to the fixed and moveable mirrors and then recombines the beams after being reflected at each mirror. The FT is named after its inventor, the French geometrician and physicist Baron Jean Baptiste Joseph Fourier, born in 1830.

The FT-IR spectra of amorphous forms are often less well defined and can be used to characterize various polymorphic forms. Heating experiments are also possible by using IRS, where the variable-temperature IRS is conducted to confirm that a solid–solid transition takes place on heating various forms of the compounds.

The disadvantages of the conventional IRS, such as the need to compress the samples, is overcome when the *diffuse reflectance Fourier transform* (*DRIFT*) technique is used, whereby a few milligrams of the compound are dispersed in approximately 250 mg of KBr, and the spectrum is obtained by reflection from the surface.

Many substances in their natural states (e.g., powders and rough surface solids) exhibit DR; that is, the incident light is scattered in all directions, as opposed to specular (mirror-like) reflection, where the angle of incidence equals the angle of reflection. In practice, the DR spectra are complex and are strongly dependent on the conditions under which they are obtained. These spectra can exhibit both absorbance and reflectance features as a result of the contributions from transmission, internal and specular reflectance components, and scattering phenomena in the collected radiation. The DR spectra are further complicated by sample preparation, particle size, sample concentration, and optical geometry effects, to name a few. Specular reflection, whether it occurs from a glossy sample surface or from a crystal surface, produces inverted bands ("Reststrahlen bands") in the DR spectrum, which reduces the usefulness of traditional transmission reference spectra. For highly absorbing samples, these Reststrahlen bands are strong. Grinding and diluting the sample with nonabsorbing powder, such as KBr, KCl, Ge, and Si, can minimize or eliminate these effects. Grinding reduces the contribution of reflection from large particle faces. Diluting ensures deeper penetration of the incident beam, thus increasing the contribution to the spectrum of the transmission and internal reflection component. The resulting spectra have an appearance more similar to that of the transmittance spectra than bulk reflectance spectra. If sample dilution is not feasible, the spectra may still be improved by using an optical geometry that employs a low incident angle and an offline collection angle.

The DR spectrum of a dilute sample of "infinite depth" (i.e., up to 3 mm) is usually calculated with reference to the diffuse reflectance of the pure diluent to yield the reflectance, $R_{i\text{Å}}$. $R_{i\text{Å}}$ is related to the concentration of the sample, c, by the Kubelka–Munk (K–M) equation:

$$f(R_{i\text{Å}}) = (1 - R_{i\text{Å}})^2 / 2R_{i\text{Å}} = 2.303 \, ac/s \qquad (6.1)$$

where a is the absorptivity and s is the scattering coefficient. The scattering coefficient depends on both particle size and degree of sample packing. Thus, the K–M function can be used for accurate quantitative analysis, provided the particle size and packing method are strictly controlled. For good diffuse reflectors, plots of the K–M function, $f(R_{i\text{Å}})$, are analogous to absorbance plots for transmission spectra. Care must be taken in applying the K–M equation when $R_{i\text{Å}}$ is much less than about 30%, because deviations from linearity can occur when the sample concentration is high.

A modification of the aforementioned DR model is the *praying mantis model*, where the preferred offline type incorporates two 6:1 90-degree off-axis ellipsoidal mirrors. One of the ellipsoids focuses the incident beam on the sample, whereas the second collects the radiation diffusely reflected by the sample. Both ellipsoidal mirrors are tilted forward; therefore, the specular component is deflected behind the collecting ellipsoid and permits the collection of primarily the diffusely reflected component. Another advantage of the "praying mantis" design is the ability to expand the available sampling area indefinitely by rotating the ellipsoids and positioning the sampling point above the optical plane. This accessory may also be used for specular reflectance at a 41.50-degree angle of incidence. This is achieved by tilting the sample angle as the alignment mirror. Specular sample holders are available for this purpose. Although diffuse reflection spectroscopy primarily measures the spectrum of the bulk, it can be very sensitive to the nature of the sample, for example, powders with a high surface area. Thus, it is valuable for catalysis and oxidation studies. In this application, it is important to measure the spectrum under controlled atmospheres and at high or low temperatures. The "praying mantis" model has a large sampling space between the ellipsoids for additional accessories, such as vacuum chambers. This cell is specially designed to conduct diffuse reflection spectroscopy studies in controlled atmospheres at high (up to 750°C) or low (liquid nitrogen) temperatures and under vacuum or high pressure (e.g., up to 1500 psi).

6.9.8 X-Ray Powder Diffraction

X-rays are part of the electromagnetic spectrum lying between the ultraviolet and gamma rays, and they are expressed in angstrom units (Å). Diffraction is a scattered phenomenon, and when X-rays are incident on crystalline solids, they are scattered in all directions. Scattering occurs as a result of the radiation wavelength being in the same order of magnitude as the interatomic distances within the crystal structure. X-rays are extensively used to characterize a crystal. In Figure 6.8, the relationship

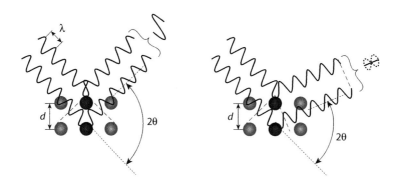

FIGURE 6.8 Bragg's diffraction.

between the interplanar spacing and the angle of an incident beam is described by Bragg's equation.

The interference is constructive when the phase shift is proportional to 2π; this condition can be expressed by Bragg's law:

$$n\lambda = 2d \sin(\theta) \tag{6.2}$$

where n is an integer, λ is the wavelength of X-rays and moving electrons, protons, and neutrons, d is the spacing between the planes in the atomic lattice, and θ is the angle between the incident ray and the scattering planes.

Bragg's equation gives an easy way to understand XRPD. Powder X-ray diffraction data collected on crystalline samples give information about peak intensities and peak positions. Peak intensities are determined by the contents of unit cells, and peak positions are closely related to the cell constants. Interplanar spacing is a function of Miller indices and cell constants. Therefore, if the cell constants are known for a crystalline compound, peak positions corresponding to Miller indices can be obtained from the Bragg's equation: the wavelength, λ, is machine-specific. The determination of cell parameters in structure determination of XRPD pattern is a reverse process to find cell constants from peak positions. Here, note that the cell constants for a unit cell are not affected by the contents in the unit cell. The contents in the unit cell have effects on the peak intensities.

The X-ray diffraction experiment requires an X-ray source, the sample under investigation, and a detector to pick up the diffracted X-rays. Figure 6.9 is a schematic diagram of a powder X-ray diffractometer.

The X-ray radiation most commonly used is that emitted by copper, whose characteristic wavelength for the K radiation is 1.5418 Å. When the incident beam strikes a powder sample, diffraction occurs in every possible orientation of 2θ. The diffracted beam may be detected by using a moveable detector, such as a Geiger counter, which is connected to a chart recorder. In normal use, the counter is set to scan over a range of 2θ values at a constant angular velocity. Routinely, a 2θ range of $5°–70°$ is sufficient to cover the most useful part of the powder pattern. The scanning speed of the counter is usually 2θ of $2°$ per min and, therefore, about 30 minutes are needed to obtain a trace.

An X-ray diffractometer is made up of an X-ray tube generating X-rays from, for example, Cu, Ka, and Co source, and a detector. The most common arrangement in

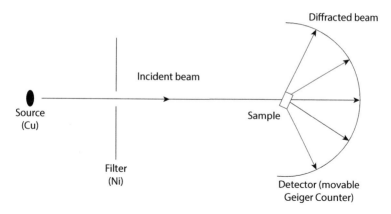

FIGURE 6.9 Design plan of a typical X-ray powder diffractometer.

pharmaceutical powder studies is the Bragg–Brentano θ–θ configuration. In this arrangement, the X-ray tube is moved through angle θ, and the detector is moved through angle θ. The sample is fixed between the detector and the X-ray, shown in Figure 6.3.

The powder pattern consists of a series of peaks that have been collected at various scattering angles, which are related to d-spacing, so that the unit cell dimensions can be determined. In most cases, the measurement of the d-spacing will suffice to positively identify a crystalline material. If the sample is of amorphous nature, that is, does not show long-range order, the X-rays are not coherently scattered, and no peaks will be observed.

Although XRPD analysis is a relatively straightforward technique for the identification of solid-phase structures, there are sources of error, including the following:

- *Variations in particle size.* Large particle sizes can lead to nonrandom orientation, and hence, particles <10 μm should be used; that is, the sample should be carefully ground. However, if the size is too small, for example, 1 μm, it leads to the broadening of the diffraction peaks. Indeed, if the crystal sizes are too small, then the sample may appear to be amorphous.
- *Preferred orientation.* If a powder consists of needle- or plate-shaped particles, these tend to become aligned parallel to the specimen axis, and thus, certain planes have a greater chance of reflecting the X-rays. To reduce the errors caused by this source, the sample is usually rotated. Alternatively, the sample can be packed into a capillary.
- *Statistical errors.* The magnitude of statistical errors depends on the number of photons counted. To keep this number small, scanning should be carried out at an appropriately slow speed.
- *Sample height.* The sample should be at the same level as the top of the holder. If the sample height is too low, the pattern shifts down the 2θ scale, and if it is too high, it moves up the 2θ scale.
- *Sample preparation procedures.* The greatest potential source of problems is grinding, which can introduce strain, amorphism, and polymorphic changes. Even the contamination from the process of grinding (e.g., in a mortar) can significantly affect the diffraction pattern. Furthermore, the atmosphere

surrounding the sample can create problems as a result of the loss or gain of moisture or carbon dioxide. This is particularly true if a heating stage is used, particularly when a compound undergoes a solid-state transition from a low-melting form to a high-melting form; this can be detected by a change in the diffraction pattern. Using the Anton Parr TTK-450 temperature attachment, the compound can be investigated between subambient temperature and several hundred degrees. In cases where desolvation occurs on micronization, heating the sample makes the peaks shaper and stronger, indicating an increase in crystallinity. This is analogous to the annealing exotherm observed in the DSC thermogram. In a similar way, the sample can be exposed to varying degrees of humidity in situ, and the diffraction pattern can be determined.

- *Irradiation effects.* Sample exposure can result in solid-state reactions, cabonization, polymorphic changes, and the like, as a result of high-energy exposure of the sample.

- *Size of sample.* The limited amount of compound available can be problematic. However, modern diffractometers can use the so-called zero-background holders (ZBH). These are made from a single crystal of silicon that has been cut along a nondiffracting plane and then polished to an optically flat finish. Thus, X-rays incident on this surface will be negated by the Bragg extinction. In this technique, a thin layer of grease is placed on the ZBH surface, and the sample of ground compound is placed on the surface. The excess is removed, such that only a monolayer is examined. The total thickness of the sample and grease should be of the order of a few microns. It is important that the sample is deagglomerated, so that the monolayer condition is met. Using this technique, the diffraction pattern of approximately 10 mg of the compound can be obtained. One disadvantage of the ZBH is that weak reflections may not be readily detectable because of the small sample size used.

- *Calibration.* The XRPD should be properly calibrated using the standards available from reliable sources, such as the Laboratory of the Government Chemist (LGC) in the United Kingdom or the National Institute of Standards and Technology (NIST) in the United States. The analysis of one or two peaks of LaB6 (line-broadening calibrator), at least weekly, should give confidence in the diffractometer performance and alert the user of any problems that may develop. The common external standards are silicon, a-quartz, gold, and silicon (SRM 640b). The primary standards for internal d-spacing include silicon (SRM 640b) and fluorophlogopite (SRM 675), and the secondary standards for internal d-spacing are tungsten, silver, quartz, and diamond. The internal quantitative intensity standards are Al_2O_3 (SRM 676); α- and β-silicon nitride (SRM 656); oxides of Al, Ce, Cr, Ti, and Zn (SRM 674a); α-silicon dioxide (SRM 1878a); and cristobalite (SRM 1879a). A typical external sensitivity standard is Al_2O_3 (SRM 1976).

6.9.9 Phase Solubility Analysis

Solubility is generally estimated by visual observation. The solubility of a compound is initially determined by weighing out 10 mg (or other suitable amount) of the compound. To this is added 10 μL of the solvent of interest. If the compound does not dissolve, a further 40 µL of the solvent is added, and its effect is noted. Successive amounts of the solvent are then added until the compound is observed to dissolve. This procedure should give an approximate value of the solubility. This method does not take into account the kinetic aspects of the dissolution processes involved in solubility measurements. To determine more accurately the concentration of a saturated solution of a compound, the following procedure can be used. A known volume of the solvent, water, or buffer is taken into a scintillation vial, and the compound is added until saturation is observed. The solution is then stirred or shaken, and the experiment is restarted. It is recommended that the experiment be conducted at least overnight or longer, for low-solubility compounds. Depending on the amount of the compound available, replicate experiments should be carried out. After stirring or shaking, the solvent should be separated from the suspension by centrifugation or by filtration, using polytetrafluoroethylene (PTFE) filters. The filtrate is then assayed preferably by HPLC; however, ultraviolet (UV)–visible spectroscopy can also be used to determine the solubility, if compound stability or impurities are not an issue. This is termed the thermodynamic solubility. It is also useful to measure the pH of the filtrate and to characterize any undissolved material by DSC to detect any phase changes that might have occurred.

For high-throughput screening (HTS) of solubility, where the amount of the compound might be severely restricted, reporting kinetic solubility might be adequate. This can be accomplished by using techniques such as a 96-well microtiter technique with an integral nephelometer, where aliquots of the aqueous solution are placed in the microtiter wells, to which 1 µL of the compounds in dimethylsulfoxide (DMSO) is added, and the plate is shaken. The turbidity of the solutions is then measured using the nephelometer. The process is repeated up to 10 times. If turbidity is detected in a cell, the experiment is terminated; that is, solution additions are stopped, and the solutions are ranked in terms of the number of additions that caused turbidity. This method is suitable to rank the compounds in terms of their solubility and not to measure solubility accurately. A transformation of the amorphous form to a crystalline form would decrease the dissolution rate in most instances. Once the presence of polymorphs is established, the solubility of the polymorphs and the thermodynamic quantities involved in the transition from a metastable to stable polymorph can be calculated. Experimentally, the solubility of the polymorphs is determined at various temperatures, and subsequently, the log of the solubility is plotted against the reciprocal of the temperature (the van't Hoff method), from which the enthalpy of solution can be calculated from the slope. If the lines intersect, it is known as the transition temperature, and one consequence of this is that there may be a transition from one polymorph to another, depending on the storage conditions.

6.9.10 Dynamic Vapor Sorption

Measurement of the hygroscopic properties of a compound can be conveniently carried out on small quantities of compound by using a DVS system (10) from Surface Measurement Systems (U.K.) that allows highly accurate measurements under different conditions and materials. The IGA_{sorp} is designed to measure accurately the magnitude and kinetics of moisture sorption onto materials. It is fully automated and combines an ultrasensitive microbalance with precise measurement and control of both humidity and temperature. The IGA® (11) series of instruments uniquely utilizes the IGA method to intelligently determine the equilibrium uptakes and kinetics, and the fully automated system is capable of isothermal, isochoric, and temperature programmed determinations. The RH is generated by bubbling nitrogen through a water reservoir, where it is saturated with moisture. Using a mixing chamber, the moist nitrogen is mixed with dry nitrogen in a fixed ratio, thus producing the required RH. The moist nitrogen is then passed over the sample, and the instrument is programmed, such that the increase in weight caused by moisture is monitored with time, using an ultrasensitive microbalance. The compound takes up moisture and reaches equilibrium, at which point the next RH stage is programmed to start. The adsorption and desorption of moisture can be studied using this instrument, and the effect of temperature can be investigated as well. Using this technique, a quantity as small as 1 mg can be assessed (12).

The SGA-100 Symmetrical Gravimetric Analyzer is a continuous vapor flow sorption instrument for obtaining water and organic vapor isotherms at temperatures ranging from 0°C to 80°C at ambient pressure. As a result of its symmetrical design (both the sample and the reference side of the microbalance are subjected to identical temperature, RH, and flow rate), this instrument achieves great accuracy and stability. Another benefit of this design is the ability to perform absolute or differential adsorption experiments. In addition to isotherms, maintaining constant humidity and equilibrating the sample to a series of temperatures, heats and kinetics of adsorption, hydrate formation can also be studied. The core of the instrument is an isothermal aluminum block containing the sample chamber, which permits very tight control of temperature and RH at the sample. The temperature within the block is kept stable by a constant temperature bath capable of temperature control within 0.01°C. Because of the easy access to the sample and the absence of glass hang-down tubes, this instrument is very easy to operate and highly reliable. The SGA-100 is also very compact, with a footprint of only 18″ × 20″ (13). The MB-300G-HP from VTI Corp is specifically designed to obtain adsorption–desorption isotherms at values above the atmospheric pressures. A stainless-steel microbalance head is integrated with a constant-temperature bath or cryostat for optimal temperature control, a 5000 torr or higher pressure transducer, and our high-quality hardware and Microsoft™ Windows™-based software. The design of the MB-300G-HP provides very easy access to the sample. When a cryostat is used, the experimental temperature range is between −190°C and 600°C. The user can also select a constant temperature bath for experimental temperatures of 0°C–80°C and can integrate a furnace for temperatures up to 500°C. The standard configuration is for up to six atmospheres of pressure; however, higher pressures can be achieved by integrating optional equipment. Isobars can also be obtained effortlessly.

The Rubotherm system provides gravimetric sorption measurements carried out in a closed measuring cell completely thermostated up to 700 K or down to 77 K without temperature differences or corrosive parts inside the whole measuring cell with pressures up to 100 MPa and a mass sensitivity down to 1 μg, using a magnetic suspension balance to measure mass transfer under controlled environments (14).

Normally, the moisture sorption–desorption profile of the compound is investigated. This can reveal a range of phenomena associated with the solid. For example, on reducing the RH from a high level, hysteresis (separation of the sorption–desorption curves) may be observed. There are two types of hysteresis loops: an open hyteresis loop, where the final moisture content is higher than the starting moisture content owing to the so-called ink-bottle pores, where condensed moisture is trapped in pores with a narrow neck, and the closed hysteresis loop, which may be closed owing to compounds having capillary pore sizes.

A large uptake of moisture often indicates a phase change. In this case, the desorption phase is characterized by only small decreases in the moisture content (depending on the stability of the hydrate formed), until at low RH, when the moisture is lost. In some cases, hydrated amorphous forms are formed on desorption of the hydrate formed on the sorption phase. In this case, the sorption of moisture causes the sample to crystallize as a hydrate, which at higher RH crystallizes into a higher hydrate. The higher hydrates are generally more stable to decreasing RH until the humidity level reaches to less than 10%, when most of the sorbed moisture can be lost to regenerate the amorphous forms.

In terms of salt selection procedure, the critical relative humidity (CRH) of each salt should be identified. This is defined as the point at which the compound starts to sorb moisture. Clearly, compounds or salts that exhibit excessive moisture uptake should be rejected. The level of this uptake is debatable, but those exhibiting deliquescence (where the sample dissolves in the moisture that has been sorbed) should be automatically excluded from further consideration.

The automation of moisture sorption measurements is a relatively recent innovation. Prior to this, moisture sorption of compounds (~10 mg) was determined by exposing weighed amounts of compound in dishes placed in sealed desiccators containing saturated solutions of salts. Saturated solutions of salts that give defined RH (as a function of temperature) have long been in use. The RH of a saturated solution at 25°C ranges between 0% for silica gel and 100% for water, potassium acetate (20%), calcium chloride (32%), sodium bromide (58%), potassium bromide (84%), and dipotassium hydrogen phosphate (92%). The test samples are placed in chambers containing these salts and then, after saturation sorption, analyzed using methods such as TGA, HPLC, and so on, to ascertain if there had been any phase change owing to sorption in the solid state; this may require additional testing using scanning electron microscopy (SEM), DSC, or XRPD.

6.9.11 Dissolution Testing

During the preformulation stage, an understanding of the dissolution rate of the drug candidate is necessary, as this property of the compound is recognized as a significant factor involved in drug bioavailability. Dissolution of a solid usually takes place in two stages: salvation of the solute molecules by the solvent molecules, followed by transport of these molecules from the interface into the bulk medium by convection or diffusion. The major factor that determines the dissolution rate is the aqueous solubility of the compound; however, other factors, such as particle size, crystalline state (polymorphs, hydrates), pH, and buffer concentration, can affect the rate. Moreover, physical properties, such as viscosity and wettability, can also influence the dissolution process.

Ideally, dissolution should simulate in vivo conditions. To do this, it should be carried out in a large volume of dissolution medium, or there must be some mechanism whereby the dissolution medium is constantly replenished by fresh solvent. Provided this condition is met, the dissolution testing is defined as taking place under sink conditions. Conversely, if there is a concentration increase during dissolution testing, such that the dissolution is retarded by a concentration gradient, the dissolution is said to be nonsink. While the use of the USP paddle dissolution apparatus is mandatory when developing a tablet, the rotating disc method has a great utility with regard to preformulation studies. The intrinsic dissolution rate is the dissolution rate of the compound under the condition of constant surface area. The rationale for the use of a compressed disc of pure material is that the intrinsic tendency of the test material to dissolve can be evaluated without formulation excipients.

Intrinsic dissolution rates of compounds obtained from rotating discs can be theoretically determined. Under hydrodynamic conditions, the intrinsic dissolution rate is usually proportional to the solubility of the solid. However, the dissolution rate obtained will depend on the rotation speed. Several modifications of rotating disc apparatus have been introduced to force zero intercepts. A disc is generally prepared by compressing about 200 mg of the candidate drug in a hydraulic press; the IR press often proves useful, as it gives a disc with a diameter of 1.3 cm. It should be noted that some compounds do not compress well and may exhibit elastic compression properties; that is, the disc may be very weak, rendering the experiment impossible. In addition to poor compression properties, another complication is that some compounds can undergo polymorphic transformations because of the application of pressure. This should therefore be borne in mind if there is insufficient compound to perform, for example, XRPD postcompaction.

If the disc has reasonable compression properties, it is then attached to a holder and set in motion in the dissolution medium (water, buffer, or simulated gastric fluid): we use a rotation speed of 100 rpm. A number of analytical techniques can be used to follow the dissolution process; however, UV–visible spectrophotometry and HPLC with fixed- or variable-wavelength detectors (or diode array) appear to be the most common. The UV system employs a flow through system and does not require much attention; however, if HPLC is used, then any aliquot taken should be replaced by an equal amount of solvent. The intrinsic dissolution rate is given by the slope of the linear portion of the concentration versus time curve, divided by the area of the disc, and has the units of mg/min cm².

6.9.12 High-Performance Liquid Chromatography

High-performance liquid chromatography is used to assess the degradation compounds in testing the stability of new drugs, since in these studies, the identification of degradation products is very important. Combined with mass spectrometer and the newer instrumentation, liquid chromatography/tandem mass spectroscopy (LC/MS/MS) and so on offer powerful tools for the elucidation of degradation mechanism.

Isocratic elution is often the most desirable method, as it does not require postequilibration phase for the next analysis; this can be an important consideration if a matrix of factors and excipients are studied for interaction. Gradient elution offers the advantage of sharper peaks, increased sensitivity, greater peak capacity, and selectivity (increased resolving power).

The type of detector to be used is usually dictated by the chemical structure of the compound under investigations. As most compounds of pharmaceutical interest contain aromatic rings, UV detection is the most common detection method. When using this technique, the most appropriate wavelength is selected from the UV spectrum of the pure compound and that of the system suitability sample. Usually, the λ_{max} is chosen; however, in order to remove unwanted interference, it may be necessary to move away from this value. Where possible, the use of wavelength <250 nm should be avoided because of the high level of background interference and solvent adsorption. In practical terms, this requires the use of far-UV-grade solvents and the avoidance of organic buffers.

Other types of detection include refractive index, fluorescence, and mass selective detectors. The use of other types of detectors, such as those based on fluorescence, may be used for assaying compounds that can be specifically detected at low concentrations in the present of nonfluorescent species. However, as few compounds are naturally fluorescent, they require chemical modification, assuming they have a suitable reactive group, to give a fluorescent derivative.

During the early stage of development, the amount of method validation carried out is likely to be limited because of compound availability. However, a calibration curve should be obtained using either an internal or external standard procedure. The latter procedure is commonly employed by injecting a fixed volume of standard samples containing a range of known concentrations of the compound of interest. Plots of peak height and/or area versus concentration are checked for linearity by subjecting the data to linear regression analysis. If more extensive validation is required, other tests, such as the limit of detection, precision of the detector response, accuracy, reproducibility, specificity, and ruggedness, may be carried out.

WEB REFERENCES

1. http://www.brukeraxs.de/index.php?id=home0
2. http://www.accelrys.com/products/cerius2/
3. http://pharmquest.com
4. http://www.transformpharma.com/te_platforms.htm
5. http://www.symyx.com
6. http://www.avantium.nl
7. http://www.solvias.com/
8. http://www.accelrys.com/products/cerius2/
9. http://www.cclrc.ac.uk/Activity/DL
10. http://www.smsuk.co.uk/index.php
11. http://www.metpowerin.com/moisure_sorption_analysis.htm
12. http://www.hidenisochema.com/products/IGAsorp.html
13. http://www.vticorp.com/products/sga100.htm
14. http://www.rubotherm.de/ENGL/MAINFR031.HTM

RECOMMENDED READING

Al-Nimry, S. S. and K. A. Alkhamis (2018). "Effect of moisture content of chitin-calcium silicate on rate of degradation of cefotaxime sodium." *AAPS Pharm Sci Tech* 19(3):1337–1343.

Assessment of incompatibilities between active pharmaceutical ingredient and pharmaceutical excipients is an important part of preformulation studies.

The objective of the work was to assess the effect of moisture content of chitin calcium silicate of two size ranges (two specific surface areas) on the rate of degradation of cefotaxime sodium. The surface area of the excipient was determined using adsorption method. The effect of moisture content of a given size range on the stability of the drug was determined at 40°C in the solid state. The moisture content was determined at the beginning and the end of the kinetic study using TGA. The degradation in solution was studied for comparison. Increasing the moisture content of the excipient of size range 63–180 µm (surface area 7.2 m(2)/g) from 3.88% to 8.06% increased the rate of degradation of the drug more than two times (from 0.0317 to 0.0718 h(−1)). While an opposite trend was observed for the excipient of size range <63 µm (surface area 55.4 m(2)/g). The rate of degradation at moisture content <3% was 0.4547 h(−1), almost two times higher than that (0.2594 h(−1)) at moisture content of 8.54%, and the degradation in solid state at both moisture contents was higher than that in solution (0.0871 h(−1)). In conclusion, the rate of degradation in solid should be studied taking into consideration the specific surface area and moisture content of the excipient at the storage condition and it may be higher than that in solution.

Alsenz, J. et al. (2016). "Miniaturized INtrinsic DISsolution Screening (MINDISS) assay for preformulation." *Eur J Pharm Sci* 87:3–13.

This study describes a novel Miniaturized INtrinsic DISsolution Screening (MINDISS) assay for measuring disk intrinsic dissolution rates (DIDR). In MINDISS, compacted mini disks of drugs (2–5 mg/disk) are prepared in custom made holders with a surface area of 3 mm(2). Disks are immersed, pellet side down, into 0.35 mL of appropriate dissolution media per well in 96-well microtiter plates, media are stirred, and disk-holders are transferred to new wells after defined periods of time. After filtration, drug concentration in dissolution media is quantified by Ultra Performance Liquid Chromatography (UPLC) and solid-state property of the disk is characterized by Raman spectroscopy. MINDISS was identified as an easy-to-use tool for rapid, parallel determination of DIDR of compounds that requires only small amounts of compound and of dissolution medium. Results obtained with marketed drugs in MINDISS correlate well with large scale DIDR methods and indicate that MINDISS can be used for (1) rank-ordering of compounds by intrinsic dissolution in late phase discovery and early development, (2) comparison of polymorphic forms and salts, (3) screening and selection of appropriate dissolution media, and (4) characterization of the intestinal release behavior of compounds along the gastro intestinal tract by changing biorelevant media during experiments.

Antovska, P. et al. (2013). "Solid-state compatibility screening of excipients suitable for development of indapamide sustained release solid-dosage formulation." *Pharm Dev Technol* 18(2):481–489.

Differential scanning calorimetry and Fourier transform infrared spectroscopy were applied as screening analytical methods to assess the solid-state compatibility of indapamide (4-chloro-N-(2-methyl-2,3-dihydroindol-1-yl)-3-sulfamoyl-benzamide) with several polymers aimed for development of 24 hours sustained release solid-dosage formulation. After the initial research phase which was directed towards selection of suitable polymer matrices, based on their solid-state compatibility with the studied pharmaceutical active ingredient, the second phase of evaluation was intended for compatibility selection of other excipients required to complete a sustained release formulation. The preformulation studies have shown that polyvinylpyrrolidone/polyvinyl acetate might be considered incompatible with indapamide, and the implementation of this polymer career should be avoided in the case of the entitled development. The experimental data additionally have revealed that sorbitol is incompatible with indapamide. The obtained results afforded deeper insight in to the solid-state stability of the studied binary systems and pointed out directions for further development of indapamide sustained release solid-dosage formulation.

Baertschi, S. W. et al. (2015). "Implications of in-use photostability: Proposed guidance for photostability testing and labeling to support the administration of photosensitive pharmaceutical products, Part 2: Topical drug product." *J Pharm Sci* 104(9):2688–2701.

Although essential guidance to cover the photostability testing of pharmaceuticals for manufacturing and storage is well-established, there continues to be a significant gap in guidance regarding testing to support the effective administration of photosensitive drug products. Continuing from Part 1, (Baertschi SW, Clapham D, Foti C, Jansen PJ, Kristensen S, Reed RA, Templeton AC, Tonnesen HH. *J Pharm Sci*. 2013;102:3888–3899) where the focus was drug products administered by injection, this commentary proposes guidance for testing topical drug products in order to support administration. As with the previous commentary, the approach taken is to examine "worst case" photoexposure scenarios in comparison with ICH testing conditions to provide practical guidance for the safe and effective administration of photosensitive topical drug products.

Baghel, S. et al. (2016). "Polymeric amorphous solid dispersions: A review of amorphization, crystallization, stabilization, solid-state characterization, and aqueous solubilization of biopharmaceutical classification system Class II drugs." *J Pharm Sci* 105(9):2527–2544.

Poor water solubility of many drugs has emerged as one of the major challenges in the pharmaceutical world. Polymer-based amorphous solid dispersions have been considered as the major advancement in overcoming limited aqueous solubility and oral absorption issues. The principle drawback of this approach is that they can lack necessary stability and revert to the crystalline form on storage. Significant upfront development is, therefore, required to generate stable amorphous formulations. A thorough understanding of the processes occurring at a molecular level is imperative for the rational design of amorphous solid dispersion products. This review attempts to address the critical molecular and thermodynamic aspects governing the physicochemical properties of such systems. A brief introduction to Biopharmaceutical Classification System, solid dispersions, glass transition, and solubility advantage of amorphous drugs is provided. The objective of this review is to weigh the current understanding of solid dispersion chemistry and to critically review the theoretical, technical, and molecular aspects of solid dispersions (amorphization and crystallization) and potential advantage of polymers (stabilization and solubilization) as inert, hydrophilic, pharmaceutical carrier matrices. In addition, different preformulation tools for the rational selection of polymers, state-of-the-art techniques for preparation and characterization of polymeric amorphous solid dispersions, and drug supersaturation in gastric media are also discussed.

Barrio, M. et al. (2017). "Pressure-temperature phase diagram of the dimorphism of the anti-inflammatory drug nimesulide." *Int J Pharm* 525(1):54–59.

Understanding the phase behavior of active pharmaceutical ingredients is important for formulations of dosage forms and regulatory reasons. Nimesulide is an anti-inflammatory drug that is known to exhibit dimorphism; however up to now its stability behavior was not clear, as few thermodynamic data were available. Therefore, calorimetric melting data have been obtained, which were found to be TI-L = 422.4 ± 1.0 K, DeltaI→LH = 117.5 ± 5.2 Jg(–1),TII-L = 419.8 ± 1.0 K and DeltaII→LH = 108.6 ± 3.3 Jg(–1). In addition, vapor-pressure data, high-pressure melting data, and specific volumes have been obtained. It is demonstrated that form II is intrinsically monotropic in relation to form I and the latter would thus be the best polymorph to use for drug formulations. This result has been obtained by experimental means, involving high-pressure measurements. Furthermore, it has been shown that with very limited experimental and statistical data, the same conclusion can be obtained, demonstrating that in first instance topological pressure-temperature phase diagrams can be obtained without necessarily measuring any high-pressure data. It provides a quick method to verify the phase behavior of the known phases of an active pharmaceutical ingredient under different pressure and temperature conditions.

Beg, S. et al. (2013). "Development of solid self-nanoemulsifying granules (SSNEGs) of ondansetron hydrochloride with enhanced bioavailability potential." *Colloids Surf B Biointerfaces* 101:414–423.

The current work aims to prepare the solid self-nanoemulsifying granules (SSNEGs) of ondansetron hydrochloride (ONH) to enhance its oral bioavailability by improving its aqueous solubility and facilitating its absorption though lymphatic pathways. Preformulation studies including screening of excipients for solubility and pseudoternary phase diagrams suggested the suitability of Capmul MCM as lipid, Labrasol as surfactant, and Tween 20 as cosurfactant for preparation of self-emulsifying formulations. Preliminary composition of the SNEDDS formulations were selected from the phase diagrams and subjected to thermodynamic stability studies and dispersibility tests. The prepared liquid SNEDDS formulations were characterized for viscosity, refractive index, droplet size and zeta potential. The TEM study confirmed the formation of nanoemulsion following dilution of liquid SNEDDS. The optimized liquid SNEDDS were transformed into free-flowing granules by adsorption on the porous carriers like Sylysia (350, 550, and 730) and Neusilin US2. Solid state characterization employing the FTIR, DSC and powder XRD studies indicated lack of any significant interaction of drug with the lipidic and emulsifying excipients, and porous carriers. In vitro drug release studies indicated faster solubilization of the drug by optimized SSNEGs (over 80% within 30 minutes) vis-a-vis the pure drug (only 35% within 30 minutes). In vivo pharmacokinetic studies in Wistar rats observed significant increase in C(max) (3.01-fold) and AUC (5.34-fold) using SSNEGs compared to pure drug, whereas no significant difference (p > 0.1) was observed with the liquid SNEDDS. Thus, the present studies ratify the bioavailability enhancement potential of SSNEGs of ONH prepared using porous carriers.

Chadha, R. and S. Bhandari (2014). "Drug-excipient compatibility screening—Role of thermoanalytical and spectroscopic techniques." *J Pharm Biomed Anal* 87:82–97.

Estimation of drug-excipient interactions is a crucial step in preformulation studies of drug development to achieve consistent stability, bioavailability and manufacturability of solid dosage forms. The advent of thermoanalytical and spectroscopic methods like DSC, isothermal microcalorimetry, HSM, SEM, FT-IR, solid-state NMR, and PXRD into preformulation studies have contributed significantly to early prediction, monitoring and characterization of the active pharmaceutical ingredient incompatibility with pharmaceutical excipients to avoid expensive material wastage and considerably reduce the time required to arrive at an appropriate formulation. Concomitant use of several thermal and spectroscopic techniques allows an in-depth understanding of physical or chemical drug-excipient interactions and aids in selection of the most appropriate excipients in dosage form design. The present review focuses on the techniques for compatibility screening of active pharmaceutical ingredient with their potential merits and demerits. Further, the review highlights the applicability of these techniques using specific drug-excipient compatibility case studies.

Dutta, A. K. et al. (2011). "Physicochemical characterization of NPC 1161C, a novel antimalarial 8-aminoquinoline, in solution and solid state." *AAPS Pharm Sci Tech* 12(1):177–191.

NPC 1161C is a novel antimalarial drug of interest because of its superior curative and prophylactic activity, and favorable toxicity profile against in vivo and in vitro models of malaria, pneumocystis carinii pneumonia, and leishmaniasis. The preformulation studies performed included determination of $pK(a)s$, aqueous and pH solubility, cosolvent solubility, log P, pH stability, thermal analysis, and preliminary hygroscopicity studies. The mean $pK(a1)$, $pK(a2)$, and $pK(a3)$ were determined to be 10.12, 4.07, and 1.88, respectively. The aqueous solubility was found to be $2.4 \times 10(-4)$ M having a saturated solution pH of 4.3–5.0 and a low intrinsic solubility of $1.6 \times 10(-6)$ M. A mathematical model of the pH-solubility profile was derived from pH 2.2 to 8.0. An exponential decrease in solubility was observed with increasing pH. The excess solid phase in equilibrium with the solution in aqueous buffers was determined to be the free-base form of the drug. A significant increase in solubility was observed with all the cosolvents studied, in both unbuffered and buffered systems. Mean log P of the salt and the free base were estimated to be 2.18 and 3.70, respectively. The compound had poor stability at pH 7.0 at 37°C, with a t (90) of 3.58 days. Thermal analysis of the drug using DSC and TGA revealed that the drug is present as a semi-crystalline powder, which transformed into the amorphous state after melting. The drug was also found to sublime at higher temperatures. Determination of physicochemical properties of NPC 1161C provided useful information for the development of a dosage form and preclinical evaluation.

Erxleben, A. (2016). "Application of vibrational spectroscopy to study solid-state transformations of pharmaceuticals." *Curr Pharm Des* 22(32):4883–4911.

Understanding the properties, stability and transformations of the solid-state forms of an active pharmaceutical ingredient (API) in the development pipeline is of crucial importance for process-development, formulation development and FDA approval.

Investigation of the polymorphism and polymorphic stability is a routine part of the preformulation studies. Vibrational spectroscopy allows the real-time in situ monitoring of phase transformations and probes intermolecular interactions between API molecules, between API and polymer in amorphous solid dispersions or between API and coformer in cocrystals or coamorphous systems and thus plays a major role in efforts to gain a predictive understanding of the relative stability of solid-state forms and formulations. Infrared (IR), near-infrared (NIR) and Raman spectroscopies, alone or in combination with other analytical methods, are important tools for studying transformations between different crystalline forms, between the crystalline and amorphous form, between hydrate and anhydrous form and for investigating solid-state cocrystal formation. The development of simple-to-use and cost-effective instruments on the one hand and recent technological advances such as access to the low-frequency Raman range down to 5 cm^{-1}, on the other, have led to an exponential growth of the literature in the field. This review discusses the application of IR, NIR and Raman spectroscopies in the study of solid-state transformations with a focus on the literature published over the last eight years.

Fan, Y. et al. (2015). "Preformulation characterization and in vivo absorption in beagle dogs of JFD, a novel anti-obesity drug for oral delivery." *Drug Dev Ind Pharm* 41(5):801–811.

JFD (N-isoleucyl-4-methyl-1,1-cyclopropyl-1-(4-chlorine)phenyl-2-amylamine. HCl) is a novel investigational anti-obesity drug without obvious cardiotoxicity. The objective of this study was to characterize the key physicochemical properties of JFD, including solution-state characterization (ionization constant, partition coefficient, aqueous and pH-solubility profile), solid-state characterization (particle size, thermal analysis, crystallinity and hygroscopicity) and drug-excipient chemical compatibility. A supporting in vivo absorption study was also carried out in beagle dogs. JFD bulk powders are prismatic crystals with a low degree of crystallinity, particle sizes of which are within 2–10 μm. JFD is highly hygroscopic, easily deliquesces to an amorphous glass solid and changes subsequently to another crystal form under an elevated moisture/temperature condition. Similar physical instability was also observed in real-time CheqSol solubility assay. pK(a) (7.49 ± 0.01), log P (5.10 ± 0.02) and intrinsic solubility (S0) (1.75 μg/mL) at 37°C of JFD were obtained using potentiometric titration method. Based on these solution-state properties, JFD was estimated to be classified as BCS II, thus its dissolution rate may be an absorption-limiting step. Moreover, JFD was more chemically compatible with dibasic calcium phosphate, mannitol, hypromellose and colloidal silicon dioxide than with lactose and magnesium stearate. Further, JFD exhibited an acceptable pharmacokinetic profiling in beagle dogs and the pharmacokinetic parameters T(max), C(max), AUC(0-t) and absolute bioavailability were 1.60 ± 0.81 hours, 0.78 ± 0.47 μg/mL, 3.77 ± 1.85 μg.h/ mL and 52.30% ± 19.39%, respectively. The preformulation characterization provides valuable information for further development of oral administration of JFD.

Gajdziok, J. and B. Vranikova (2015). "Enhancing of drug bioavailability using liquisolid system formulation." *Ceska Slov Farm* 64(3):55–66.

One of the modern technologies of how to ensure sufficient bioavailability of drugs with limited water solubility is represented by the preparation of liquisolid systems. The functional principle of these formulations is the sorption of a drug in a liquid phase to a porous carrier (aluminometasilicates, microcrystalline cellulose, etc.). After addition of further excipients, in particular a coating material (colloidal silica), a powder is formed with the properties suitable for conversion to conventional solid unit dosage forms for oral administration (tablets, capsules). The drug is subsequently administered to the GIT already in a dissolved state, and moreover, the high surface area of the excipients and their surface hydrophilization by the solvent used, facilitates its contact with and release to the dissolution medium and GI fluids. This technology, due to its ease of preparation, represents an interesting alternative to the currently used methods of bioavailability improvement. The article follows up, by describing the specific aspects influencing the preparation of liquid systems, on the already published papers about the bioavailability of drugs and the possibilities of its technological improvement. Key words: liquisolid systems bioavailability porous carrier coating material preformulation studies.

Kim, M. S. et al. (2013). "Supersaturatable formulations for the enhanced oral absorption of sirolimus." *Int J Pharm* 445(1–2):108–116.

The purpose of this study was to develop supersaturatable formulations for the enhanced solubility and oral absorption of sirolimus. Supersaturatable formulations of hydrophilic polymers and/or surfactants were screened by formulation screening, which is based on solvent casting. The solid dispersion particles in the optimized formulations were prepared by spray drying. The particles were characterized in vitro and in vivo. The most effective supersaturatable formulation found in the formulation screening process was hydroxypropylmethyl cellulose (HPMC)-D-alpha-tocopheryl polyethylene glycol 1000 succinate (TPGS), followed by HPMC-Sucroester. In addition, the supersaturated state generated from HPMC-TPGS and HPMC-Sucroester 15 particles prepared by spray drying significantly improved the oral absorption of sirolimus in rats. Based on the pharmacokinetic parameters and supporting in vitro supersaturated dissolution data, the enhanced supersaturation properties of sirolimus led to enhanced in vivo oral absorption. In addition, the experimental results from the formulation screening used in our study could be useful for enhancing the bioavailability of sirolimus in preformulation and formulation studies.

Kumar, L. et al. (2013). "Effect of counterion on the solid state photodegradation behavior of prazosin salts." *AAPS Pharm Sci Tech* 14(2):757–763.

The effect of counterion was evaluated on the photodegradation behavior of six prazosin salts, viz., prazosin hydrochloride anhydrous, prazosin hydrochloride polyhydrate, prazosin tosylate anhydrous, prazosin tosylate monohydrate, prazosin oxalate dihydrate, and prazosin camsylate anhydrous. The salts were subjected to UV-Visible irradiation in a photostability test chamber for 10 days. The samples were analyzed for chemical changes by a specific stability-indicating high-performance liquid chromatography method. pH of the microenvironment was determined in 10%w/v aqueous slurry of the salts. The observed order of photostability was: prazosin hydrochloride anhydrous > prazosin camsylate anhydrous ~ prazosin-free base > prazosin hydrochloride polyhydrate > prazosin tosylate anhydrous > prazosin oxalate dihydrate ~ prazosin tosylate monohydrate. Multivariate analysis of the photodegradation behavior suggested predominant contribution of the state of hydration and also intrinsic photosensitivity of the counterion. Overall, hydrated salts showed higher photodegradation compared to their anhydrous counterparts. Within the anhydrous salts, aromatic and carbonyl counterion-containing salts showed higher susceptibility to light. The pH of microenvironment furthermore contributed to photodegradation of prazosin salts, especially for drug counterions with inherent higher pH. The study reveals importance of selection of a suitable drug salt form for photosensitive drugs during preformulation stage of drug development.

Liltorp, K. et al. (2011). "Solid state compatibility studies with tablet excipients using non thermal methods." *J Pharm Biomed Anal* 55(3):424–428.

Compatibility between two new active pharmaceutical ingredients (API) and several pharmaceutical excipients used in solid formulations has been investigated by FT-IR and HPLC following storage under two different conditions. Compatibility was investigated by storage at isothermal stress conditions for (i) 3 days and subsequently analysed by FT-IR and (ii) 12 weeks of storage and analysis by HPLC. For the majority of the examined excipients a large degradation measured by HPLC after 12 weeks storage was also detected by FT-IR following storage at isothermal stress conditions for 3 days, i.e. there was a general agreement between the results obtained by the two protocols. Further, the FT-IR method showed clear incompatibility with three excipients where no degradation products were detected by HPLC, but where a significant decrease in the API quantified by the HPLC assay, was observed. The accelerated method thus showed a clear advantage: incompatibility found after 12 weeks using HPLC was seen after 3 days with FT-IR. Furthermore, FT-IR provides an insight into structural changes not seen with HPLC. This is exemplified by the desalting of a hydrogen bromide salt of one of the two compounds, which might lead to changes of the intrinsic dissolution rate and potentially affect the bioavailability of the API.

Madsen, C. M. et al. (2016). "Supersaturation of zafirlukast in fasted and fed state intestinal media with and without precipitation inhibitors." *Eur J Pharm Sci* 91:31–39.

Poor water solubility is a bottle neck in the development of many new drug candidates, and understanding and circumventing this are essential for a more effective drug development. Zafirlukast (ZA) is a leukotriene antagonist marketed for the treatment of asthma (Accolate(R)). ZA is poorly water soluble and is formulated in an amorphous form (aZA) to improve its solubility and oral bioavailability. It has been shown that upon dissolution of aZa, the concentration of ZA in solution is supersaturated with respect to its stable crystalline form (ZA monohydrate), and thus, in theory, the bioavailability increases upon amorphization of ZA. The polymers hydroxypropylmethylcellulose (HPMC) and polyvinylpyrrolidone (PVP), often used as stabilizers of the supersaturated state, are in the excipient list of Accolate(R). It is not recommended to take Accolate(R) with food, as this reduces the bioavailability by 40%. The aim of this study was to investigate the effect of simulated fasted and fed state intestinal media as well as the effect of HPMC and PVP on the supersaturation and precipitation of ZA in vitro. Supersaturation of aZA was studied in vitro in a small-scale setup using the muDiss Profiler. Several media were used for this study: One medium simulating the fasted state intestinal fluids and three media simulating different fed state intestinal fluids. Solid state changes of the drug were investigated by small angle X-ray scattering. The duration wherein aZA was maintained at a supersaturated state was prolonged in the presence of HPMC and lasted more than 20 hours in the presence of PVP in a fasted state intestinal medium. The presence of PVP increased the concentration of drug dissolved in the supersaturated state.

The duration of supersaturation was shorter in fed than in a fasted state simulated intestinal media, but the concentration during supersaturation was higher. It was thus not possible to predict any positive or negative food effects from the dissolution/precipitation curves from different media. Lipolysis products in the fed state simulated media seemed to cause both a negative effect on the duration of supersaturation, and an increased drug concentration during supersaturation. In contrast, when testing the effect of a fed state simulated medium compared to the fasted state medium, in the presence of PVP, a clear negative effect was seen on the dissolution/precipitation curved of the fed state medium. The drug concentration during supersaturation was marginally different in the two media, but a precipitation of ZA was seen in the fed state medium, which was not observed in the fasted state medium. Solid state transformation from aZA to ZA monohydrate (mhZA) upon precipitation of the supersaturated solutions was confirmed by small angle X-ray scattering. All of these results can explain the described in vivo behavior of ZA. For ZA simple dissolution experiments in vitro can be used to examine supersaturation, effectiveness of PI and potential food effects on these.

Malaj, L. et al. (2011). "Characterization of nicergoline polymorphs crystallized in several organic solvents." *J Pharm Sci* 100(7):2610–2622.

Nicergoline (NIC), a poorly water-soluble semisynthetic ergot derivative, was crystallized from several organic solvents, obtaining two different polymorphic forms, the triclinic form I and the orthorhombic form II. NIC samples were then characterized by several techniques such as (13)C cross-polarization magic angle spinning solid-state spectroscopy, room-temperature and high-temperature X-ray powder diffraction, differential scanning calorimetry, and by analysis of weight loss, solvent content, powder density, morphology, and particle size. Solubility and intrinsic dissolution rates determined for the two polymorphic forms in water and hydrochloride solutions (HCl 0.1 N) were always higher for form II than for form I, which is actually the form used for the industrial preparation of NIC medicinal products. Preformulation studies might encourage industry for the evaluation of polymorph II, as it is more suitable for pharmaceutical applications. Results in drug delivery, as well as those obtained by the above-mentioned techniques, and the application of Burger-Ramberger rules make it possible to conclude that there is a thermodynamic relation of monotropy between the two polymorphs. This last assumption may help formulators in predicting the relative stability of the two forms.

Moriyama, K. et al. (2017). "Visualization of protonation/deprotonation of active pharmaceutical ingredient in solid state by vapor phase amine-selective alkyne tagging and Raman imaging." *J Pharm Sci* 106(7):1778–1785.

Here, we report a simple and direct method to visualize the protonation/deprotonation of an amine active pharmaceutical ingredient (API) in the solid state using a solid-vapor reaction with propargyl bromide and Raman imaging for the assessment of the API during the manufacturing process of solid formulations. An alkyne tagging occurred on the free form of solid haloperidol by the vapor phase reaction, and a distinct Raman signal of alkyne was detected. Alkyne signal monitoring by Raman imaging enabled us to visualize the distribution of the free-form haloperidol in a solid formulation. On the other hand, haloperidol hydrochloride did not react with propargyl bromide in the solid-vapor reaction, and the alkyne signal was not observed. Using the difference in reactivity, the protonation/deprotonation of the amine API in the solid state could be visualized. As an example of application, we tried to visually assess the protonation/deprotonation state when the free-form haloperidol was ground with acids using the solid-vapor reaction and Raman imaging and found that haloperidol was partially protonated when ground with 2 equivalents of hydrogen chloride. Furthermore, we demonstrated the relationship between the degree of protonation and the amount of water added as a medium for grinding haloperidol with succinic acid.

Mortko, C. J. et al. (2010). "Risk assessment and physicochemical characterization of a metastable dihydrate API phase for intravenous formulation development." *J Pharm Sci* 99(12):4973–4981.

(1S,5R)-2-{[(4S)-azepan-4-ylamino]carbonyl}-7-oxo-2,6-diazabicyclo[3.2.0] heptane-6-sulfonic acid (Compound 1) is a beta-lactamase inhibitor for intravenous administration. The objective of this preformulation study was to determine the most appropriate form of the API for development. Compound 1 can exist as an amorphous solid and four distinct crystalline phases A, B, C, and D in the solid state. Slurry experiments along with analysis of physicochemical properties were used to construct a phase diagram and select the most suitable form of the API for development. In aqueous formulations, the dihydrate form of the API was predominant and, due to the more favorable solubility and dissolution profile required for preclinical and clinical studies, a metastable form of the API was selected, and the risks associated with developing this form were evaluated.

Nie, H. et al. (2016). "Impact of metallic stearates on disproportionation of hydrochloride salts of weak bases in solid-state formulations." *Mol Pharm* 13(10):3541–3552.

Excipient-induced salt disproportionation (conversion from salt form to free form) in the solid state during storage or manufacturing is a severe formulation issue that can negatively influence product performance. However, the role of excipient properties on salt disproportionation and mechanisms of proton transfer between salt and excipients are still unclear. Moreover, knowledge about the formation of disproportionation products and the consequent impact of these reactions products on the disproportionation process is still inadequate. In the present study, three commonly used lubricants (sodium stearate, calcium stearate, and magnesium stearate) were mixed with a hydrochloride salt as binary mixtures to examine their different capabilities for inducing salt disproportionation at a stressed storage condition (40°C/65% RH). The overall objective of this research is to explore factors influencing the kinetics and extent of disproportionation including surface area, alkalinity, hygroscopicity, formation of new species, etc. In addition, we also aim to clarify the reaction mechanism and proton transfer between the model salt and stearates to provide insight into the in situ formed reaction products. We found that the properties of stearates significantly affect the disproportionation process in the initial stage of storage, while properties of the reaction products negatively affect the hygroscopicity of the powder mixture promoting disproportionation during longer-term storage. In addition, lubrication difference among three stearates was evaluated by performing compaction studies. The findings of this study provide an improved understanding of the proton transfer mechanism between the ionized form of an active pharmaceutical ingredient and excipients in solid dosage forms. It also provides pragmatic information for formulation scientists to select appropriate lubricants and other excipients, and to design robust formulations.

Nie, H. et al. (2017). "Crystalline solid dispersion-a strategy to slowdown salt disproportionation in solid state formulations during storage and wet granulation." *Int J Pharm*
517(1–2):203–215.

Salt disproportionation (a conversion from the ionized to the neutral state) in solid
formulations is a potential concern during manufacturing or storage of products
containing a salt of the active pharmaceutical ingredient (API) due to the negative
ramifications on product performance. However, it is challenging to find an effective approach to prevent or mitigate this undesirable reaction in formulations. Hence,
the overall objective of this study is to explore novel formulation strategies to reduce
the risk of salt disproportionation in pharmaceutical products. Crystals of pioglitazone hydrochloride salt were dispersed into polymeric matrices as a means of
preventing the pharmaceutical salt from direct contact with problematic excipients.
It was found that the level of salt disproportionation could be successfully reduced
during storage or wet granulation by embedding a crystalline salt into a polymeric
carrier. Furthermore, the impact of different polymers on the disproportionation process of a salt of a weakly basic API was investigated herein. Disproportionation of
pioglitazone hydrochloride salt was found to be significantly affected by the physicochemical properties of different polymers including hygroscopicity and acidity of
substituents. These findings provide an improved understanding of the role of polymeric carriers on the stability of a salt in solid formulations. Moreover, we also found
that introducing acidifiers into granulation fluid can bring additional benefits to retard
the disproportionation of pioglitazone HCl during the wet granulation process. These
interesting discoveries offer new approaches to mitigate disproportionation of API
salt during storage or processing, which allow pharmaceutical scientists to develop
appropriate formulations with improved drug stability.

Paczkowska, M. et al. (2015). "Complex of rutin with beta-cyclodextrin as potential delivery system." *PLoS One* 10(3):e0120858.

This study aimed to obtain and characterize an RU-beta-CD complex in the context
of investigating the possibility of changes in the solubility, stability, antioxidative and
microbiological activity as well as permeability of complexated rutin as against its free
form. The formation of the RU-beta-CD complex via a co-grinding technique was confirmed by using DSC, SEM, FT-IR, and Raman spectroscopy, and its geometry was
assessed through molecular modeling. It was found that the stability and solubility of
the so-obtained complex were greater compared to the free form; however, a slight
decrease was observed in its antibacterial potency. An examination of changes in the
EPR spectra of the complex excluded any reducing effect of complexation on the anti-
oxidative activity of rutin. Considering the prospect of preformulation studies involving
RU-beta-CD complexes, of significance is also the observed possibility of prolongedly
releasing rutin from the complex at a constant level over period of 20 hours, and the fact
that twice as much complexated rutin was able to permeate compared to its free form.

Paudel, A. et al. (2015). "Raman spectroscopy in pharmaceutical product design." *Adv
Drug Deliv Rev* 89:3–20.

Almost 100 years after the discovery of the Raman scattering phenomenon, related
analytical techniques have emerged as important tools in biomedical sciences.
Raman spectroscopy and microscopy are frontier, non-invasive analytical techniques

amenable for diverse biomedical areas, ranging from molecular-based drug discovery, design of innovative drug delivery systems and quality control of finished products. This review presents concise accounts of various conventional and emerging Raman instrumentations including associated hyphenated tools of pharmaceutical interest. Moreover, relevant application cases of Raman spectroscopy in early and late phase pharmaceutical development, process analysis and micro-structural analysis of drug delivery systems are introduced. Finally, potential areas of future advancement and application of Raman spectroscopic techniques are discussed.

Penumetcha, S. S. et al. (2016). "Hot melt extruded Aprepitant-Soluplus solid dispersion: Preformulation considerations, stability and in vitro study." *Drug Dev Ind Pharm* 42(10):1609–1620.

CONTEXT: Solubility limitation of BCS class II drugs pose challenges to in vitro release. OBJECTIVE: To investigate the miscibility of Aprepitant (APR) and Soluplus® (SOL) for hot melt extrusion (HME) viability and improved in vitro release of APR. METHODS: Solubility parameters of APR and SOL from group contribution methods were evaluated. Heat-cool-heat differential scanning calorimetry (DSC) scans were assessed for determining the glass forming ability (GFA) and glass stability (GS) of APR. An optimum HME temperature was selected based on melting point depression in physical mixtures. Moisture sorption isotherms were collected using a dynamic vapor sorption (DVS) analyzer at 25°C. A 1:4 APR:SOL physical mixture was extruded in a co-rotating 12 mm twin screw extruder and in vitro release was assessed in fasted state simulated intestinal fluid (FaSSIF) with 0.25% SLS. Extrudates were analyzed using TGA, DSC, XRD and FTIR. RESULTS: APR was classified as a class II glass former. APR and SOL had composition dependent miscibility based on Gibb's free energy of mixing. Extrudate prepared using HME had an amorphous as well as a crystalline phase that showed good stability in accelerated stability conditions. Smaller particle size extrudates exhibited a higher % moisture uptake and in vitro release compared to larger particle size extrudates. Enhanced in vitro release of APR from extrudates was attributed to amorphization of APR, solubilization as well as crystal growth inhibition effect of SOL due to H-bond formation with APR. CONCLUSIONS: A solid dispersion of APR with improved in vitro release was successfully developed using HME technology.

Purohit, H. S. et al. (2017). "Insights into nano- and micron-scale phase separation in amorphous solid dispersions using fluorescence-based techniques in combination with solid state nuclear magnetic resonance spectroscopy." *Pharm Res* 34(7):1364–1377.

PURPOSE: Miscibility between the drug and the polymer in an amorphous solid dispersion (ASD) is considered to be one of the most important factors impacting the solid-state stability and dissolution performance of the active pharmaceutical ingredient (API). The research described herein utilizes emerging fluorescence-based methodologies to probe (im)miscibility of itraconazole (ITZ)-hydroxypropyl methylcellulose (HPMC) ASDs. METHODS: The ASDs were prepared by solvent evaporation with varying evaporation rates and were characterized by steady-state fluorescence spectroscopy, confocal imaging, differential scanning calorimetry (DSC), and solid state nuclear magnetic resonance (ssNMR) spectroscopy. RESULTS: The size of the phase separated domains for the ITZ-HPMC ASDs was affected by the solvent evaporation rate. Smaller domains (<10 nm) were observed in spray-dried

ASDs, whereas larger domains (>30 nm) were found in ASDs prepared using slower evaporation rates. Confocal imaging provided visual confirmation of phase separation along with chemical specificity, achieved by selectively staining drug-rich and polymer-rich phases. ssNMR confirmed the results of fluorescence-based techniques and provided information on the size of phase separated domains. CONCLUSIONS: The fluorescence-based methodologies proved to be sensitive and rapid in detecting phase separation, even at the nanoscale, in the ITZ-HPMC ASDs. Fluorescence-based methods thus show promise for miscibility evaluation of spray-dried ASDs.

Saal, W. et al. (2018). "The quest for exceptional drug solubilization in diluted surfactant solutions and consideration of residual solid state." *Eur J Pharm Sci* 111:96–103.

Solubility screening in different surfactant solutions is an important part of pharmaceutical profiling. A particular interest is in low surfactant concentrations that mimic the dilution of an oral dosage form. Despite of intensive previous research on solubilization in micelles, there is only limited data available at low surfactant concentrations and generally missing is a physical state analysis of the residual solid. The present work therefore studied 13 model drugs in 6 different oral surfactant solutions (0.5%, w/w) by concomitant X-ray diffraction (XRPD) analysis to consider effects on solvent-mediated phase transformations. A particular aspect was potential occurrence of exceptionally high drug solubilization. As a result, general solubilization correlations were observed especially between surfactants that share chemical similarity. Exceptional solubility enhancement of several hundred-fold was evidenced in case of sodium dodecyl sulfate solutions with dipyridamole and progesterone. Furthermore, carbamazepine and testosterone showed surfactant-type dependent hydrate formation. The present results are of practical relevance for an optimization of surfactant screenings in preformulation and early development and provide a basis for mechanistic modeling of surfactant effects on solubilization and solid-state modifications.

Sadou Yaye, H. et al. (2017). "Investigating therapeutic usage of combined Ticagrelor and Aspirin through solid-state and analytical studies." *Eur J Pharm Sci* 107:62–70.

The mainstay treatment for patients with acute coronary syndrome is an oral route dual antiplatelet therapy with a P2Y12-receptor antagonist and Aspirin (ASA). To improve patient adherence to such treatments, combination therapies (polypill) are envisioned. Physicochemical solid-state studies have been carried out to develop a preformulation strategy of ASA with the P2Y12-receptor antagonist Ticagrelor (TIC). The investigations were carried out using differential scanning calorimetry, liquid chromatography-high resolution-multistage mass spectrometry (LC-HR-MS(n)) and as complementary techniques Fourier transform infrared measurements and thermogravimetric analysis. A simple eutectic transition at 98°C with a mole fraction for the eutectic liquid of 0.457 has been observed and the mixing of ASA and TIC molecules in each other's crystal structures appears to be limited. No cocrystals of TIC and ASA have been found. The appearance of the eutectic liquid was linked with a clear onset of chemical instability of the two pharmaceuticals. The decomposition mechanism in the liquid phase involves prior decomposition of ASA, whose residues react with well-identified TIC interaction sites. Seven interaction products were observed by LC-HR-MS(n) linked to corresponding degradation products. The most important degradation pathway is N-dealkylation. In conclusion, polypills of ASA and TIC are a viable approach, but the decomposition of ASA should be avoided by eliminating high temperatures and high humidity.

Saha, S. C. et al. (2013). "Physicochemical characterization, solubilization, and stabilization of 9-nitrocamptothecin using pluronic block copolymers." *J Pharm Sci* 102(10):3653–3665.

Solid-state properties and physicochemical characteristics of 9-nitrocamptothecin (9NC) were investigated with a view of molecular and bulk level understanding of its poor aqueous solubility and hydrolytic instability that prevent efficient drug delivery and pharmacological activity. 9NC bulk drug substance was found to be a nonhygroscopic, yellowish crystalline solid with long rectangular prism-shaped particle morphology and a sharp melting point at 264°C. Hydrolysis of 9NC-lactone occurs above pH 4, whereas complete conversion of lactone to carboxylate was recorded above pH 8. At saturated conditions, appreciable concentrations of 9NC-lactone were detected at pH as high as 11. 9NC undergoes oxidation in the presence of dimethyl sulfoxide with formation of 9NC-N-oxide. The total solubility of lactone and carboxylate forms of 9NC in deionized water was found to be less than 5 µg/mL, whereas the solubility of 9NC-lactone in aqueous acidic media was determined to be approximately 2.5 µg/mL. Incorporation of 10% pluronic copolymers P123, F127, and F68 in 10 mM HCl increased 9NC solubility by 13-fold, eightfold, and fivefold, respectively. The thermodynamic stability of drug-loaded pluronic micelles was evaluated under isothermal variable volume conditions and found F127, among all poloxamers, to offer the best hydrolytic protection efficacy for 9NC.

Sigfridsson, K. et al. (2018). "Salt formation improved the properties of a candidate drug during early formulation development." *Eur J Pharm Sci* 120:162–171.

The purpose of this study was to investigate if AZD5329, a dual neurokinin NK1/2 receptor antagonist, is a suitable candidate for further development as an oral immediate release (IR) solid dosage form as a final product. The neutral form of AZD5329 has only been isolated as amorphous material. In order to search for a solid material with improved physical and chemical stability and more suitable solid-state properties, a salt screen was performed. Crystalline material of a maleic acid salt and a fumaric acid salt of AZD5329 were obtained. X-ray powder diffractiometry, thermogravimetric analysis, differential scanning calorimetry and dynamic vapor sorption were used to investigate the physicochemical characteristics of the two salts. The fumarate salt of AZD5329 is anhydrous, the crystallization is reproducible and the hygroscopicity is acceptable. Early polymorphism assessment work using slurry technique did not reveal any better crystal modification or crystallinity for the fumarate salt. For the maleate salt, the form isolated originally was found to be a solvate, but an anhydrous form was found in later experiments; by suspension in water or acetone, by drying of the solvate to 100°C–120°C or by subjecting the solvate form to conditions of 40°C/75%RH for 3 months. The dissolution behavior and the chemical stability (in aqueous solutions, formulations and solid-state) of both salts were also studied and found to be satisfactory. The compound displays sensitivity to low pH, and the salt of the maleic acid, which is the stronger acid, shows more degradation during stability studies, in line with this observation. The presented data indicate that the substance fulfils basic requirements for further development of an IR dosage form, based on the characterization on crystalline salts of AZD5329.

Sigfridsson, K. et al. (2015). "A small structural change resulting in improved properties for product development." *Drug Dev Ind Pharm* 41(5):866–873.

AZD9343 is a water-soluble gamma amino butyric acid (GABA) agonist intended for symptomatic relief in gastroesophageal reflux disease (GERD) patients.

The compound has good chemical stability in aqueous solutions, as well as in the solid state. Only one crystal modification has been observed to date. This polymorph is slightly hygroscopic (1.5% water uptake at 80% RH), which is an improvement compared to the structurally similar agonist lesogaberan (AZD3355), which liquefies at 65% RH. Since the substance is very polar and lacks a UV chromophore, conventional separation and detection techniques cannot be used to characterize the substance and its impurities. The analytical techniques are described, focusing on the capillary electrophoresis method with indirect UV detection for assay and purity, the liquid chromatographic method for enantiomeric separation with derivatization with UV chromophore and three complementary nuclear magnetic resonance (NMR) approaches ((31)P-NMR, (13)C-NMR and (1)H-NMR) for impurities. For oral solutions, it was important to select the right concentration of phosphate buffer for the specific drug concentration and routinely use small additions of EDTA. I.V. solutions containing physiological saline as tonicity modifier could not be stored frozen at $-20°C$. Properties of AZD9343 will be discussed in light of experiences from the structurally similar lesogaberan and (2R)-(3-amino-2-fluoropropyl)sulphinic acid (AFPSiA).

Sigfridsson, K. and K. E. Carlsson (2017). "A preformulation evaluation of a photosensitive surface active compound, explaining concentration dependent degradation." *Eur J Pharm Sci* 109:650–656.

A candidate drug within the cardiovascular area was identified during early research and evaluated for further development. The aim was to understand and explain the degradation mechanisms for the present compound. The stability of the active pharmaceutical ingredient (API) in solution and solid state was studied during different conditions. The bulk compound was exposed to elevated temperatures, increased RH and stressed light conditions. Degradation of the drug in solutions was followed in the presence versus absence of ethylenediaminetetraacetic acid (EDTA), during aerobic versus anaerobic conditions, stored protected from light versus exposed to light and as a function of pH and concentration. It was possible to improve the stability by adding EDTA and completely abolish degradation by storing dissolved compound at anaerobic conditions. Solutions of API were stable between pH3 and 7, with some degradation at pH1, when stored protected from light and at 22°C but degrade rapidly when exposed to ambient light conditions. The degradation products were identified by mass spectroscopy. Degradation schemes were drawn. There was concentration dependence in the degradation of dissolved drug when exposed to light, showing a titration behavior that concurred with the measured critical micelle/aggregation concentration (CMC/CAC) of the compound. The compound was stable in solution during the investigated time period, at concentrations above CMC/CAC, where the molecule was protected from photodegradation when the compound aggregated. Below CMC/CAC, a significant degradation of the API occurred. This may be a potential explanation why other surface-active compounds show concentration dependent degradation. The photosensitivity was also observed for the neutral compound in crystalline and amorphous form, as well as for the crystalline chloride salt of the drug. However, the degradation of amorphous form was faster compared to crystalline material. No difference was observed in the degradation pattern between the neutral form of the compound and the salt form of the drug.

Sigfridsson, K. et al. (2017). "Preformulation investigation and challenges; salt formation, salt disproportionation and hepatic recirculation." *Eur J Pharm Sci* 104:262–272.

A compound, which is a selective peroxisome proliferator activated receptor (PPAR) agonist, was investigated. The aim of the presented studies was to evaluate the potential of the further development of the compound. Fundamental physicochemical properties and stability of the compound were characterized in solution by liquid chromatography and NMR and in solid-state by various techniques. The drug itself is a lipophilic acid with tendency to form aggregates in solution. The neutral form was only obtained in amorphous form with a glass-transition temperature of approximately 0°C. The intrinsic solubility at room temperature was determined to 0.03 mg/mL. Chemical stability studies of the compound in aqueous solutions showed good stability for at least two weeks at room temperature, except at pH1, where a slight degradation was already observed after one day. The chemical stability in the amorphous solid-state was investigated during a period of three months. At 25°C/60% RH (RH) and 40°C/75% RH no significant degradation was observed. At 80°C, however, some degradation was observed after four weeks and approximately 3% after three months. In an accelerated photostability study, degradation of approximately 4% was observed. Attempts to identify a crystalline form of the neutral compound were unsuccessful, however, salt formation with tert-butylamine, resulted in crystalline material. Results from stability tests of the presented crystalline salt form indicated improved chemical stability at conditions whereas the amorphous neutral form degraded. However, the salt form of the drug dissociated under certain conditions. The drug was administered both per oral and intravenously, as amorphous nanoparticles, to conscious dogs. Plasma profiles showed curves with secondary absorption peaks, indicating hepatic recirculation following both administration routes. A similar behavior was observed in rats after oral administration of a pH-adjusted solution. The observed double peaks in plasma exposure and the dissociation tendency of the salt form, were properties that contributed to make further development of the candidate drug challenging. Options for development of solid dosage forms of both amorphous and crystalline material of the compound are discussed.

Toscani, S. et al. (2016). "Stability hierarchy between Piracetam forms I, II, and III from experimental pressure-temperature diagrams and topological inferences." *Int J Pharm* 497(1–2):96–105.

The trimorphism of the active pharmaceutical ingredient piracetam is a famous case of polymorphism that has been frequently revisited by many researchers. The phase relationships between forms I, II, and III were ambiguous because they seemed to depend on the heating rate of the DSC and on the history of the samples or they have not been observed at all (equilibrium II-III). In the present paper, piezo-thermal analysis and high-pressure differential thermal analysis have been used to elucidate the positions of the different solid-solid and solid-liquid equilibria. The phase diagram, involving the three solid phases, the liquid phase and the vapor phase, has been constructed. It has been shown that form III is the high-pressure, low-temperature form and the stable form at room temperature. Form II is stable under intermediary conditions and form I is the low pressure, high temperature form, which possesses a stable melting point. The present paper demonstrates the strength of the topological approach based on the Clapeyron equation and the alternation rule when combined with high-pressure measurements.

Trivedi, M. K. et al. (2017). "In-depth investigation on physicochemical and thermal properties of magnesium (II) gluconate using spectroscopic and thermoanalytical techniques." *J Pharm Anal* 7(5):332–337.

Magnesium gluconate is a classical organometallic pharmaceutical compound used for the prevention and treatment of hypomagnesemia as a source of magnesium ion. The present research described the in-depth study on solid state properties viz. physicochemical and thermal properties of magnesium gluconate using sophisticated analytical techniques like PXRD, PSA, FT-IR, UV-Vis spectroscopy, TGA/DTG, and DSC. Magnesium gluconate was found to be crystalline in nature along with the crystallite size ranging from 14.10 to 47.35 nm. The particle size distribution was at d(0.1) = 6.552 microm, d(0.5) = 38.299 microm, d(0.9) = 173.712 microm, and d(4,3) = 67.122 microm along with the specific surface area of 0.372 m(2)/g. The wavelength for the maximum absorbance was at 198.0 nm. Magnesium gluconate exhibited 88.51% weight loss with three stages of thermal degradation process up to 895.18°C from room temperature. The TGA/DTG thermograms of the analyte indicated that magnesium gluconate was thermally stable up to around 165°C. Consequently, the melting temperature of magnesium gluconate was found to be 169.90°C along with the enthalpy of fusion of 308.7 J/g. Thus, the authors conclude that the achieved results from this study are very useful in pharmaceutical and nutraceutical industries for the identification, characterization and qualitative analysis of magnesium gluconate for preformulation studies and also for developing magnesium gluconate based novel formulation.

Yamashita, M. et al. (2015). "Vapor phase alkyne coating of pharmaceutical excipients: Discrimination enhancement of Raman chemical imaging for tablets." *J Pharm Sci* 104(12):4093–4098.

Raman chemical imaging has become a powerful analytical tool to investigate the crystallographic characteristics of pharmaceutical ingredients in tablet. However, it is often difficult to discriminate some pharmaceutical excipients from each other by Raman spectrum because of broad and overlapping signals, limiting their detailed assessments. To overcome this difficulty, we developed a vapor phase coating method of excipients by an alkyne, which exhibits a distinctive Raman signal in the range of 2100–2300 cm(−1). We found that the combination of two volatile reagents, propargyl bromide and triethylamine, formed a thin and nonvolatile coating on the excipient and observed the Raman signal of the alkyne at the surface. We prepared alkyne-coated cellulose by this method and formed a tablet. The Raman chemical imaging of the tablet cross-section using the alkyne peak area intensity of 2120 cm(−1) as the index showed a much clearer particle image of cellulose than using the peak area intensity of 1370 cm(−1), which originated from the cellulose itself. Our method provides an innovative technique to analyze the solid-state characteristics of pharmaceutical excipients in tablets.

7

Dosage Form Considerations in Preformulation

I'm not interested in being Wonder Woman in the delivery room. Give me drugs.

Madonna Ciccone

7.1 Introduction

Preformulation studies inevitably extend beyond the basic characterization of the lead compound, because what is considered an acceptable characteristic of a lead compound will largely depend on the intended or anticipated dosage form. For example, the solubility issues will largely determine the route of administration; conversely, if a particular route of administration is the only desired route, then preformulation studies should attempt to find out the structural changes necessary for the candidate molecule.

In most instances, the choice of a prospective dosage form will depend on a variety of factors:

1. Rate of entry to body tissues desired
2. Onset of action desired
3. Aqueous and nonaqueous solubility
4. Irritability of solution of drug
5. Stability of drug at the site of administration
6. Storage and handling requirements for the dosage form
7. Shelf life desired
8. Patient acceptance vis-à-vis the customary routes for the defined class

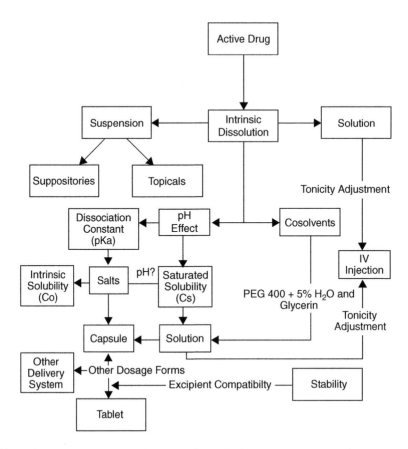

SCHEME 7.1 Selection criteria for dosage form selection. (From http://www.pharmquest.com/default.html; Courtesy of Pharmquest Corporation, Mountain View, CA.)

Scheme 7.1 lists some of the pivotal factors that go into the selection of an appropriate drug delivery system, particularly with reference to the first and foremost requirement, the dissolution of drug.

It is noteworthy that the dissolution rate considerations play a pivotal role in the selection of a dosage form and hence the time spent on studying this at the preformulation stages. Although it may be too early to set dissolution rate criteria for the dosage forms, preformulation studies can be very useful where a definite dosage form is envisioned. Schemes 7.2 through 7.4 show the decision-making

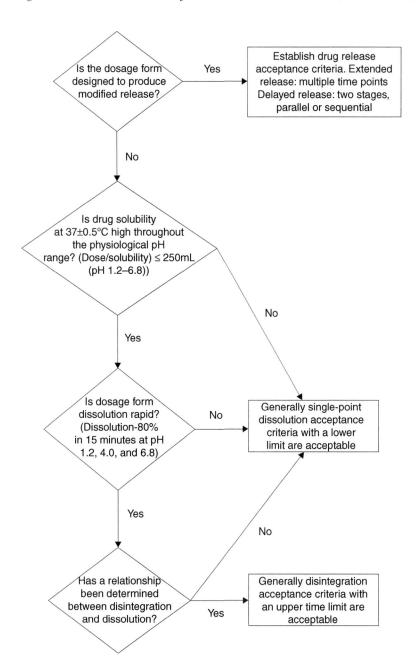

SCHEME 7.2 Setting acceptance criteria for drug product dissolution; that is, which types of drug release acceptance criteria are acceptable? (Courtesy of Pharmquest Corporation, Mountain View, CA.)

process for setting the acceptance criteria for dissolution rates. Following three questions need to be addressed at this stage:

1. What types of drug release acceptance criteria are appropriate (Scheme 7.2)?
2. What specific test conditions and acceptance criteria are appropriate for immediate-release products (Scheme 7.3)?
3. What are the appropriate acceptable ranges for extended-release dosage forms (Scheme 7.4)?

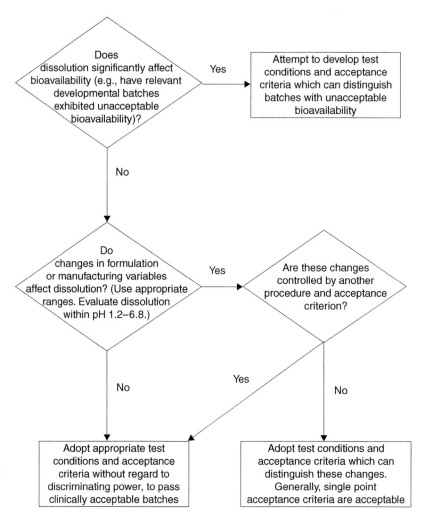

SCHEME 7.3   Setting acceptance criteria for drug product dissolution; that is, which specific test conditions and acceptance criteria are needed for the immediate release of dosage forms? (Courtesy of Pharmquest Corporation, Mountain View, CA.)

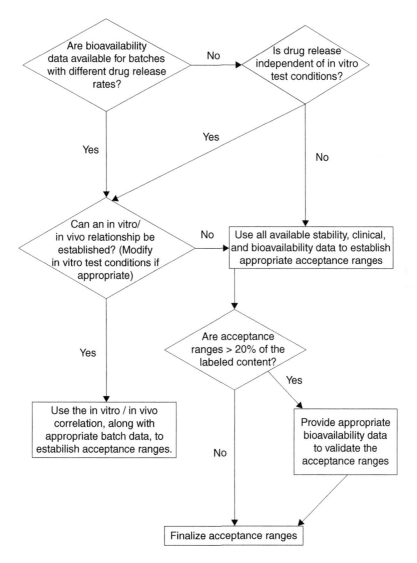

SCHEME 7.4 Setting acceptance criteria for drug product dissolution; that is, the appropriate acceptance ranges for extended-release dosage forms. (Courtesy of Pharmquest Corporation, Mountain View, CA.)

7.2 Solid Dosage Form Considerations

Most pharmaceutical companies would rather have their new molecule enter the market as a tablet or a capsule for a variety of safety, cost, and marketing considerations. As a result, almost 70% of all drugs administered today are in solid dosage forms. When so intended, the default form should be a solid dosage form (unless it is predetermined in the case of therapeutic proteins or other drugs that must be administered by parenteral route or other specific routes for specificity of the desired activity). The typical parameter studies for solid dosage forms relate to the ability of a powder mix to flow well in manufacturing machines and to the intrinsic characteristics that make it compressible. Some examples of properties studied include crystal structures (polymorphs), external shapes (habits), compression properties, cohesion, powder flow, micromeritics, crystallization, yield strengths, effects of moisture and hygroscopicity, particle size, true bulk and tapped density, and surface area.

7.2.1 Particle Size Studies

The particle size of a new drug substance is a critical parameter, as it affects every phase of formulation and its effectiveness. Appropriate particle size is required to achieve the optimal dissolution rate in solid dosage forms and to control sedimentation and flocculation in suspensions. Small particle size (2–5 μm) is required for inhalation therapy. The content uniformity and compressibility are governed by the particle size. As a result, the preformulation studies must develop a specification of particle size as early as possible in the course of the studies and develop specifications that need to be adhered to, throughout the studies.

Conventional methods of grinding in mortar or ball milling (where sample quantity is sufficient; generally, it is not sufficient and is limited to about 25–100 mg) or micronization techniques are used to reduce the particle size. The method used can have significant effect on the crystallinity, polymorphic structures (often to amorphous forms), and drug substance stability and can range from discoloration to significant chemical degradation. Changes in polymorphic forms can be determined by performing X-ray powder diffraction (XRPD) before and after milling.

Micronization, where possible, allows an increase in the surface area to the maximum, which can have an impact on the solubility, dissolution, and, as a result, bioavailability. As the aim of most preformulation studies is to determine if a solid dosage form can be administered, knowing that the reduction of the particle size, where it changes the dissolution rates, can be pivotal in decision-making for the selection of dosage forms. In the process of micronization, the drug substance is fed into a confined circular chamber, where it is suspended in a high-velocity stream of air. Interparticulate collisions result in a size reduction. Smaller particles are removed from the chamber by the escaping air stream toward the center of the mill, where they are discharged and collected. Larger particles recirculate until their particle size is reduced. Micronized particles are typically less than 10 μm in diameter. In some instances, micronization can prove counterproductive, where it results in increased aggregation (leading to reduced surface area) or alteration of crystallinity, which must be studied by using methods such as microcalorimetry, dynamic vapor sorption (DVS), and inverse gas chromatography (IGC).

The introduction of DVS in 1994 revolutionized the world of gravimetric moisture sorption measurement, bringing the use of outdated, time-intensive, and labor-intensive desiccator into the modern world of cutting-edge instrumentation and overnight vapor sorption isotherms. With a resolution down to 0.1 μg, a 1% change in the mass of a 10-mg sample on exposure to the humidity-controlled gas flow is both easily discernable and reproducible. The DVS is a valued tool for studies related to polymorphism, compound stability, and bulk and surface adsorption effects of water and organic vapors. The DVS studies would typically show percent mass increases, but often, a hysteresis loop relationship is observed, where there is crystallization of compound that results in the expelling of excess moisture. This effect can be important in some formulations, such as dry powder inhaler devices, as it can cause agglomeration of the powders and variable flow properties. The DVS is a useful study when amorphous forms are involved on size reduction. In many cases, a low level of amorphous character cannot be detected by techniques such as XRPD; microcalorimetry can detect <10% amorphous content (the limit of detection is 1% or less). The amorphous content of a micronized drug can be determined by measuring the heat output caused by the water vapor inducing the crystallization of the amorphous regions.

Figure 7.1 shows a typical DVS chart for microcrystalline cellulose, and Figure 7.2 shows the chart for lactose. The reaction to moisture is dramatically represented in this study.

Excellent instrumentation support and advice are available through Surface Measurement Systems (SMS) (1), manufacturer of DVS-Advantage and DVS-1000 and 2000 series of equipment for dynamic vapor interaction studies. The DVS-HT represents the first new generation of gravimetric vapor sorption analyzers for more than a decade by Surface Measurement Systems (5 Wharfside, Rosemont Road, Alperton, Middlesex, HA0 4PE, U.K.). The DVS-HT is recommended for stability

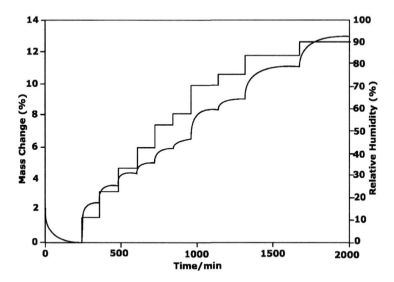

FIGURE 7.1 The dynamic vapor sorption chart for microcrystalline cellulose. The percentage mass change is based on a 10-mg sample of microcrystalline cellulose reference material. Steps refer to relative humidity changes. (Courtesy of Surface Measurement Systems; From http://www.smsuk.co.uk/index.php.)

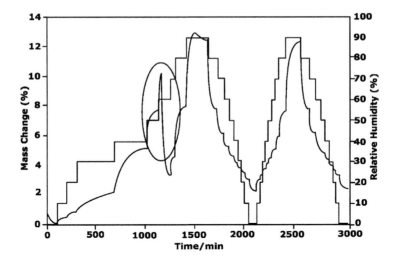

FIGURE 7.2   The dynamic vapor sorption chart for lactose. A humidity-induced recrystallization event of spray-dried lactose is marked. Steps refer to relative humidity changes. (Courtesy of Surface Measurement Systems; From http://www.smsuk.co.uk/index.php.)

studies to select the optimal drug and excipient combinations. The DVS-HT features the following:

- Rapid screens of salts, solvates, hydrates, polymorphs, and cocrystals
- Large-scale preformulation and *formulation* studies
- Characterization of polymers, food ingredients, and fine particles
- Process optimization monitoring of surface and bulk chemistry
- Quality control of incoming raw materials
- Investigation of batch-to-batch variations in material formulations
- At-line process analytical technology (PAT) support of production performance to specifications

Although microcalorimetery remains the workhorse of studies, the use of IGC is becoming more popular to determine the changes to drug substances on micronization. The IGC differs from traditional gas chromatography (GC) insofar as the stationary phase is the powder under investigation. The behavior of pharmaceutical solids, during either processing or use, can be noticeably affected by the surface energetics of the constituent particles. Several techniques exist to measure the surface energy, for example, sessile drop, and dynamic contact angle measurements. The IGC is an alternative technique where the powder surface is characterized by the retention behavior of minute quantities of well-characterized vapors that are injected into a column containing the material of interest. Recently published articles using IGC on pharmaceutical powders have ranged from linking surface energetic data with triboelectric charging to studying the effect of surface moisture on surface energetics. Molecular modeling has also recently been used to explore the links between IGC data and the structural and chemical factors that influence the surface properties, thereby achieving predictive knowledge regarding powder behavior during processing. In this type of study, a range of nonpolar and polar adsorbates (probes) is used, for example, alkanes, from hexane to decane; acetone; diethyl ether; and ethyl acetate. The retention volume, that is, the net volume of carrier gas (nitrogen) required to elute the probe, is then measured.

The IGC is a gas-phase technique for characterizing the surface and bulk properties of solid materials. The principles of IGC are very simple, being the reverse of a conventional GC experiment. A cylindrical column is uniformly packed with the solid material of interest, typically a powder, fiber, or film. A pulse or constant concentration of gas is then injected down the column at a fixed carrier gas flow rate, and the time taken for the pulse or concentration front to elute down the column is measured by a detector. A series of IGC measurements with different gas-phase probe molecules then allows access to a wide range of physicochemical properties of the solid sample. The flow and retention of gas are shown in Figure 7.3.

The injected gas molecules passing over the material adsorb on the surface with a partition coefficient K_s:

$$K_s = V_N/W_s \tag{7.1}$$

where V_N is the net retention volume—the volume of carrier gas required for eluting the injection through the column, and W_s is the mass of the sample. V_N is a measure of extent of the interaction of the probe gas with the solid sample and is the fundamental data obtained from an IGC experiment. A wide range of surface and bulk properties can be calculated from it. The surface partition coefficient (K_s) of the probes between carrier gas and surfaces of test powder particles can then be calculated. From this, a free energy can be calculated, which can show that one batch may favorably adsorb the probes when compared with another, implying a difference in the surface energetics. The experimental parameter measured in IGC experiments is the net retention volume, V_N. This parameter is related to the surface partition coefficient, K_s,

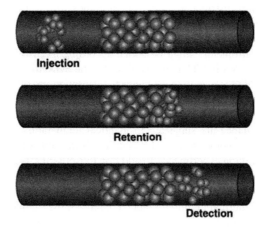

Injection

Retention

Detection

FIGURE 7.3 Inverse gas chromatography principles.

which is the ratio between the concentration of the probe molecule in the stationary and the mobile phases shown by:

$$K_s = \frac{V_s}{m} \times A_{sp}$$ (7.2)

where m is the weight of the sample in the column, and A_{sp} is the specific surface of the sample in the column.

From K_s, the free energy of adsorption ($-\Delta G_A$) is defined by:

$$\Delta G_A = RT \ln\left(K_s \times \frac{P_{sg}}{P} \right) a^{(\gamma_s^{LD})^{1/2}}$$ (7.3)

where P_{sg} is the standard vapor state (101 KN/m^2), and P is the standard surface pressure, which has a value of 0.338 mN/m.

In a typical experiment, the samples are micronized to various particle sizes, and γ_s^{LD} is measured and plotted against the median particle size. This will show that as the particle size decreases, the surface of the particles become more energetic. Depending on which functional groups are exposed more on micronization, there can be an increase or decrease in electron donation, as the particle size decreases. Therefore, by using moisture sorption, microcalorimetry, IGC, molecular modeling, and other techniques, the consequences of the particle size reduction process can be assessed. Moreover, surface energetics can be measured directly and predictions made about the nature of the surface, which ultimately could affect properties such as the flow of powders and adhesion of particles. The IGC is a useful tool, and the newer IGC chromatographs are advanced instruments for the characterization of particulates, fibers, and thin films. This opens up a whole new world of sorption solutions. Some of the applications reported include surface energetics (as described earlier), heat of sorption, sorption isotherms, phase transitions, diffusion kinetics, and so on. The new revolutionary IGC from SMS is the world's first commercial IGC. The unique SMS flow control technology provides accurate and reproducible humidity control. The standard instrument configuration comes with a thermal conductivity detector (TCD) and a flame ionization detector (FID). This combination allows the differentiation between the moisture and the organic solvent elutants. Further detectors (e.g., mass spectrometer) might be added according to customer requirements. Another supplier of DVS is VTI Technologies (2). The SGA-100 symmetrical gravimetric analyzer of VTI is a continuous vapor flow sorption instrument for obtaining water and organic vapor isotherms at temperatures ranging from 0°C to 80°C at ambient pressure. As a result of its symmetrical design (both the sample and the reference side of the microbalance are subjected to identical temperature, relative humidity [RH], and flow rate). Another benefit of this design is the ability to perform absolute or differential adsorption experiments. In addition to isotherms, isohumes, maintaining constant humidity and equilibrating the sample to a series of temperatures, heats, and kinetics of adsorption, hydrate formation can also be studied. The core of the instrument is an isothermal aluminum block containing the sample chamber, which permits very tight control of temperature and RH at the sample. The temperature within the block is kept stable by a constant temperature bath capable of temperature control within 0.01°C.

7.2.2 Particle Size Distribution

Particle size reduction particularly mandates the study of particle size distribution by using techniques such as sieving, optical microscopy in conjunction with image analysis, electron microscopy, the Coulter counter, and laser diffractometers, depending on the anticipated size of the particles. Although the size characterization is simple for spherical particles, the study of irregular particles requires specialized methods. The Malvern Mastersizer series (3) is an example of an instrument that measures particle size by laser diffraction. The use of this technique is based on light scattered through various angles, which is directly related to the diameter of the particle. Thus, by measuring the angles and intensity of scattered light from the particles, a particle size distribution can be deduced. It should be noted that the particle diameters reported are the same as those produced by spherical particles under similar conditions. In the former, each particle is treated as spherical and essentially opaque to the impinging laser light. Figure 7.4 shows different methods of detection and the size of the particles.

Two different light scattering (DLS) methodologies can be used to characterize particles. The classical, also known as "static" or "Rayleigh" scattering or multiple-angle laser light scattering, provides a direct measure of mass.

The DLS, which is also known as "photon correlation spectroscopy" (PCS) or "quasi-elastic light scattering" (QELS), uses the scattered light to measure the rate of diffusion of the particles. This motion data is conventionally processed to derive a size distribution for the sample, where the size is given by the "Stokes radius" or "hydrodynamic radius" of the protein particle. This hydrodynamic size depends on

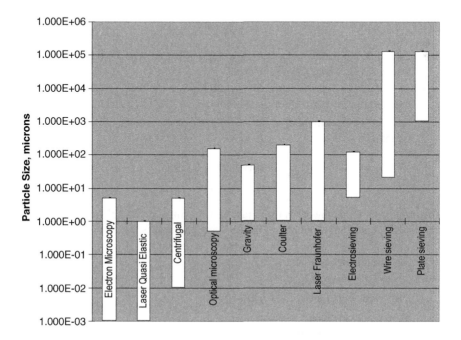

FIGURE 7.4 Techniques of particle size detection and their limits.

both mass and shape (conformation). Dynamic scattering is particularly good at sensing the presence of very small amounts of aggregated particles and studying samples containing a very large range of masses. It can be quite valuable for comparing the stability of different formulations, including real-time monitoring of changes at elevated temperatures. For submicron materials, particularly colloidal particles, QELS is the preferred technique. Two theories dominate the theory of light scattering—the Fraunhofer and Mie. According to the Fraunhofer theory, the particles are spherical, nonporous, and opaque; diameter is greater than wavelength; particles are distant enough from each other and have random motion; and all particles diffract light with the same efficiency, regardless of size and shape. The Mie theory takes into account the differences in refractive indices between the particles and the suspending medium. If the diameter of the particles is >10 μm, then the size produced by utilizing each theory is essentially the same. However, discrepancies may occur when the diameter of the particles approaches that of the wavelength of the laser source.

The following are the values reported from diffraction experiments:

- $D(v, 0.1)$ is the size of particles for which 10% of the sample is below this size.
- $D(v, 0.5)$ is the volume (v) median diameter, of which 50% of the sample is below and above this size.
- $D(v, 0.9)$ is the size of the particle for which 90% of the sample is below this size.
- $D[4, 4]$ is the equivalent volume mean diameter calculated using:

$$D[4,3] = \frac{\Sigma d4}{\Sigma d3} \qquad (7.4)$$

- $D[3, 2]$ is the surface area mean diameter, also known as the Sauter mean, where d is the diameter of each unit.
- Log difference represents the difference between the observed light energy data and the calculated light energy data for the derived distribution.
- Span is the measurement of the width of the distribution and is calculated using:

$$\text{Span} = \frac{D(v,0.9) - D(v,0.1)}{D(v,0.5)} \qquad (7.5)$$

The dispersion of the powder is important in achieving reproducible results. Ideally, the dispersion medium should have the following characteristics:

- Have a suitable absorbancy
- Not swell the particles
- Disperse a wide range of particles
- Slow sedimentation of particles
- Allow homogeneous dispersion of the particles
- Be safe and easy to use

In terms of sample preparation, it is necessary to deggregate the samples, so that the primary particles are measured. To achieve this, the sample may be sonicated; however, there is a potential problem of the sample being disrupted by the ultrasonic vibration. To check for this, it is recommended that the particle dispersion be examined by optical microscopy.

Although laser light diffraction is a rapid and highly repeatable method in determining the particle size distributions of pharmaceutical powders, the results obtained can be affected by the particle shape. The laser light scattering generally reports broader size distribution compared with image analysis. In addition, the refractive index of the particles can introduce an error of 10% under most circumstances and should be accounted for. Another laser-based instrument, relying on light scattering, is the aerosizer. The aerosizer measures particles one at a time in the range of 0.20–700 μm. The particles may be in the form of a dry powder or may be sprayed from a liquid suspension as an aerosol. The particles are blown through the system and dispersed in air to a preset count rate. The aerosizer operates on the principle of aerodynamic time of flight. The particles are accelerated by a constant, known force caused by the airflow and are forced through a nozzle at nearly sonic velocity. Smaller particles are accelerated at a greater rate than large particles as a result of a greater force-to-mass ratio. Two laser beams measure the time of flight through the measurement region by detecting the light scattered by the particles. Statistical methods are used to correlate the start and stop times of each particle in a particular size range (channel) through the measurement zone. The time of flight is used in conjunction with the density of the particles, and calibration curves are established to determine the size distribution of the sample.

7.2.3 Surface Area

As the surface area exposed to the site of administration determines the speed with which a particle dissolves in accordance with the Noyes–Whitney equation, these determinations are important. In addition, in those instances where the particle size is difficult to measure, a gross estimation of the surface area is the second best parameter to characterize the drug. The most common methods of surface area measurement, including gas adsorption (nitrogen or krypton), based on what is most commonly described as the Braunauer, Emmet, and Teller (BET) method, are applied either as a multipoint or single-point determination.

Adsorption is defined as the concentration of gas molecules near the surface of a solid material. The adsorbed gas is called *adsorbate*, and the solid where adsorption takes place is known as the *adsorbent*. Adsorption is a physical phenomenon (usually called physisorption) that occurs at any environmental condition (pressure and temperature), but it becomes measurable only at very low temperatures. Thus, physisorption experiments are performed at very low temperatures, usually at the boiling temperature of liquid nitrogen at atmospheric pressure. Adsorption takes place because of the presence of an intrinsic surface energy. When a material is exposed to a gas, an attractive force acts between the exposed surface of the solid and gas molecules. The result of these forces is characterized as physical (or van der Waals) adsorption, in contrast to the stronger chemical attractions associated with chemisorption. The surface area of a solid includes both the external surface and the internal surface of the pores.

Because of the weak bonds involved between the gas molecules and the surface (<15 KJ/mol), adsorption is a reversible phenomenon. Gas physisorption is considered nonselective, thus filling the surface step by step (or layer by layer), depending on the available solid surface and the relative pressure. Filling the first layer enables the measurement of the surface area of the material, because the amount of gas adsorbed when the monolayer is saturated is proportional to the entire surface area of the sample. The complete adsorption–desorption analysis is called an adsorption isotherm. The six International Union for Physical and Applied Chemistry (IUPAC) standard adsorption isotherms are shown in Figure 7.5; they differ because the systems demonstrate different gas–solid interactions (4).

Once the isotherm is obtained, a number of calculation models can be applied to different regions of the adsorption isotherm to evaluate the specific surface area (i.e., BET, Dubinin, Langmuir, and the like) or the micro- and mesopore volume and size distributions (i.e., Barett–Joyner–Halenda, Dubinin–Radushkevich, Horvath and Kawazoe, Saito and Foley, and the like).

The surface area of a solid material is the total surface of the sample that is in contact with the external environment. It is expressed as square meters per gram of dry sample. This parameter is strongly related to the pore size and the pore volume; that is, the larger the pore volume, the greater the surface area, and the smaller the pore size, the greater the surface area. The surface area results from the contribution of the internal surface area of the pores along with the external surface area of the solid or the particles (in case of powders). Whenever a significant porosity is present, the fraction of the external surface area to the total surface area is small.

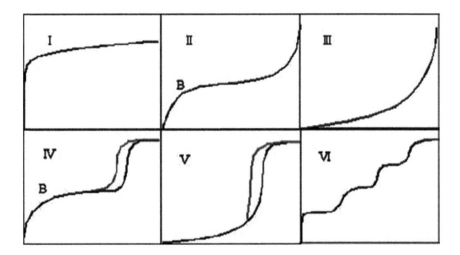

FIGURE 7.5   The six types of International Union for Physical and Applied Chemistry isotherms. The type I isotherm is typical of microporous solids and chemisorption isotherms. Type II is shown by finely divided nonporous solids. Types III and V are typical of vapor adsorption (i.e., water vapor on hydrophobic materials). Types V and VI feature a hysteresis loop generated by the capillary condensation of the adsorbate in the mesopores of the solid. The rare type VI, the step-like, isotherm is shown by nitrogen adsorbed on special carbon.

The BET isotherm for type II adsorption processes (typical for pharmaceutical powders) is given by:

$$\frac{P}{V(P_o - P)} = \frac{1}{cV_{mon}} + \left\{\frac{c-1}{cV_{mon}}\right\}\left\{\frac{P}{P_o}\right\} \tag{7.6}$$

where P is the partial pressure of the adsorbate, V is the volume of gas adsorbed at pressure p, V_{mon} is the volume of the gas at monolayer coverage, P_o is the saturation pressure, and c is related to the intercept. Thus, by plotting $P/V(P_o - P)$ versus P/P_o, a straight line of slope $c - 1/cV_{mon}$ and intercept $1/cV_{mon}$ will be obtained. The total surface area is thus:

$$S_t = \frac{V_{mon}NA_{CS}}{M} \tag{7.7}$$

where N is the Avogadro's number, A_{CS} is the cross-sectional area of the adsorbate, and M is the molecular weight (MW) of the adsorbate. It follows that the specific surface area is given by S_t/m, where m is the mass of the sample. According to the U.S. Pharmacopeia (USP), the data are considered to be acceptable, if, on linear regression, the correlation coefficient is not <0.9975; that is, r^2 is not <0.995.

It should be noted that, experimentally, it is necessary to remove gases and vapors that may be present on the surface of the powder. This is usually achieved by drawing a vacuum or purging the sample in a flowing stream of nitrogen. Raising the temperature may not always be advantageous, as often, it is found that the specific surface area of the sample decreases with an increase in temperature. Thermal degassing can therefore affect the results. From other measurements using differential scanning calorimetry (DSC) and thermogravimetric analysis (TGA), it was found that raising the temperature changed the nature of the samples. Hence, it was recommended that magnesium stearate should not be degassed at elevated temperature.

7.2.4 Porosity

Most solid powders contain a certain void volume of empty space. This is distributed within the solid mass in the form of pores, cavities, and cracks of various shapes and sizes. The total sum of the void volume is called the porosity. Porosity strongly determines the important physical properties of materials, such as durability, mechanical strength, permeability, adsorption properties, and so on. The knowledge of pore structure is an important step in characterizing materials and predicting their behavior.

There are two main and important typologies of pores: closed and open pores. Closed pores are completely isolated from the external surface, not allowing the access of external fluids in either liquid phase or gaseous phase. Closed pores influence parameters such as density and the mechanical and thermal properties. Open pores are connected to the external surface and are therefore accessible to fluids, depending on the pore nature or size and the nature of fluid. Open pores can be further divided into dead-end or interconnected pores. Further classification is related to the pore shape, whenever is possible to determine it. The characterization of solids in terms of porosity consists in determining the following parameters:

- *Pore size*: Pore dimensions cover a very wide range. Pores are classified according to three main groups depending on the access size:
  - Micropores: <2 nm diameter
  - Mesopores: between 2 nm and 50 nm diameter
  - Macropores: >50 nm diameter
- *Specific pore volume and porosity*: The internal void space in a porous material can be measured. It is generally expressed as a void volume (in cc or mL) divided by a mass unit (g).
- *Pore size distribution*: It is generally represented as the relative abundance of the pore volume (as a percentage or a derivative) as a function of the pore size.
- *Bulk density*: Bulk density (or envelope density) is calculated by the ratio between the dry sample mass and the external sample volume.
- *Percentage porosity*: The percentage porosity is represented by the ratio between the total pore volume and the external (envelope) sample volume, multiplied by 100.
- *Surface area*: See Section 7.2.5.

7.2.5 Instrumentation for Particle Size, Surface Area, and Porosity

The following discussion lists some of the most widely used instruments; this by no means represents a comprehensive list or constitutes an endorsement of one instrument over another.

The *Sorptomatic 1990* (5) is a completely computerized instrument based on a static volumetric principle to characterize solid samples by the technique of gas adsorption. It is designed to perform physisorption measurements to determine the specific surface area and mesopore size distribution of porous materials by using inert gases, such as nitrogen, argon, carbon dioxide, and so on. This instrument can also perform chemisorption measurements on activated solids such as catalysts and acid/basic materials (as zeolites), using reactive gases (i.e., hydrogen, carbon monoxide, or oxygen) or corrosive gases (i.e., gaseous dry ammonia). It has a specially designed pretreatment unit, and hence, it is possible to connect up to six gases to the special flow gas burette to properly activate the catalyst before the experiment. The software enables the determination of metal-specific surface area and dispersion in supported catalysts from chemisorption isotherms.

Static volumetric gas adsorption requires a high-vacuum pumping system to be able to generate a good vacuum over the sample of at least 10^{-4} torr. The system features stainless-steel plumbing with high-vacuum fittings to ensure precise results, as the experiment is carried out starting from high vacuum, increasing the pressure step by step up to the *adsorbate* saturation pressure. A schematic of the instrument is shown in Figure 7.6.

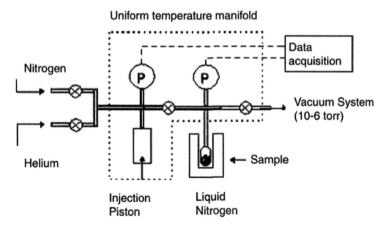

FIGURE 7.6 Static volumetric gas adsorption system.

The principle behind this method consists of introducing consecutive known amounts of *adsorbate* to the sample holder, which is kept at liquid nitrogen temperature (77 K). Adsorption of the injected gas onto the sample causes the pressure to decrease slowly, until an equilibrium pressure is established in the manifold. The injection system of the Sorptomatic 1990 consists of a calibrated piston, where both the pressure and the injection volume can be automatically varied by the system according to the adsorption rate and the required resolution. The piston method is advantageous over other methods, as it does not increase the manifold dead volume, even as the system waits for pressure equilibration. A small dead volume over the sample makes the instrument very sensitive to the amount of gas adsorbed. The equilibrium pressure is measured by a transducer chosen according to the pressure range, where adsorption is established during the experiment. The raw experimental data are the equilibrium pressures and the amount of gas adsorbed for each step. The gas uptake is calculated directly from the equilibrium pressure values, but a dead volume calibration has to be performed before or after the measurement by a "blank run" (i.e., an analysis using an inert gas, typically helium, not adsorbed on the sample in the analytical conditions).

The static volumetric method is very precise and is considered a very accurate technique to evaluate the surface area and the pore size in the region of micro- and mesopores. However, it is not advisable whenever a fast measurement of surface area is required, because this method involves a long analysis time to produce highly accurate and reliable results.

The *QSurf quick surface area analyzers* (5) offer a simple, straightforward analytical layout, enabling easy and rapid operations, and is tailored to increase lab productivity. QSurf is a fast surface area analyzer designed for determining specific surface area and total pore volume in porous and nonporous materials by dynamic gas adsorption and desorption. Available in four different configurations, single- and multipoint BET analyses, and with one to three analytical ports, QSurf is capable of accommodating the vast diversity in analytical and throughput requirements of modern laboratories. Based on flow technique, these new instruments are fully auto-mated, thus allowing unattended operations.

The QSurf analyzers are based on the dynamic method for the determinations of specific surface area and total pore volume in porous and nonporous materials. The gas adsorbed and desorbed by the samples under test is measured by a TCD. The sample under test is submitted to a flow (at atmospheric pressure) in a gas mix-ture between helium and nitrogen in different percentages. Helium is generally not adsorbed, and it is called the carrier gas. The carrier gas first flows through the ref-erence channel of a TCD, then through the sample holder, and finally through the analytical channel of the TCD. At the start of the experiment, the sample is kept at room temperature; thus, adsorption does not take place. In this situation, the thermal conductivity of the carrier in the two TCD channels is the same, as the gas composi-tion is the same before and after the sample. Subsequently, the system immerses the sample in a liquid nitrogen bath, cooling the sample at a very low temperature. In this condition, adsorption begins, but only nitrogen is adsorbed. Therefore, the gas com-position after the sample holder is now changed, and the carrier thermal conductivity in the reference and analysis channels is different. The TCD generates a signal that is proportional to the amount of nitrogen adsorbed. When the signal returns to the starting baseline, the sample is saturated by the adsorbate at a certain partial pressure. The next step consists in removing the sample holder from the coolant. When the sample temperature rises to room temperature, the phenomenon of desorption takes place, and nitrogen is released from the sample surface. In addition, in this case, the composition of the carrier in the two TCD channels is different, because the sample is releasing the adsorbate. The TCD again generates a signal (of opposite polarity with respect to adsorption) that is proportional to the amount of gas desorbed. The Qsurf integrates the aforementioned peaks and compares the resulting integrals to a calibration peak determined previously by injecting a known dose of pure adsor-bate (calibration step is performed by an automatic loop valve). The desorption peak integration thus provides the amount of gas adsorbed by the sample, and the gas mix percentage permits to calculate the partial pressure of nitrogen over the sample during the adsorption–desorption stages.

Micromeritics offers a comprehensive line of instrumentation for particle size, surface, and porosity analysis (6). The *TriStar 3000* gas adsorption analyzer is a fully automated, three-station surface area and porosimetry analyzer that delivers high-quality surface area data (and more) at an affordable price. It can increase the speed and efficiency of routine QC analyses, yet has the accuracy, resolution, and data reduction capability to meet most research requirements. Designed with the user in mind, the TriStar 3000 provides versatility in analysis methods and data reduction, allowing one to optimize analyses for a wide range of applications. The *ASAP 2020* accelerated surface area, and porosimetry analyzer uses gas sorption techniques for research and quality control applications. Also available is the chemical adsorption ("chemisorption") option, which uses the static volumetric technique to determine the percent metal dispersion, active metal surface area, the size of active particles, and the surface acidity of catalyst materials. The Micromeritics Gemini V Series of surface area analyzers rapidly and reliably produces accurate and repeatable sur-face area and porosity determinations of the sample material. Its simplicity of use and ruggedness have earned the Gemini its place in laboratories worldwide as an essential tool in both research and quality control environments. The *FlowSorb III* is an entry-level single- and multipoint BET surface area instrument. The FlowSorb measures the surface area by using the flowing gas method, which involves the continuous flow of an adsorptive and inert gas mixture over the sample at atmospheric pressure. It is ruggedly constructed and is ideal for demanding analytical environments.

7.2.6 True Density

Density is the ratio of the mass of an object to its volume, and for solids, this term describes the arrangement of molecules. The study of compaction of powders is described by the Heckel equation:

$$\ln\left[\frac{1}{1-D}\right] = KP + A \tag{7.8}$$

where D is the relative density, which is the ratio of the apparent density to the true density, K is determined from the linear portion of the Heckel plot, and P is the pressure. The densities of molecular crystals can be increased by compression. Information about the true density of a powder can be used to predict whether a compound will cream or sediment in a suspension, such as metered dose inhaler (MDI) formulation. Therefore, suspensions of compounds that have a true density less than these figures will cream (rise to the surface), and those that are denser will sediment. It should be noted, however, that the physical stability of a suspension is not merely a function of the true density of the material. The true density is thus a property of the material and is independent of the method of determination. In this respect, the true density can be determined using three methods: displacement of a liquid, displacement of a gas (pycnometry), and floatation in a liquid. The liquid displacement is tedious and tends to underestimate the true density. Displacement of a gas is more accurate but needs relatively expensive instrumentation. As an alternative, the floatation method is simple to use and inexpensive.

Gas pycnometry is probably the most commonly used method in the pharmaceutical industry for measuring true density. Gas pycnometers rely on the measurement of pressure changes, as a reference volume of gas, typically helium, added to, or deleted, from the test cell.

7.2.7 Flow and Compaction of Powders

The flow properties of a powder will determine the nature and quantity of excipients needed to prepare a compressed or powder dosage form. This refers mainly to factors such as the ability to process the powder through machines. To make a quick evaluation, the compound is compressed using an infrared (IR) press and die under 10 torr of pressure, with variable dwell times, and the resulting tablets are tested with regard to their crushing strength after storing them for about 24 hours. If longer dwell times result in higher crushing strength, then the material is likely to be plastic. Elastic material will show capping at low dwell times, and the brittle material will not show any effect of dwell times. It is recommended that the compressed tablets be subjected to XPRD to record any changes in the polymorphic forms.

There appears to be a relationship between indentation hardness and the molecular structure of organic materials. However, a prerequisite for predicting indentation hardness is the knowledge of the crystal structure. As a result, highly sophisticated computational methods and extensive crystallography libraries have recently become available to study the properties of powders. For example, Pfizer Research relies on the Cambridge Structural Database (CSD) (7), which is one of the largest repository of small-molecule crystal structures. The CSD is the principal product of the Cambridge Crystallographic Data Centre (CCDC). It is the central focus of the CSD system, which also comprises software for database access, structure visualization, and data analysis and structural knowledge bases derived from the CSD. The CSD records bibliographic, chemical, and crystallographic information for organic molecules and metal-organic compounds, whose three-dimensional (3D) structures have been determined using X-ray diffraction (XRD) or neutron diffraction. The CSD records results of single-crystal studies and powder diffraction studies, which yield 3D atomic coordinate data for at least all non-H atoms. In some cases, the CCDC is unable to obtain coordinates, and incomplete entries are archived to the CSD. The CSD is distributed as part of the CSD system, which includes software for search and information retrieval (ConQuest), structure visualization (Mercury), numerical analysis (Vista), and database creation (PreQuest). The CSD system also incorporates IsoStar, a knowledge base of intermolecular interactions containing data derived from both the CSD and the Protein Data Bank. Some software listed here are available for free use.

X-ray microtomography, such as the one available from Skyscan (8), is used to analyze the effect of compaction on powder particles. It allows for the noninvasive 3D analysis of resulting structures and has shown that the structure may be controlled by the choice of porogen and the method of solvent removal. Simple seeding of the substrate surface with drug crystals can be used initially, with a view to incorporating more sophisticated substrate polymorph approaches. The Skyscan-1172 represents a new generation in desktop X-ray micro-CT systems. A novel architecture in which both the sample stage and the X-ray camera are moveable allows an unprecedented combination of image resolution, sample size accommodation, scan speed, and sample throughput. This innovative flexible scanner geometry of the Skyscan-1172 is particularly advantageous over intermediate resolution levels, where scans are around 10 times faster (to obtain the same or better image quality) compared with previous scanners with a fixed source-detector design. The Skyscan-1172 features two X-ray camera options: the high-performance 10-megapixel option and the economy 1.3-megapixel option. The former, 10-megapixel camera, allows the maximum scanning versatility, with an image field width of 68 mm (in dual-image camera shift mode) or 3 mm (in standard single camera image mode). A nominal resolution (pixel size) of <1 μm is attainable. A scannable height of around 70 mm allows for either large samples or automatic batch scanning of a column of smaller samples. The system obtains multiple X-ray "shadow" transmission images of the object from different angular views, as the object rotates on a high-precision stage. From these shadow images, cross-section images of the object are reconstructed by a modified Feldkamp cone-beam algorithm, creating a complete 3D representation of internal microstructure and density over a selected range of heights in the transmission images. The best micro-CT images are obtained from objects in which microstructure coincides with contrast in X-ray absorption of the sample's constituent materials.

7.2.8 Color

The color of a powder sample is used to indicate the presence of solvents, distribution of particle size, and other possible differences in the different lots of a new lead compound. In some instances, degradation of drug can be correlated with color changes to such a degree that accurate color measurements can be used as a tool to provide product specification. The compendia often describe the color of the substances but mostly in subjective terms. Historically, the color evaluation has been a subjective measurement; however, newer quantitative measurement systems make this a more objective process. There are two basic methods for measuring the colors of surfaces:

- The first is to imitate the analysis made by the eye in terms of responses to three stimuli. This technique, known as "tristimulus colorimetry," sets out to measure X, Y, and Z directly.
- The second method is to determine the reflectance (R) for each wavelength band across the range of the spectrum to which the eye is sensitive and then calculate the visual responses by summing the products of R and the standard values for the distribution of the sensitivity of the three-color responses.

The tristimulus method has theoretical advantages, where the materials to be measured are fluorescent, but there are serious practical problems in assuming that a tristimulus colorimeter exactly matches human vision, that is, in eliminating color blindness from the instrument.

Two commonly used types of color measurement equipment are colorimeter and spectrophotometer. A tristimulus colorimeter has three main components:

- A source of illumination (usually a lamp functioning at a constant voltage)
- A combination of filters used to modify the energy distribution of the incident or reflected light
- A photoelectric detector that converts the reflected light into an electrical output

Each color has a fingerprint reflectance pattern in the spectrum. The colorimeter measures color through three wide-band filters corresponding to the spectral sensitivity curves. Measurements made on a tristimulus colorimeter are normally comparative, the instrument being standardized on glass or ceramic standards. To achieve the most accurate measurements, it is necessary to use calibrated standards of similar colors to the materials to be measured. This "hitching post" technique enables reasonably accurate tristimulus values to be obtained, even when the colorimeter is demonstrably color blind. Tristimulus colorimeters are most useful for quick comparison of near-matching colors. They are not very accurate. Large differences are evident between the various instrument manufacturers. However, colorimeters are less expensive than spectrophotometers.

To get a precise measurement of color, it is advisable to use a spectrophotometer. A spectrophotometer measures the reflectance for each wavelength and allows to calculate the tristimulus values. The advantage over tristimulus colorimetry is that adequate information is obtained for the calculation of color values for any illuminant and that metamerism is detected automatically. Metamerism is a psychophysical phenomenon commonly defined incompletely as "two samples which match when illuminated by a particular light source and then do not match when illuminated by a different light source." In actuality, there are several types of metamerism, of which the sample metamerism and illuminant metamerism are the most common. In sample metamerism, two color samples appear to match under a particular light source and then do not match under a different light source. Illuminant metamerism appears when different light sources illuminate the same sample and the differences are revealed. The observer metamerism refers to the spot where each individual perceives color slightly differently. The geometric metamerism arises when identical colors appear different when viewed at different angles, distances, light positions, and so on.

In a spectrophotometer, the light is usually split into a spectrum by a prism or a diffraction grating before each wavelength band is selected for measurement. Instruments in which narrow bands are selected by interference filters have also been developed. The spectral resolution of the instrument depends on the narrowness of the bands utilized for each successive measurement. In theory, a spectrophotometer could be set up to compare the reflected light directly with the incident light, but it is more usual to calibrate against an opal glass standard that has been calibrated by an internationally recognized laboratory. Checks must also be made on the optical zero, for example, by measurements with a black light trap, because dust or other problems can give rise to stray light in an instrument (which would give false readings). Spectrophotometers contain monochromators and photodiodes that measure the reflectance curve of color every 10 nm or less. The analysis generates typically 30 or more data points, with which a precise color composition can be calculated.

A large number of suppliers provide colorimeters, including a large array of equipment from Hunter Lab's Labscan XE with special adapter for small quantity of powders, offering an excellent choice in preformulation work. The instrument has a 3-mm port and requires 0.4-cc powder to perform the testing (9).

7.2.9 Electrostaticity

When subjected to attrition, powders can acquire an electrostatic charge, the intensity of which is often proportional to the physical force applied, as static electrification of two dissimilar materials occurs by the making and breaking of surface contacts (triboelectrification or friction electrification). Electrostatic charges are often used to induce adhesive character to bind drugs to carrier systems, for example, glass beads coated with hydroxypropylmethyl cellulose–containing drugs. The net charge on a powder may be either electropositive or electronegative, depending on the direction of electron transfer. The mass charge density can vary from 10^{-5} to 100 μC/kg, depending on the stress, ranging from gentle sieving to micronization process. This can be done using electric detectors to determine the polarity and the electrostatic field. The electrostaticity results in significant changes in the powder flow properties.

Studies on triboelectrification and potential charge buildup on equipment and particle surfaces and the subsequent adhesion caused by static charge often overlook the fact that all materials (whether they have a net surface charge or not) exhibit surface energy forces that are very short in range but come into play once the surfaces are "touching." These van der Waals forces are caused by the dispersive and polar surface energies inherent at material boundaries. Dry powders with mass-median particle sizes larger than around 100–200 µm seldom exhibit strong "cohesive" powder behavior, and such powders are usually described as "free flowing." However, as the particle size decreases, the amount of surface area per unit mass increases, and surface energy forces have a greater influence on bulk powder flow characteristics. For contacting particles smaller than 2–20 µm, such forces can be strong enough to cause small amounts of plastic deformation on the particle surfaces near the points of contact—even with no applied external loads. The bulk behavior of such fine powders can be dominated by their "cohesivity." It is well known that powders composed of finer particles are more cohesive, and, when very cohesive powders are placed in a rotating drum, they neither usually flow easily nor do they form a smooth top surface. Instead, cohesive powders build up large overhanging "chunks" that can break off and collapse or cascade in random avalanches onto the material further down the slope. Placing the rotating drum in a centrifuge at an elevated g-level can cause a "nonflowable" cohesive powder to flow.

7.2.10 Caking

Powders cake as a result of agglomeration, owing to factors such as static electricity, hygroscopicity, particle size, impurities of the powder, storage conditions, stress temperature, RH, storage time, and so on. The mechanisms involved in caking are based on the formation of five types of interparticle bonds, such as bonding resulting from mechanical tangling, bonding resulting from steric effects, bonds via static electricity, bonds as a result of free liquid, and bonds caused by solid bridges. During the process of micronization, the formation of localized amorphous zones can lead to caking, as these zones are more reactive to factors described earlier, especially when exposed to moisture. The mechanisms involve moisture sorption as a result of surface sintering and recrystallization at well below the critical RH. In most instances, the increase in RH begins to show some impact at values >20%, resulting in most dramatic effects above 75%–80% RH for powders that are subject to humidity effects.

7.2.11 Polymorphism

Because polymorphism can have an effect on so many aspects of drug development, it is important to fix the polymorph (usually the stable form) as early as possible in the development cycle. Although it is not necessary to create additional solid-state forms by techniques or conditions unrelated to the synthetic process for the purpose of clinical trials, regulatory submission of a thorough study of the effects of solvent, temperature, and possibly pressure on the stability of the solid-state forms is advised. A conclusion that polymorphism does not occur with a compound must be substantiated by crystallization experiments, from a range of solvents. This should also include solvents that may be involved in the manufacture of the drug product, for example, during granulation.

As it is hoped that the issue of polymorphism is resolved during prenomination and early development, it can remain a concern when the synthesis of the drug is scaled up into a larger reactor or transferred to another production site. It is not unlikely that a metastable form identified in prenomination may not be reproduced in later batch products because of some unrecorded conditions in the early phases of development. Related substances, whether identified or not, can significantly alter the predominance of a specific polymorph. To develop a reliable commercial recrystallization process, the following scheme should be followed in the production of candidate drugs:

1. Selection of solvent system
2. Characterization of the polymorphic forms
3. Optimization of process times, temperature, solvent compositions, and the like
4. Examination of the chemical stability of the drug during processing
5. Manipulation of the polymorphic form, if necessary

Many analytical techniques have been used to quantitate mixtures of polymorphs; for example, XRPD has been used to quantify the various polymorphs. Assay development requires the creation of calibration curves and validation, which can be a difficult task where mixed polymorphs are present, and also requires a study to prove that there is no polymorphic transformation during analysis or change in the hydration of crystals, if that is also a concomitant problem. Although at the preformulation stage, the dosage form considerations are still developing, there is a need to answer questions such as how would a polymorph change and should this be subjected to manufacturing equipment stress, such as granulation or drying of granules, wet or dry granulation, and compression? In addition to the polymorphism of active drugs, the excipients, such as magnesium stearate, can be present in various polymorphic forms that can significantly alter the behavior of active drug in the formulation stages. Studies using XRPD, IR, or scanning electron microscopy (SEM) should be made for excipients and the active drug.

7.3 Solution Formulations

Solution dosage forms offer several advantages, particularly the resolution of bioavailability problems and instant administration as injectable forms (though nonsolution forms are also given parenterally). At the preformulation stage, more important factors are the solubility (and any pH dependence) and stability of the new compound.

7.3.1 Solubility

In case a solution form is desired and the compound has low solubility, there are several techniques—some very simple and some very complex—to achieve the desirable property of the lead drug, including pH manipulation, use of cosolvents and surfactants, emulsion formation, and addition of complexing agents. In a more complex stage, the liposomes or similar drug delivery systems can be used.

As many compounds are weak acids or bases, their solubilities become a function of pH. However, the ionic strength of the medium plays a significant role, and as a result, most parenteral formulations are buffered to prevent the crystallization of drugs.

The use of cosolvents improves the solubility as a result of the polarity of the cosolvent mixture being closer to the drug than it is in water:

$$\log S_m = f \log S_c + (1 - f) \log S_w \tag{7.9}$$

where S_m is the solubility of the compound in the solvent mix, S_w is the solubility in water, S_c is the solubility of the compound in pure cosolvent, f is the volume fraction of the cosolvent, and σ is the slope of the plot of $\log(S_m/S_w)$ versus f. There is a definite correlation between the s value and indices of the cosolvent polarity, such as the dielectric constant, solubility parameter, surface tension, interfacial tension, and octanol–water partition coefficient. The aprotic cosolvents give a much higher degree of solubility than the amphiprotic cosolvents. This means that if a cosolvent can donate a hydrogen bond, it might be an important factor in determining whether it is a good cosolvent. Use of cosolvents with polar drugs can reduce the solubility.

On formulating parenteral dosage forms, the use of cosolvents to prevent precipitation can be hampered by the quantity of the allowed cosolvents in the formulation for toxicity and hemolysis considerations. Other considerations such as dilution prior to administration and the rate of administration (dilution factor) should also be simulated using in vitro techniques. Although cosolvents can increase the solubility of compounds, on certain occasions, they can have a detrimental effect on their stability. One point that is often overlooked when considering cosolvents is their influence on buffers or salts. As these are conjugate acid–base systems, it is not surprising that by introducing solvents into the solution, a shift in the pK_a of the buffer or salt can result. These effects are important in formulation terms, as many injectable formulations that contain cosolvents also contain a buffer to control the pH.

7.4 Emulsion Formulations

For drugs with poor water solubility, emulsion formulation, such as oil-in-water (O/W), where the drug has good partitioning in the oil phase chosen, often offers an excellent choice. The particle size of the emulsion and its stability (physical and chemical) then become significant factors, as larger globule sizes may lead to phlebitis. To achieve smaller particle size, the technique of microfluidization is often used, among other available homogenization methods. The phospholipids added stabilize emulsions through surface charge changes and provide a good mechanical barrier.

The particle size of an emulsion is governed by the method used. Figure 7.7 shows the various particle sizes achieved by using different methods.

The particle size is measured using PCS (10), a technique for measuring particle size distributions. When fine particles are suspended in a fluid, they are constantly in random motion as a result of collisions with the molecules of the fluid. This is known as "Brownian motion" and was first observed in the 1820s. When the suspension is irradiated by a beam of laser light, some of the light is scattered by the particles. Very fine particles exhibit wavelength smaller than that of light (typically 500–700 nm), and as they move relative to the light beam, the phase of the light scattered from each particle will vary. The intensity of the scattered light, measured at some fixed point, is the sum of the light scattered from all the individual particles, formed by constructive

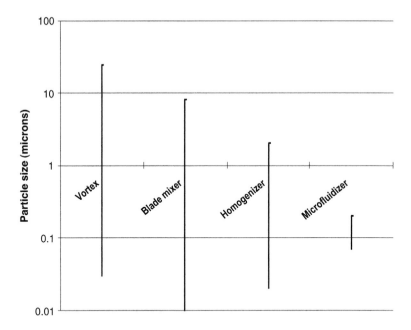

FIGURE 7.7 Emulsion particle size dependence on the method of manufacture.

and destructive interference. This intensity will therefore vary as the particles move, and the rate of variation will depend on the speed of the movement of the particles, which is in turn related to their size. This is why PCS is also known as "dynamic light scattering." The advantages of the use of PCS include the following:

- Direct measurement of particle size in the submicron range
- Particles are observed in situ in the fluid matrix
- Broad range: 1–5000 nm (5 microns)
- Reasonably fast

The disadvantages of the use of PCS include the following:

- Requires very dilute dispersions and careful sample preparation
- Low resolution: provides only limited detail of the distributions
- Expensive equipment
- Skill required to interpret results

A large variety of instruments are available for PCS (11).

Also useful are the measurements of zeta potential. Particles in suspensions typically acquire a surface charge by the adsorption of ions on the surface, dissolution of the material, chemical reaction, or preferential adsorption of a specific additive or impurity ions from the solution. Surface charge of colloidal particles can be inferred through the measurement of the zeta potential (the particle charge at the shear plane). The zeta potential is an important particle property that affects interparticle forces,

particle adhesion, suspension stability, and polymer or surfactant adsorption characteristics. A large zeta potential, either positive or negative, promotes a stable dispersion, while a small zeta potential signifies poor stability or an unstable dispersion.
The zeta potential of the particles can be determined by measuring the mobility of the
particles in an applied direct electric field (termed as electrophoretic mobility) or its
sonic response to an alternating electric field (electrokinetic sonic amplitude effect).
For large particles or flat surfaces, streaming potential measurements can be utilized
to determine the zeta potential. In streaming potential measurements, the flow of
electrolyte induces an electric field that can be measured. The reverse electro-osmosis
phenomena can be used to determine the charge on large particles or surfaces that
cannot be measured by electrophoretic methods. Other methods, such as atomic force
microscope (AFM) measurements, can be used to measure the surface forces between
particles and surfaces.

From these data, the surface charge on the particles can often be determined.
The AFM is one of about two dozen types of scanned-proximity probe microscopes.
All of these microscopes work by measuring a local property, such as the height,
optical absorption, and magnetism, with a probe or "tip" placed very close to the
sample. The small probe-sample separation (on the order of the instrument's resolution) makes it possible to take measurements over a small area. To acquire an image,
the microscope raster scans the probe over the sample, at the same time as measuring
the local property in question. The resulting image resembles an image on a televi-
sion screen in that both consist of many rows or lines of information placed one above
the other. Unlike traditional microscopes, scanned-probe systems do not use lenses;
hence, the size of the probe, rather than diffraction effects, generally limits their
resolution. The AFM operates by measuring attractive or repulsive forces between
a tip and the sample. In its repulsive "contact" mode, the instrument lightly touches
a tip at the end of a leaf spring or "cantilever" to the sample. As a raster scan drags the
tip over the sample, some sort of detection apparatus measures the vertical deflection
of the cantilever, which indicates the local sample height. Thus, in contact mode, the
AFM measures hard-sphere repulsion forces between the tip and the sample. In non-
contact mode, the AFM derives topographic images from measurements of attractive
forces; the tip does not touch the sample. The AFM can achieve a resolution of 10 Å
and, unlike electron microscopes, can image samples in air and under liquids. In principle, AFM resembles the record player and the stylus profilometer. However, AFM
incorporates a number of refinements that enable it to achieve atomic-scale resolution:

- Sensitive detection
- Flexible cantilevers
- Sharp tips
- High-resolution tip-sample positioning
- Force feedback

Several vendors provide additional details on the refined features of AFM (12–14).

The physical instability of emulsions involves creaming, flocculation, coalescence,
or breaking, whereas the chemical instability can be a result of hydrolysis of the stabilizing moieties. In order to assess the stability of the emulsion, heating and freezing
cycles, centrifugation, and steam sterilization can be employed. Generally, emulsions

with a high negative zeta potential do not show any change in their particle-size distribution after autoclaving. Emulsions with a lower negative value, on the other hand, would generally separate into two phases during autoclaving. Because the stability of phospholipid-stabilized emulsions is dependent on the surface charge, these emulsions are normally autoclaved at pH 8–9.

7.4.1 Stability Considerations

Newer drug molecules appear to be more reactive and potent in their response. As a result, they are also more reactive in the dosage forms, and when the dosage forms are liquids, the stability becomes a serious challenge to overcome. This is one reason why solid dosage forms are preferred by formulation scientists. A basic matrix to evaluate stability potential can take scores of permutations and combinations of pH, ionic strength, dielectric constant, temperature, and the like. Given the small quantity of substance available at the preformulation stage, it is unlikely to complete these studies with sufficient vigor.

The degradation kinetics of drugs in solution state has been a broad subject dealt with in major textbooks and in a large number of detailed review articles. What needs to be understood at the preformulation level are gross observations as to whether a drug would sustain the solution or liquid environment for any significant length of time. Quick pH and accelerated testing is required, where the quantity of the substance available is sufficient for the purpose. At this stage, stability may be tested with most likely cosolvents, particularly those used in pediatric or geriatric dosage forms.

For parenteral formulations, sterility can be maintained either by sterile filtration or by autoclaving. It is noteworthy that there is no history of any significant recalls of products that were autoclaved, and thus, manufacturers prefer to use this method of sterilization, where possible; obviously, it cannot be used where drugs are inherently unstable to heat, such as the biological products. Autoclaving (usually 15–20 minutes at 121°C) at various pH values is a good test to study the impact on impurities, color, pH, and other degradation products. The autoclave cycle should ideally represent a real-time manufacturing process, with its common fill, heat-up, peak-dwell, and cooldown steps.

7.4.2 Oxidation

Oxygen sensitivity is common for many molecules. Oxidation reactions are the most difficult reactions to understand, let alone prevent. As a result, oxidation-prone compounds are combined with antioxidants. In a solution form, the degradation is fast, particularly in the presence of trace metals.

The common antioxidants, such as water-soluble sodium bisulfate, sodium sulfite, sodium metabisulfite, sodium thiosulfate, sodium formaldehyde sulfoxylate, L- and D-ascorbic acid, acetylcysteine, cysteine, thioglycerol, thioglycollic acid, thiolactic acid, thiourea, dithithreitol or oil-soluble propyl gallate, butylated hydroxyanisole, butylated hydroxytoluene, ascorbyl palmitate, nordihydroguaiaretic acid, and *a*-tocopherol are widely used in pharmaceutical formulations. Oxygen-sensitive substances should be screened for their compatibility with a range of antioxidants. One of the most commonly used antioxidants is metabisulfite. It should be noted that bisulfite has also been known to catalyze hydrolysis reactions. The reaction of bisulfate with dissolved oxygen is given by:

$$2HSO_3^- + O_2 \rightarrow 2SO^{-4} + 2H^+ \tag{7.10}$$

Several newer techniques, such as cyclic voltammetry (CV), are now used to identify a proper choice of an antioxidant. The CV is an electrolytic method that uses microelectrodes and an unstirred solution, so that the measured current is limited by analyte diffusion at the electrode surface. The electrode potential is ramped linearly to a more negative potential and then ramped in reverse, back to the starting voltage. The forward scan produces a current peak for any analyte that can be reduced through the range of the potential scan. The current will increase as the potential reaches the reduction potential of the analyte but then fall off as the concentration of the analyte is depleted close to the electrode surface. As the applied potential is reversed, it will reach a potential that will reoxidize the product formed in the first reduction reaction and produce a current of reverse polarity from the forward scan. This oxidation peak will usually have a similar shape to the reduction peak. The peak current, i_p, is described by the Randles–Sevcik equation:

$$i_p = (2.69 \times 10^5)\, n^{3/2} A C D^{1/2} v^{1/2} \tag{7.11}$$

where n is the number of moles of electrons transferred in the reaction, A is the area of the electrode, C is the analyte concentration (in mol/cm^3), D is the diffusion coefficient, and v is the scan rate of the applied potential.

The potential difference between the reduction and the oxidation peaks is theoretically 59 mV for a reversible reaction. In practice, the difference is typically 70–100 mV. Larger differences, or nonsymmetric reduction and oxidation peaks, are an indication of a nonreversible reaction. These parameters of cyclic voltammograms make CV most suitable for the characterization and mechanistic studies of redox reactions at the electrodes.

The basic components of a modern electroanalytical system for voltammetry are a potentiostat, a computer, and an electrochemical cell. In some cases, the potentiostat and the computer are bundled into one package, whereas in other systems, the computer and the converters and microcontrollers are separate, and the potentiostat can operate independently.

7.4.3 Trace Metals

Trace metal ions can affect the stability and can arise from the bulk drug, formulation excipients, or glass containers. Metal ions can also act as degradation catalysts by their involvement in the production of highly reactive free radicals, especially in the presence of oxygen. The formation of these radicals can be initiated by the action of light or heat and propagate the reaction until they are destroyed by inhibitors or by side reactions that break the chain. Free-radical oxygen species can be generated by transition metals in solutions, such that reactions can be initiated. Because of the involvement of metal ions in degradation reactions, the inclusion of a chelating agent is often advocated.

Chelating agents are frequently used to protect substances from undergoing oxidation by removing metallic contaminants. A chelate is a chemical compound composed of a metal ion and a chelating agent. A chelating agent is a substance whose molecules can form several bonds to a single metal ion. In other words, a chelating agent is a multidentate ligand. An example of a simple chelating agent is ethylenediamine. A single molecule of ethylenediamine can form two bonds to a transition metal ion, such as nickel (II), Ni^{2+}. The bonds form between the metal ion and the nitrogen atoms of ethylenediamine. The nickel (II) ion can form six such bonds; hence, a maximum of three ethylenediamine molecules can be attached to one Ni^{2+} ion. A chelating agent of particular economic significance is ethylenediaminetetraacetic acid (EDTA). It is a versatile chelating agent; it can form four or six bonds with a metal ion and forms chelates with both transition metal ions and main group ions. It is frequently used in pharmaceutical products. In addition to EDTA, β-hydroxyethylenediaminetri acetic acid (HEDTA), diethylenetriaminepentaacetic acid and isoniazid solutions are also used.

Ethylenediaminetetraacetic acid has pK_a values of $pK_1 = 2.0$, $pK_2 = 2.7$, $pK_3 = 6.2$, and $pK_4 = 10.4$ at 20°C. Generally, the reaction of EDTA with metal ions can be described by:

$$M^{n+} + Y^{4-} \longrightarrow MY^{(4-n)+} \tag{7.12}$$

In practice, however, the disodium salt is used because of its greater solubility, hence:

$$M^+ + H_2Y \longrightarrow MY^{(4-n)+} + 2H^+ \tag{7.13}$$

The dissociation (or equilibrium) is sensitive to the pH of the solution; therefore, this will have implications for the formulation. The stability of the complex formed by EDTA–metal ions is characterized by the stability or formation constant, K. This is derived from the reaction equation and is given by:

$$K = \frac{[(MY)_{(n-4)+}]}{[M^+]} \tag{7.14}$$

Equation 7.14 assumes that the fully ionized form of $EDTA^{4-}$ is present in solution; however, at low pH, other species, that is, $HEDTA^{3-}$, H_2EDTA^{2-}, and H_2EDTA^{2-}, and the undissociated H_4EDTA will be present. Thus, the stability constants become conditional on pH.

The ratio can be calculated for the total uncombined EDTA (in all forms) to the form $EDTA^{4-}$. Thus, the apparent stability constant becomes K/α_L, such that:

$$\alpha_L = \frac{[EDTA] \text{ all forms}}{[EDTA_{4-}]} \tag{7.15}$$

Thus,

$$K_H = \frac{K}{\alpha_L} \quad \text{or} \quad K_H = \log K - \alpha_L \tag{7.16}$$

where log K_H is known as the conditional stability constant. Fortunately, α_L can be calculated from the known dissociation constants of EDTA, and its value can be calculated from:

$$\alpha_L = \left\{1 + \frac{[H+]}{K_4} + \frac{[H+]}{K_4 K_3} + \cdots \right\} = 1 + 10^{(pK_4 - pH)} + 10^{(pK_4 + pK_3\, pH)} + \cdots \qquad (7.17)$$

Thus at pH = 4, the conditional stability constants of some metal–EDTA complexes are calculated as follows:

$$\log K_H \text{ EDTA Ba}^{2+} = 0.6 \qquad (7.18)$$

$$\log K_H \text{ EDTA Mg}^{2+} = 1.5 \qquad (7.19)$$

$$\log K_H \text{ EDTA Ca}^{2+} = 3.4 \qquad (7.20)$$

$$\log K_H \text{ EDTA Zn}^{2+} = 9.5 \qquad (7.21)$$

$$\log K_H \text{ EDTA Fe}^{2+} = 17.9 \qquad (7.22)$$

Thus, at pH = 4, the zinc and ferric complexes will exist; however, calcium, magnesium, and barium will be only weakly complexed, if at all.

The inclusion of EDTA is occasionally not advantageous, as there are a number of reports of EDTA catalyzing the decomposition of drugs. Citric acid, tartaric acid, glycerin, and sorbitol can also be considered complexing agents; however, these are often ineffective. Interestingly, some Japanese formulators often resort to amino acids or tryptophan, because of a ban on EDTA in a particular country.

7.4.4 Photostability

For drug substances, photostability testing should consist of two parts: forced degradation testing and confirmatory testing. The purpose of forced degradation testing studies is to evaluate the overall photosensitivity of the material for method development purposes and/or degradation pathway elucidation. This testing may involve the drug substance alone and/or in simple solutions or suspensions to validate the analytical procedures. In these studies, the samples should be in chemically inert and transparent containers. In these forced degradation studies, a variety of exposure conditions may be used, depending on the photosensitivity of the drug substance involved and the intensity of the light sources used. For development and validation purposes, it is appropriate to limit the exposure and end the studies if extensive decomposition occurs. Under forced conditions, decomposition products that are unlikely to be formed under the conditions used for confirmatory studies may be observed. This information may be useful in developing and validating suitable analytical methods. If in practice it is demonstrated that they are not formed in the confirmatory studies, these degradation products need not be examined further. The forced degradation studies should be designed to provide suitable information to develop and validate test methods for the confirmatory studies. These test methods should be capable of resolving and detecting photolytic degradants that appear during the confirmatory studies.

When evaluating the results of these studies, it is important to recognize that they form a part of the stress testing and are not therefore designed to establish qualitative or quantitative limits for change.

Confirmatory studies should then be undertaken to provide the information necessary for handling, packaging, and labeling. Normally, only one batch of drug substance is tested during the development phase, and subsequently, the photostability characteristics should be confirmed on a single batch selected, as described in the parent guideline, if the drug is clearly photostable or photolabile. If the results of the confirmatory study are equivocal, testing of up to two additional batches should be conducted. Care should be taken to ensure that the physical characteristics of the samples under test are taken into account, and efforts, such as cooling and/or placing the samples in sealed containers, should be made to ensure that the effects of the changes in physical states, such as sublimation, evaporation, and melting, are minimized. All such precautions should be chosen to provide minimal interference with the exposure of samples under test. Possible interactions between the samples and any material used for containers or for the general protection of the sample should also be considered and eliminated, wherever not relevant to the test being carried out. The confirmatory studies should identify precautionary measures needed in manufacturing or in the formulation of the drug product and if light-resistant packaging is needed. When evaluating the results of confirmatory studies to determine whether the change caused by exposure to light is acceptable, it is important to consider the results from other formal stability studies, in order to ensure that the drug will be within the justified limits at the time of use.

As a direct challenge for samples of solid drug substances, an appropriate amount of sample should be taken and placed in a suitable glass or plastic dish and protected with a suitable transparent cover, if considered necessary. Solid drug substances should be spread across the container to give a thickness of typically not more than 3 mm. In cases where solid drug substance samples are involved, sampling should ensure that a representative portion is used in individual tests. Similar sampling considerations, such as homogenization of the entire sample, apply to other materials that may not be homogeneous after exposure. The analysis of the exposed sample should be performed concomitantly with that of any protected samples used as dark control, if these are used in the test.

Drug substances that are liquids should be exposed in chemically inert and transparent containers. At the end of the exposure period, the samples should be examined for any changes in physical properties (e.g., appearance, clarity, and color of solution) and for assay. The degradants must be examined by a method suitably validated for products likely to arise from photochemical degradation processes.

Protection from light often offers excellent solutions to stabilize liquids; the use of amber-colored vials and ampuls is one example of precaution taken in reducing the effect of light waves.

7.4.5 Surface Activity

Many drugs show surface-active behavior, because they have the correct mixture of chemical groups that are characteristic of surfactants. The surface activity of drugs can be important if they show a tendency to, for example, adhere to surfaces, or if solutions foam. Not all surface-active drugs form micelles, because of steric hindrances. The surface activity of compounds can be determined using a variety of techniques, such as surface tension measurements using a Du Nouy tensiometer (15), Wilhelmy plate, and conductance measurements. Sigma 703 is a simple, reliable instrument for the measurement of surface and interfacial tension by Du Nouy ring or Wilhelmy plate methods (16).

7.4.6 Osmolality

A 0.9% w/v NaCl solution is iso-osmotic with blood. The commonly used unit to express osmolality is the ion, and this is defined as the weight in grams per solute, existing in a solution as molecules, ions, macromolecules, and the like, and is osmotically equivalent to the gram MW of an ideally behaving nonelectrolyte. This is an important consideration for parenteral and ophthalmic products. Extreme discomfort in the use of ophthalmic preparations is experienced when the osmolality is too high or too low. Osmolality is determined using a cryoscopic osmometer, which is calibrated with deionized water and solutions of sodium chloride of known concentrations (17). Using this technique, the sodium chloride equivalents and freezing point depressions for a large number of substances have been determined and reported.

7.5 Freeze-Dried Formulations

The stability of the solution forms intended for parenteral administration can be significantly improved by lyophilizing the solutions to dryness, without the use of heat. The solution is frozen to a very low temperature, and vacuum is applied to remove water through sublimation. The cake left is easily dispersible and thus offers a highly desirable dosage form that is reconstituted just prior to administration. Examples of lyophilized drugs include erythromycin, vancomycin, bacitracin, cyclophosphamide, cefazolin, infliximab, somatropin, trimetrexate glucuronate multivitamin injection (MVI), and doxorubicin. The Food and Drug Administration (FDA) classification for lyophilized products is as follows:

713   injection, powder, lyophilized, for liposomal suspension
705   injection, powder, lyophilized, for solution
706   injection, powder, lyophilized, for suspension
712   injection, powder, lyophilized, for suspension, extended release

Another advantage of lyophilization is that it allows the formulation without any additives; however, some are often added to increase the bulk. As a result, each drug must be formulated with a highly specific temperature and a vacuum cycle that is highly dependent on the nature of the drug, the quantity used, and the nature of the additives. The science of lyophilization is complex, and specialized training is needed to evaluate this potential of new molecules. If during freezing, the solutes crystallize, the first thermal event detected using DSC will be the endotherm that corresponds to the melting of the eutectic formed between ice and the solute. This is usually followed by an endothermic event, corresponding to the melting of ice. Normally, freeze-drying of these systems is carried out below the eutectic melting temperature. Another way of detecting whether a solute or formulation crystallizes on freezing is to conduct subambient XRD. If there is no crystallization on cooling the solution of the drug, the supercooled liquid becomes more concentrated and viscous, leading to glass formation at a temperature known as the glass transition temperature (T_g). Generally, the freeze drying should take place below this temperature to avoid the collapsing of the cake, wherein high residual water remains and requires prolonged reconstitution time. There is an increased degradation as a result of increased mobility of molecules above T_g.

Testing of lead compound would preferably involve freezing and studying using DSC. In some cases, an endotherm caused by stress relaxation may be superimposed on the glass transition. It is possible to resolve these events using the related technique, modulated DSC (MDSC), or dynamic DSC (DDSC). The DSC is used to determine a wide range of physical properties of materials, including the glass transition temperature T_g, the melting temperature T_m, and solid–solid transitions. In this technique, a sample and a reference material are subjected to a controlled temperature program. When a phase transition, such as melting, occurs in the sample, an input of energy is required to keep the sample and the reference at the same temperature. This difference in energy is recorded as a function of temperature to produce the DSC trace. The MDSC provides the same qualitative and quantitative information about the physical and chemical changes as the conventional DSC and, in addition, provides unique thermochemical data that are unavailable from the conventional DSC. The effects of baseline slope and curvature are reduced, increasing the sensitivity of the system. Overlapping events, such as molecular relaxation and glass transitions, can be separated. Heat capacity can be measured directly with MDSC in a minimum number of experiments. Both MDSC and DSC measure the difference in heat flow to a sample and to an inert reference. The sample and reference cells are identical. However, MDSC uses a different heating profile. The DSC measures the heat flow as a function of a constant rate of change in temperature, whereas the MDSC superimposes a sinusoidal temperature modulation on this rate. The sinusoidal change in temperature permits the measurement of heat capacity effects simultaneously with the kinetic effect. Typical experimental procedure for an initial MDSC experiment includes a heating rate from isothermal to 5°C/min and a modulation amplitude from 0.01°C to 10°C. The modulation period can vary from 10 to 100 seconds or is expressed as a frequency, from 10 to 100 MHz.

The method of DDSC, such as using the PerkinElmer DSC 7 (18), along with the Pyris software platform, creates a modulated temperature profile applied to the sample, rather than a straight heating ramp, and the response of the sample is analyzed by Fourier transformation. The DDSC is particularly useful for separating overlapping thermal events, such as melting and recrystallization. Subambient operation of the DSC 7 normally employs a PerkinElmer Intracooler II, which allows reliable data to be acquired down to approximately −40°C; for even lower temperatures, a liquid nitrogen bath can be employed, which allows the collection of data down to approximately −150°C.

7.6 Suspensions

When the lead compound has limited solubility and the efforts to enhance it fail and when there is a tendency for fast crystallization from solutions, or even when chemical stability is a problem, often formulating suspension dosage forms obviates some of these drawbacks. However, suspensions, by nature, must have higher viscosity to prevent the settling of particles and thus create problems in pourability, syringability, and so on. Appropriate selection of a vehicle that provides an ideal compromise among all characteristics thus becomes a critical factor, because the intent is to have as little solubility in the vehicle as possible to prevent crystallization from the solution that surrounds the suspended particles. As a result, weak acids and bases appear as poor choices for suspension formulation. In some instances, it may be possible to prepare a derivative with larger hydrophobic groups or salt formation that would have lower solubility, if preparing a suspension dosage form was particularly desired. Compounds that can form hydrates when in suspension state can create stability problems. A significant thermodynamic problem in suspension formulation comes from Ostwald ripening and crystal growth, not because of phase change but as a result of the differences in the solubility as a function of crystal size:

$$\frac{RT}{M} \ln\left(\frac{S_2}{S_1}\right) = \frac{2\sigma}{\rho}\left(\frac{1}{r_1} - \frac{1}{r_2}\right) \tag{7.23}$$

where R is the gas constant, T is the absolute temperature, S_1 and S_2 are the solubilities of crystals of radii r_1 and r_2, respectively, σ is the specific surface energy, ρ is the density, and M is the MW of the solute molecules. Temperature fluctuation is obviously one factor that promotes Ostwald ripening. Although phase changes can be studied using standard techniques, such as DSC, hot-stage microscopy, and XRPD, Ostwald ripening is best studied using microscopic methods. The art of suspension formulation is complex, as a large number of factors, including additives, can have a significant influence on the crystal growth; for example, dye molecules often attach to high-energy points on crystals, affecting their growth. Similarly, it is reported that polyvinyl pyrrolidine (PVP), a common ingredient of many suspension formulations, inhibits crystal growth. Albumin is also known to have a similar impact. The choice of additives is also governed by the final form of suspension. If it has to be sterilized, the additives must be able to sustain autoclave temperatures; besides, autoclaving can affect both the physical and chemical stabilities of the drug. Zeta potential measurements of suspensions often prove useful.

Shelf-life specifications of a suspension dosage form include redispersability on storage. However, there is no official method to test this, and most manufacturers design their own methods, chiefly requiring some type of subjective shaking. The stability of the suspensions is partly dependent on the particle size in suspension. This can be measured using techniques such as laser diffraction and Malvern Mastersize (19). As the stabilized suspension is mostly in a flocculated form, owing to the electrolytes added to it, it may be necessary to apply sonification in the study of particle sizes.

7.7 Topical

Topical delivery of drugs using semisolid, controlled release patches, and many other dosage forms offers advantages, including reduced blood level fluctuation, obviating the first-pass effect and protection from the gastrointestinal pH. In cases where localized action is desired, this dosage form offers remarkable opportunity for drug action. However, skin is a poor medium to deliver drugs, because, by its very design, it is supposed to prevent the entry of chemicals (though it fails miserably, as we know from the chemical warfare agents). Generally, large polar molecules do not penetrate the stratum corneum well. The intrinsic physicochemical properties of candidate drugs important in expediting delivery across the skin include MW, volume, aqueous solubility, melting point, and log P. For weakly acidic or basic drugs, the skin pH will play a strong role in their transport. Drugs that form zwitter ions can be made more penetrable by using appropriate salt forms.

The formulation additives strongly impact transdermal delivery, as a variety of dosage forms, such as creams, ointments, lotions, gels, and patches, offer a wide variety of formulation additives. The problems related to the crystallization of drugs, as discussed under suspension dosage forms, also apply here, just as the considerations that optimize the physical and chemical stabilities. The entire textbook has been dedicated to the formulation of semisolid and topical delivery dosage forms that describe in detail how the choice of basic drug structure and additives affects the stability. Where salt forms are available, it is often difficult to predict the stability profile, including factors such as photostability, a test that must be conducted for all dosage forms. It is known that different salt forms can show differences in their photostability profile.

7.8 Pulmonary Delivery

The pressurized MDIs in the use of environmentally friendly propellants mean the choice of hydrofluoroalkanes, wherein the dosage form can be a suspension of the solution form. The problems of formulating suspensions, as discussed earlier, apply here as well but particularly with respect to interactions with the formulation components specific to pressurized inhaler systems.

Solution dosage forms require the selection of propellants, wherein the drug can dissolve without crystallizing, and may require the addition of surfactants and cosolvents. However, there are toxicological issues with the use of surfactants. The solubility of drugs in solvents is determined by filtering the suspension in a pressurized can into another can and then evaporating the clear solution (bringing to room temperature), followed by the determination of the amount of drug in it. High solubility in propellants can lead to crystal growth, as propellants evaporate. Ostwald ripening, common to suspensions, applies to inhalation suspensions. The changes in the property of suspension can be studied by using microscopy and observing the changes in the axial ratio of crystal.

Drugs for inhalation therapy in a powder form require a particular particle size, which is achieved by the process of micronization between 1 and 6 μm, to allow deep penetration through the lung alveoli system. There are a number of devices that can deliver drugs to the lungs as dry powders, for example, Turbuhaler™ and Diskhaler™.

These dosage forms rely on a larger carrier particle, such as *a*-lactose monohydrate, to which the drug is attached. The lactose is usually fractionated, such that it lies in the size range of 63–90 μm. On delivery, the drug detaches from the lactose, and because the drug is micronized, it is delivered to the lung, while the lactose is eventually swallowed. It should be realized that the polymorphic form of the lactose used could affect the aerosolization properties of the formulation. The *β*-forms were easily entrained but held onto the drug particles most strongly when the flow properties were studied. The anhydrous *α*-form shows an opposite behavior, and the monohydrate *α*-form demonstrates an intermediate behavior. Interactions with packaging materials can also alter the powder characteristics; for example, long contact times with poly-vinyl chloride, polyethylene, or aluminum should be avoided, because the adhesion force between the drug and these surfaces is much higher than that between it and the lactose carrier. Thus, detachment and loss of drug in the formulation could occur. As lactose is widely used as a carrier, its compatibility with the new drugs should be studied in detail, especially if there are any amino groups in the structure. The surface property of lactose is also important. With increasing specific surface area and roughness, the effective index of inhalation decreases as a result of the drug being held more tightly in the inhaled airstreams. Therefore, characterization of the carrier particles by, for example, surface area measurements, SEM, and other solid-state techniques, is a recommended preformulation activity.

The recent approval of Exubera, an inhalation form of insulin, by the U.S. FDA is a classical example where the dosage form is an integral part of drug action. Using the Nektar company's delivery system to create a fine powder mist, insulin in Exubera is absorbed, as the mist of fine powder reaches into the deep portions of the lung structure, without getting impacted. Although reduction in particle size is pivotal to the pulmonary delivery of drugs, micronization makes powders difficult to flow, and these changes should be studied using techniques such as DVS, microcalorimetry, and IGC. The high energy at the surface of micronized powders can often be relieved by exposing it to air of higher humidity, which can crystallize the amorphous high-energy regions. As a result, the common preformulate stage evaluations include the measurements of the micromeritic, RH, and electrostatic properties of the powder. Different salt forms show variant flow properties; for example, stearate salts are generally better for aerosol formulation.

Nebulizer formulations are normally solutions, but suspensions (particle size of <2 μm) are also used. Important preformulation considerations include stability, solubility, viscosity, and surface tension of the solution of suspension.

7.9 General Compatibility

Some excipients are universal to specific dosage forms. General compatibility testing with components such as lactose and other fillers, lubricants such as magnesium stearate, and suspending agents such as PVP and the like can be done at the preformulation level if a sufficient quantity of drug is available. In cases where a specific dosage form, such as a pulmonary delivery aerosol, is definitely desired, this testing becomes more important. Generally, chemical reactivity known between prominent function groups can be put to test in projecting the likely excipients. The testing involves making a binary mixture of the drug with the excipient in the ratio 1:1 or other similar ratios, followed by moistening and sealing into ampoules. Storage at suitable temperatures, such as 50°C, and analysis at various time points—preferably after 3 weeks, using HPLC, DSC, and TGA, as appropriate—provide gross incompatibility profile. In cases where a larger number of excipients are to be tested, a factorial design can be used to minimize the testing samples. The purpose of testing at this stage is to determine if there were any phase changes, changes in the crystallinity, and so on.

WEB REFERENCES

1. http://www.smsuk.co.uk/index.php
2. http://www.vticorp.com/products/sga100.html
3. http://www.malvern.co.uk/home/index.html
4. http://www.iupac.org/reports/2001/colloid_2001/manual_of_s_and_t.pdf
5. http://www.thermo.com/com/cda/product/detail/1,1055, 12967,00.html
6. http://micromeritics.com
7. http://www.ccdc.cam.ac.uk/
8. http://www.skyscan.be/next/home.html
9. http://www.hunterlab.com/
10. http://www.pcs-instruments.com/
11. http://www.pcs-instruments.com/products.shtml
12. http://www.veeco.com
13. http://www.microphotonics.com
14. http://www.asylumresearch.com/
15. http://www.thomassci.com/catalog/product/25667
16. http://www.ksvinc.com/tensiometers.html
17. http://www.rlinstruments.com/osmometer.html
18. http://www.princeton.edu/~polymer/dsc.html
19. http://www.malvern.co.uk
20. http://www.pharmquest.com/default.html

RECOMMENDED READING

Allen, L. V., Jr. (2008). "Dosage form design and development." *Clin Ther* 30(11):2102–2111.

BACKGROUND: Drugs must be properly formulated for administration to patients, regardless of age. Pediatric patients provide some additional challenges to the formulator in terms of compliance and therapeutic efficacy. Due to the lack of sufficient drug products for the pediatric population, the pharmaceutical industry and compounding pharmacies must develop and provide appropriate medications designed for children. OBJECTIVE: The purpose of this article was to review the physical, chemical, and biological characteristics of drug substances and pharmaceutical ingredients to be used in preparing a drug product. In addition, stability, appearance, palatability, flavoring, sweetening, coloring, preservation, packaging, and storage are discussed. METHODS: Information for the current article was gathered from a literature review; from presentations at professional and technical meetings; and from lectures, books, and publications of the author, as well as from his professional experience. Professional society meetings and standards-setting bodies were also used as a resource. RESULTS: The proper design and formulation of a dosage form requires consideration of the physical, chemical, and biological characteristics of all of the drug substances and pharmaceutical ingredients (excipients) to be used in fabricating the product. The drug and pharmaceutical materials utilized must be compatible and produce a drug product that is stable, efficacious, palatable, easy to administer, and well tolerated. Preformulation factors include physical properties such as particle size, crystalline structure, melting point, solubility, partition coefficient, dissolution, membrane permeability, dissociation constants, and drug stability. CONCLUSIONS: Successful development of a formulation includes multiple considerations involving the drug, excipients, compliance, storage, packaging, and stability, as well as patient considerations of taste, appearance, and palatability.

Baghel, S. et al. (2016). "Polymeric amorphous solid dispersions: A review of amorphization, crystallization, stabilization, solid-state characterization, and aqueous solubilization of biopharmaceutical classification system class II drugs." *J Pharm Sci* 105(9):2527–2544.

Poor water solubility of many drugs has emerged as one of the major challenges in the pharmaceutical world. Polymer-based amorphous solid dispersions have been considered as the major advancement in overcoming limited aqueous solubility and oral absorption issues. The principle drawback of this approach is that they can lack necessary stability and revert to the crystalline form on storage. Significant upfront development is, therefore, required to generate stable amorphous formulations. A thorough understanding of the processes occurring at a molecular level is imperative for the rational design of amorphous solid dispersion products. This review attempts to address the critical molecular and thermodynamic aspects governing the physicochemical properties of such systems. A brief introduction to Biopharmaceutical Classification System, solid dispersions, glass transition, and solubility advantage of amorphous drugs is provided. The objective of this review is to weigh the current understanding of solid dispersion chemistry and to critically review the theoretical, technical, and molecular aspects of solid dispersions (amorphization and crystallization) and potential advantage of polymers (stabilization and solubilization) as inert, hydrophilic, pharmaceutical carrier matrices. In addition, different preformulation tools for the rational selection of polymers, state-of-the-art techniques for preparation and characterization of polymeric amorphous solid dispersions, and drug supersaturation in gastric media are also discussed.

Chadha, R. and S. Bhandari (2014). "Drug-excipient compatibility screening—Role of thermoanalytical and spectroscopic techniques." *J Pharm Biomed Anal* 87:82–97.

Estimation of drug-excipient interactions is a crucial step in preformulation studies of drug development to achieve consistent stability, bioavailability and manufacturability of solid dosage forms. The advent of thermoanalytical and spectroscopic methods like DSC, isothermal microcalorimetry, HSM, SEM, FT-IR, solid state NMR and PXRD into pre-formulation studies have contributed significantly to early prediction, monitoring and characterization of the active pharmaceutical ingredient incompatibility with pharmaceutical excipients to avoid expensive material wastage and considerably reduce the time required to arrive at an appropriate formulation. Concomitant use of several thermal and spectroscopic techniques allows an in-depth understanding of physical or chemical drug-excipient interactions and aids in selection of the most appropriate excipients in dosage form design. The present review focuses on the techniques for compatibility screening of active pharmaceutical ingredient with their potential merits and demerits. Further, the review highlights the applicability of these techniques using specific drug-excipient compatibility case studies.

Darji, M. A. et al. (2018). "Excipient stability in oral solid dosage forms: A review." *AAPS Pharm Sci Tech* 19(1):12–26.

The choice of excipients constitutes a major part of preformulation and formulation studies during the preparation of pharmaceutical dosage forms. The physical, mechanical, and chemical properties of excipients affect various formulation parameters, such as disintegration, dissolution, and shelf life, and significantly influence the final product. Therefore, several studies have been performed to evaluate the effect of drug-excipient interactions on the overall formulation. This article reviews the information available on the physical and chemical instabilities of excipients and their incompatibilities with the active pharmaceutical ingredient in solid oral dosage forms, during various drug-manufacturing processes. The impact of these interactions on the drug formulation process has been discussed in detail. Examples of various excipients used in solid oral dosage forms have been included to elaborate on different drug-excipient interactions.

Gajdziok, J. and B. Vranikova (2015). "Enhancing of drug bioavailability using liquisolid system formulation." *Ceska Slov Farm* 64(3):55–66.

One of the modern technologies of how to ensure sufficient bioavailability of drugs with limited water solubility is represented by the preparation of liquisolid systems. The functional principle of these formulations is the sorption of a drug in a liquid phase to a porous carrier (aluminometasilicates, microcrystalline cellulose, etc.). After addition of further excipients, in particular a coating material (colloidal silica), a powder is formed with the properties suitable for conversion to conventional solid unit dosage forms for oral administration (tablets, capsules). The drug is subsequently administered to the GIT already in a dissolved state, and moreover, the high surface area of the excipients and their surface hydrophilization by the solvent used, facilitates its contact with and release to the dissolution medium and GI fluids. This technology, due to its ease of preparation, represents an interesting alternative to the currently used methods of bioavailability improvement. The article follows up, by describing the specific aspects influencing the preparation of liquid systems, on the already published papers about the bioavailability of drugs and the possibilities of its technological improvement. Key words: liquisolid systems bioavailability porous carrier coating material preformulation studies.

Kawakami, K. (2012). "Modification of physicochemical characteristics of active pharmaceutical ingredients and application of supersaturatable dosage forms for improving bioavailability of poorly absorbed drugs." *Adv Drug Deliv Rev* 64(6):480–495.

New chemical entities are required to possess physicochemical characteristics that result in acceptable oral absorption. However, many promising candidates need physicochemical modification or application of special formulation technology. This review discusses strategies for overcoming physicochemical problems during the development at the preformulation and formulation stages with emphasis on overcoming the most typical problem, low solubility. Solubility of active pharmaceutical ingredients can be improved by employing metastable states, salt forms, or cocrystals. Since the usefulness of salt forms is well recognized, it is the normal strategy to select the most suitable salt form through extensive screening in the current developmental study. Promising formulation technologies used to overcome the low solubility problem include liquid-filled capsules, self-emulsifying formulations, solid dispersions, and nanosuspensions. Current knowledge for each formulation is discussed from both theoretical and practical viewpoints, and their advantages and disadvantages are presented.

Lagrange, F. (2010). "Current perspectives on the repackaging and stability of solid oral doses." *Ann Pharm Fr* 68(6):332–358.

Which are the guidelines and scientific aspects for repackaged oral solid medications in France in 2010 whereas it develops? The transient or definitive displacement of the solid oral form from the original atmosphere to enter a repackaging process, sometimes automated, is likely to play a primary role in the controversy. However, the solid oral dose is to be repackaged in materials with defined quality. Considering these data, a review of the literature for determination of conditions for repackaged drug stability according to different international guidelines is presented in this paper. Attention is also paid to the defined conditions ensuring the conservation and handling of these drugs throughout the repackaging process. However, there is lack of scientific published stability data. Nevertheless, recent alternatives may be proposed to overcome the complexity of studying stability in such conditions. Then, the comparison of the moisture barrier properties of the respective package, a galenic model of hygroscopic molecules, or light sensitive molecules or stability data obtained during the industrial preformulation phase could also secure the list of drugs to be reconditioned. Similarly, a wise precaution will be to get stability data for the industrial blisters and unit doses undergoing the real conditions of the medication use process in hospitals and other healthcare settings. By now, reduction of dispensing errors and improvement of the compliance aid put a different perspective on the problem of repackaged drugs. To date, the pharmacist is advised to carry out its analysis of the risks.

Narayan, P. (2011). "Overview of drug product development." *Curr Protoc Pharmacol* Chapter 7: Unit 7.3.1–29.

The process for developing drug delivery systems has evolved over the past two decades with more scientific rigor, involving a collaboration of various fields, i.e., biology, chemistry, engineering, and pharmaceutics. Drug products, also commonly known in the pharmaceutical industry as formulations or "dosage forms," are used for administering the active pharmaceutical ingredient (API) for purposes of assessing safety in preclinical models, early- to late-phase human clinical trials, and for routine clinical/commercial use. This overview discusses approaches for creating small-molecule API dosage forms, from preformulation to commercial manufacturing.

8

Chemical Drug Substance Characterization

Characterization is integral to the theatrical experience.

Robert Ludlum

8.1 Introduction

Lead drug substances might be derived from three sources: chemical, biological, and botanical (including minerals). These compounds (or a mixture of compounds) may be delivered to the preformulation team at a myriad of characterization stages. Although the drug discovery group has, by this time, established the pharmacological activity, the synthesis or extraction group has, by this time, not necessarily fully characterized the lead compound. There is also a proposal on the table regarding the prospective drug delivery systems and their routes of administration. The task of the preformulation group therefore starts with the development of a detailed plan for the complete characterization of the lead compound. The depth and breadth of the characterization would depend on the type and source of the compound as well as its destination—the dosage form. Although the formulation part is yet to come, the preformulation group must provide lead suggestions on the choice of the excipients through preliminary interaction trials. These studies must be conducted using analytical methods that are established, though not necessarily fully validated at this stage.

The regulatory impact of preformulation studies is very significant, as in one format or another, the key component of all regulatory filings involves the complete characterization of the drug substance. These details are provided in the guidance provided by the U.S. Food and Drug Administration (FDA) on the preparation of the chemistry, manufacturing, and control package or in the Common Technical Document package, as required by the European Agency for Evaluation of Medicinal Products. Although the full scope of these documents covers the drug substance and the drug product, the studies conducted at the drug substance level are pivotal to further development. The aim of pharmaceutical development is to design a quality product and a manufacturing process to deliver the product in a reproducible manner. The information and knowledge gained from pharmaceutical development studies provide scientific understanding to support the establishment of specifications and manufacturing controls. Of greatest importance in the development of pharmaceutical studies are the sections devoted to the characterization of drug substances.

The physicochemical and biological properties of the drug substance that can influence the performance of the drug product and its manufacturability, or those that are specifically designed into the drug substance (e.g., crystal engineering, botanical extraction conditions, and protein yields at folding stages) should be identified and discussed. However, the type of properties of the drug substance to be studied is highly dependent on the source of the drug. While most of the new drugs are still derived by chemical synthesis, more drugs are now beginning to be sourced from biological sources, particularly through recombinant DNA manufacturing, and the recent acknowledgment by the regulatory authorities that botanical (herbal in Europe) drugs should be controlled has resulted in an organized sourcing through botanical means as well. This chapter describes the characterization of drug substances derived by chemical synthesis, wherein the molecules are well defined. The general characteristics described here may also apply to biological and botanical drugs; the specific differences will be discussed in a later chapter devoted to those drugs.

8.2 Scheme of Characterization

Systematic development cycles are more likely to be efficient and should result in a definite specification for the lead compound. Scheme 8.1 shows a typical flow chart for the characterization that leads to the development of specifications for the lead compound.

Examples of properties that are routinely examined include solubility, water content, particle size, crystal properties, biological structure, chirality, and so on. The compatibility of the drug substance with excipients should be discussed. For products that contain more than one drug substance, the compatibility of the drug substances with each other should also be evaluated. Although the dosage form considerations are still to evolve, based on a prospective dosage form, the specifications should include those parameters that may be relevant. For example, if the final dosage form intended is an injectable product, solubility and thermal stability (to autoclaving) are important considerations. Table 8.1 lists some common study protocols for different dosage forms.

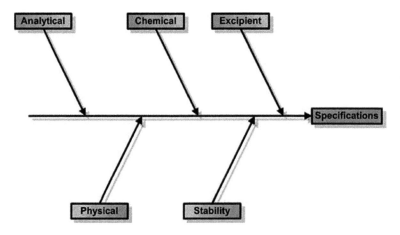

SCHEME 8.1   Steps that lead to the development of specifications for new lead compounds.

TABLE 8.1

Study Factors for Various Prospective Dosage Forms

Prospective Dosage Form	Study Factors
Parenteral	Solubility, micellization, thermal stability, chemical stability, packaging component interaction (glass and stoppers), photostability, physical stress (particularly for protein drugs), buffer interactions, and viscosity
Oral solids	Solubility, dissolution, polymorphism, chirality, particle size, powder flow, chemical stability, photostability, compressibility, hygroscopicity, and excipient interactions
Oral liquids	Solubility, polymorphic conversions, chirality, excipient interactions, chemical stability, photostability, pH effects, and container interactions (e.g., type III glass)
Semisolids	Solubility, dissolution, particle size, polymorphism, chirality, chemical stability, photostability, viscosity, and excipient interactions

The experience and data accumulated during the preformulation stage prove pivotal to the development of the dosage form, based on the specifications developed. A specification is defined as a list of tests, references to analytical procedures, and appropriate acceptance criteria that are numerical limits, ranges, or other criteria for the tests described. It establishes the set of criteria to which a new drug substance or new drug product should conform to be considered acceptable for its intended use. Conformance to specifications means that the drug substance and/or drug product, when tested according to the listed analytical procedures, will meet the listed acceptance criteria. Specifications are critical quality standards that are proposed and justified by the manufacturer and approved by regulatory authorities as conditions of approval. It is possible that, in addition to release tests, a specification may list in-process tests, periodic or skip tests, and other tests that are not always conducted on a batch-by-batch basis. When a specification is first proposed, justification should be presented for each procedure and each acceptance criterion included. The justification should refer to relevant development data, pharmacopoeia standards, test data for drug substances and drug products used in toxicology and clinical studies, and results from accelerated and long-term stability studies, as appropriate. In addition, a reasonable range of expected analytical and manufacturing variability should be considered. Test results from stability and scale-up/validation batches, with emphasis on the primary stability batches, should be considered in setting and justifying specifications.

The U.S. FDA recommends the initiative process analytical technology (PAT), which applies to both drug substances and drug products (1). The PAT is a system for designing, analyzing, and controlling the manufacture through timely measurements (i.e., during processing) of critical quality and performance attributes of raw and in-process materials and processes, with the goal of ensuring the final product quality. The goal of PAT is to understand and control the manufacturing process, which is consistent with our current drug quality system: *quality cannot be tested into products; it should be built in or should be by design*. It is important to note that the term *analytical* in PAT is viewed broadly to include chemical, physical, microbiological, mathematical, and risk analysis conducted in an integrated manner. There are many current and new tools available that enable scientific, risk-managed pharmaceutical development, manufacture, and quality assurance (QA). These tools, when used within a system, can provide effective and efficient means for acquiring information to facilitate process understanding, develop risk-mitigation strategies, achieve continuous improvement, and share information and knowledge. In the PAT framework, these tools can be categorized as follows:

- Multivariate data acquisition and analysis tools
- Modern process analyzers or process analytical chemistry tools
- Process and endpoint monitoring and control tools
- Continuous improvement and knowledge management tools

An appropriate combination of some, or all, of these tools may be applicable to a single-unit operation or to an entire manufacturing process and its QA. A variety of sophisticated software, such as RAPID-Pharma (2), are now available to consolidate many functions required to manage the initiatives related to PAT.

8.2.1 Specifications

The following tests and acceptance criteria are considered generally applicable to all new drug substances.

8.2.1.1 Description

Description is a qualitative statement about the state (e.g., solids and liquids) and color of the new drug substance. If any of these characteristics changes during storage, this change should be investigated, and appropriate action needs to be taken.

8.2.1.2 Identification

Identification testing should optimally be able to discriminate between compounds of closely related structures that are likely to be present. Identification tests should be specific for the new drug substance, for example, infrared (IR) spectroscopy. Identification solely by a single chromatographic retention time, for example, is not regarded as being specific. However, the use of two chromatographic procedures, where the separation is based on different principles or a combination of tests into a single procedure, such as high-pressure liquid chromatography (HPLC)/ultraviolet (UV) diode array, HPLC/mass spectroscopy (MS), and gas chromatography (GC)/MS, is generally acceptable. If the new drug substance is a salt, identification testing should be specific for the individual ions. An identification test that is specific for the salt should suffice.

8.2.1.3 Chirality

New drug substances that are optically active may also need specific identification testing or performance of a chiral assay. For chiral drug substances that are developed as a single enantiomer, control of the other enantiomer should be considered in the same manner as for other impurities. However, technical limitations may preclude the

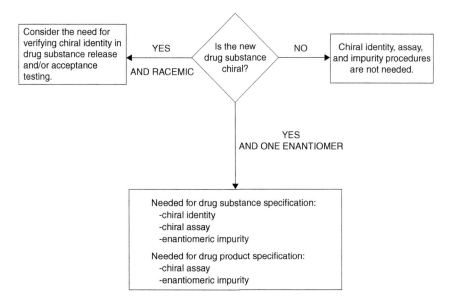

SCHEME 8.2   Decision tree for chiral compound resolution. (Courtesy of Pharmquest Corporation, Mountain View, CA.)

same limits of quantification or qualification from being applied. Assurance of control could also be given by appropriate testing of a starting material or intermediate, with suitable justification. An enantioselective determination of the drug substance should be part of the specification. It is considered acceptable in order to achieve this, either through the use of a chiral assay procedure or by the combination of an achiral assay and appropriate methods for controlling the enantiomeric impurity. For a drug substance developed as a single enantiomer, the identity test(s) should be capable of distinguishing both enantiomers and the racemic mixture. For a racemic drug substance, there are generally two situations where a stereospecific identity test is appropriate for the release/acceptance testing: one, where there is a significant possibility that the enantiomer might be substituted for the racemate, and second, when there is evidence that preferential crystallization may lead to unintentional production of a nonracemic mixture. Scheme 8.2 shows a decision-making tree on the studies that are needed when a chiral substance is suspected.

8.2.2 Assay

A specific, stability-indicating procedure should be developed to determine the content of the new drug substance. In many cases, it is possible to employ the same procedure (e.g., HPLC) for both the assay of the new drug substance and the quantification of the impurities. In cases where use of a nonspecific assay is justified, other supporting analytical procedures should be used to achieve the overall specificity. For example, where titration is adopted to assay the drug substance, the combination of the assay and a suitable test for impurities should be used. Assay methods clearly

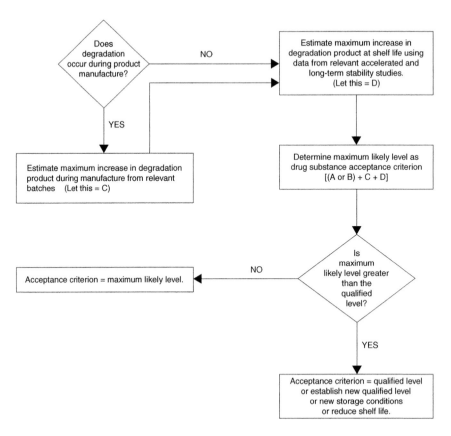

SCHEME 8.3 Decision tree for the disposition of degradation products. (Courtesy of Pharmquest Corporation, Mountain View, CA.)

define the degradation products and their limits. Scheme 8.3 shows a decision tree for handling the degradation products in the drug substance.

8.2.2.1 Impurities

Organic and inorganic impurities and residual solvents are included in this category. Scheme 8.4 shows a decision tree that can be used to decide the disposition of impurities in the drug substance.

8.2.3 Physicochemical Properties

Physicochemical properties are properties, such as the pH of an aqueous solution, melting point/range, and refractive index. The procedures used for the measurement of these properties are usually unique and do not need much elaboration, for example, capillary melting point and Abbe refractometry. The tests performed in this

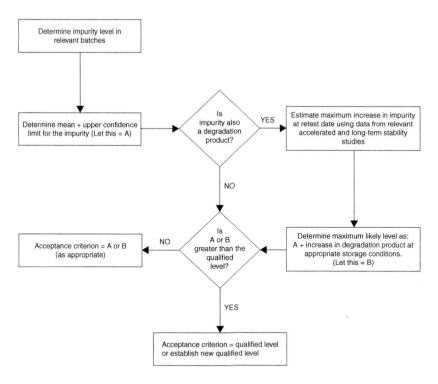

SCHEME 8.4 Decision tree for the disposition of impurities in the drug substances. (Courtesy of Pharmquest Corporation, Mountain View, CA.)

category should be determined by the physical nature of the new drug substance and its intended use.

8.2.3.1 Particle Size

For some new drug substances intended for use in solid or suspension drug products, particle size can have a significant effect on dissolution rates, bioavailability, and/or stability. In such instances, testing for particle size distribution should be carried out using an appropriate procedure, and acceptance criteria should be provided. Scheme 8.5 is a decision tree for the disposition of particle size variations in the drug substances.

8.2.3.2 Polymorphic Forms

Some new drug substances exist in different crystalline forms that differ in their physical properties. Polymorphism may also include solvation or hydration products (also known as pseudopolymorphs) and amorphous forms. Differences in these forms could, in some cases, affect the quality or performance of the new drug products.

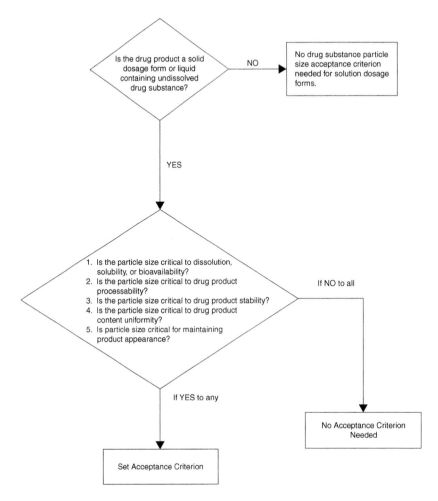

SCHEME 8.5   Decision tree for the disposition of particle size variation. (Courtesy of Pharmquest Corporation, Mountain View, CA.)

In such cases, the bioavailability stability can be altered, requiring the choice of specific stable solid dosage forms (Scheme 8.6).

8.2.3.3 *Microbiology*

Microbiological attributes are required where preparation and storage can significantly compromise microbiological quality. Scheme 8.7 shows a decision tree for the disposition of microbiologically related attributes.

8.2.3.4 *Excipients*

The excipients chosen, their concentration, and the characteristics that can influence the drug product performance (e.g., stability and bioavailability), or manufacturability

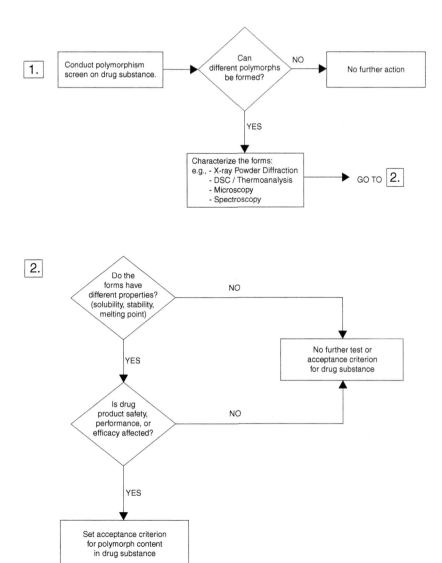

SCHEME 8.6 Decision tree for the disposition of polymorphism. (Courtesy of Pharmquest Corporation, Mountain View, CA.)

should be discussed relative to the respective function of each excipient. Compatibility of excipients with other excipients, where relevant (e.g., combination of preservatives in a dual preservative system), should be established. The ability of excipients (e.g., antioxidants, penetration enhancers, disintegrants, and release-controlling agents) to provide their intended functionality, and the intended drug product shelf life that is needed for performance throughout, should also be demonstrated. The information on excipient performance can be used, as appropriate, to justify the choice and quality attributes of the excipient and to support the justification of the drug product

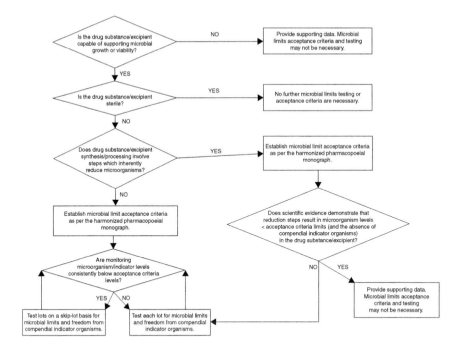

SCHEME 8.7 Decision tree for the disposition of microbiological attributes. (Courtesy of Pharmquest Corporation, Mountain View, CA.)

specification. Information to support the safety of excipients, when appropriate, should be cross-referenced.

8.2.4 Stability Evaluation

The International Conference on Harmonization (ICH) guidelines regarding the quality of drug substances are specific and require frequent referral to keep the preformulation activities current with the regulatory requirements. The pertinent guidelines are listed in the following:

- Q1A(R2) Stability Testing of New Drug Substances and Products (issued 11/2003, posted 11/20/2003)
- Q1B Photostability Testing of New Drug Substances and Products (issued 11/1996, reposted 7/7/1998)
- Q1D Bracketing and Matrixing Designs for Stability Testing of New Drug Substances and Products (issued 1/2003, posted 1/15/2003)
- Q1E Evaluation of Stability Data (issued 6/2004, posted 6/7/2004)
- Q3A Impurities in New Drug Substances (issued 2/10/2003, posted 2/10/2003)

- Q3B(R) Impurities in New Drug Products (issued 11/2003, posted 11/13/2003)
- Q5C Quality of Biotechnological Products: Stability Testing of Biotechnological/ Biological Products
- Q6A ICH; Guidance on Q6A Specifications: Test Procedures and Acceptance Criteria for New Drug Substances and New Drug Products: Chemical Substances (12/29/2000)
- Q6B Specifications: Test Procedures and Acceptance Criteria for Biotechnological/Biological Products (issued 8/1999, posted 12/14/2001)
- Q7A Good Manufacturing Practice Guidance for Active Pharmaceutical Ingredients (issued 8/2001, posted 9/24/2001); ICH, "Q3A Impurities in New Drug Substances," 1996

Knowledge about the chemical and physical stabilities of a candidate drug in the solid and liquid states is extremely important in drug development for a number of reasons. In the longer term, the stability of the formulation will dictate the shelf life of the marketed product; however, to achieve this stable formulation, careful preformulation work would have characterized the drug substance, such that a rational choice of conditions and excipients is available to the formulation team.

Candidate drugs being evaluated for development are often one of a series of related compounds that may have similar chemical properties; that is, similar paths of degradation may be deduced. However, this rarely tells us the rate at which they decompose, which is of more importance to pharmaceutical development terms. To elucidate their stability with respect to temperature, pH, light, and oxygen, a number of experiments need to be performed. The major objectives of the preformulation team are, therefore, to identify conditions to which the compound is sensitive and to identify degradation profiles under these conditions.

The major routes of drug degradation in solution are via hydrolysis, oxidation, or photochemical degradation.

8.2.4.1 Hydrolysis

Hydrolysis is a two-stage process, where a nucleophile, such as water or the hydroxyl ion, adds to, for example, an acyl carbon, to form an intermediate from which the leaving group breaks away in the second stage. The structure of the compound affects the hydrolysis rate; the stronger the conjugate acid that leaves, the faster the reaction.

Many drugs contain the functional groups, which are extremely prone to hydrolysis; the replacement of the X group with the hydroxyl moiety from water takes place, as shown in the following to yield the two types of hydrolysis reactions:

$$\begin{array}{c} R \\ \diagdown \\ \diagup C = O \\ X \end{array}$$ where $X = OR$ (ester), NR^1R^2 (amide)

or related systems (Type I)

$$\begin{array}{c} R \\ \diagdown \\ \diagup C = O \\ X \end{array}$$ where $X =$ halogen or good leaving group (Type II)

The hydrolysis of type I compounds can be catalyzed both by acids and bases; hence, pH control of formulations has a strong influence on the rates of decomposition. An example of acid-catalyzed hydrolysis is expressed as follows:

$$(8.1)$$

The base-catalyzed hydrolysis takes place as follows:

$$(8.2)$$

Common examples of drugs with hydrolysis-prone function groups are shown in Table 8.2.

The common examples are ester (aspirin), thiol ester (spirolactone), amide (chloramphenicol), sulfonamide (sulfapyrazine), imide (phenobarbital), lactam (methicillin), lactone (spiranolactone), and halogenated aliphatic (chlorambucil).

Examples of hydrolysis include drugs, such as atropine, procaine, and so on. Atropine undergoes hydrolysis at pH values higher than four, as shown in the following:

$$(8.3)$$

TABLE 8.2

Common Functional Groups of Drugs

Functional Group	Name	Example
—C—	Alkane	$CH_3CH_2CH_3$ (propane)
C=C	Alkene	$CH_3CH=CH_2$ (propene)
C≡C	Alkyne	CH_3CCH (propyne)
F, Cl, Br, or I	Alkyl halide	CH_3Br (methyl bromide)
—OH	Alcohol	CH_3CH_2OH (ethanol)
—O—	Ether	CH_3OCH_3 (dimethyl ether)
—NH₂	Amine	CH_3NH_2 (methyl amine)
—C(=O)—H	Aldehyde	CH_3CHO (acetaldehyde)
—C(=O)—	Ketone	CH_3COCH_3 (acetone)
—C(=O)—Cl	Acyl chloride	CH_3COCl (acetyl chloride)
—C(=O)—OH	Carboxylic acid	CH_3CO_2H (acetic acid)
—C(=O)—O—	Ester	$CH_3CO_2CH_3$ (methyl acetate)
—C(=O)—NH₂	Amide	CH_3NH_2 (acetamide)

This decomposition can be accounted for the base-catalyzed hydrolysis. At pH values less than four, the acid-catalyzed decomposition that causes acceleration in hydrolysis is observed owing to dehydration of the alcoholic portion of the molecule, followed by hydrolysis.

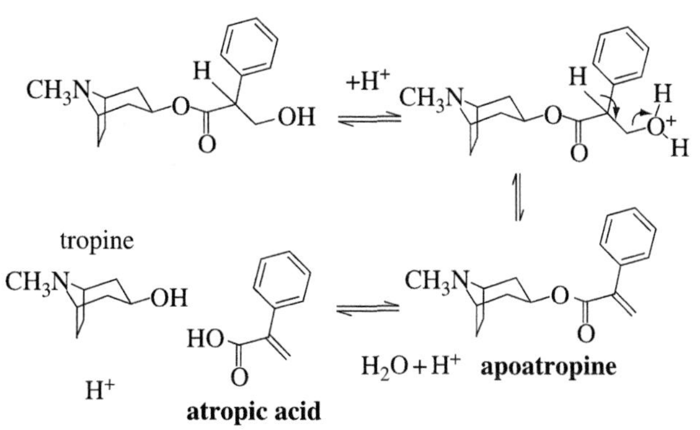

(8.4)

As a consequence, it is recommended to preserve aqueous atropine solutions buffered at around pH 3.5–4. If stored in lime glass, the stability is reduced as a result of the alkalinity of the glass.

Another good example of hydrolysis reaction is the anesthetic procaine, which is prone to specific acid-catalyzed decomposition (of the protonated form) at a pH value less than 2.5, a specific base-catalyzed hydrolysis between pH 5.5 and 8.5, titration around pH 8.5–11.0, and, finally, the base-catalyzed hydrolysis of the free base at a pH value greater than 12.0. Maximum stability occurs at pH 3.5.

$$
\text{(8.5)}
$$

Commercial preparations of procaine are limited to injectable forms. As water is the solvent of choice for injectable drugs, procaine can be protected from hydrolysis by increasing the solubility of procaine in a nonaqueous environment and by protecting (shielding) the drug from hydrolysis by employing surfactants to micellize the drug.

Degradation by hydrolysis is affected by a number of factors, including solution pH, buffer salts, ionic strength, and so on. In addition, in the presence of cosolvents, complexing agent's surfactant can also affect this type of degradation. The most important factor is the solution pH, as the hydroxyl ions are stronger nucleophiles than water; thus, degradation reactions are usually faster in alkaline solution than in water. At low pH, protons can also catalyze hydrolysis reactions as a result of specific acid–base catalysis. Besides these two ions, buffer ions such as acetate and citric acid can also catalyze degradation, where the effect is known as general acid–base degradation. Therefore, pH adjustment should make the right choice of buffers and, where possible, in smallest quantities (strength).

8.2.4.2 Oxidation

The second most common way in which a compound can decompose in solution is via oxidation. Reduction–oxidation (redox) reactions involve either the transfer of oxygen or hydrogen atoms or the transfer of electrons. Oxidation is promoted by the presence of oxygen, and the reaction can be initiated by the action of heat, light, or trace metal ions that produce organic free radicals. These radicals propagate the oxidation reaction, which proceeds until inhibitors destroy the radicals or until side reactions eventually break the chain. A simple test to see if a drug substance is prone to oxidation is to bubble air or oxygen or treat with hydrogen peroxide and estimate the level of degradation.

The sensitivity of each new drug entity to atmospheric oxygen must be evaluated to establish if the final product should be packaged under inert atmospheric conditions and if it should contain an antioxidant. Sensitivity to oxidation of a solid drug can be ascertained by investigating its stability in an atmosphere of high oxygen tension.

Usually, a 40% oxygen atmosphere allows for a rapid evaluation. Results should be compared against those obtained under inert or ambient atmospheres.

To test whether a compound is sensitive to oxygen, simply bubble air through the solution or add hydrogen peroxide, and assess the amount of degradation that takes place.

Focusing on the functional groups in a molecule allows us to recognize patterns in the behavior of related compounds. As an example, consider what we know about the reaction between sodium metal and water.

$$2Na(s) + 2H_2O(l) \rightarrow H_2(g) + 2Na^+(aq) + 2OH^-(aq) \qquad (8.6)$$

We can divide this reaction into two half reactions. One involves the oxidation of sodium metal to form sodium ions.

Oxidation:

$$Na \rightarrow Na^+ + e^- \qquad (8.7)$$

The other involves the reduction of an H^+ ion in water to form a neutral hydrogen atom that combines with another hydrogen atom to form a hydrogen molecule.

Reduction:

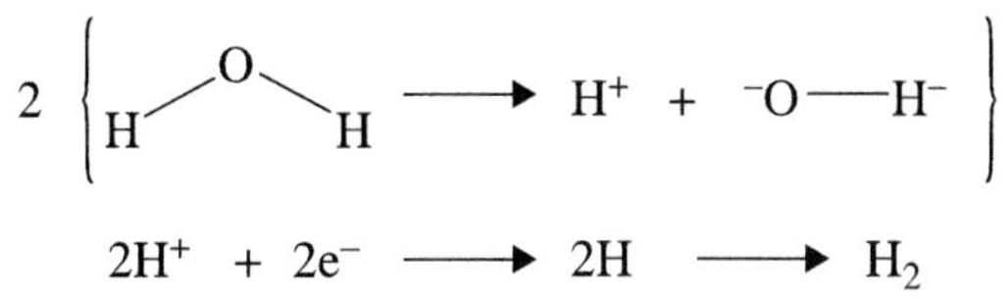

$$2H^+ + 2e^- \longrightarrow 2H \longrightarrow H_2$$

(8.8)

Once we recognize that water contains an —OH functional group, we can predict what might happen when sodium metal reacts with an alcohol that contains the same functional group. Sodium metal reacts with methanol (CH_3OH), for example, to give hydrogen gas and a solution of the Na^+ and CH_3O^- ions dissolved in this alcohol.

$$2Na(s) + 2CH_3OH(l) \rightarrow H_2(g) + 2Na^+(alc) + 2CH_3O^-(alc) \qquad (8.9)$$

Because of the involvement of transfer of electrons, the reactions between sodium metal and either water or an alcohol are examples of oxidation–reduction reactions. But what about the following reaction, in which hydrogen gas reacts with an alkene in the presence of a transition metal catalyst to form an alkane?

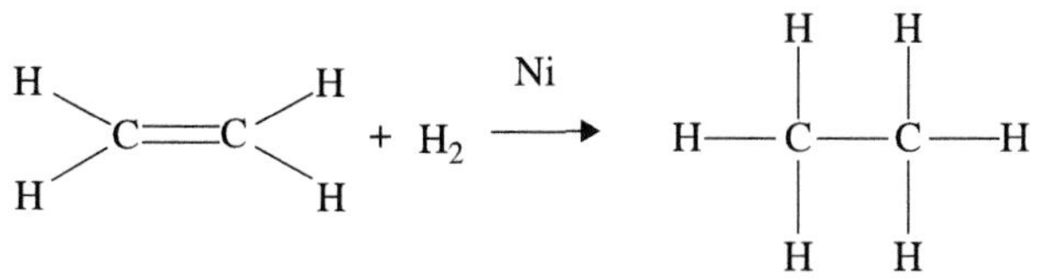

(8.10)

There is no change in the number of valence electrons in any of the atoms in this reaction. Both before and after the reaction, each carbon atom shares a total of eight valence electrons, and each hydrogen atom shares two electrons. Instead of electrons, this reaction involves the transfer of atoms—in this case, the hydrogen atoms. There are so many atom-transfer reactions that chemists developed the concept of *oxidation number* to extend the idea of oxidation and reduction to reactions in which electrons are not necessarily gained or lost. Oxidation involves an increase in the oxidation number of an atom, whereas reduction occurs when the oxidation number of an atom decreases.

During the transformation of ethene into ethane, there is a *decrease* in the oxidation number of the carbon atom. This reaction therefore involves the *reduction* of ethene to ethane.

$$\text{(8.11)}$$

Reactions in which none of the atoms undergo a change in oxidation number are called *metathesis reactions*. Consider the reaction between a carboxylic acid and an amine, for example.

$$CH_3CO_2H + CH_3NH_2 \longrightarrow CH_3CO_2^- + CH_3NH_3^+ \tag{8.12}$$

Or the reaction between an alcohol and hydrogen bromide.

$$CH_3CH_2OH + HBr \longrightarrow CH_3CH_2Br + H_2O \tag{8.13}$$

These are metathesis reactions, because there is no change in the oxidation number of any atom in either reaction.

The oxidation numbers of the carbon atoms in a variety of compounds are given in Table 8.3.

The oxidation numbers given in Table 8.3 can be used to classify organic reactions as either oxidation–reduction reactions or metathesis reactions. Because electrons are neither created nor destroyed, oxidation cannot occur in the absence of reduction, or vice versa. It is often useful, however, to focus attention on one component of the reaction and ask: Is that substance oxidized or reduced? Assigning oxidation numbers to the individual carbon atoms in a complex molecule can be difficult. Fortunately, there is another way to recognize oxidation–reduction reactions in organic chemistry.

Oxidation occurs when hydrogen atoms are removed from a carbon atom or when an oxygen atom is added to a carbon atom. Reduction occurs when hydrogen atoms are added to a carbon atom or when an oxygen atom is removed from a carbon atom.

TABLE 8.3

Typical Oxidation Numbers of Carbon

Functional Group	Example	Oxidation Number of Carbon in the Example
Alkane	CH_4	−4
Alkyl lithium	CH_3Li	−4
Alkene	$H_2C=CH_2$	−2
Alcohol	CH_3OH	−2
Ether	CH_3OCH_3	−2
Alkyl halide	CH_3Cl	−2
Amine	CH_3NH_2	−2
Alkyne	HC CH	−1
Aldehyde	H_2CO	0
Carboxylic acid	HCO_2H	2
Carbon dioxide	CO_2	4

An alkene is reduced, for example, when it reacts with hydrogen to form the corresponding alkane.

$$CH_2=CHCH_3 + H_2 \xrightarrow{Ni} CH_3CH_2CH_3 \tag{8.14}$$

The scheme that follows Equation 8.15 provides a useful guide to the oxidation–reduction reactions of organic compounds. Each of the arrows in this figure involves a two-electron oxidation of a carbon atom along the path toward carbon dioxide. A line is drawn through the first arrow, because it is impossible to achieve this transformation in a single step.

$$
\begin{array}{ccccccccc}
& & & & O & & O & & \\
& & & & \parallel & & \parallel & & \\
CH_4 & \not\longrightarrow & CH_3OH & \longrightarrow & HCH & \longrightarrow & HCOH & \longrightarrow & CO_2 \\
-4 & & -2 & & 0 & & +2 & & +4
\end{array}
\tag{8.15}
$$

8.2.4.2.1 Kinetics of Degradation

In real-time stability tests, a product is stored at recommended storage conditions and monitored for a period of time (t_{test}). The product will degrade below its specification, at some time, denoted t_s, and it must also be ensured that t_s is less than or equal to t_{test}. The estimated value of t_s can be obtained by modeling the degradation pattern. Good experimental design and practices are needed to minimize the risk of biases and reduce the amount of random error during data collection. Testing should be performed at time intervals that encompass the target shelf life and must be continued for a period after the product degrades below specification. It is also required that at least three lots of material be used in stability testing to capture lot-to-lot variation, which is an important source of product variability.

The true degradation pattern of a certain product, assuming that it degrades via a first-order reaction, can be described as follows:

$$D = \alpha \exp(-\delta t) \qquad (8.16)$$

The observed result (Y) of each has a random component ϕ associated with it, and a random experimental error, ε.

$$Y = D + \phi + \varepsilon = \alpha \exp(-\delta t) + \phi + \varepsilon \qquad (8.17)$$

Both α and δ represent the fixed parameters of the model that need to be estimated from the data, while ϕ and ε are assumed to be normally distributed, with mean $= 0$ and standard deviations of $\sigma\phi$ and $\sigma\varepsilon$, respectively. Equation 8.17 is a nonlinear mixed model.

Let C represent a critical level, where the essential performance characteristics of the product are within the specification. A product is considered to be stable when $Y \geq C$. The product is not stable when $Y < C$, while $Y < C$ occurs at t_s. The manufacturer determines the value of C. The estimated time during which the product is stable is calculated as:

$$t_s = \{\ln C - \ln a\}/{-}d \qquad (8.18)$$

where a and d are the estimated values of the intercept and the degradation rate. The standard error of the estimated time can be obtained from the Taylor series approximation method and is used to calculate confidence limits. The labeled shelf life of the product is the lower confidence limit of the estimated time.

In accelerated stability testing, a product is stored at elevated stress conditions. Degradation at recommended storage conditions could be predicted based on the degradation at each stress condition and known relationships between the acceleration factor and the degradation rate. A product may be released based on accelerated stability data, but the real-time testing must be done in parallel to confirm the shelf life prediction. Sometimes, the amount of error of the predicted stability is so large that the prediction itself is not useful. The experiments have to be designed carefully to reduce this error. It is recommended that several products should be stored at various acceleration levels to reduce prediction error. Increasing the number of levels is a good strategy for reducing the error.

Temperature is probably the most common acceleration factor used for chemicals, pharmaceuticals, and biological products, as its relationship with the degradation rate is well characterized by the Arrhenius equation. This equation describes a relationship between temperature and the degradation rate, as in Equation 8.19.

$$\delta = A\exp\left(\frac{-E_a}{RT}\right) \qquad (8.19)$$

where A is the Arrhenius factor, E_a is the activation energy, R is the gas constant, and T is the temperature.

This relationship can be used in accelerated stability studies when the following conditions are met:

- A zero- or first-order kinetic reaction takes place at each elevated temperature and at the recommended storage temperature.
- The same model is used to fit the degradation patterns at each temperature.

These requirements do not fully guarantee that the Arrhenius equation can be used to predict the degradation rate at the storage temperature, but they are a good start. The analytical accuracy should not be compromised during the course of the study to distinguish between the degradation rates at each temperature.

Temperature levels should be selected based on the nature of the product and the recommended storage temperature. The selected temperatures should stimulate relatively fast degradation and quick testing but not destroy the fundamental characteristics of the product. It is not reasonable to test at very high temperatures for a very short period of time, as the mechanisms of degradation at high temperatures may be very different than those at the recommended storage temperature. The adjacent levels should be chosen appropriately, so that degradation trends are larger than experimental variability.

The choice of levels depends on the nature of the product and analytical accuracy, but other practical implications also need to be considered. Testing should be performed at time intervals that encompass the target stability at each elevated temperature. Some data below C should be acquired, so that the degradation trend can be determined. Humidity and pH can be used along with temperature to accelerate degradation, but modeling of multifactor degradation is very complex.

Assuming that the degradation pattern follows a first-order reaction, as described in Equation 8.17, the Arrhenius equation (Equation 8.19) can be used to predict the degradation rate at the recommended storage temperature. First, an acceleration factor, l, is calculated as the ratio of the degradation rate at an elevated temperature to the degradation rate at the storage temperature. This ratio, which can be worked out easily from Equation 8.17, can be expressed as:

$$\lambda = \exp\left(\frac{E_a}{0.00199}\left(\frac{1}{T_s} - \frac{1}{T_e}\right)\right) \tag{8.20}$$

where T_e is the elevated temperature, and T_s is the storage temperature.

The true degradation pattern at the storage temperature can be expressed as:

$$D = \alpha \exp(-\delta \lambda t) \tag{8.21}$$

where λ is obtained from accelerated stability tests. The testing result (Y) will include random components representing a lot-to-lot variability and experimental error. Once the estimates of α and δ are obtained, stability time is calculated in a similar fashion as in real-time stability testing. Shelf life is the lower confidence limit of the estimated time.

Activation energy is usually estimated from the accelerated stability data. However, when the activation energy is known, the degradation rate at the storage temperature may be predicted from data collected at only one elevated temperature. This practice is sometimes preferred in the industry, as it reduces the size and time of accelerated stability tests. Experience indicates that some pharmaceutical analytes have activation energies in the range of 10–20 kcal/mol, but it is unlikely you will have precise information or be able to make assumptions about the activation energy of a certain product.

The bracket method is a straightforward application of the Arrhenius equation that can be used if the value of the activation energy is known. Assuming that the stability of a product at 50°C is 32 days, and it will be stored at 25°C, then, $t_e = 32$ days, $T_e = 273 + 50°C = 323$ K, and $T_s = 273 + 25°C = 298$ K. We know that activation energy is $E_a = 10$ kcal/mol. Stability at recommended storage temperature is calculated as:

$$t_s = \lambda t_e = \exp\left[\frac{E_a}{0.00199}\left(\frac{1}{T_s} - \frac{1}{T_e}\right)\right]$$

$$t_e = \exp\left[\frac{10}{0.00199}\left(\frac{1}{298} - \frac{1}{323}\right)\right](32) = 118 \text{ days}$$

(8.22)

Calculated stability is highly dependent on the value of the activation energy. A stability of 435 days results when $E_a = 20$ kcal/mol.

The bracket method should not be confused with bracketing, which is an experimental design that allows one to test a minimum number of samples at extremes of certain factors, such as strength, container size, and container fill. Bracketing assumes that the stability of any intermediate level is represented by the stability of the extremes, and testing at those extremes is performed at all time points.

The Q-rule states that the degradation rate decreases by a constant factor when temperature is lowered by certain degrees. The value of Q is typically set at two, three, or four. This factor is proportional to the temperature change Q_n, where n equals the temperature change in °C, divided by 10°C. As 10°C is the baseline temperature, the Q-rule is sometimes referred to as Q_{10}.

To illustrate the application of the Q-rule, let us assume that the stability of a product at 50°C is 32 days. The recommended storage temperature is 25°C, and $n = (50 - 25)/10 = 2.5$. Let us set an intermediate value of $Q = 3$. Thus, $Q_n = (3)2.5 = 15.6$. The predicted shelf life is 32 days $\times$ 15.6 = 500 days. This approach is more conservative when lower values of Q are used. Both Q-rule and the bracket methods are rough approximations of stability. They can be effectively used to plan elevated temperature levels and the duration of testing in the accelerated stability testing protocol.

Theoretically, the Arrhenius equation does not apply when more than one kind of molecule are involved in the reactions. However, if the degradation rate and temperature are linearly related, the prediction of shelf life can be approximated by the Arrhenius equation. In a polynomial model to fit the degradation,

$$D = \beta_0 + (\beta_1 + \beta_2 t)t$$

(8.23)

where β_0, β_1, and β_2 are the parameters of the second-degree polynomial, and t is the time. The degradation rate is a function of time, which is not constant in this case.

$$\delta = \beta_1 + \beta_2 t \tag{8.24}$$

Degradation at the storage temperature can be predicted from the degradation at elevated temperatures as:

$$D = \beta_0 + (\beta_1 + \beta_2 t)t\lambda \tag{8.25}$$

The acceleration factor, λ, is based on the Arrhenius equation. Statistical tests indicated that the use of this equation was appropriate in this case. Shelf life predictions were also verified by real-time stability testing results.

8.2.4.2.2 Similar Products

When most of the assumptions required to use the Arrhenius equation are not satisfied, comparisons with a product of a known stability are performed to assess shelf life. This approach requires having a similar product with a known shelf life to be used as a control. The new or test product is expected to demonstrate a similar behavior to the control, as they belong to the same family and have the same kinetics of degradation. Side-by-side testing of the control and test products at different elevated temperatures is then performed. It is necessary to assume that the same model can represent the degradation pattern at each elevated and storage temperature.

If the degradation patterns of the test and control samples at the same elevated temperatures are not statistically different, it can be assumed that they will degrade similarly at the storage temperatures. The closer the elevated temperatures are to the storage temperatures, the more confident we can be in making this statement. The experimental protocols used are similar to the protocols used with the Arrhenius equation. Degradation patterns of a family of products at certain elevated temperatures can be modeled and used to check the behavior of a new product that belongs to the family.

The complications in calculations arise mainly because of the degradation models that are usually nonlinear mixed models, where a lot-to-lot variability is the random component. Estimation of the parameters of the models is important for the accuracy of shelf life predictions. It is recommended to use the maximum likelihood (ML) approach to estimate these parameters. As no closed-form solutions for ML estimates exist, an iterative procedure is performed, starting with some initial values for the parameters and updating them until differences between consecutive iterations are minimal and the estimates converge to their final value. Initial values are usually chosen by experience. The closer these values are to the final values, the faster the model will converge. A suitable program is nonlinear mixed model procedure of statistical analysis system for data analysis (3). Values of the real-time stability model converge relatively quickly, while several initial values for the parameters of the accelerated model are tried before they converge. Statistical theory and the applicability of ML estimation are common in the literature, and many computer routines are available to facilitate data analysis. However, experience with the modeling and estimation processes is necessary, as any unexpected results must be interpreted appropriately. It is quite easy to get useless numbers from a computer run.

Owing to insufficient drug quantity, it will probably not be possible to construct a complete degradation profile during prenomination studies, but it should be possible to assess the stability of the candidate drug at a few pH values (acid, alkaline, and neutral) to establish the approximate stability of the compound with respect to hydrolysis. To accelerate the reaction, temperature elevation will probably be necessary to generate the data. Although it is difficult to assign a definite temperature for these studies, 50°C–90°C in the first instance is a reasonable compromise. This should be followed by extrapolation via the Arrhenius equation to 25°C. Hydrolytic stability of more than 100 days at 25°C should be taken as a goal of these studies. In terms of candidate drug selection, if all other factors are equal, the compound that is most stable should be the one taken forward into development.

Normally, the stability of solutions is assessed using HPLC to determine the amount of decomposition of a compound with time. However, microcalorimetry can determine decomposition reactions with an annual degradation rate of 0.03%, that is, a half-life of 2200 years. However, the nature and form of the reaction and the calorimetric output need to be assessed extremely carefully, and this can require careful workup of the technique to bring it into routine use.

8.2.4.2.3 Solid-State Stability

The solid-state degradation of candidate drugs, particularly in the candidate selection phase, is an important consideration, as degradation rates as slow as 0.5% per year at 25°C may affect the development of the compound. Solid-state degradation reactions can be complex and can involve both oxidation and hydrolysis together. As with solutions, solids can also exhibit instability owing to the effects of light. This is further complicated by the fact that in solids, these reactions usually occur only on the surface. Three phases have been identified in solid-state degradation: the lag, acceleration, and deceleration phases. Depending on the conditions of temperature and the humidity to which the solid is exposed, the acceleration phase may follow zero, first, or higher order. A general equation has been proposed to describe the process:

$$\frac{d[D]}{dt} = k\alpha 1 - x(1-\alpha)1 - y \tag{8.26}$$

where a is the fraction of the reaction that has occurred at time t, such that $\alpha = 0$ when $t = 0$, and $a = 1$ at $t = \infty$; k is the rate constant; and x and y are constants, characteristic of the reaction rate law, that is, when $x = y = 1$, the reaction is of zero order. If, however, $x = 1$ and $y = 0$, the reaction is of first order. If x and y have fractional values, the reaction will be autocatalytic.

To accelerate the degradation so that the amount degraded becomes quantifiable in a typical calculation using the Arrhenius equation, the assumption made during these studies is that the degradation mechanism at a higher temperature is the same as that at 25°C. However, this need not be the case, and a nonlinear Arrhenius plot may be an indication of change of mechanism as the temperature is increased. Furthermore, many compounds are hydrates that dehydrate at a higher temperature, which can change the degradation mechanism in the solid state.

The effect of moisture uptake in solid stability state depends on the extent of available water. Where the quantity is limited, water is used up during the degradation reaction, and there is not enough present to degrade the compound completely. Where there is adequate water, the degradation can be significant, and where there is excess water, that is, greater than what is needed to dissolve the drug, solution degradation kinetics is observed.

With regard to crystallinity, it should be noted that amorphous materials are generally less stable than the corresponding crystalline forms. Often, amorphous phases crystallize on exposure to moisture. In amorphous solids, the net effect of water sorption is to lower the glass transition temperature, T_g, and hence plasticize the material. In turn, this increases the molecular mobility and, therefore, the chemical reactivity.

In prenomination studies, a useful protocol to assess the effects of these factors is as follows: The compound is accurately weighed into each of six open glass vials. These are then placed (in duplicate if possible) under the following conditions: light stress (5000 lux, 25°C), 40°C/75% relative humidity (RH), and 30°C/60% RH. Typically, the sample would be sampled, as necessary, up to 3 months to determine its stability. After each time point, all samples are assessed visually and with a suitable HPLC (or liquid chromatography tandem mass spectroscopy method that can detect degradation products). In addition, differential scanning calorimetry and X-ray powder diffraction can be used to detect phase changes.

8.2.4.2.4 Photostability

A wide range of drug types undergo photochemical degradation. Theoretically, candidate drugs with absorption maxima greater than 280 nm may decompose in sunlight. However, instability due to light will probably be a problem only if the drug significantly absorbs light with a wavelength greater than 330 nm and, even then, only if the reaction proceeds at a significant rate. Light instability is a problem in both the solid and solution states, and formulations therefore need to be designed to protect the compound from its deleterious effects. There are a number of chemical groups that might be expected to give rise to decomposition. These include the carbonyl group, the nitroaromatic group, the N-oxide group, the C=C bond, the aryl chloride group, groups with a weak C—H bond, sulfides, alkenes, polyenes, and phenols. The first evidence that compounds are light-sensitive is usually discovered during lead optimization studies. Thus, candidate drugs should be assessed in the prenomination phase with respect to light stability, to alert the formulation team whether special measures are needed to protect the drug from light. Indeed, this could be used as a selection criterion in many cases to reject unsuitable candidate drugs.

The ICH guideline on photostability testing is a good document to follow, wherein it is suggested that photostability testing should consist of forced degradation and confirmatory testing. The forced degradation experiments can involve the candidate drug alone, in solution, or in suspension, using exposure conditions that reflect the nature of the compound and the intensity of the light sources used. The samples are then analyzed at various time points by using appropriate techniques (e.g., HPLC). In addition, changes in physical properties, such as appearance, clarity, or color, should be noted. Confirmatory studies involve exposing the compound to light whose total output is not less than 1.2 million lux hours and has a near-UV energy of not less than 200 watt h/m^2. Light sources for testing photostability include artificial daylight tubes, xenon lamps, tungsten–mercury lamps, laboratory light, and natural light. Instruments from Thermometric (4) are useful in measuring solid-state stability. Up to four independent calorimeter units can be used simultaneously with thermal activity monitor (TAM) III. A unit can be a 4-mL nanocalorimeter for measurements that require very high sensitivity, a 20-mL standard microcalorimeter, a multicalorimeter consisting of six minicalorimeters, or the semi-adiabatic solution calorimeter. The multicalorimeter increases sample throughput considerably and is used for applications where microwatt, rather than nanowatt, sensitivity is sufficient. TAM III also exists in a 48-channel version for screening applications or, in general, when high sample throughput is required. TAM III can be operated in isothermal, step-isothermal, or temperature scanning mode. The isothermal mode is the classical mode for microcalorimetric experiments. In the isothermal mode, the liquid thermostat is maintained at a constant temperature (± 50 μK). Any heat generated or absorbed by the sample as a consequence of any chemical or physical process is measured continuously as a function of time. Step-isothermal mode is used to perform isothermal experiments at a number of temperatures in one single experiment. This is of particular interest for extracting temperature-dependent kinetic behavior for different kinds of processes. In the scanning mode, the temperature is scanned linearly over a certain interval. As the scanning rate is very slow, the sample can be considered to be in virtual thermal, chemical, and physical equilibria during measurement. For sample handling, a variety of ampoules and microreaction systems can be inserted in the calorimetric units, the type of which is determined by the experimental application.

The terahertz pulsed imaging (TPI)™ spectra 1000 system exploits the spectroscopic information within each TPI™ waveform to determine the chemical composition and the structural features of a sample (5) by using terahertz technology. Terahertz data are complementary to Raman spectroscopy. It also provides information on both high-frequency (just below IR) and low-frequency vibrational modes; the latter are difficult to assess in Raman spectroscopy, owing to the proximity to the visible excitation line. Terahertz spectral interpretation and instrumentation are similar to basic IR and are therefore easy to understand. The sample preparation techniques are the same as those used in IR and Raman spectroscopy. The unique spectral imaging characteristics of combining TPI and terahertz pulsed spectroscopy (TPS) can be used to investigate the applications of proteomics in the pharmaceutical industry. The TPI™ spectra 1000 can assist pharmaceutical companies in the rapid characterization of the stability and polymorphic forms of drugs. Many drug molecules after purification can crystallize in many different forms. These are known as polymorphs. Terahertz technology provides a rapid technique to identify different polymorphs.

In terms of the kinetics, light degradation in dilute solution is of first order; however, in more concentrated solutions, decomposition approaches pseudo-zero order. The reason for this is that as the solution becomes more concentrated, degradation becomes limited owing to the limited number of incident quanta and quenching reactions between the molecules. It should be noted that ionizable compounds, for example, ciprofloxacin, can show large differences in photostability between the ionized and unionized forms.

8.2.5 Regulatory Consideration in Stability Testing

The purpose of stability testing is to provide evidence on how the quality of a drug substance or drug product varies with time under the influence of a variety of environmental factors, such as temperature, humidity, and light, and to establish a retest period for the drug substance or a shelf life for the drug product and recommended storage conditions.

The choice of test conditions defined in this guidance is based on an analysis of the effects of climatic conditions in the three regions of the European Union, Japan, and the United States. The mean kinetic temperature in any part of the world can be derived from climatic data, and the world can be divided into four climatic zones, I–IV. This guidance addresses climatic zones I and II. The principle has been established that stability information generated in any one of the three regions of the European Union, Japan, and the United States would be mutually acceptable to the other two regions, provided that the information is consistent with this guidance and the labeling is in accordance with the national/regional requirements. Information on the stability of the drug substance is an integral part of the systematic approach to stability evaluation.

8.2.5.1 Stress Testing

Stress testing of the drug substance can help to identify the likely degradation products, which can, in turn, help to establish the degradation pathways and the intrinsic stability of the molecule and validate the stability, indicating the power of the analytical procedures used. The nature of the stress testing will depend on the individual drug substance and the type of the drug product involved.

Stress testing is likely to be carried out on a single batch of the drug substance. The testing should include the effect of temperatures (in 10°C increments [e.g., 50°C–60°C] above that for accelerated testing), humidity (e.g., 75% RH or greater), oxidation, and photolysis, where appropriate, on the drug substance. The testing should also evaluate the susceptibility of the drug substance to hydrolysis across a wide range of pH values when in solution or suspension. Photostability testing should be an integral part of stress testing. The standard conditions for photostability testing are described in ICH *Q1B Photostability Testing of New Drug Substances and Products.*

Examination of degradation products under stress conditions is useful in establishing degradation pathways and developing and validating suitable analytical procedures. However, such examination may not be necessary for certain degradation products if it has been demonstrated that they are not formed under accelerated or long-term storage conditions.

Results from these studies will form an integral part of the information provided to regulatory authorities.

8.2.5.2 Selection of Batches

Data from formal stability studies should be provided on at least three primary batches of the drug substance. The batches should be manufactured to a minimum of pilot scale by the same synthetic route as production batches and using a method of manufacture and procedure that simulates the final process to be used for production batches. The overall quality of the batches of drug substance placed on formal stability studies should be representative of the quality of the material to be made on a production scale. Other supporting data can be provided.

8.2.5.3 Container Closure System

The stability studies should be conducted on the drug substance packaged in a container closure system that is the same as or simulates the packaging proposed for storage and distribution.

8.2.5.4 Specifications

Specification, which is a list of tests, references to analytical procedures, and proposed acceptance criteria, is addressed in ICH *Q6A Specifications: Test Procedures and Acceptance Criteria for New Drug Substances and New Drug Products: Chemical Substances* and *Q6B Specifications: Test Procedures and Acceptance Criteria for New Drug Substances and New Drug Products: Biotechnological/Biological Products.* In addition, specification for degradation products in a drug substance is discussed in ICH *Q3A Impurities in New Drug Substances.*

Stability studies should include testing of those attributes of the drug substance that are susceptible to change during storage and are likely to influence quality, safety, and/or efficacy. The testing should cover, as appropriate, the physical, chemical, biological, and microbiological attributes. Validated stability-indicating analytical procedures should be applied. Whether and to what extent replication should be performed should depend on the results from validation studies.

8.2.5.5 Testing Frequency

For the long-term studies, frequency of testing should be sufficient to establish the stability profile of the drug substance. For drug substances with a proposed retest period of at least 12 months, the frequency of testing at the long-term storage condition should normally be every 3 months over the first year, every 6 months over the second year, and annually thereafter throughout the proposed retest period.

At the accelerated storage condition, a minimum of three time points, including the initial and final time points (e.g., 0, 3, and 6 months), from a 6-month study is recommended. Where an expectation (based on development experience) exists such that the results from accelerated studies are likely to approach significant change criteria, increased testing should be conducted either by adding samples at the final time point or by including a fourth time point in the study design.

When testing at the intermediate storage condition is called for as a result of significant change at the accelerated storage condition, a minimum of four time points, including the initial and final time points (e.g., 0, 6, 9, and 12 months), from a 12 month study is recommended.

8.2.5.5.1 Storage Conditions

In general, a drug substance should be evaluated under the storage conditions (with appropriate tolerances) that test its thermal stability and, if applicable, its sensitivity to moisture. The storage conditions and the duration of studies chosen should be sufficient to cover storage, shipment, and subsequent use.

TABLE 8.4

General Case of Study, Storage Condition, and Time Covered

Study	Storage Condition	Minimum Time Period Covered by Data at Submission
Long-term[a]	25°C ± 2°C/60% RH ± 5% RH or 30°C ± 2°C/65% RH ± 5% RH	12 months
Intermediate[b]	30°C ± 2°C/65% RH ± 5% RH	6 months
Accelerated	40°C ± 2°C/75% RH ± 5% RH	6 months

[a] It is up to the applicant to decide whether long-term stability studies are performed at 25°C ± 2°C/60% RH ± 5% RH or 30°C ± 2°C/65% RH ± 5% RH.

[b] If 30°C ± 2°C/65% RH ± 5% RH is the long-term condition, there is no intermediate condition.

The long-term testing should cover a minimum of 12 months' duration on at least three primary batches at the time of submission and should be continued for a period of time sufficient to cover the proposed retest period. Additional data accumulated during the assessment period of the registration application should be submitted to the authorities, if requested. Data from the accelerated storage condition and, if appropriate, from the intermediate storage condition can be used to evaluate the effect of short-term excursions outside the label storage conditions (for example, it might occur during shipping).

Long-term, accelerated, and, where appropriate, intermediate storage conditions for drug substances are detailed in Table 8.4. The general case should apply if the drug substance is not specifically covered by a subsequent section. Alternative storage conditions can be used if justified (Table 8.4).

If long-term studies are conducted at 25°C ± 2°C/60% RH ± 5% RH and *significant change* occurs at any time during the 6 months' testing at the accelerated storage condition, additional testing at the intermediate storage condition should be conducted and evaluated against significant change criteria. Testing at the intermediate storage condition should include all tests, unless otherwise justified. The initial application should include a minimum of 6 months' data from a 12-month study at the intermediate storage condition. *Significant change* for a drug substance is defined as failure to meet its specification (Table 8.5).

Data from refrigerated storage should be assessed according to the evaluation section of this guidance, except where explicitly noted in Table 8.6.

If significant change occurs between 3 months' and 6 months' testing at the accelerated storage condition, the proposed retest period should be based on the real-time data available during the long-term storage condition.

If significant change occurs within the first 3 months' testing at the accelerated storage condition, a discussion should be provided to address the effect of short-term excursions outside the label storage condition (e.g., during shipping or handling). This discussion can be supported, if appropriate, by further testing on a single batch of the drug substance for a period shorter than 3 months, but with more frequent testing than usual. It is considered unnecessary to continue to test

TABLE 8.5

Storage and Minimum Time Covered for Drug Substances Intended for Storage in a
Refrigerator

Study	Storage Condition	Minimum Time Period Covered by Data at Submission
Long-term	5°C ± 3°C	12 months
Accelerated	25°C ± 2°C/60% RH ± 5% RH	6 months

TABLE 8.6

Storage Conditions and Minimum Time for Drug Substances Intended for Storage in a
Freezer

Study	Storage Condition	Minimum Time Period Covered by Data at Submission
Long-term	−20°C ± 5°C	12 months

a drug substance through 6 months when a significant change has occurred within
the first 3 months.

For drug substances intended for storage in a freezer, the retest period should
be based on the real-time data obtained at the long-term storage condition. In the
absence of an accelerated storage condition for drug substances intended to be stored
in a freezer, testing on a single batch at an elevated temperature (e.g., 5°C ± 3°C and
25°C ± 2°C) for an appropriate time period should be conducted to address the effect
of short-term excursions outside the proposed label storage condition (e.g., during
shipping or handling). Drug substances intended for storage below −20°C should be
treated on a case-by-case basis.

8.2.5.6 Stability Commitment

When available long-term stability data on primary batches do not cover the proposed
retest period granted at the time of approval, a commitment should be made to continue the stability studies postapproval to firmly establish the retest period.

Where the submission includes long-term stability data on three production batches
covering the proposed retest period, a postapproval commitment is considered unnecessary. Otherwise, one of the following commitments should be made:

- If the submission includes data from stability studies on at least three production batches, a commitment should be made to continue these studies
  through the proposed retest period.
- If the submission includes data from stability studies on fewer than three
  production batches, a commitment should be made to continue these studies through the proposed retest period and to place additional production

batches, to a total of at least three, on long-term stability studies through the proposed retest period.

- If the submission does not include stability data on production batches, a commitment should be made to place the first three production batches on long-term stability studies through the proposed retest period.

The stability protocol used for long-term studies for the stability commitment should be the same as that for the primary batches, unless otherwise scientifically justified.

8.2.5.6.1 Evaluation

The purpose of the stability study is to establish, based on testing a minimum of three batches of the drug substance and evaluating the stability information (including, as appropriate, the results of the physical, chemical, biological, and microbiological tests), a retest period applicable to all future batches of the drug substance manufactured under similar circumstances. The degree of variability of individual batches affects the confidence that a future production batch will remain within specification throughout the assigned retest period.

The data may show very little degradation and so little variability that it is apparent from looking at the data that the requested retest period will be granted. Under these circumstances, it is normally unnecessary to go through the formal statistical analysis; providing a justification for the omission should be sufficient.

An approach for analyzing the data on a quantitative attribute that is expected to change with time is to determine the time at which the 95%, one-sided confidence limit for the mean curve intersects the acceptance criterion. If the analysis shows that the batch-to-batch variability is small, it is advantageous to combine the data into one overall estimate. This can be done by applying appropriate statistical tests (e.g., P values for the level of significance of rejection of >0.25) to the slopes of the regression lines and zero time intercepts for the individual batches. If it is inappropriate to combine data from several batches, the overall retest period should be based on the minimum time for which a batch can be expected to remain within the acceptance criteria.

The nature of any degradation relationship will determine whether the data should be transformed for linear regression analysis. Usually, the relationship can be represented by a linear, quadratic, or cubic function on an arithmetic or logarithmic scale. Statistical methods should be employed to test the goodness of fit of the data on all batches and combined batches (where appropriate) to the assumed degradation line or curve.

Limited extrapolation of the real-time data from the long-term storage condition beyond the observed range to extend the retest period can be undertaken at the approval time, if justified. This justification should be based, for example, on what is known about the mechanism of degradation, the results of testing under accelerated conditions, the goodness of fit of any mathematical model, batch size, and/or existence of supporting stability data. However, this extrapolation assumes that the same degradation relationship will continue to apply beyond the observed data.

Any evaluation should cover not only the assay but also the levels of degradation products and other appropriate attributes.

8.2.5.7 Statements/Labeling

A storage statement should be established for the labeling, in accordance with relevant national and/or regional requirements. The statement should be based on the stability evaluation of the drug substance. Where applicable, specific instructions should be provided, particularly for drug substances that cannot tolerate freezing. Terms such as *ambient conditions* and *room temperature* should be avoided.

A retest period should be derived from the stability information, and a retest date should be displayed on the container label, if appropriate (Table 8.7).

If long-term studies are conducted at 25°C ± 2°C/60% RH ± 5% RH and *significant change* occurs at any time during 6 months' testing at the accelerated storage condition, additional testing at the intermediate storage condition should be conducted and evaluated against significant change criteria. The initial application should include a minimum of 6 months' data from a 12-month study at the intermediate storage condition.

In general, *significant change* for a drug product is defined as one or more of the following (as appropriate for the dosage form):

- A 5% change in assay from its initial value or failure to meet the acceptance criteria for potency when using biological or immunological procedures.
- Any degradation product exceeding its acceptance criterion.
- Failure to meet the acceptance criteria for appearance, physical attributes, and functionality test (e.g., color, phase separation, resuspendibility, caking, hardness, and dose delivery per actuation). However, some changes in physical attributes (e.g., softening of suppositories and melting of creams) may be expected under accelerated conditions.
- Failure to meet the acceptance criterion for pH.
- Failure to meet the acceptance criteria for dissolution for 12 dosage units.

8.2.5.7.1 Photostability Testing

The *ICH Harmonized Tripartite Guideline on Stability Testing of New Drug Substances* notes that light testing should be an integral part of stress testing.

TABLE 8.7

Retest Study, Storage Condition, and Minimum Time Period

Study	Storage Condition	Minimum Time Period Covered by Data at Submission
Long-term[a]	25°C ± 2°C/60% RH ± 5% RH	12 months
	or	
	30°C ± 2°C/65% RH ± 5% RH	
Intermediate[b]	30°C ± 2°C/65% RH ± 5% RH	6 months
Accelerated	40°C ± 2°C/75% RH ± 5% RH	6 months

[a] It is up to the applicant to decide whether long-term stability studies are performed at 25°C ± 2°C/60% RH ± 5% RH or 30°C ± 2°C/65% RH ± 5% RH.

[b] If 30°C ± 2°C/65% RH ± 5% RH is the long-term condition, there is no intermediate condition.

The intrinsic photostability characteristics of new drug substances should be evaluated to demonstrate that, as appropriate, light exposure does not result in unacceptable change. Normally, photostability testing is carried out on a single batch of material. Under some circumstances, these studies should be repeated if certain variations and changes are made to the product (e.g., formulation and packaging). Whether these studies should be repeated depends on the photostability characteristics determined at the time of initial filing and the type of variation and/or change made.

A systematic approach to photostability testing is recommended, covering, as appropriate, studies such as light sources and the procedures used. The light sources described next may be used for photostability testing, while maintaining the temperature to avoid these effects to confound light effects. Any light source that is designed to produce an output similar to the D65/ID65 emission standard, such as an artificial daylight fluorescent lamp combining visible (VIS) and UV outputs, xenon, or metal halide lamp can be used. D65 is the internationally recognized standard for outdoor daylight, as defined in ISO 10977 (1993). ID65 is the equivalent indoor indirect daylight standard. For a light source emitting a significant radiation below 320 nm, an appropriate filter(s) may be fitted to eliminate such radiation. An alternate source of light is a cool white fluorescent lamp designed to produce an output similar to that specified in ISO 10977 (1993) and a near-UV fluorescent lamp having a spectral distribution from 320 nm to 400 nm, with a maximum energy emission between 350 nm and 370 nm; a significant proportion of UV should be in both bands of 320–360 nm and 360–400 nm.

For confirmatory studies, samples should be exposed to light providing an overall illumination of not less than 1.2 million lux hours and an integrated near-UV energy of not less than 200 watt h/m^2 to allow direct comparisons to be made between the drug substance and the drug product. Samples may be exposed side by side with a validated chemical actinometric system to ensure that the specified light exposure is obtained or for the appropriate duration of time when conditions have been monitored using calibrated radiometers/lux meters. If protected samples (e.g., wrapped in aluminum foil) are used as dark controls to evaluate the contribution of thermally induced change to the total observed change, these should be placed alongside the authentic sample.

The photostability testing should consist of two parts: forced degradation testing and confirmatory testing. The purpose of forced degradation testing studies is to evaluate the overall photosensitivity of the material for method development purposes and/or degradation pathway elucidation. This testing may involve the drug substance alone and/or in simple solutions/suspensions to validate the analytical procedures. In these studies, the samples should be in chemically inert and transparent containers. In these forced degradation studies, a variety of exposure conditions may be used, depending on the photosensitivity of the drug substance involved and the intensity of the light sources used. For development and validation purposes, it is appropriate to limit exposure and end the studies if extensive decomposition occurs. For photostable materials, studies may be terminated after an appropriate exposure level has been used. The design of these experiments is left to the applicant's discretion; however, the exposure levels used should be justified.

Under forced conditions, decomposition products that are unlikely to be formed under the conditions used for confirmatory studies may be observed. This information may be useful in developing and validating suitable analytical methods.

If, in practice, it has been demonstrated that they are not formed in the confirmatory studies, these degradation products need not be examined further. Confirmatory studies should then be undertaken to provide the information necessary for handling, packaging, and labeling. Normally, only one batch of drug substance is tested during the development phase, and then, the photostability characteristics should be confirmed on a single batch selected, as described in the parent guideline, if the drug is clearly photostable or photolabile. If the results of the confirmatory study are equivocal, testing of up to two additional batches should be conducted. Samples should be selected as described in the parent guideline.

Care should be taken to ensure that the physical characteristics of the samples under test are taken into account and efforts, such as cooling and/or placing the samples in sealed containers, should be made to ensure that the effects of the changes in physical states, such as sublimation, evaporation, and melting, are minimized. All such precautions should be chosen to provide minimal interference with the exposure of samples under test. Possible interactions between the samples and any material used for containers or for general protection of the sample should also be considered and eliminated wherever not relevant to the test being carried out.

As a direct challenge for samples of solid drug substances, an appropriate amount of sample should be taken and placed in a suitable glass or plastic dish and protected with a suitable transparent cover, if considered necessary. Solid drug substances should be spread across the container to give a thickness of typically not more than 3 mL. Drug substances that are liquids should be exposed in chemically inert and transparent containers.

At the end of the exposure period, the samples should be examined for any changes in physical properties (e.g., appearance, clarity, or color of the solution) and for assay and degradants by a method suitably validated for products likely to arise from photochemical degradation processes. Where solid drug substance samples are involved, sampling should ensure that a representative portion is used in individual tests. Similar sampling considerations, such as homogenization of the entire sample, apply to other materials that may not be homogeneous after exposure. The analysis of the exposed sample should be performed concomitantly with that of any protected samples used as dark control if these are used in the test.

The forced degradation studies should be designed to provide suitable information to develop and validate test methods for the confirmatory studies. These test methods should be capable of resolving and detecting photolytic degradants that appear during the confirmatory studies. When evaluating the results of these studies, it is important to recognize that they form part of the stress testing and are not therefore designed to establish qualitative or quantitative limits for change.

The confirmatory studies should identify precautionary measures needed in the manufacturing or formulation of the drug product and whether light-resistant packaging is needed. When evaluating the results of confirmatory studies to determine whether change due to exposure to light is acceptable, it is important to consider the results from other formal stability studies in order to ensure that the drug will be within the justified limits at the time of use.

8.2.5.7.2 Bracketing

For the study of drug substances, matrixing is of limited utility, and bracketing is generally not applicable.

8.3 Impurities

Impurities can be classified into the following categories:

- Organic impurities (process- and drug-related)
- Inorganic impurities
- Residual solvents

Organic impurities can arise during the manufacturing process and/or storage of the new drug substance. They can be identified or unidentified, volatile or nonvolatile, and include the following:

- Starting materials
- By-products
- Intermediates
- Degradation products
- Reagents, ligands, and catalysts

There is a need to summarize the actual and potential impurities most likely to arise during the synthesis, purification, and storage of a new drug substance. This summary should be based on sound scientific appraisal of the chemical reactions involved in the synthesis, impurities associated with raw materials that could contribute to the impurity profile of the new drug substance, and the possible degradation products. This discussion can be limited to those impurities that might reasonably be expected based on the knowledge of the chemical reactions and the conditions involved.

In addition, the applicant should summarize the laboratory studies conducted to detect impurities in the new drug substance. This summary should include test results of batches manufactured during the development process and of batches from the proposed commercial process, as well as the results of stress testing (see ICH Q1A(R) on stability) used to identify potential impurities that arise during storage. The impurity profile of the drug substance batches intended for marketing should be compared with those used in development, and any differences should be discussed.

The studies conducted to characterize the structure of actual impurities present in a new drug substance at a level greater than the identification threshold calculated using the response factor of the drug substance are described separately. Note that any impurity at a level greater than the identification threshold in any batch manufactured by the proposed commercial process should be identified. In addition, any degradation product observed in stability studies at recommended storage conditions at a level greater than the identification threshold should be identified. When identification of an impurity is not feasible, a summary of the laboratory studies demonstrating the unsuccessful effort should be included in the application. Where attempts have been made to identify the impurities present at levels of not more than the identification thresholds, it is also useful to report the results of these studies.

Identification of impurities present at an apparent level of not more than the identification threshold is generally not considered necessary. However, analytical procedures should be developed for those potential impurities that are expected to be unusually potent, producing toxic or pharmacological effects at a level not more than the identification threshold. All impurities described as follows should be qualified:

- Each specified, unidentified impurity
- Any unspecified impurity with an acceptance criterion of not more than the identification threshold
- Total impurities

Inorganic impurities can result from the manufacturing process. They are normally known and identified and include the following:

- Reagents, ligands, and catalysts
- Heavy metals or other residual metals
- Inorganic salts
- Other materials (e.g., filter aids and charcoal)

Inorganic impurities are normally detected and quantified using pharmacopoeial or other appropriate procedures. Carryover of catalysts to a new drug substance should be evaluated during development. The need for the inclusion or exclusion of inorganic impurities in a new drug substance specification should be discussed. Acceptance criteria should be based on pharmacopoeial standards or known safety data.

Solvents are inorganic or organic liquids used as vehicles for the preparation of solutions or suspensions in the synthesis of a new drug substance. As these are generally of known toxicity, the selection of appropriate controls is easily accomplished (see ICH Q3C on Residual Solvents). The control of residues of the solvents used in the manufacturing process for a new drug substance should be discussed and presented according to ICH *Q3C Impurities: Residual Solvents.*

A registration application should include documented evidence that the analytical procedures are validated and suitable for the detection and quantification of impurities (see ICH Q2A and Q2B on Analytical Validation). Technical factors (e.g., manufacturing capability and control methodology) can be considered as part of the justification for the selection of alternative thresholds based on manufacturing experience with the proposed commercial process. The use of two decimal places for thresholds does not necessarily reflect the precision of the analytical procedure used for routine quality control (QC) purposes. Thus, the use of lower-precision techniques (e.g., thin-layer chromatography) can be appropriate where justified and appropriately validated. Differences in the analytical procedures used during development and those proposed for the commercial product should be discussed in the registration application. The quantification limit for the analytical procedure should be not more than the reporting threshold.

Organic impurity levels can be measured by a variety of techniques, including those that compare an analytical response of an impurity with that of an appropriate reference standard or with the response of the new drug substance itself.

Reference standards used in the analytical procedures for control of impurities should be evaluated and characterized according to their intended uses. The drug substance can be used as a standard to estimate the levels of impurities. In cases where the response factors of a drug substance and the relevant impurity are not close, this practice can still be appropriate, provided a correction factor is applied or the impurities are, in fact, being overestimated. Acceptance criteria and analytical procedures used to estimate the identified or unidentified impurities can be based on analytical assumptions (e.g., equivalent detector response). These assumptions should be discussed in registration applications.

The specification for a new drug substance should include a list of impurities. Stability studies, chemical development studies, and routine batch analyses can be used to predict those impurities that are likely to occur in the commercial product. The selection of impurities in a new drug substance specification should be based on the impurities found in batches manufactured by the proposed commercial process. Those individual impurities with specific acceptance criteria included in the specification for a new drug substance are referred to as *specified impurities* in this guidance. Specified impurities can be identified or unidentified.

A rationale for the inclusion or exclusion of impurities in a specification should be presented. The rationale should include a discussion of the impurity profiles observed in the safety and clinical development batches, together with a consideration of the impurity profile of batches manufactured by the proposed commercial process. Specified, identified impurities should be included, along with the specified, unidentified impurities estimated to be present at a level greater than the identification threshold given. For the impurities known to be unusually potent or that produce toxic or unexpected pharmacological effects, the quantification/detection limit of the analytical procedures should be commensurate with the level at which the impurities should be controlled. For the unidentified impurities, the procedure used and the assumptions made in establishing the level of the impurity should be stated clearly. Specified, unidentified impurities should be referred to by an appropriate qualitative analytical descriptive label (e.g., "unidentified A" and "unidentified with relative retention of 0.9"). A general acceptance criterion of not more than the identification threshold for any unspecified impurity and an acceptance criterion for total impurities should be included.

Acceptance criteria should be set no higher than the level that can be justified by the safety data and should be consistent with the level achievable by the manufacturing process and the analytical capability. Where there is no safety concern, impurity acceptance criteria should be based on the data generated on batches of a new drug substance manufactured by the proposed commercial process, allowing sufficient latitude to deal with normal manufacturing and analytical variations and the stability characteristics of the new drug substance. Although normal manufacturing variations are expected, significant variation in batch-to-batch impurity levels can indicate that the manufacturing process of the new drug substance is not adequately controlled and validated (see ICH Q6A guidance on specifications, decision tree #1, for establishing an acceptance criterion for a specified impurity in a new drug substance). The use of two decimal places for thresholds does not necessarily indicate the precision of the acceptance criteria for the specified impurities and total impurities.

Qualification is the process of acquiring and evaluating the data that establishes the biological safety of an individual impurity or a given impurity profile at the level(s) specified. The applicant should provide a rationale for establishing impurity acceptance criteria that include safety considerations. The level of any impurity present in a new drug substance that has been adequately tested in safety and/or clinical studies would be considered qualified. The impurities that are also significant metabolites present in animal and/or human studies are generally considered qualified. A level of a qualified impurity higher than that present in a new drug substance can also be justified based on an analysis of the actual amount of impurity administered in previous relevant safety studies.

If data are unavailable to qualify the proposed acceptance criterion of an impurity, studies to obtain such data can be appropriate when the usual qualification thresholds given are exceeded.

Higher or lower thresholds for the qualification of impurities can be appropriate for some individual drugs based on the scientific rationale and level of concern, including drug class effects and clinical experience. For example, qualification can be especially important when there is evidence that such impurities in certain drugs or therapeutic classes have previously been associated with adverse reactions in patients. In these instances, a lower qualification threshold can be appropriate. Conversely, a higher qualification threshold can be appropriate for individual drugs when the level of concern for safety is less than the usual, based on similar considerations (e.g., patient population, drug class effects, and clinical considerations). Proposals for alternative thresholds would be considered on a case-by-case basis.

The "decision tree for identification and qualification" (Scheme 8.8) describes considerations for the qualification of impurities when thresholds are exceeded. In some cases, decreasing the level of impurity to not more than the threshold can be simpler than providing the safety data. Alternatively, adequate data could be available in the scientific literature to qualify an impurity. If neither is the case, additional safety testing should be considered. The studies considered appropriate to qualify an impurity will depend on a number of factors, including the patient population, daily dose, and the route and duration of drug administration. Such studies can be conducted on the new drug substance containing the impurities to be controlled; however, studies using isolated impurities can sometimes be appropriate.

Although this guidance is not intended to apply during the clinical research stage of development, in the later stages of development, the thresholds in this guidance can be useful in evaluating new impurities observed in drug substance batches prepared by the proposed commercial process. Any new impurity observed in later stages of development should be identified if its level is greater than the identification threshold. Similarly, the qualification of the impurity should be considered if its level is greater than the qualification threshold (Table 8.8). Safety assessment studies to qualify an impurity should compare the new drug substance containing a representative amount of the new impurity with previously qualified material. Safety assessment studies using a sample of the isolated impurity can also be considered.

If considered desirable, a minimum screen (e.g., genotoxic potential) should be conducted. A study to detect point mutations and one to detect chromosomal aberrations, both in vitro, are considered an appropriate minimum screen. If general toxicity studies are desirable, one or more studies should be designed to allow comparison of unqualified and qualified materials. The study duration should be based on the

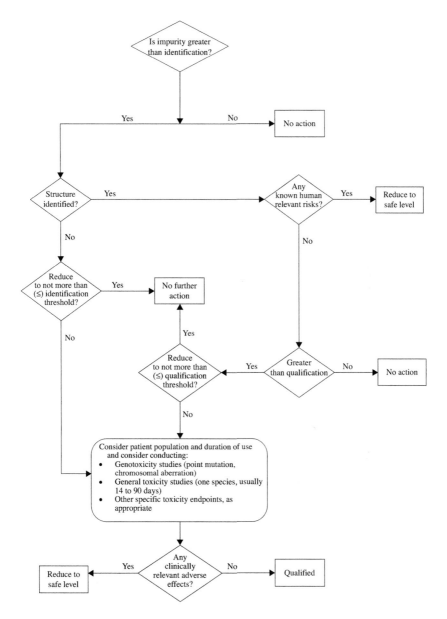

SCHEME 8.8 Decision tree for impurities in drug substances. (Courtesy of Pharmquest Corporation, Mountain View, CA.)

available relevant information and performed in the species most likely to maximize the potential to detect the toxicity of an impurity. On a case-by-case basis, single-dose studies can be appropriate, especially for single-dose drugs. In general, a minimum duration of 14 days and a maximum duration of 90 days would be considered appropriate. Lower thresholds can be appropriate if the impurity is unusually toxic.

TABLE 8.8

Thresholds of Impurities

Maximum Daily Dose[a]	Reporting Threshold[b,c]	Identification Threshold[c]	Qualification Threshold[c]
≤2 g/day	0.05%	0.10% or 1.0 mg/day intake (whichever is lower)	0.15% or 1.0 mg/day intake (whichever is lower)
>2 g/day	0.03%	0.05%	0.05%

[a] The amount of drug substance administered per day.
[b] Higher reporting thresholds should be scientifically justified.
[c] Lower thresholds can be appropriate if the impurity is unusually toxic.

For example, does known safety data for this impurity or its structural class preclude human exposure at the concentration present?

8.3.1 Good Manufacturing Practice

The term *manufacturing* is defined as one that includes all operations of receipt of materials, production, packaging, repackaging, labeling, relabeling, QC, release, storage, and distribution of active pharmaceutical ingredients (APIs) and the related controls. An API starting material is a raw material, an intermediate, or an API that is used in the production of an API and that is incorporated as a significant structural fragment into the structure of the API. The API starting materials normally have defined chemical properties and structure.

The company should designate and document the rationale for the point at which the production of the API begins. For synthetic processes, this is known as the point at which API starting materials are entered into the process. For other processes (e.g., fermentation, extraction, and purification), this rationale should be established on a case-by-case basis. Table 8.9 gives guidance on the point at which the API starting material is normally introduced into the process.

From this point on, appropriate good manufacturing practice (GMP), as defined in this guidance, should be applied to these intermediate and/or API manufacturing steps. This would include the validation of critical process steps determined to impact the quality of the API. However, it should be noted that the fact that a company chooses to validate a process step does not necessarily define that step as critical.

The guidance in this document would normally be applied to the steps shown in gray in Table 8.9. However, all steps shown may not need to be completed. The stringency of GMP in API manufacturing should increase as the process proceeds from early API steps to the final steps, purification, and packaging. Physical processing of APIs, such as granulation, coating, and physical manipulation of particle size (e.g., milling and micronizing), should be conducted according to this guidance. This GMP guidance does not apply to steps prior to the introduction of the defined API starting material.

TABLE 8.9

Application of Good Manufacturing Practice to Active Pharmaceutical Ingredient Manufacturing

Type of Manufacturing	Application Zone in Gray				
Chemical manufacturing	Production of the API starting material	Introduction of the API starting material into the process	Production of intermediate(s)	Isolation and purification	Physical processing and packaging
API derived from animal sources	Collection of organ, fluid, or tissue	Cutting, mixing, and/or initial processing	Introduction of the API starting material into the process	Isolation and purification	Physical processing and packaging
API extracted from plant sources	Collection of plant	Cutting and initial extraction(s)	Introduction of the API starting material into the process	Isolation and purification	Physical processing and packaging
Herbal extracts used as API	Collection of plants	Cutting and initial extraction		Further extraction	Physical processing and packaging
API consisting of comminuted or powdered herbs	Collection of plants and/or cultivation and harvesting	Cutting/comminuting			Physical processing and packaging
Biotechnology: fermentation/cell culture	Establishment of master cell bank and working cell bank	Maintenance of working cell bank	Cell culture and/or fermentation	Isolation and purification	Physical processing and packaging
"Classical" fermentation to produce an API	Establishment of cell bank	Maintenance of the cell bank	Introduction of the cells into fermentation	Isolation and purification	Physical processing and packaging

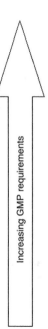

Increasing GMP requirements

Abbreviation: API, *active* pharmaceutical ingredient.

8.3.2 Quality Management

The system for managing quality should encompass the organizational structure, procedures, processes, and resources, as well as the activities to ensure confidence that the API will meet its intended specifications for quality and purity. All quality-related activities should be defined and documented. There should be a quality unit(s) that is independent of production and that fulfills both the QA and QC responsibilities. The quality unit can be in the form of separate QA and QC units or a single individual or group, depending on the size and structure of the organization. The persons authorized to release intermediates and APIs should be specified. All quality-related activities should be recorded at the time at which they are performed. Any deviation from the established procedures should be documented and explained. Critical deviations should be investigated, and the investigation and its conclusions should be documented.

No materials should be released or used before the satisfactory completion of evaluation by the quality unit(s), unless there are appropriate systems in place to allow for such use or the use of raw materials or intermediates pending completion of evaluation.

Procedures should exist for notifying responsible management in a timely manner of regulatory inspections, serious GMP deficiencies, product defects, and related actions (e.g., quality-related complaints, recalls, and regulatory actions).

Equipment used in the manufacture of intermediates and APIs should be of appropriate design and adequate size and suitably located for its intended use, cleaning, sanitation (where appropriate), and maintenance. Equipment should be constructed so that surfaces that contact the raw materials, intermediates, or APIs do not alter the quality of the intermediates and APIs beyond the official or other established specifications. Production equipment should be used only within its qualified operating range. Major equipment (e.g., reactors and storage containers) and permanently installed processing lines used during the production of an intermediate or an API should be appropriately identified.

Any substance associated with the operation of the equipment, such as lubricants, heating fluids, and coolants, should not contact the intermediates or APIs so as to alter the quality of APIs or intermediates beyond the official or other established specifications. Any deviations from this practice should be evaluated to ensure that there are no detrimental effects on the material's fitness for use. Wherever possible, food-grade lubricants and oils should be used.

Closed or contained equipment should be used whenever appropriate. Where open equipment is used, or equipment is opened, appropriate precautions should be taken to minimize the risk of contamination. A set of current drawings should be maintained for equipment and critical installations (e.g., instrumentation and utility systems).

For each batch of intermediate and API, appropriate laboratory tests should be conducted to determine conformance to specifications. An impurity profile describing the identified and unidentified impurities present in a typical batch produced by a specific controlled production process should normally be established for each API. The impurity profile should include the identity or some qualitative analytical designation (e.g., retention time), the range of each impurity observed, and the classification of each identified impurity (e.g., inorganic, organic, and solvent). The impurity profile is normally dependent on the production process and the origin of the API. Impurity profiles are normally not necessary for APIs from herbal or animal tissue origin. Biotechnology considerations are covered in ICH guidance Q6B. The impurity profile should be compared at appropriate intervals against the impurity profile in the regulatory submission or against historical data to detect changes to the API resulting from modifications in raw materials, equipment-operating parameters, or the production process. Appropriate microbiological tests should be conducted on each batch of the intermediate and API where microbial quality is specified.

A documented, on-going testing program should be established to monitor the stability characteristics of APIs, and the results should be used to confirm appropriate storage conditions and retest or expiry dates. The test procedures used in stability testing should be validated and should be indicative of stability.

Stability samples should be stored in containers that simulate the market container. For example, if the API is marketed in bags within fiber drums, stability samples can be packaged in bags of the same material and in small-scale drums of similar or identical material composition to the market drums.

Normally, the first three commercial production batches should be placed on the stability-monitoring program to confirm the retest or expiry date. However, where data from previous studies show that the API is expected to remain stable for at least 2 years, fewer than three batches can be used. Thereafter, at least one batch per year of API manufactured (unless none is produced that year) should be added to the stability-monitoring program and tested at least annually to confirm the stability.

For APIs with short shelf lives, testing should be done more frequently. For example, for those biotechnological or biologic and other APIs with shelf lives of 1 year or less, stability samples should be obtained and tested monthly for the first 3 months and at 3-month intervals later. When the data exist that confirm that the stability of the API is not compromised, the elimination of specific test intervals (e.g., 9-month testing) can be considered. Where appropriate, the stability storage conditions should be consistent with the ICH guidance on stability.

When an intermediate is intended to be transferred outside the control of the manufacturer's material management system and an expiry or retest date is assigned, supporting stability information (e.g., published data and test results) should be available.

An API expiry or retest date should be based on an evaluation of the data derived from stability studies. Common practice is to use a retest date, not an expiration date.

Preliminary API expiry or retest dates can be based on pilot-scale batches if: (*i*) the pilot batches employ a method of manufacture and procedure that simulates the final process to be used on a commercial manufacturing scale and (*ii*) the quality of the API represents the material to be made on a commercial scale.

A representative sample should be taken for the purpose of performing a retest. The company's overall policy, intentions, and approach to validation, including the validation of production processes, cleaning procedures, analytical methods, in-process control test procedures, computerized systems, and persons responsible for design, review, approval, and documentation of each validation phase, should be documented. The critical parameters and attributes should normally be identified during the development stage or from historical data, and the necessary ranges for the reproducible operation should be defined. This should include the following:

- Defining the API in terms of its critical product attributes
- Identifying process parameters that could affect the critical quality attributes of the API
- Determining the range for each critical process parameter expected to be used during routine manufacturing and process control

Validation should extend to those operations determined to be critical to the quality and purity of the API.

Before initiating process validation activities, appropriate qualification of critical equipment and ancillary systems should be completed. Qualification is usually carried out by conducting the following activities, individually or combined:

- *Design qualification*: Documented verification that the proposed design of the facilities, equipment, or systems is suitable for the intended purpose
- *Installation qualification*: Documented verification that the equipment or systems, as installed or modified, comply with the approved design, the manufacturer's recommendations, and/or user requirements
- *Operational qualification*: Documented verification that the equipment or systems, as installed or modified, perform as intended throughout the anticipated operating ranges
- *Performance qualification*: Documented verification that the equipment and ancillary systems, as connected together, can perform effectively and reproducibly based on the approved process method and specifications

WEB REFERENCES

1. http://www.fda.gov/cder/OPS/PAT.htm
2. http://www.automsoft.com/products/solutionsforpat.asp
3. http://www.sas.com/
4. http://www.thermometric.se
5. http://www.brukeroptics.com/terahertz/

RECOMMENDED READING

Allen, L. V., Jr. (2008). "Dosage form design and development." *Clin Ther* 30(11):2102–2111.

BACKGROUND: Drugs must be properly formulated for administration to patients, regardless of age. Pediatric patients provide some additional challenges to the formulator in terms of compliance and therapeutic efficacy. Due to the lack of sufficient drug products for the pediatric population, the pharmaceutical industry and compounding pharmacies must develop and provide appropriate medications designed for children. OBJECTIVE: The purpose of this article was to review the physical, chemical, and biological characteristics of drug substances and pharmaceutical ingredients to be used in preparing a drug product. In addition, stability, appearance, palatability, flavoring, sweetening, coloring, preservation, packaging, and storage are discussed. METHODS: Information for the current article was gathered from a literature review; from presentations at professional and technical meetings; and from lectures, books, and publications of the author, as well as from his professional experience. Professional society meetings and standards-setting bodies were also used as a resource. RESULTS: The proper design and formulation of a dosage form requires consideration of the physical, chemical, and biological characteristics of all of the drug substances and pharmaceutical ingredients (excipients) to be used in fabricating the product. The drug and pharmaceutical materials utilized must be compatible and produce a drug product that is stable, efficacious, palatable, easy to administer, and well tolerated. Preformulation factors include physical properties such as particle size, crystalline structure, melting point, solubility, partition coefficient, dissolution, membrane permeability, dissociation constants, and drug stability. CONCLUSIONS: Successful development of a formulation includes multiple considerations involving the drug, excipients, compliance, storage, packaging, and stability, as well as patient considerations of taste, appearance, and palatability.

Baertschi, S. W. et al. (2015). "Implications of in-use photostability: Proposed guidance for photostability testing and labeling to support the administration of photosensitive pharmaceutical products, Part 2: Topical drug product." *J Pharm Sci* 104(9):2688–2701.

Although essential guidance to cover the photostability testing of pharmaceuticals for manufacturing and storage is well-established, there continues to be a significant gap in guidance regarding testing to support the effective administration of photosensitive drug products. Continuing from Part 1, (Baertschi SW, Clapham D, Foti C, Jansen PJ, Kristensen S, Reed RA, Templeton AC, Tonnesen HH. 2013. *J Pharm Sci* 102: 3888–3899) where the focus was drug products administered by injection, this commentary proposes guidance for testing topical drug products in order to support administration. As with the previous commentary, the approach taken is to examine "worst case" photo-exposure scenarios in comparison with ICH testing conditions to provide practical guidance for the safe and effective administration of photosensitive topical drug products.

Baghel, S. et al. (2016). "Polymeric amorphous solid dispersions: A review of amorphization, crystallization, stabilization, solid-state characterization, and aqueous solubilization of biopharmaceutical classification system Class II drugs." *J Pharm Sci* 105(9):2527–2544.

Poor water solubility of many drugs has emerged as one of the major challenges in the pharmaceutical world. Polymer-based amorphous solid dispersions have been considered as the major advancement in overcoming limited aqueous solubility and oral absorption issues. The principle drawback of this approach is that they can lack necessary stability and revert to the crystalline form on storage. Significant upfront development is, therefore, required to generate stable amorphous formulations. A thorough understanding of the processes occurring at a molecular level is imperative for the rational design of amorphous solid dispersion products. This review attempts to address the critical molecular and thermodynamic aspects governing the physicochemical properties of such systems. A brief introduction to Biopharmaceutical Classification System, solid dispersions, glass transition, and solubility advantage of amorphous drugs is provided. The objective of this review is to weigh the current understanding of solid dispersion chemistry and to critically review the theoretical, technical, and molecular aspects of solid dispersions (amorphization and crystallization) and potential advantage of polymers (stabilization and solubilization) as inert, hydrophilic, pharmaceutical carrier matrices. In addition, different preformulation tools for the rational selection of polymers, state-of-the-art techniques for preparation and characterization of polymeric amorphous solid dispersions, and drug supersaturation in gastric media are also discussed.

Bergstrom, C. A. et al. (2014). "Early pharmaceutical profiling to predict oral drug absorption: Current status and unmet needs." *Eur J Pharm Sci* 57:173–199.

Preformulation measurements are used to estimate the fraction absorbed in vivo for orally administered compounds and thereby allow an early evaluation of the need for enabling formulations. As part of the Oral Biopharmaceutical Tools (OrBiTo) project, this review provides a summary of the pharmaceutical profiling methods available, with focus on in silico and in vitro models typically used to forecast active pharmaceutical ingredient's (APIs) in vivo performance after oral administration. An overview of the composition of human, animal and simulated gastrointestinal (GI) fluids is provided and state-of-the art methodologies to study API properties impacting on oral absorption are reviewed. Assays performed during early development, i.e. physicochemical characterization, dissolution profiles under physiological conditions, permeability assays and the impact of excipients on these properties are discussed in detail and future demands on pharmaceutical profiling are identified. It is expected that innovative computational and experimental methods that better describe molecular processes involved in vivo during dissolution and absorption of APIs will be developed in the OrBiTo. These methods will provide early insights into successful pathways (medicinal chemistry or formulation strategy) and are anticipated to increase the number of new APIs with good oral absorption being discovered.

Bharate, S. S. and R. A. Vishwakarma (2013). "Impact of preformulation on drug development." *Expert Opin Drug Deliv* 10(9):1239–1257.

INTRODUCTION: Preformulation assists scientists in screening lead candidates based on their physicochemical and biopharmaceutical properties. This data is useful for selection of new chemical entities (NCEs) for preclinical efficacy/toxicity studies which is a major section under investigational new drug application. A strong collaboration between discovery and formulation group is essential for selecting right NCEs in order to reduce attrition rate in the late stage development. AREAS COVERED: This article describes the significance of preformulation research in drug discovery and development. Various crucial preformulation parameters with case studies have been discussed. EXPERT OPINION: Physicochemical and biopharmaceutical characterization of NCEs is a decisive parameter during product development. Early prediction of these properties helps in selecting suitable physical form (salt, polymorph, etc.) of the candidate. Based on pharmacokinetic and efficacy/toxicity studies, suitable formulation for Phase I clinical studies can be developed. Overall these activities contribute in streamlining efficacy/toxicology evaluation, allowing pharmacologically effective and developable molecules to reach the clinic and eventually to the market. In this review, the magnitude of understanding preformulation properties of NCEs and their utility in product development has been elaborated with case studies.

Chadha, R. and S. Bhandari (2014). "Drug-excipient compatibility screening—Role of thermoanalytical and spectroscopic techniques." *J Pharm Biomed Anal* 87:82–97.

Estimation of drug-excipient interactions is a crucial step in preformulation studies of drug development to achieve consistent stability, bioavailability and manufacturability of solid dosage forms. The advent of thermoanalytical and spectroscopic methods like DSC, isothermal microcalorimetry, HSM, SEM, FT-IR, solid state NMR and

PXRD into pre-formulation studies have contributed significantly to early prediction, monitoring and characterization of the active pharmaceutical ingredient incompatibility with pharmaceutical excipients to avoid expensive material wastage and considerably reduce the time required to arrive at an appropriate formulation. Concomitant use of several thermal and spectroscopic techniques allows an in-depth understanding of physical or chemical drug-excipient interactions and aids in selection of the most appropriate excipients in dosage form design. The present review focuses on the techniques for compatibility screening of active pharmaceutical ingredient with their potential merits and demerits. Further, the review highlights the applicability of these techniques using specific drug-excipient compatibility case studies.

Darji, M. A. et al. (2018). "Excipient stability in oral solid dosage forms: A review." *AAPS Pharm Sci Tech* 19(1):12–26.

The choice of excipients constitutes a major part of preformulation and formulation studies during the preparation of pharmaceutical dosage forms. The physical, mechanical, and chemical properties of excipients affect various formulation parameters, such as disintegration, dissolution, and shelf life, and significantly influence the final product. Therefore, several studies have been performed to evaluate the effect of drug-excipient interactions on the overall formulation. This article reviews the information available on the physical and chemical instabilities of excipients and their incompatibilities with the active pharmaceutical ingredient in solid oral dosage forms, during various drug-manufacturing processes. The impact of these interactions on the drug formulation process has been discussed in detail. Examples of various excipients used in solid oral dosage forms have been included to elaborate on different drug-excipient interactions.

Egart, M. et al. (2016). "Application of instrumented nanoindentation in preformulation studies of pharmaceutical active ingredients and excipients." *Acta Pharm* 66(3):303–330.

Nanoindentation allows quantitative determination of a material's response to stress such as elastic and plastic deformation or fracture tendency. Key instruments that have enabled great advances in nanomechanical studies are the instrumented nanoindenter and atomic force microscopy. The versatility of these instruments lies in their capability to measure local mechanical response, in very small volumes and depths, while monitoring time, displacement and force with high accuracy and precision. This review highlights the application of nanoindentation for mechanical characterization of pharmaceutical materials in the preformulation phase (primary investigation of crystalline active ingredients and excipients). With nanoindentation, mechanical response can be assessed with respect to crystal structure. The technique is valuable for mechanical screening of a material at an early development phase in order to predict and better control the processes in which a material is exposed to stress such as milling and compression.

Erxleben, A. (2016). "Application of vibrational spectroscopy to study solid-state transformations of pharmaceuticals." *Curr Pharm Des* 22(32):4883–4911.

Understanding the properties, stability and transformations of the solid-state forms of an active pharmaceutical ingredient (API) in the development pipeline is of crucial importance for process-development, formulation development and FDA approval. Investigation of the polymorphism and polymorphic stability is a routine part of the preformulation studies. Vibrational spectroscopy allows the real-time in situ monitoring of phase transformations and probes intermolecular interactions between API molecules, between API and polymer in amorphous solid dispersions or between API and coformer in cocrystals or coamorphous systems and thus plays a major role in efforts to gain a predictive understanding of the relative stability of solid-state forms and formulations. Infrared (IR), near-infrared (NIR) and Raman spectroscopies, alone or in combination with other analytical methods, are important tools for studying transformations between different crystalline forms, between the crystalline and amorphous form, between hydrate and anhydrous form and for investigating solid-state cocrystal formation. The development of simple-to-use and cost-effective instruments on the one hand and recent technological advances such as access to the low-frequency Raman range down to 5 cm-1, on the other, have led to an exponential growth of the literature in the field. This review discusses the application of IR, NIR and Raman spectroscopies in the study of solid-state transformations with a focus on the literature published over the last eight years.

Gajdziok, J. and B. Vranikova (2015). "Enhancing of drug bioavailability using liquisolid system formulation." *Ceska Slov Farm* 64(3):55–66.

One of the modern technologies of how to ensure sufficient bioavailability of drugs with limited water solubility is represented by the preparation of liquisolid systems. The functional principle of these formulations is the sorption of a drug in a liquid phase to a porous carrier (aluminometasilicates, microcrystalline cellulose, etc.). After addition of further excipients, in particular a coating material (colloidal silica), a powder is formed with the properties suitable for conversion to conventional solid unit dosage forms for oral administration (tablets, capsules). The drug is subsequently administered to the GIT already in a dissolved state, and moreover, the high surface area of the excipients and their surface hydrophilization by the solvent used, facilitates its contact with and release to the dissolution medium and GI fluids. This technology, due to its ease of preparation, represents an interesting alternative to the currently used methods of bioavailability improvement. The article follows up, by describing the specific aspects influencing the preparation of liquid systems, on the already published papers about the bioavailability of drugs and the possibilities of its technological improvement. Key words: liquisolid systems bioavailability porous carrier coating material preformulation studies.

Hageman, M. J. (2010). "Preformulation designed to enable discovery and assess developability." *Comb Chem High Throughput Screen* 13(2):90–100.

Physicochemical properties of drug molecules impact many aspects of both in vivo and in vitro behavior. Poor physicochemical properties can often create a significant impediment to establishing reliable SAR, establishing proof of principle type studies using in vivo models, and eventually leading to added performance variability and costs throughout the development life cycle; in the worst-case scenario, even preventing execution of the desired development plan. Understanding the fundamental physicochemical properties provides the basis to dissect and deconvolute experimental observations in such a way that modification or mitigation of poor molecular properties can be impacted at the design phase, insuring design and selection of a molecule which has a high probability of making it through the arduous development cycle. This review will discuss the key physicochemical properties and how they can be assessed and how they are implicated in both discovery enablement and in final product developability of the selected candidate.

Hofmann, M. and H. Gieseler (2018). "Predictive screening tools used in high-concentration protein formulation development." *J Pharm Sci* 107(3):772–777.

This review examines the use of predictive screening approaches in high-concentration protein formulation development. In addition to the normal challenges associated with protein formulation development, for high-concentration formulations, solubility, viscosity, and physical protein degradation play major roles. To overcome these challenges, multiple formulation conditions need to be evaluated such that it is desirable to have predictive but also low-volume and high-throughput methods in order to identify optimal formulation conditions very early in development without time- and material-consuming setups. Many screening techniques have been reported for use in high-concentration formulation development, but not all fulfill the requirements mentioned previously. This review summarizes the advantages and disadvantages of different screening approaches currently used in formulation development and the correlation of predictive data to protein solubility, viscosity, and stability at high protein concentrations.

Kawakami, K. (2012). "Modification of physicochemical characteristics of active pharmaceutical ingredients and application of supersaturatable dosage forms for improving bioavailability of poorly absorbed drugs." *Adv Drug Deliv Rev* 64(6):480–495.

New chemical entities are required to possess physicochemical characteristics that result in acceptable oral absorption. However, many promising candidates need physicochemical modification or application of special formulation technology. This review discusses strategies for overcoming physicochemical problems during the development at the preformulation and formulation stages with emphasis on overcoming the most typical problem, low solubility. Solubility of active pharmaceutical ingredients can be improved by employing metastable states, salt forms, or cocrystals. Since the usefulness of salt forms is well recognized, it is the normal strategy to select the most suitable salt form through extensive screening in the current developmental study. Promising formulation technologies used to overcome the low solubility problem include liquid-filled capsules, self-emulsifying formulations, solid dispersions, and nanosuspensions. Current knowledge for each formulation is discussed from both theoretical and practical viewpoints, and their advantages and disadvantages are presented.

Kerns, E. H. et al. (2008). "In vitro solubility assays in drug discovery." *Curr Drug Metab* 9(9):879–885.

The solubility of a compound depends on its structure and solution conditions. Structure determines the lipophilicity, hydrogen bonding, molecular volume, crystal energy and ionizability, which determine solubility. Solution conditions are affected by pH, co-solvents, additives, ionic strength, time and temperature. Many drug discovery experiments are conducted under "kinetic" solubility conditions. In drug discovery, solubility has a major impact on bioassays, formulation for in vivo dosing, and intestinal absorption. A good goal for the solubility of drug discovery compounds is >60 ug/mL. Equilibrium solubility assays can be conducted in moderate throughput, by incubating excess solid with buffer and agitating for several days, prior to filtration and HPLC quantitation. Kinetic solubility assays are performed in high throughput with shorter incubation times and high throughput analyses using plate readers. The most frequently used of these are the nephelometric assay and direct UV assay, which begin by adding a small volume of DMSO stock solution of each test compound to buffer. In nephelometry, this solution is serially diluted across a microtiter plate and undissolved particles are detected via light scattering. In direct UV, undissolved particles are separated by filtration, after which the dissolved material is quantitated using UV absorption. Equilibrium solubility is useful for preformulation. Kinetic solubility is useful for rapid compound assessment, guiding optimization via structure modification, and diagnosing bioassays. It is often useful to customize solubility experiments using conditions that answer specific research questions of drug discovery teams, such as compound selection and vehicle development for pharmacology and PK studies.

Knopp, M. M. et al. (2016). "Recent advances and potential applications of modulated differential scanning calorimetry (mDSC) in drug development." *Eur J Pharm Sci* 87:164–173.

Differential scanning calorimetry (DSC) is frequently the thermal analysis technique of choice within preformulation and formulation sciences because of its ability to provide detailed information about both the physical and energetic properties of a substance and/or formulation. However, conventional DSC has shortcomings with respect to weak transitions and overlapping events, which could be solved by the use of the more sophisticated modulated DSC (mDSC). mDSC has multiple potential applications within the pharmaceutical field and the present review provides an up-to-date overview of these applications. It is aimed to serve as a broad introduction to newcomers, and also as a valuable reference for those already practicing in the field. Complex mDSC was introduced more than two decades ago and has been an important tool for the quantification of amorphous materials and development of freeze-dried formulations. However, as discussed in the present review, a number of other potential applications could also be relevant for the pharmaceutical scientist.

Lagrange, F. (2010). "Current perspectives on the repackaging and stability of solid oral doses." *Ann Pharm Fr* 68(6):332–358.

Which are the guidelines and scientific aspects for repackaged oral solid medications in France in 2010 whereas it develops? The transient or definitive displacement of the solid oral form from the original atmosphere to enter a repackaging process, sometimes automated, is likely to play a primary role in the controversy. However, the solid oral dose is to be repackaged in materials with defined quality. Considering these data, a review of the literature for determination of conditions for repackaged drug stability according to different international guidelines is presented in this paper. Attention is also paid to the defined conditions ensuring the conservation and handling of these drugs throughout the repackaging process. However, there is lack of scientific published stability data. Nevertheless, recent alternatives may be proposed to overcome the complexity of studying stability in such conditions. Then, the comparison of the moisture barrier properties of the respective package, a galenic model of hygroscopic molecules, or light sensitive molecules or stability data obtained during the industrial preformulation phase could also secure the list of drugs to be reconditioned. Similarly, a wise precaution will be to get stability data for the industrial blisters and unit doses undergoing the real conditions of the medication use process in hospitals and other healthcare settings. By now, reduction of dispensing errors and improvement of the compliance aid put a different perspective on the problem of repackaged drugs. To date, the pharmacist is advised to carry out its analysis of the risks.

Narayan, P. (2011). "Overview of drug product development." *Curr Protoc Pharmacol* Chapter 7: Unit 7.3.1–29.

The process for developing drug delivery systems has evolved over the past two decades with more scientific rigor, involving a collaboration of various fields, i.e., biology, chemistry, engineering, and pharmaceutics. Drug products, also commonly known in the pharmaceutical industry as formulations or "dosage forms," are used for administering the active pharmaceutical ingredient (API) for purposes of assessing safety in preclinical models, early- to late-phase human clinical trials, and for routine clinical/commercial use. This overview discusses approaches for creating small-molecule API dosage forms, from preformulation to commercial manufacturing.

Paudel, A. et al. (2015). "Raman spectroscopy in pharmaceutical product design." *Adv Drug Deliv Rev* 89:3–20.

Almost 100 years after the discovery of the Raman scattering phenomenon, related analytical techniques have emerged as important tools in biomedical sciences. Raman spectroscopy and microscopy are frontier, non-invasive analytical techniques amenable for diverse biomedical areas, ranging from molecular-based drug discovery, design of innovative drug delivery systems and quality control of finished products. This review presents concise accounts of various conventional and emerging Raman instrumentations including associated hyphenated tools of pharmaceutical interest. Moreover, relevant application cases of Raman spectroscopy in early and late phase pharmaceutical development, process analysis and micro-structural analysis of drug delivery systems are introduced. Finally, potential areas of future advancement and application of Raman spectroscopic techniques are discussed.

Razinkov, V. I. et al. (2015). "Accelerated formulation development of monoclonal antibodies (mAbs) and mAb-based modalities: Review of methods and tools." *J Biomol Screen* 20(4):468–483.

More therapeutic monoclonal antibodies and antibody-based modalities are in development today than ever before, and a faster and more accurate drug discovery process will ensure that the number of candidates coming to the biopharmaceutical pipeline will increase in the future. The process of drug product development and, specifically, formulation development is a critical bottleneck on the way from candidate selection to fully commercialized medicines. This article reviews the latest advances in methods of formulation screening, which allow not only the high-throughput selection of the most suitable formulation but also the prediction of stability properties under manufacturing and long-term storage conditions. We describe how the combination of automation technologies and high-throughput assays creates the opportunity to streamline the formulation development process starting from early preformulation screening through to commercial formulation development. The application of quality by design (QbD) concepts and modern statistical tools are also shown here to be very effective in accelerated formulation development of both typical antibodies and complex modalities derived from them.

Talaczynska, A. et al. (2016). "Benefits and limitations of polymorphic and amorphous forms of active pharmaceutical ingredients." *Curr Pharm Des* 22(32):4975–4980.

Active pharmaceutical ingredients (APIs) can exist in different polymorphic forms as well as in amorphous state. Polymorphic and amorphous forms of APIs can differ in physicochemical properties which in turn can significantly influence their therapeutic safety and effectiveness of the treatment. This review focuses on benefits and limitations of polymorphic and amorphous forms of APIs used in preformulation and formulation studies. Authors present their work on safety precautions for the use of polymorphic and amorphous forms of APIs, analytical techniques used for their identification as well as methods of their preparation especially in regard to limitations of labile APIs.

9

Characterization of Biopharmaceuticals

Any fool can know. The point is to understand.

Albert Einstein

9.1 Background

Biopharmaceuticals are complex, large-molecular-weight, variable-structure, dynamic protein and antibody molecules as compared with pharmaceutical products, wherein a fixed structure is always present. Some prominent examples include cytokines, antibodies, and hormones.

Cytokines are a broad and loose category of small proteins (~5–20 kDa) that are important in cell signaling. They are released by cells and affect the behavior of other cells. Cytokines can also be involved in autocrine signaling. Cytokines include chemokines, interferons, interleukins, lymphokines, and tumor necrosis factor but generally not hormones or growth factors (despite some terminology overlap). Cytokines are produced by a broad range of cells, including immune cells such as macrophages, B lymphocytes, T lymphocytes, and mast cells, as well as endothelial cells, fibroblasts, and various stromal cells. A given cytokine may be produced by more than one type of cell. Cytokines act through receptors and are especially important in the immune system. They modulate the balance between the humoral and cell-based immune responses, and they regulate the maturation, growth, and responsiveness of particular cell populations. Some cytokines enhance or inhibit the action of other cytokines in complex ways. They are different from hormones, which are also important cell signaling molecules, in that hormones circulate in much lower concentrations and hormones tend to be made by specific kinds of cells.

An antibody, also known as an immunoglobulin (Ig), is a large, Y-shaped protein produced by plasma cells that are used by the immune system to identify and neutralize pathogens such as bacteria and viruses. The antibody recognizes an antigen, via the variable region. Each tip of the "Y" of an antibody contains a paratope that is specific for one particular epitope (similarly analogous to a key) on an antigen, allowing these two structures to bind together with precision. Using this binding mechanism, an antibody can tag a microbe or an infected cell for attack by other parts of the immune system or can neutralize its target directly (e.g., by blocking a part of a microbe that is essential for its invasion and survival). The ability of an antibody to communicate with the other components of the immune system is mediated via its Fc region (located at the base of the "Y"), which contains a conserved glycosylation site involved in these interactions. The production of antibodies is the main function of the humoral immune system.

Though the general structure of all antibodies is very similar, a small region at the tip of the protein is extremely variable, allowing millions of antibodies with slightly different tip structures, or antigen-binding sites, to exist. This region is known as the hypervariable region. Each of these variants can bind to a different antigen. This enormous diversity of antibody paratopes on the antigen-binding fragments allows the immune system to recognize an equally wide variety of antigens.

Hormones are a class of signaling molecules produced by glands in multicellular organisms; these are transported by the circulatory system to target distant organs to regulate physiology and behavior. Hormones have diverse chemical structures, including eicosanoids, steroids, amino acid derivatives, peptides, and proteins. The glands that secrete hormones include the endocrine signaling system. The term *hormone* is sometimes extended to include chemicals produced by cells that affect the same cell (autocrine or intracrine signaling) or the nearby cells (paracrine signaling).

The protein hormones are synthesized in cells from amino acids according to messenger RNA (mRNA) transcripts, which are synthesized from DNA templates inside the cell nucleus. Preprohormones, or peptide hormone precursors, are then processed in several stages, typically in the endoplasmic reticulum, including the removal of the *N*-terminal signal sequence and sometimes glycosylation, resulting in prohormones. The prohormones are then packaged into membrane-bound secretory vesicles, which can be secreted from the cell by exocytosis in response to specific stimuli (e.g., an increase in Ca^{2+} and cyclic adenosine monophosphate [cAMP] concentration in the cytoplasm). These prohormones often contain superfluous amino acid residues that were needed to direct folding of the hormone molecule into its active configuration but have no function once the hormone folds. Specific endopeptidases in the cell cleave the prohormone just before it is released into the bloodstream, generating the mature hormone form of the molecule. Mature peptide hormones then travel through the blood to all cells of the body, where they interact with specific receptors on the surfaces of their target cells (Figure 9.1).

The Food and Drug Administration (FDA) expects the sponsors to come up with a high level of scientific evaluation of their biosimilar candidate products, and it all begins with a full understanding of proteins, as it is relevant to their development as biosimilar products. This chapter is not a primer in protein science, which I assume, would be well understood by the sponsor, but is a description of what is relevant to the development of biosimilars, as the FDA views it.

The first leg of establishing biosimilarity is a demonstration of structural similarity between a biosimilar candidate and the originator product. In this chapter, I would describe the nature of the structural variants that are common, not necessarily always relevant, and the techniques available to establish this basic level of similarity. This is the step where we begin collecting evidence that will lead us to the totality of the evidence.

9.1.1 Developing Biosimilars

If a new biological product development is akin to a horse running wild and reaching the goal post, biosimilar development is like running a horse on exactly the same

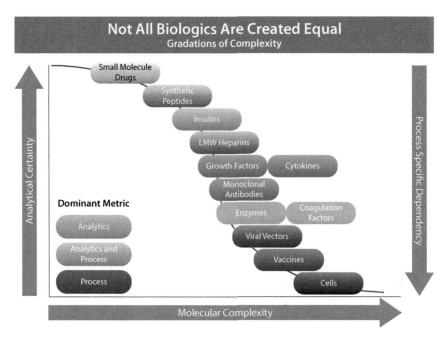

FIGURE 9.1 Analytics and process metrics. (From http://www.fda.gov/downloads/Advisory Committees/CommitteesMeetingMaterials/Drugs/AdvisoryCommitteeforPharmaceutical ScienceandClinicalPharmacology/UCM315764.pdf.)

track without any fences around the track; in one case, it is it is uncertain, while in the other, it is extremely onerous. This chapter provides details of the critical aspects of protein and antibody structure that are relevant to establishing biosimilarity. This is not a primer to protein chemistry, as only those elements that are relevant to a regulatory development of biosimilar are provided here.

The nature of products that a biosimilar product developer will face vary greatly in their nature, even though they are all proteins. Our body cells exploit an enormous array of proteins, approximately 2000, to perform nearly every functional and structural role to stay alive. As of date, more than 130 genuine and a similar number of modified therapeutic proteins are approved for clinical use in the European Union and the United States, with sales reaching more than $100 billion; the monoclonal antibodies (mAbs) account for almost half of the sales volume.

Based on their pharmacological activity, therapeutic proteins can be divided into five groups: (a) replacing a protein that is deficient or abnormal; (b) augmenting an existing pathway; (c) providing a novel function or activity; (d) interfering with a molecule or organism; and (e) delivering other compounds or proteins, such as a radionuclide, a cytotoxic drug, or an effector protein. Therapeutic proteins can also be grouped based on their molecular types that include antibody-based drugs, Fc fusion proteins, anticoagulants, blood factors, bone morphogenetic proteins, engineered protein scaffolds, enzymes, growth factors, hormones, interferons, interleukins, and thrombolytics. They can also be classified based on their molecular mechanism of activity as (a) binding noncovalently to target, for example, mAbs; (b) affecting covalent bonds, for example, enzymes; and (c) exerting activity without specific interactions, for example, serum albumin. Most protein therapeutics currently on the market are recombinant, and hundreds of them are in clinical trials for the therapy of cancers, immune disorders, infections, and other diseases. New engineered proteins, including bispecific mAbs and multispecific fusion proteins, mAbs conjugated with small-molecule drugs, and proteins with optimized pharmacokinetics, are currently under development. Despite the remarkable growth in this category of drugs, the technology for their production remains genetic-engineering-based recombinant production. Perhaps novel techniques of the future may make it possible to synthesize these drugs, which may reduce some complexity, but that seems far; the next generation of biosimilars, as reported in Chapter 2, will likely be recombinant proteins expressed in prokaryotic and eukaryotic systems, the living systems that inevitably and invariably introduce significant variability in the primary, secondary, tertiary, and quaternary structures of these proteins. A keen understanding of the possible differences and their source is essential to develop biosimilars; this chapter provides this discussion.

9.2 Protein Structure

9.2.1 Building Elements

The 20 different naturally occurring amino acids give a staggering number of different possible proteins, 20^n to be exact, where n is the number of amino acid units or *residues* (Figures 9.2 and 9.3).

Each amino acid has a carboxylic group and an amine group, and amino acids link to one another to form a chain by a dehydration reaction by joining the carboxyl group of one amino acid with the amino group of the next. Thus, polypeptide chains have an end with an unbound carboxyl group, the *C*-terminus, and a beginning with an amine group, the *N*-terminus.

9.2.2 Translation

When a protein is translated from nRNA, it is created from the *N*-terminus to the *C*-terminus. The amino end of an amino acid (on a charged transfer RNA [tRNA]) during the elongation stage of translation attaches to the carboxyl end of the growing chain. Since the start codon of the genetic code codes for the amino acid methionine, most protein sequences start with a methionine (or, in bacteria, mitochondria, and chloroplasts, the modified version *N*-formylmethionine [fMet]). However, some proteins are modified posttranslationally, for example, by cleavage from a protein precursor, and, therefore, they may have different amino acids at their *N*-terminus.

Amino acid	Three-latter code	Single-latter code	Structure
Alanine	Ala	A	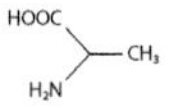 HOOC—CH$_3$, H$_2$N
Arginine	Arg	R	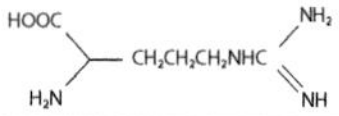 HOOC—CH$_2$CH$_2$CH$_2$NHC(NH$_2$)=NH, H$_2$N
Asparagine	Asn	N	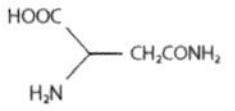 HOOC—CH$_2$CONH$_2$, H$_2$N
Aspartic Acid	Asp	D	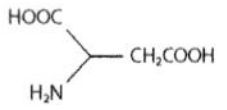 HOOC—CH$_2$COOH, H$_2$N
Cysteine	Cys	C	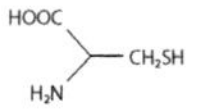 HOOC—CH$_2$SH, H$_2$N
Glutamic Acid	Glu	E	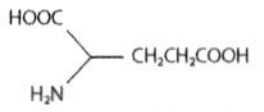 HOOC—CH$_2$CH$_2$COOH, H$_2$N
Glutamine	Gln	Q	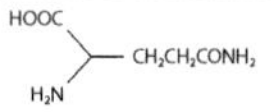 HOOC—CH$_2$CH$_2$CONH$_2$, H$_2$N
Glycine	Gly	G	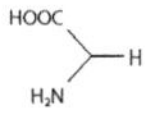 HOOC—H, H$_2$N
Histidine	His	H	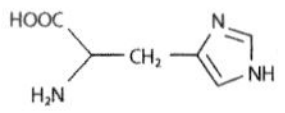 HOOC—CH$_2$-imidazole, H$_2$N
Isoleucine	Ile	I	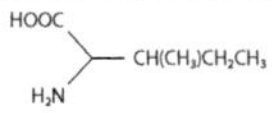 HOOC—CH(CH$_3$)CH$_2$CH$_3$, H$_2$N
Leucine	Leu	L	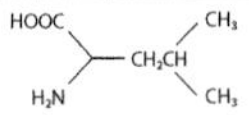 HOOC—CH$_2$CH(CH$_3$)$_2$, H$_2$N
Lysine	Lys	K	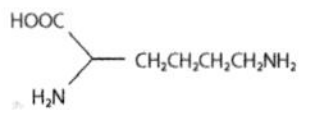 HOOC—CH$_2$CH$_2$CH$_2$CH$_2$NH$_2$, H$_2$N
Methionine	Met	M	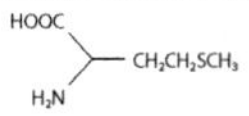 HOOC—CH$_2$CH$_2$SCH$_3$, H$_2$N
Phenylalanine	Phe	F	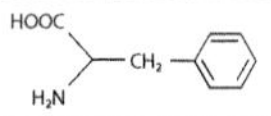 HOOC—CH$_2$-phenyl, H$_2$N
Proline	Pro	P	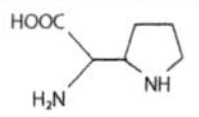 HOOC-pyrrolidine (NH), H$_2$N
Serine	Ser	S	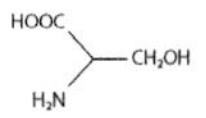 HOOC—CH$_2$OH, H$_2$N
Threonine	Thr	T	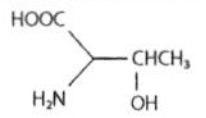 HOOC—CHCH$_3$(OH), H$_2$N
Tryptophan	Trp	W	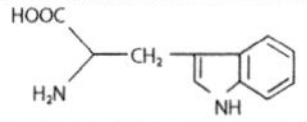 HOOC—CH$_2$-indole (NH), H$_2$N
Tyrosine	Tyr	Y	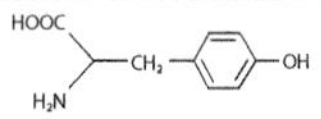 HOOC—CH$_2$-phenyl-OH, H$_2$N
Valine	Val	V	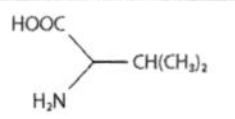 HOOC—CH(CH$_3$)$_2$, H$_2$N

FIGURE 9.2 The structure of the 20 essential amino acids.

Formula	MW	Niddle unit residue (–H₂O) Formula	MW	Charge at pH 6.0–7.0	Hydrophobic (non-polar)	Uncharged (polar)	Hydrophilic (polar)
$C_3H_7NO_2$	89.1	C_3H_5NO	71.1	Neutral	■		
$C_6H_{14}N_4O_2$	174.2	$C_6H_{12}N_4O$	156.2	Basic(+ve)			■
$C_4H_8N_2O_3$	132.1	$C_4H_6N_2O_2$	114.1	Neutral		■	
$C_4H_7NO_4$	133.1	$C_4H_5NO_3$	115.1	Acidic(-ve)			■
$C_3H_7NO_2S$	121.2	C_3H_5NOS	103.2	Neutral		■	
$C_5H_9NO_4$	147.1	$C_5H_7NO_3$	129.1	Acidic(-ve)			■
$C_5H_{10}N_2O_3$	146.1	$C_5H_8N_2O_2$	128.1	Neutral		■	
C_2H_5NO	275.1	C_2H_3NO	57.1	Neutral		■	
$C_6H_9N_3O_2$	155.2	$C_6H_7N_3O$	137.2	Basic(+ve)			■
$C_6H_{13}NO_2$	131.2	$C_6H_{11}NO$	113.2	Neutral	■		
$C_6H_{13}NO_2$	131.2	$C_6H_{11}NO$	113.2	Neutral	■		
$C_6H_{14}N_2O_2$	146.2	$C_6H_{12}N_2O$	128.2	Basic(+ve)			■
$C_5H_{11}NO_2S$	149.2	C_5H_9NOS	131.2	Neutral	■		
$C_9H_{11}NO_2$	165.2	C_9H_9NO	147.2	Neutral	■		
$C_5H_9NO_2$	115.1	C_5H_7NO	97.1	Neutral	■		
$C_3H_7NO_3$	105.1	$C_3H_5NO_2$	87.1	Neutral		■	
$C_4H_9NO_3$	119.1	$C_4H_7NO_2$	101.1	Neutral		■	
$C_{11}H_{12}N_2O_2$	204.2	$C_{11}H_{10}N_2O$	186.2	Neutral	■		
$C_9H_{11}NO_3$	181.2	$C_9H_9NO_2$	163.2	Neutral		■	
$C_5H_{11}NO_2$	117.1	C_5H_9NO	99.1	Neutral	■		

FIGURE 9.3 Properties of the 20 essential amino acids.

9.2.3 Peptide Bond

The chemical link between amino acid is called a *peptide bond*. It is formed between the carbonyl oxygen and carbon, α-carbons on each side of the peptide bond, and the amide nitrogen and hydrogen, which is due to the partial-double-bond character that exists between the carbonyl carbon and the amide nitrogen atoms (Figure 9.4). The peptide bond has a planar structure that produces restrictions in the angular range of bond rotation around the $C\alpha-N$, expressed by ϕ (phi), and $C-C\alpha$, expressed by Ψ (psi) bonds. These restrictions are summarized in a two-dimensional graphical plot called the Ramachandran plot; the plot graphically shows how certain structural features of proteins can only exist within limited ranges of angles, for example, α-helix.

The ω angle at the peptide bond is normally 180°, since the partial-double-bond character keeps the peptide planar. Because dihedral angle values are circular, and 0° is the same as 360°, the edges of the Ramachandran plot "wrap" right to left and bottom to top (Figure 9.5).

The higher-order structure (HOS) of proteins includes secondary, tertiary, and quaternary structures, as shown in Figure 9.6.

Figure 9.7 shows the three-dimensional (3D) structure of a filgrastim, a recombinant protein widely used for the treatment of neutropenia.

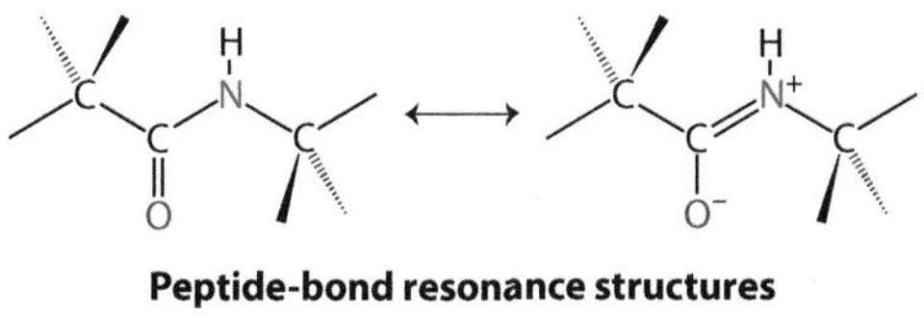

Peptide-bond resonance structures

FIGURE 9.4 Peptide bond; the double-bond character is about 40%, owing to resonance. (From Stryer, L. et al., *Biochemistry*, 9th ed., W. H. Freeman & Co., 2019.)

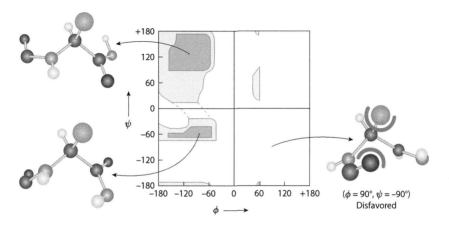

FIGURE 9.5 Ramachandran plot. (From Stryer, L. et al., *Biochemistry*, 9th ed., W. H. Freeman & Co., 2019.)

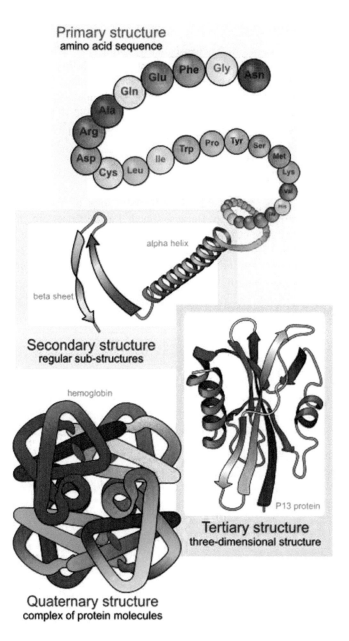

FIGURE 9.6   The four levels of protein structure.

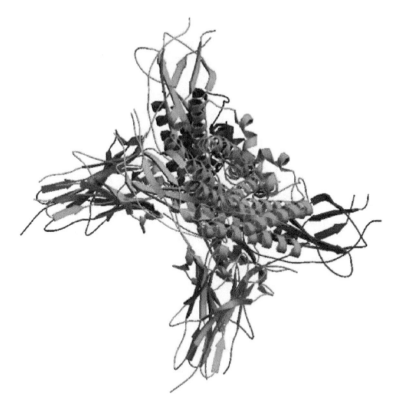

FIGURE 9.7   The three-dimensional structure of filgrastim.

9.3 Motifs and Domains

The primary and secondary structures are involved in a single polypeptide chain, the rest of the interactions take place between two or more identical or different polypeptide chains. The secondary structure leads to the formation of α-helix and β-sheets (Figure 9.6), which give rise to 3D structures, which are referred to as tertiary structures that provide the unique physicochemical and biological properties to proteins. The tertiary structures may acquire one or more peculiar folding patterns called *motifs* or super-secondary structure or complex folds, which are essentially "local tertiary structures" and should not be confused with the final or global tertiary structure. The same applies to groups of *motifs* called domains, which are one or more independent compact regions of a protein. While motifs are structural elements, domains are functional elements, regardless of their size (Figure 9.8).

Proteins containing two or more domains are called multidomain proteins, wherein the domains may be covalently linked by highly flexible bonds called linkers. Despite the complexity of various HOS, small changes in the amino acid sequence may not necessarily affect the HOS, a protein demonstrating same activity. There can be more

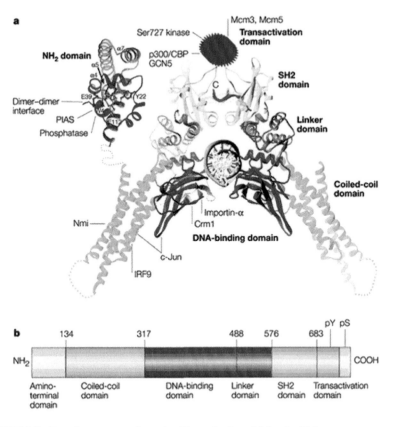

FIGURE 9.8 Domain structures of proteins. Nature Reviews, Molecular Biology.

than one polypeptide chain, in which case more than one tertiary structure are bonded together to produce quaternary structures. Proteins can aggregate to form dimers, trimers, and tetramers; there is some confusion regarding the label used to describe these; a tetramer can be four polypeptide chains bonded through sulfur bonds but that does not make a new monomer.

One domain may appear in a variety of different proteins. Molecular evolution uses domains as building blocks, and these may be recombined in different arrangements to create proteins with different functions. Domains vary in length from about 25 amino acids up to 500 amino acids in length. The shortest domains such as zinc fingers are stabilized by metal ions or disulfide bridges. Domains often form functional units, such as the calcium-binding EF hand domain of calmodulin.

Because they are independently stable, domains can be "swapped" by genetic engineering between one protein and another to make chimeric proteins. It is independent because domains may often be cloned, expressed, and purified independently of the rest of the protein, and they may even show activity if there is any known activity associated with them. Some proteins contain only a single domain, while others may contain several domains. A protein domain is assigned a certain type of fold. Domains with the same fold may or may not be related to each other functionally, because nature has used and reused the same fold many times in different contexts. The currently available Protein Data Bank (PDB; http://www.wwpdb.org/) is a repository for the 3D structural data of large biological molecules, such as proteins and nucleic acids.

The domains can be divided into four main classes based on the secondary structural content of the domain:

- All-α domains have a domain core built exclusively from α-helices. This class is dominated by small folds, many of which form a simple bundle of helices running up and down.
- All-β domains have a core composed of antiparallel β-sheets, usually two sheets packed against each other. Various patterns can be identified in the arrangement of the strands, often giving rise to the identification of recurring motifs, for example, the Greek key motif.
- The $\alpha+\beta$ domains are a mixture of all-α and all-β motifs. Classification of proteins into this class is difficult because of the overlaps between the other three classes and, therefore, is not used in the CATH domain database.
- The α/β domains are made from a combination of $\beta-\alpha-\beta$ motifs that predominantly form a parallel β-sheet surrounded by amphipathic α-helices.

Domains have limits on the size and vary from 36 residues in E-selectin to 692 residues in lipoxygenase-1, but the majority, 90%, have less than 200 residues, with an average of approximately 100 residues. Very short domains, less than 40 residues, are often stabilized by metal ions or disulfide bonds. Larger domains, greater than 300 residues, are likely to consist of multiple hydrophobic cores.

9.4 Association and Aggregation

The HOS is stabilized through a large number of weak and strong bonds, including weak noncovalent bonds formed ionic, dipoles (hydrogen bonds), nonpolar (hydrophobic), and van der Waals interactions. These bonds involve the interaction of amino acid side chains and the polypeptide chain. Since the transition from a polypeptide chain to HOS requires a significant loss of entry (structuring), it must be compensated by enthalpy released from the forming of bond (energy is released when a bond is formed); as a result, the protein structure can remain a dynamic state of structuring that may affect its activity and stability. In most instances, the changes are transitory, and the protein returns to its native structure. However, the possibility of dynamic changes to protein structure makes it possible for a molecule to have a different activity if its physicochemical properties are altered; in addition, if there is aggregation, a loss of activity and a likely increase in the immunogenicity of the protein may occur. Protein aggregation is caused by two factors: colloidal and conformational stability. The attractions on the surface of proteins can make colloidal dispersions that can be dynamic and significantly affect the safety and effectiveness of proteins under stress conditions; the conformational changes are brought about by the hydrophobic interactions of the buried functional groups. There is a likelihood of both types of aggregates, and, in some instances, one leads to another. So far, the regulatory authorities have not focused on these differentiations, but over time, it is likely that these would be included as part of risk analysis of the manufacturing process.

There is also a likelihood of aggregation owing to molecular crowding when the drug is exposed to high concentration of other proteins in plasma. Would it ever be a requirement to study the nature of circulating protein drug? This remains to be seen. However, a recent trend in reformulation of proteins such as adalimumab and rituximab in high-concentration formulations is alarming. Motivated by IP protection as these drugs come off patent, the originators are reformulating their products, without fully realizing that the molecular crowding at the site of administration, if not in the vial or syringe, is likely to increase aggregation potential. The regulatory agencies should require the demonstration of safety at this level when a formula change request is made. This aspect of safety consideration is a topic of a citizen's petition filed by the author with the FDA.

The HOS that a protein takes is intrinsically dictated by its primary structure and posttranslational modifications (PTMs). In the 1960s, Cyrus Levinthal proposed an interesting observation regarding protein folding. In a 100-residue protein, if 5×10^{47} possible conformations are allowed and if each conformation takes 1 picosecond, it will take 10^{18} times the age of the universe. It is truly amazing how a protein HOS is repeatedly formed approximately the same, even if there are a few defects left in the primary structure. It is this possibility of variability that makes the development of biosimilar products challenging. Misfolded proteins often reach a stage of energy level that may be difficult to overcome and it may be difficult to return them to their native state—the conditions under which proteins are manufactured can significantly alter this profile.

Protein synthesis involves a complex array of cellular machinery, primarily ribosomes. Proteins are synthesized from the N-terminus to the C-terminus in a sequential manner at a rate of 50–300 amino acids per minute; the folding begins once the chain has acquired 50–60 amino acids—cotranslational protein folding that constraints and limits the pathways that a protein can take into HOS, and this may explain why Levinthal calculations come short.

Chaperones are proteins that help other proteins fold correctly in additional to proteolytic apparatus available in the cells.

There are some proteins that have no well-defined HOS. These are disordered or unstructured random coils, such as the synthetic polymer chains and denatured proteins. This state may be a transitory state during the binding process and may be responsible for a multitude of protein actions in the cell. This intrinsic disorder creates a challenge to demonstrate structure–functional relationship, and although these aspects are not yet recognized by the regulatory authorities, it is only a matter of time when the biosimilar product developers may be required to demonstrate the disordered state comparisons as well—that will significantly raise the bar on the development of biosimilar products.

There are two types of proteins that can be labeled as "unnatural" construction—the fusion proteins or the conjugate (e.g., pegylated) proteins and very large assembly or virus particles or nanoparticle delivery systems. The fusion of an Fc (fragment crystallizable) part of an antibody (typically an IgGI antibody) with that of another pharmaceutically relevant protein through recombinant genetic technology results in fusion proteins. The Fc portion of an antibody increases the circulation time, just as does the pegylation; examples include fusion of Fc to the blood-clotting Factor VIII and Factor IX. In June 2014, the U.S. FDA approved Eloctate, Antihemophilic Factor (Recombinant), Fc Fusion Protein, for use in adults and children who have hemophilia A. Eloctate is the first hemophilia A treatment designed to require less frequent injections when used to prevent or reduce the frequency of bleeding. In March 2014, FDA approved Alprolix Coagulation Factor IX (Recombinant), Fc Fusion Protein, which is a recombinant DNA-derived, coagulation Factor IX concentrate. It temporarily replaces the missing coagulation Factor IX needed for effective hemostasis. Etanercept is a fusion protein produced by recombinant DNA technology. It fuses the tumor necrosis factor (TNF) receptor to the constant end of the IgG1 antibody. First, the developers isolated the DNA sequence that codes the human gene for soluble TNF receptor 2, which is a receptor that binds to TNF-α. Second, they isolated the DNA sequence that codes the human gene for the Fc end of IgG1. Third, they linked the DNA for TNF receptor 2 to the DNA for IgG1 Fc. Finally, they expressed the linked DNA to produce a protein that links the protein for TNF receptor 2 to the protein for IgG1 Fc.

Fusion of two relatively large proteins, each being over 50 kDa, raises the question whether this would impact the functionality of either protein. While a potential variance is possible, the existing science reveals no significant impact. This comment is important, as in the future, the regulatory authorities may raise this question.

The utility of pegylation is well understood and appreciated, as the popular products such as Neulasta (pegylated GCSF) have established their safety and effectiveness, while prolonging their disposition half-life. The two PEG molecules protect the molecule from degradation in the body, as well as reduce the immunogenicity.

9.5 Posttranslational Modification

Biological products are complex structures, not only because of their basic protein structure but also because of other modifications that they undergo during their maturation, generating a "final form" that is not a "single" and monomolecular entity (as could be expected of a chemical molecule with 99.9% purity) but rather a complex mix of the same protein molecule under various structurally close isoforms.

A protein is characterized by its primary to the quaternary structure and also by its additional characteristics acquired *during* the cellular process of protein synthesis. These are called "posttranslational modifications," owing to the fact that they occur once the gene (nucleic acids sequence) has been translated into the corresponding protein sequence (the amino acid chain). These modifications are also designated as "maturation phase," essential before the release and secretion of cell proteins. These modifications consist of the grafting on defined amino acids of one or several chemical and biological groups such as phosphate and sulfate groups or sugars (when it will be termed glycosylation) that modify the global charge and physicochemical or biological characteristics of these "mature" proteins as the final active forms.

Figure 9.9 shows the process of PTM.

Figure 9.10 shows the various PTMs that are frequently encountered.

The impact of PTM on stability risk and functionality risk is demonstrated in Figure 9.11.

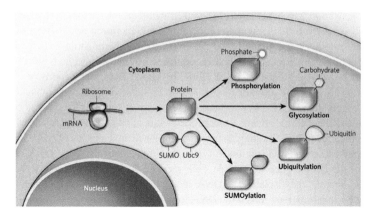

FIGURE 9.9   Posttranslational modification of proteins.

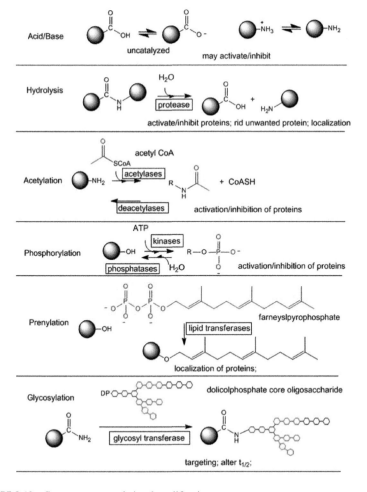

FIGURE 9.10   Common posttranslational modifications.

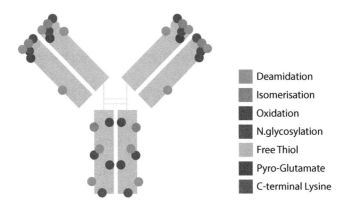

Deamidation
Isomerisation
Oxidation
N.glycosylation
Free Thiol
Pyro-Glutamate
C-terminal Lysine

FIGURE 9.11 Possible sites of various posttranslational modifications.

These PTMs that take place on specific sites of the protein are not controlled by the gene that expresses the protein sequence; instead, it is specific to each cellular kind that presents a unique combination of milieu interior, such as the presence of enzymes and the thermodynamic conditions during the reaction; it is for this reason that often these complex chemical reactions are not controllable by any alteration of the gene sequence but only by mastering the production conditions during expression. However, this is not relevant to expression inside prokaryotic organisms (bacteria) or very simple inferior eukaryotes such as yeasts as it is indigenous to a "mammalian" cells such as Chinese hamster ovary (CHO) cells.

Examples of PTMs include the following:

- PTMs involving addition of an enzyme in vivo
  - PTMs involving addition of hydrophobic groups for membrane localization
    – Myristoylation, attachment of myristate, a C14 saturated acid
    – Palmitoylation, attachment of palmitate, a C16 saturated acid
    – Isoprenylation or prenylation, the addition of an isoprenoid group (e.g., farnesol and geranylgeraniol)
      – Farnesylation
      – Geranylgeranylation
    – Glypiation, glycosylphosphatidylinositol (GPI) anchor formation via an amide bond to C-terminal tail
  - PTMs involving addition of cofactors for enhanced enzymatic activity
    – Lipoylation, an attachment of a lipoate (C8) functional group
    – Flavin moiety (FMN or FAD) may be covalently attached
    – Heme C attachment via thioether bonds with cysteine
    – Phosphopantetheinylation, the addition of a 4′-phosphopantetheine moiety from coenzyme A, as in fatty acid, polyketide, nonribosomal peptide, and leucine biosynthesis
    – Retinylidene Schiff base formation

- PTMs involving unique modifications of translation factors
    - Diphthamide formation (on a histidine found in eEF2)
    - Ethanolamine phosphoglycerol attachment (on glutamate found in eEF1α)
    - Hypusine formation (on conserved lysine of eIF5A [eukaryotic] and aIF5A [archeal])
- PTMs involving addition of smaller chemical groups
    - Acylation, for example, *O*-acylation (esters), *N*-acylation (amides), and *S*-acylation (thioesters)
        - Acetylation, the addition of an acetyl group, either at the *N*-terminus of the protein or at lysine residues. The reverse is called deacetylation
        - Formylation
    - Alkylation, the addition of an alkyl group, for example, methyl and ethyl
        - Methylation by the addition of a methyl group, usually at lysine or arginine residues. The reverse is called demethylation
    - Amide bond formation
        - Amidation at *C*-terminus
        - Amino acid addition
            - Arginylation, a tRNA-mediation addition
            - Polyglutamylation, covalent linkage of glutamic acid residues in the *N*-terminus of tubulin and some other proteins (see tubulin polyglutamylase)
            - Polyglycylation, covalent linkage of one to more than 40 glycine residues in the tubulin *C*-terminal tail
    - Butyrylation
    - Gamma-carboxylation dependent on Vitamin K
    - Glycosylation, the addition of a glycosyl group to either arginine, asparagine, cysteine, hydroxylysine, serine, threonine, tyrosine, or tryptophan, resulting in a glycoprotein; distinct from glycation, which is regarded as a nonenzymatic attachment of sugars
        - Polysialylation, the addition of polysialic acid (PSA) to NCAM
    - Malonylation
    - Hydroxylation
    - Iodination (e.g., of thyroglobulin)
    - Nucleotide addition, such as ADP-ribosylation
    - Oxidation
    - Phosphate ester (O-linked) or phosphoramidate (N-linked) formation
        - Phosphorylation, the addition of a phosphate group, usually to serine, threonine, and tyrosine (O-linked) or histidine (N-linked)
        - Adenylylation, the addition of an adenylyl moiety, usually to tyrosine (O-linked) or histidine and lysine (N-linked)

- – Propionylation
- – Pyroglutamate formation
- – S-glutathionylation
- – S-nitrosylation
- – Succinylation, the addition of a succinyl group to lysine
- – Sulfation, the addition of a sulfate group to a tyrosine
- • PTMs involving nonenzymatic additions in vivo
  - • Glycation, the addition of a sugar molecule to a protein without the controlling action of an enzyme
- • PTMs involving nonenzymatic additions in vitro
  - • Biotinylation, the acylation of conserved lysine residues with a biotin appendage
  - • Pegylation
- • PTMs involving addition of other proteins or peptides
  - • ISGylation, the covalent linkage to the ISG15 protein (interferon-stimulated gene 15)
  - • SUMOylation, the covalent linkage to the SUMO protein (small ubiquitin-related modifier)
  - • Ubiquitination, the covalent linkage to the protein ubiquitin
  - • Neddylation, the covalent linkage to Nedd
  - • Pupylation, the covalent linkage to the Prokaryotic ubiquitin-like protein
- • PTMs involving changing the chemical nature of amino acids
  - • Citrullination, or deimination, the conversion of arginine to citrulline
  - • Deamidation, the conversion of glutamine to glutamic acid or asparagine to aspartic acid
  - • Elimination, the conversion of an alkene by beta-elimination of phosphothreonine and phosphoserine or dehydration of threonine and serine, as well as by decarboxylation of cysteine
  - • Carbamylation, the conversion of lysine to homocitrulline
- • PTMs involving structural changes
  - • Disulfide bridges, the covalent linkage of two cysteine amino acids
  - • Proteolytic cleavage, cleavage of a protein at a peptide bond
  - • Racemization
  - • Of proline by prolyl isomerase
  - • Of serine by a protein-serine epimerase
  - • Of alanine in dermorphin, a frog opioid peptide
  - • Of methionine in deltorphin, also a frog opioid peptide

9.5.1 Glycosylation

One of the more important PTM is glycosylation; this is distinct from glycans. An example of how glycosylation reaction occurs and its consequences on protein characteristics and reproducibility of recombinant protein is shown in Figure 9.12.

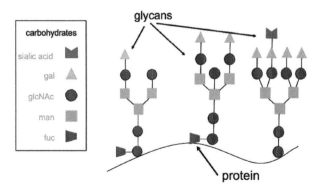

FIGURE 9.12   Schematic drawing of carbohydrate residues (or glycanic structures) present on some protein sequences.

Glycosylation is the most frequent PTM. The terms *glycan* and *polysaccharide* are defined by the International Union of Pure and Applied Chemistry (IUPAC) as synonyms meaning "compounds consisting of a large number of monosaccharides linked glycosidically." However, in practice, the term *glycan* may also be used to refer to the carbohydrate portion of a glycol conjugate, such as a glycoprotein, glycolipid, or a proteoglycan, even if the carbohydrate is only an oligosaccharide. Glycans usually consist solely of O-glycosidic linkages of monosaccharides. For example, cellulose is a glycan (or, to be more specific, a glucan) composed of β-1,4-linked D-glucose, and chitin is a glycan composed of β-1,4-linked *N*-acetyl-D-glucosamine.

Glycans can be homo- or heteropolymers of monosaccharide residues and can be linear or branched. The chemical modifications introduced are very complex owing to the glycan structures that are added to the protein skeleton. Protein glycosylation engages endoplasmic reticulum and Golgi apparatuses. A glycosylation consists of branching on the protein, on determined amino acids (for instance, for *N*-glycosylation, Asn, which is in the Asn-X-Thr sequence), and sugar groups such as mannose, fructose, or galactose, following a well-determined order. These glycosylation chemical reactions will lead to the making of "sugar chains," more or less complex and diversified, considering all the possible attaching combinations (number of antenna(e) on a glycosylation site and the nature of sugars making up this antenna), even if some mandatory sequences are found in each structure.

Finally, the end of the sugar chain is most often capped by a sialic acid in the form of neuraminic *N*-acetyl acid (NANA) in human cells, when for many mammals, a part of the sialic acid is in the form of neuraminic *N*-glycolyl acid (NGNA), because the gene that codes for the enzyme that allows the NANA form to become NGNA is muted and inactive in humans. This species specificity is important when choosing systems involving carbohydrates expression or production of the recombinant protein of interest, to ensure that the sialylation is as close as possible to the human form. The mature protein, so "glycolyzed" and more or less "sialylated," gets some characteristics that are more or less acidic, with a changed isoelectric point (pI). Consequently, at the end of PTMs, the protein appears not as a single entity but as a mix, a molecular population with the same basic protein structure (primary sequence imposed by gene sequence) on which various types of sugar chains will have been attached, giving each protein molecule its own pI. These series of isoforms are qualitatively and quantitatively studied using appropriate analytical techniques that separate the various isoforms, based on their charge, for example.

Since the glycosylation profile of a protein is important in determining its activity, proteins are characterized by their "pI" value and by a series of visible and quantifiable bandwidths, by separation methods of isoelectrofocusing.

There are four types of glycosylation links:

- *N*-linked glycosylation: *N*-linked glycosylation is the most common type of glycosidic bond and is important for the folding of some eukaryotic proteins and for cell–cell and cell–extracellular matrix attachment. The *N*-linked glycosylation process occurs in eukaryotes in the lumen of the endoplasmic reticulum and widely in archaea but very rarely in bacteria.
- *O*-linked glycosylation: *O*-linked glycosylation is a form of glycosylation that occurs in eukaryotes in the Golgi apparatus [6] but also occurs in archaea and bacteria. Xylose, fucose, mannose, and GlcNAc phosphoserine glycans have been reported in the literature.
- C-mannosylation: A mannose sugar is added to the first tryptophan residue in the sequence W-X-X-W (W indicates tryptophan and X is any amino acid). Thrombospondins are one of the most commonly C-modified proteins; however, this form of glycosylation appears elsewhere as well. C-mannosylation is unusual, because the sugar is linked to a carbon rather than a reactive atom such as nitrogen and oxygen. Recently, the first crystal structure of a protein containing this type of glycosylation has been determined—that of human complement component 8, PDB ID 3OJY.
- Formation of glycophosphatidylinositol (GPI) anchors (glypiation): A special form of glycosylation is the formation of a GPI anchor. In this kind of glycosylation, protein is attached to a lipid anchor, via a glycan chain.

Glycanic structures are obtained by combining the sugar group's nature Gal = Galactose, Man = Mannose, Fuc = Fucose, glcNAc = *N*-acetyl glucosamine and its organization in antennae (mono, bi, or even tri-antennae). Let us also note the presence of a "sialic acid" group that sometimes caps the antennae's ends. The sialic acid groups notably contribute to the protein molecule's half-life.

Posttranslational modifications, usually illustrated by the glycosylation profile, are intrinsic quality criteria of the protein, as well as critical parameters to consider during the assessment of the production process and its reproducibility, notably when changes are introduced in the production method, and a fortiori, when a new manufacturer offers a "biosimilar" version of a reference protein.

Indeed, for the new producer of a given glycosylated protein, one could fear an isoform distribution different from that of the original molecule. This different isoelectric profile, which is often difficult to distinguish by the only analytical methods offered by the manufacturer, will potentially have an impact on the pharmacokinetics or the biological activity of the therapeutic protein. Then, it will be the pharmacological and/or clinical data that will reveal the sometimes-subtle change in the isoform distribution when the quality control analytical data are detecting no noticeable difference.

Although some studies suggest that the consequence of different isoelectric profile mostly concerns the neoantigenicity risk, it seems that this phenomenon rather impacts the half-life of the molecule, which will be more or less rapidly eliminated by the receiving patient body. Indeed, the sugar chains, notably depending on their sialic acid capping, protect the protein from capture and degradation by hepatic cells.

Thus, a recombinant protein will have to have an adapted glycosylation, as well as a correct sialic acid level (in the NANA form), to not to be eliminated too quickly and keep a sufficient pharmacological activity and reduce any potential to generate in patients a defense reaction with the formation of antibodies to the protein of interest.

Whereas the molecules with PTM may have one species forming most of the protein component, the other glycans and components may be just as important in determining the final activity of the product. For example, erythropoietin (EP) specification states that it should have specific distribution ranges for its eight isoforms to be similar to the reference standard.

9.6 Protein Expression Variability

A clear understanding of how the recombinant DNA technique works is necessary for the understanding of factors that may contribute to protein structure variability, besides the inherent properties as described previously. The genes are DNA portions carrying a message that ultimately leads to the production of proteins. They are present in genomes of all living creatures and are sequences of nucleotides (A, T, G and C). Each of these genes' sequence is specific for a protein (Figure 9.13).

Cells transcribe the genes (DNA) into mRNA, which in turn are translated into proteins. These steps are represented in the sequence shown in Figure 9.14.

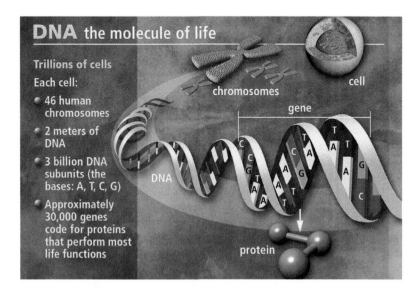

FIGURE 9.13   Structure of DNA. (From http://freepages.genealogy.rootsweb.ancestry.com/~ncscotts/ GG/DNA_Gallery.htm.)

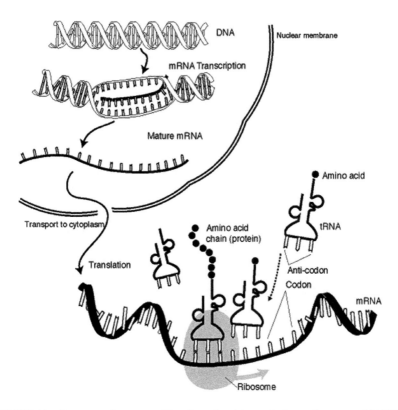

FIGURE 9.14 Gene expression system. (From https://mariakonovalenko.wordpress.com/2010/10/07/gene-expression-defined/.)

The living entities expressing cytokines and monoclonal antibodies have modified gene encoding to include the human protein sequence of interest. As the genetic code is universal, it will be read in the same way by all cellular systems of the animal, plant, or bacterial kingdom (even as the existence of dominant codons per cell system is known). This universality is the basis of the production of recombinant therapeutic proteins of the human sequence into heterologous host systems (bacteria, yeast, plant, mammalian cell, and transgenic animals) to make that host system "produce" a protein of a given sequence.

For the human protein to be correctly expressed by the producer–host organism, it is necessary to optimize the gene sequence in using, for each amino acid, the dominant codon of the species used. The optimized sequence is affixed to a promoter, which controls the protein expression by the genetically modified host system. Selecting the promoter depends on the host cell and leads to optimizing the expression yield.

For complex proteins, necessitating posttranslation specific reactions (such as specific conformations, oligomerization, proteolytic cleavages, phosphorylations, and glycosylation reactions) in a eukaryotic system is needed, wherein these reactions take place in the endoplasmic reticulum and in the Golgi apparatus. The three levels of these organisms are used:

- Lower eukaryotes such as yeasts and fungi are able to make relatively simple PTMs such as glycoproteins. Since yeasts produce *N*-glycosylations rich in mannose residues, which are strongly immunogenic for humans, the choice may be limited.
- Higher eukaryotes such as mammalian cells and insect or plant cells provide much lower yields and are more difficult to manage. Mammalian cells such as ovarian cells of Chinese hamsters (CHO cells) are commonly used to produce complex glycoproteins.
- Plant and transgenic animals produce therapeutic proteins in tissue (for the plant) or in a fluid (most often milk for transgenic animals) in large quantities and are highly practical sources of future biological products.

Given that living entities are involved in the expression of proteins, it is easy to see how a change in bioprocessing conditions can readily alter the structure of proteins. More difficult to manage are the variance in the glycan patterns, the antibody dependent cellular toxicity (ADCC), and other similar variations that might not necessarily be clinically meaningful, yet to prove it otherwise may be impossible, resulting in a biosimilar product developer to modify the bioprocessing to assure that the structure of protein expressed is as close to the originator molecule as possible.

9.7 Preformulation Considerations

An early characterization of biopharmaceuticals (proteins) is needed to evaluate the comparability of materials, which is more complicated owing to the inherently heterogeneous nature of many biologicals. This includes factors such as microheterogeneity of glycosylation, differential proteolytic processing during cellular production, and variations in PTMs, factors that are not common to small-molecule characterization and evaluation for interaction. This requires the availability of highly specific discriminating methodologies, such as spectrophotometric, chromatographic, electrophoretic methods, and mass spectroscopy (MS), often combined with liquid chromatography (LC).

Unlike small-molecule drugs, there are 3D and four-dimensional (4D) considerations (aggregates) with almost endless variations of polypeptides and proteins that make them a challenge to develop into products. Whereas in small-molecule drugs, there can be classes of drugs with common elements, this is not the case with protein drugs, as each one of them offers a unique structure, requiring techniques of production and purification specific to the protein. The same holds true for the stability profile of these compounds. Specification of biopharmaceutical drugs also includes elements not found in small molecules such as virus clearance, aggregate formation, and so on. As a result, the regulatory authorities worldwide treat biopharmaceutical drugs under separate administration, wherein a high level of expertise is inducted to evaluate these products.

Marketing authorization approvals for biological products are subject to a similar process as adopted for chemical drugs; however, the nature of these products mandates special evaluation and monitoring techniques. As a result, historically, the U.S. FDA has established separate sections for these products. Title 21 of the Code of Federal

TABLE 9.1

Parts of Title 21 of the Code of Federal Regulations Relevant to Biological Drugs

Parts	
1–99	Includes general enforcement regulations, product jurisdiction, enforcement policy, hearings, protection of human subjects, financial disclosure by clinical investigators, institutional review boards, and good laboratory practice for nonclinical laboratory studies.
200–299	Includes labeling, advertising, registration, medication guides, GMP, product official, and established names.
300–320	Includes combination drugs, new drugs, IND application, application for approval to market, orphan drugs, bioavailability, and bioequivalence.
600–680	Includes information for biological products: general, licensing, GMP for blood and blood components, establishment registration for manufacturers of blood and blood products, product standards, requirements for human blood and blood products.
800	Includes information for medical devices: general, labeling, reporting, in vitro diagnostic products, investigational device exemptions, premarket approval, postmarket surveillance, and classification procedures.
1270	Human tissue intended for transplantation.
1271	Human cells, tissues and cellular and tissue-based products.

Abbreviations: GMP, good manufacturing practices; IND, investigational new drug.

Regulations (CFR) concerns food and drugs. Table 9.1 lists those parts that particularly pertain to products under the purview of the Center for Biologics Evaluation and Research (CBER) of the U.S. FDA. The CFR (1996–2005) is available for browsing and/or searching (1).

On June 30, 2003, the FDA transferred some of the therapeutic biological products that had been reviewed and regulated by the CBER to the Center for Drug Evaluation and Research (CDER). The CDER now has regulatory responsibility, including premarket review and continuing oversight, over the transferred products. In regulating the products assigned to them, the CBER and the CDER will consult with each other regularly and whenever necessary (Table 9.2).

TABLE 9.2

Approved Products Transferred from the Center for Biologics Evaluation and Research to the Center for Drug Evaluation and Research

Product Name	Proprietary Name	Applicant Name
Abciximab	ReoPro®	Centocor B.V.
Adalimumab	Humira®	Abbott Laboratories
Agalsidase beta	Fabrazyme®	Genzyme Corp.
Aldesleukin	Proleukin®	Chiron Corp.
Alefacept	Amevive®	Biogen, Inc.
Alemtuzumab	Campath®	ILEX Pharmaceuticals LP
Alteplase	Activase®	Genentech, Inc.
Anakinra	Kineret®	Amgen, Inc.
Anistreplase	Eminase®	Wulfing Pharma GmbH

(Continued)

TABLE 9.2 (*Continued*)

Approved Products Transferred from the Center for Biologics Evaluation and Research
to the Center for Drug Evaluation and Research

Product Name	Proprietary Name	Applicant Name
Arcitumomab	CEA-Scan®	Immunomedics, Inc.
Asparaginase	Elspar®	Merck & Co., Inc.
Basiliximab	Simulect®	Novartis Pharmaceuticals Corp.
Becaplermin	Regranex®	OMJ Pharmaceuticals, Inc.
Becaplermin concentrate		Chiron Corp.
Botulinum toxin type A	Botox®	Allergan, Inc.
Botulinum toxin type B	Myobloc®	Elan Pharmaceuticals
Capromab pendetide	ProstaScint®	Cytogen Corp.
Collagenase	Santyl®	Advance Biofactures Corp.
Daclizumab	Zenapax®	Hoffmann-La Roche, Inc.
Darbepoetin alfa	Aranesp®	Amgen, Inc.
Denileukin diftitox	Ontak®	Seragen, Inc.
Dornase alfa	Pulmozyme®	Genentech, Inc.
Drotrecogin alfa	Xigris®	Eli Lilly & Co.
Epoetin alfa	Epogen®	Amgen, Inc.
Epoetin alfa	Eprex®	Ortho Biologics LLC
Etanercept	Enbrel®	Immunex Corp.
Filgrastim	Neupogen®	Amgen, Inc.
Ibritumomab tiuxetan	Zevalin®	IDEC Pharmaceuticals Corp.
Indium In-111 chloride	Indium Chloride®	In-111 Mallinckrodt Medical, Inc.
Indium In-111 chloride	Indiclor®	Medi-Physics, Inc.
Infliximab	Remicade®	Centocor, Inc.
Interferon alpha-2a	Roferon A®	Hoffmann-La Roche, Inc.
Interferon alpha-2b	Intron A®	Schering Corp.
Interferon alfacon-1	Infergen®	InterMune, Inc.
Interferon alpha-n3 (human leukocyte derived)	Alferon N Injection®	Interferon Sciences, Inc.
Interferon beta-1a	Avonex®	Biogen, Inc.
Interferon beta-1a	Rebif®	Serono, Inc.
Interferon beta-1b	Betaseron®	Chiron Corp.
Interferon gamma-1b	Actimmune®	InterMune, Inc.
Laronidase	Aldurazyme®	Biomarin Pharmaceutical, Inc.
Muromonab-CD3	Orthoclone OKT3®	Ortho Biotech Products, LP
Nofetumomab	Verluma®	Boehringer Ingelheim Pharma
Omalizumab	Xolair®	Genentech, Inc.
Oprelvekin	Neumega®	Genetics Institute, Inc.
Palivizumab	Synagis®	MedImmune, Inc.
Pegaspargase	Oncaspar®	Enzon, Inc.
Pegfilgrastim	Neulasta®	Amgen, Inc.
Peginterferon alpha-2a	Pegasys®	Hoffman-La Roche, Inc.

(*Continued*)

TABLE 9.2 (*Continued*)

Approved Products Transferred from the Center for Biologics Evaluation and Research to the Center for Drug Evaluation and Research

Product Name	Proprietary Name	Applicant Name
Peginterferon alpha-2b	Polyethylene glycol (PEG)-Intron®	Schering Corp.
Rasburicase	Elitek®	Sanofi-Synthelabo, Inc.
Reteplase	Retavase®	Centocor, Inc.
Rituximab	Rituxan®	Genentech, Inc.
Rituximab formulated bulk		IDEC Pharmaceuticals Corp.
Sargramostim	Leukine®	Berlex Laboratories, Inc.
Satumomab concentrate		LONZA Biologics PLC
Satumomab pendetide	OncoScint CR/OV®	Cytogen Corp.
Streptokinase	Streptase®	Aventis Behring GmbH
Tenecteplase	TNKase®	Genentech, Inc.
Tositumomab and iodine I 131 tositumomab	Bexxar®	Corixa Corp.
Trastuzumab	Herceptin®	Genentech, Inc.
Urokinase	Abbokinase®	Abbott Laboratories

The categories of therapeutic biological products transferred to CDER (2) are as follows:

- Monoclonal antibodies (MAbs) for in vivo use.
- Proteins intended for therapeutic use, including cytokines (e.g., interferons), enzymes (e.g., thrombolytics), and other novel proteins, except for those that are specifically assigned to CBER (e.g., vaccines and blood products). This category includes therapeutic proteins derived from plants, animals, or microorganisms, and recombinant versions of these products.
- Immunomodulators (nonvaccine and nonallergenic products intended to treat disease by inhibiting or modifying a pre-existing immune response).
- Growth factors, cytokines, and MAbs intended to mobilize, stimulate, decrease, or otherwise alter the production of hematopoietic cells in vivo.

The categories of therapeutic biological products that remain in the CBER are as follows:

- Cellular products, including products composed of human, bacterial, or animal cells (such as pancreatic islet cells for transplantation), or physical parts of those cells (such as whole cells, cell fragments, and other components intended for use as preventative or therapeutic vaccines).
- Gene therapy products. Human gene therapy/gene transfer is the administration of nucleic acids, viruses, or genetically engineered microorganisms that

mediate their effect by the transcription and/or translation of the transferred genetic material and/or by integration into the host genome. Cells may be modified in these ways ex vivo for subsequent administration to the recipient or altered in vivo by gene therapy products administered directly to the recipient.

- Vaccines (products intended to induce or increase an antigen-specific immune response for prophylactic or therapeutic immunization, regardless of the composition or method of manufacture).
- Allergenic extracts used for the diagnosis and treatment of allergic diseases and allergen patch tests.
- Antitoxins, antivenins, and venoms.
- Blood, blood components, plasma-derived products (e.g., albumin, Igs, clotting factors, fibrin sealants, and proteinase inhibitors), including recombinant and transgenic versions of plasma derivatives (e.g., clotting factors), blood substitutes, plasma volume expanders, human, or animal polyclonal antibody preparations, including radiolabeled or conjugated forms, and certain fibrinolytics, such as plasma-derived plasmin and red cell reagents.

Significant developments over the past couple of decades have resulted in the development of a new class of biopharmaceutical products based on recombinant DNA technology that has placed a greater burden on the developer to provide characterization protocols that take into account modifications induced by the recombinant techniques. Generally, the analytical precision for these molecules has not been as sophisticated as that available for small molecules; a few thousand Daltons seemed to be the limit of analytical accuracy; the characterization method essentially require biological methods that are by nature more variable. However, recent developments in both in vivo and in vitro studies needed to ensure comparable safety and efficacy; the powerful techniques, such as the high-resolution tandem mass spectrometry, circular dichroism, and chromatographic media, make it possible to provide complete covalent structure for proteins over 100,000 Da, with less than one Dalton change in proteins routinely detectable. The newer sensitive methods now detect differences in the HOS, and for all practical purposes, it is reasonable to conclude that the historic differences between characterization specifications have been removed.

9.8 Preformulation Studies

The unique nature of characteristics of biological products requires early integration of scientific activity bringing onboard protein biochemists, purification scientists, quality control and regulatory affairs personnel, clinical investigators, manufacturing technicians, marketing specialists, and managers.

The diversity of preformulation studies required to characterize biological drugs requires the application of a comprehensive array of multiple sensitive and selective analytical methods to several batches. This requires the use of orthogonal methods to study virtually every observable property of a protein, including covalent structure, conformation, pI, aggregation, charge, mass, fragmentation, surface structure, hydrophobicity, spectrophotometric, magnetic resonance, fluorescence, light scattering, sedimentation, electrophoretic properties, charge, immunological properties, enzyme activity, biological potency, substituent patterns, and so on. The methods currently available adequately characterize covalent structure, using peptide mapping with high-resolution (LC/MS) (Q-TOF) to locate every atom in peptide backbone and other sensitive methods such as circular dichroism (CD), high-performance liquid chromatography (HPLC), Fourier transform-infrared (FT-IR), fluorescence, nuclear magnetic resonance (NMR), size-exclusion chromatography (SEC), light scattering, analytical ultracentrifugation (AUC), enzyme-linked immunosorbent assay (ELISA), and surface plasmon resonance (SPR). The impurities are easily detected using HPLC, SEC, isoelectric chromatography, sodium dodecyl sulfate-polyacrylamide gel electrophoresis (SDS-PAGE), and isoelectric focusing (IEF). Multidimensional analytical methods (e.g., LC/MS and 2D NMR) provide greater information than the one-dimensional (1D) methods, particularly when combined with multivariate mathematical methods for analyzing complex mixture data. The preformulation studies further encompass the scope of studies that are required to prove equivalence of products in the new generation of biogeneric (or biosimilar or follow-on) products. The unique set of activities related to overcoming the inherent instability of the drug is referred to as formulation development and would not normally fall under preformulation exercises, but recently, the boundary between the preformulation and formulation studies of biological drugs is disappearing.

A biopharmaceutical drug often undergoes development before its mechanism of action or other properties are established. The new protein may be identified through genomics or proteomics activities or through more traditional medical research. It may initially be associated with a particular disease process or a certain metabolic event. In any case, its mechanism of action—as well as many of its structural characteristics and biochemical properties—may be unknown. One of the more challenging aspects of developing protein pharmaceuticals is dealing with and overcoming the inherent physical and chemical instabilities of proteins. This inherent instability has the potential to alter the state of the protein from the desired (native) form to an undesirable form (upon storage), compromising patient safety and drug efficacy. While there are numerous ways for a protein to lose its stability, the three most commonly encountered modes of denaturation and degradation are aggregation, oxidation, and deamidation. The commonly accepted strategy for rational formulation development relies on identifying the mechanisms of denaturation and degradation, in order to develop effective countermeasures. Once the specifics of any particular degradation pathway are understood, a more informed choice regarding excipients and formulation can be made, accelerating product development.

Preformulation is an exploratory activity that begins early in biopharmaceutical development. Preformulation studies are designed to determine the compatibility of initial excipients with the active substance for a biopharmaceutical, physicochemical, and analytical investigation in support of promising experimental formulations. Data from preformulation studies provide the necessary groundwork for formulation attempts. Successful formulations take into account a drug's interactions with the physicochemical properties of other ingredients (and their interactions with each other) to produce a safe, stable, beneficial, and marketable product. One factor that narrows the scope of studies is the route of administration, as most biological drugs are likely to be administered parenterally; this obviates the need and investment in characterization vis-à-vis other dosage form presentations. However, some other considerations become involved, such as the dosage required; for example, while many drugs are administered at the microgram level, many MAbs are given in much larger quantities (hundreds of milligrams per dose) and are normally delivered intravenously. The drive to reduce healthcare costs has created a need to administer MAb therapeutics more conveniently, at home, subcutaneously. Thus, MAbs must be available at high concentrations (~200 mg/mL) in the vial. At these high concentrations, MAb-containing solutions are viscous, making them difficult to administer conveniently. Hence, a preformulation activity that needs to be considered is a concentration study investigating the solubility behavior, the effect of concentration on viscosity, and the increased potential for aggregation. These studies have the potential to strongly influence the target product profile and the design of the clinical trial. Similarly, such questions as to whether a drug is going to be administered in a freeze-dried form or liquid form focus the studies accordingly. These considerations are mostly determined by stability considerations, as freeze-drying imparts greater stability; however, some recent studies suggest that the reconstitution process can alter the 3D structure of proteins, making them more immunogenic.

Preformulation begins with thorough characterization of proteins, including their pharmacokinetics and physicochemical characterization. Ideally, this information should be in hand at the beginning of the product development program, but this is unrealistic, as product characterization is an evolving process that involves contributions at different stages of the product life cycle.

9.8.1 Stability

The most difficult aspect of biopharmaceutical stabilization is the ease with which these products begin to show aggregation, something that is often difficult to predict. As a result, evaluation of biopharmaceutical products focuses on both physical and chemical stability studies that investigate temperature dependencies to convert in vivo to native forms (if it has denatured). Bioassays study protein activity, identity, and critical pathways. Chemical degradation changes the primary structure of a protein. Bond cleavage will create an entirely new molecule. Such chemical degradation is usually preceded by a causal physical process, typically unfolding, which makes available residues that are usually inaccessible for chemical reactions with their environment. Physical degradation changes only the HOS (secondary, tertiary, and quaternary) of the polypeptide, not necessarily creating a brand-new molecule. Such degradation includes aggregation, adsorption, unfolding, and precipitation.

Because proteins and peptides are such large molecules and exist to interact with their environment, they are somewhat fragile. They must be protected from denaturation and degradation until they can be delivered to their site of action in a patient's body.

The biopharmaceutical development process does not allow enough time to confirm stability requirements for a final formulation (which could take two years) before the company is otherwise ready to apply to market the product. Initial indications should be developed during clinical studies, so formulators must begin with 3-, 6-, and 9-month tests of their molecule's structure and innate stability by using various analytical methods. "Accelerated" stability tests subject products to various stresses: a range of pH values, heat, light, freezing and thawing conditions, additives, and surface materials and interfaces. The test for agitation-induced denaturation is performed by swirling (creating a vortex inside the vials), rotating vials at elevated temperatures, and testing the surface tension of the liquid formulation.

The stress tests form the basis of many directions in which the preformulation studies can assist in the final dosage formulation. The common tests include the shake test (agitation), surfactant test, freeze–thaw test, and heating experiments (limited because of denaturation). Each formulation configuration is shaken in a vial to determine whether it forms aggregates. Then, a surfactant (usually a polysorbate detergent, such as Tween 80®) may be selected to prevent the formation of precipitants by making it harder for proteins to aggregate. Human albumin is a frequent additive, but its use is discouraged because of supply constraints and viral clearance requirements. Formulations are checked through multiple freeze–thaw cycles (which can take about a week) to check for the effects of temperature and freezing-process stresses. Most proteins are stable around 2°C–8°C, but few are stable at room temperature. Heating experiments help scientists examine degradation at temperature extremes by heating them to 30°C (about 86°F) and maybe even to 45°C (about 113°F). At high temperatures, different mechanisms of protein denaturation may arise.

Most prominent stability reactions include oxidation, hydrolysis, and disulfide exchange. Stability of protein products can be significantly enhanced if the oxygen is removed from the headspace of the unit pack, as oxygen induces specific degradation reactions, which are complex and difficult to study. In most instances, this will speed up the development time, as fewer matrices would have to be evaluated for factors affecting stability. Certain amino acids (tryptophan, methionine, cysteine, histidine, and tyrosine) are susceptible to oxidation. Metal ions such as copper and iron can accelerate the process of oxidation, as does the higher pH, fluorescent light, and hydrogen peroxide. If the amino acids along a polypeptide chain are deformed by oxidation, the molecule can be irreversibly altered, and the new molecule will likely be inactive. Antioxidants help to protect against oxidation by scavenging oxygen for themselves. Ascorbic acid is used, but citric acid is preferred, and it can be used as a pH adjuster as well.

Hydrolysis of a side-chain amide on a polypeptide's glutamine or asparagine residues can yield a carboxylic acid. The process, called deamidation, is facilitated by elevated temperature and pH, resulting in the loss of activity. The peptide bonds that hold amino acids together in the chain can also be severed by hydrolysis—particularly where aspartic acid residues are located. This effect is usually due to heat or low pH.

Cysteine residues form disulfide bonds, which are important to protein's structural integrity. Shuffling of these bonds, where two sulfur atoms from two different amino acid molecules link up, often changes the 3D structure, causing a loss of activity.

9.8.1.1 Excipients

Salts and nonelectrolytes (such as ammonium sulfate and glycerol) help to stabilize proteins in high temperatures and low pH, when freezing is not an option, but they still require low-temperature storage. Sometimes, they must be removed before the drug is used, which can be inconvenient, time-consuming, and expensive. Also, the active ingredient must be diluted, allowing further waste and variability in the final product, just as in reconstituting freeze-dried products.

The biological drug is not likely to be stable without the addition of additives such as buffers, albumin, and surfactants, if kept in a liquid form; otherwise, an early conversion of the drug to a lyophilized form is completed. Most formulations would not include any preservative. Table 9.3 lists the recombinant products approved by the

TABLE 9.3

Composition of Approved Biological Products

Product	Composition
Abciximab is chimeric human-murine MAb at 47,615 Da.	Each single-use vial contains 2 mg/mL of Abciximab in a buffered solution (pH 7.2) of 0.01 M sodium phosphate, 0.15 M sodium chloride, and 0.001% polysorbate 80 in water for injection. No preservatives are added.
Adalimumab is a recombinant human IgG1 MAb that consists of 1330 amino acids and has a MW of approximately 148 kDa.	Each syringe delivers 0.8 mL (40 mg) of DP. Each vial contains approximately 0.9 mL of solution to deliver 0.8 mL (40 mg) of DP. Each 0.8 mL contains 40 mg of adalimumab, 4.93 mg of sodium chloride, 0.69 mg of monobasic sodium phosphate dihydrate, 1.22 mg of dibasic sodium phosphate dihydrate, 0.24 mg of sodium citrate, 1.04 mg of citric acid monohydrate, 9.6 mg of mannitol, 0.8 mg of polysorbate 80 and water for injection, USP. Sodium hydroxide added as necessary to adjust pH.
Aldesleukin is an interleukin-2 product with MW of approximately 15,300 Da. The chemical name is des-alanyl-1, serine-125 human interleukin-2.	Each milliliter contains 18 million International Unit (IU) (1.1 mg) of aldesleukin, 50 mg mannitol, and 0.18 mg sodium dodecyl sulfate, buffered with approximately 0.17 mg monobasic and 0.89 mg dibasic sodium phosphate to a pH of 7.5 (range 7.2–7.8).
Alemtuzumab is a recombinant DNA-(rDNA)-derived humanized MAb (Campath-1H) that has an approximate MW of 150 kDa.	Each single use ampule of Campath contains 30 mg Alemtuzumab, 24.0 mg sodium chloride, 3.5 mg dibasic sodium phosphate, 0.6 mg potassium chloride, 0.6 mg monobasic potassium phosphate, 0.3 mg polysorbate 80, and 0.056 mg disodium edetate. No preservatives are added.
Alteplase is a glycoprotein of 527 amino acids.	Each 100 mg vial contains alteplase (100 mg), L-arginine (3.5 g), phosphoric acid (1 g), polysorbate 80 (>11 mg); the 50 mg vial is packed under vacuum.
Anakinra is a nonglycosylated form of the human interleukin-1 and consists of 153 amino acids; it has a MW of 17.3 kDa.	Each 1 mL prefilled glass syringe contains 0.67 mL (100 mg) of anakinra in a solution (pH 6.5) containing sodium citrate (1.29 mg), sodium chloride (5.48 mg), disodium EDTA (0.12 mg), and polysorbate 80 (0.70 mg) in water for injection, USP.

(Continued)

TABLE 9.3 (*Continued*)

Composition of Approved Biological Products

Product	Composition
AHF (recombinant) is a glycoprotein consisting of multiple peptides, including an 80 kDa and various extensions of the 90 kDa.	It is formulated with sucrose (0.9%–1.3%), glycine (21–25 mg/mL), and histidine (18–23 mM) as stabilizers in the final container in place of albumin. The final product also contains calcium chloride (2–3 mM), sodium (27–36 mEq/L), chloride (32–40 mEq/L), polysorbate 80 (not more than [NMT] 35 µg/mL), imidazole (NMT 20 µg/1000 IU), tri-n-butyl phosphate (NMT 5 p.g/1000 IU), and copper (NMT 0.6 µg/1000 IU). The product contains no preservatives. The albumin formulation contains 12.5 mg/mL albumin (human), 1.5 mg/mL polyethylene glycol (PEG) (3350), 180 mEq/L sodium, 55 mM histidine, 1.5 pg/AHF IU polysorbate-80, and 0.20 mg/mL calcium.
Antihemophilic factor (recombinant), plasma/albumin-free method (rAHF-PFM), is a purified glycoprotein consisting of 2332 amino acids.	When reconstituted, the product contains the following stabilizers in maximal amounts: 38 mg/mL mannitol, 10 mg/mL trehalose, 108 mEq/L sodium, 12 mM histidine, 12 mM Tris, 1.9 mM calcium, 0.17 mg/mL polysorbate-80, and 0.10 mg/mL glutathione. In another formulation, each vial contains nominally 250, 500, or 1000 IU per vial and upon reconstitution contains sodium chloride, sucrose, L.histidine, calcium chloride, and polysorbate 80.
Arcitumomab, formulated to be labeled with Technetium Tc 99 m, is a Fab' fragment generated from IMMU-4, a murine IgG1 MAb produced in murine ascitic fluid and is of 50,000 Da.	Each vial contains the nonradioactive materials necessary to prepare one patient dose, which is a sterile, lyophilized formulation, containing 1.25 mg of Arcitumomab and 0.29 mg of stannous chloride per vial, with potassium sodium tartrate tetrahydrate, sodium acetate trihydrate, sodium chloride, acetic acid, glacial, hydrochloric acid, and sucrose. Technetium Tc 99 m Arcitumomab, is formed by reconstitution of the contents of this vial with 30 mCi of Tc 99 m sodium pertechnetate in 1 mL of sodium chloride for injection, USP.
Basiliximab is a chimeric (murine/human) MAb (also known as CD25 antigen) on the surface of activated T-lymphocytes; the calculated MW of the glycoprotein is 144 kDa.	Each vial contains 20 mg basiliximab, 7.21 mg monobasic potassium phosphate, 0.99 mg disodium hydrogen phosphate (anhydrous), 1.61 mg sodium chloride, 20 mg sucrose, 80 mg mannitol, and 40 mg glycine, to be reconstituted in 5 mL of SWFI, USP. No preservatives are added.

(Continued)

TABLE 9.3 (*Continued*)

Composition of Approved Biological Products

Product	Composition
Becaplermin has a MW of approximately 25 kDa and is a homodimer composed of two identical polypeptide chains that are bound together by disulfide bonds.	Each gram of gel contains 100 μg of becaplermin, sodium carboxymethylcellulose, sodium chloride, sodium acetate trihydrate, glacial acetic acid, water for injection, and methylparaben, propylparaben, and m-cresol as preservatives, and L-lysine hydrochloride as a stabilizer.
Capromab pendetide is the murine MAb, 7E11-C5.3, conjugated to the linker-chelator, glycyltyrosyl-(N-diethylenetriaminepentaacetic acid)-lysine hydrochloride (GYK-DTPA-HCl). Given with Indium In 111.	Each vial contains 0.5 mg of capromab pendetide in 1 mL of sodium phosphate-buffered saline solution adjusted to pH 6; the sodium acetate solution must be added to the sterile, nonpyrogenic high-purity Indium In 111 chloride solution to buffer it prior to radiolabeling.
Choriogonadotropin alpha is a water-soluble glycoprotein consisting of two noncovalently linked subunits—designated (alpha) and (beta)—consisting of 92 and 145 amino acid residues, respectively, with carbohydrate moieties linked to ASN-52 and ASN-78 (on alpha subunit) and ASN-13, ASN-30, SER-121, SER-127, SER-132, and SER-138 (on beta subunit).	Each vial contains 285 mcg of choriogonadotropin alpha, 30 mg sucrose, 0.98 mg phosphoric acid, and sodium hydroxide (for pH adjustment) which, when reconstituted with the diluent, will deliver 250 mcg of recombinant human chorionic gonadotropin. The pH of the reconstituted solution is 6.5–7.5.
Coagulation Factor IX (recombinant) is a glycoprotein with an approximate molecular mass of 55,000 Da consisting of 415 amino acids in a single chain.	Each vial contains 250, 500, or 1000 IU of Coagulation Factor IX (recombinant). After reconstitution of the lyophilized DP, the concentrations of excipients in the 500- and 1000 IU dosage strengths are 10 mM l-histidine, 1% sucrose, 260 mM glycine, and 0.005% polysorbate 80. The concentrations after reconstitution in the 250 IU dosage strength are half those of the other two dosage strengths. The 500-and 1000 IU dosage strengths are isotonic after reconstitution, and the 250 IU dosage strength has half the tonicity of the other two dosage strengths after reconstitution. All dosage strengths yield a clear, colorless solution upon reconstitution.
Coagulation Factor VIIa (rFVIIa) is a vitamin K- dependent glycoprotein consisting of 406 amino acid residues (MW is 50 kDa).	Each vial contains 1.2 mg rFVIIa, 5.85 mg sodium chloride, calcium chloride (2.94 mg), glycylglycine (2.64 mg), Tween 80 (0.14 mg), and mannitol (60 mg); the sodium content is 0.44 mEq and calcium content is 0.06 mEq.

(Continued)

TABLE 9.3 (*Continued*)

Composition of Approved Biological Products

Product	Composition
Daclizumab is humanized IgG1 MAb with MW of approximately 144 kDa.	Each milliliter contains 5 mg of Daclizumab and 3.6 mg of sodium phosphate monobasic monohydrate, 11 mg of sodium phosphate dibasic heptahydrate, 4.6 mg of sodium chloride, 0.2 mg of polysorbate 80 and may contain hydrochloric acid or sodium hydroxide to adjust the pH to 6.9. No preservatives are added.
Darbepoetin alpha is a 165-amino acid protein that differs from recombinant human erythropoietin in containing five *N*-linked oligosaccharide chains, whereas recombinant human erythropoietin contains three. The two additional *N*-glycosylation sites result from amino acid substitutions in the erythropoietin peptide backbone. The additional carbohydrate chains increase the approximate MW of the glycoprotein from 30,000 to 37,000 Da.	Two formulations contain excipients as follows: polysorbate solution contains 0.05 mg of polysorbate 80, 2.12 mg of sodium phosphate monobasic monohydrate, 0.66 mg of sodium phosphate dibasic anhydrous, and 8.18 mg of sodium chloride in water for injection, USP (per 1 mL) at pH 6.2 ± 0.2. Albumin solution contains 2.5 mg of albumin (human), 2.23 mg of sodium phosphate monobasic monohydrate, 0.53 mg of sodium phosphate dibasic anhydrous, and 8.18 mg of sodium chloride in water for injection, USP (per 1 mL) at pH 6.0 ± 0.3.
Denileukin diftitox, a rDNA-derived cytotoxic protein composed of the amino acid sequences for diphtheria toxin fragments A and B (Met 1-Thr 387)-His followed by the sequences for interleukin-2 (IL-2: Ala 1-Thr 133) and has a MW of 58 kDa.	Each 2 mL vial contains 300 mcg of recombinant denileukin diftitox in a sterile solution of citric acid (20 mM), EDTA (0.05 mM), and polysorbate 20 (<1%) in water for injection, USP. The solution has a pH of 6.9–7.2.
Dornase alpha, rhDNase, a glycoprotein that contains 260 amino acids with an approximate MW of 37,000 Da.	The aqueous solution contains 1.0 mg/mL of dornase alpha, 0.15 mg/mL of calcium chloride dihydrate, and 8.77 mg/mL of sodium chloride. The solution contains no preservative. The nominal pH of the solution is 6.3 and is used as nebulizer.
Drotrecogin alpha (activated) is a glycoprotein of approximately 55 kDa MW, consisting of a heavy chain and a light chain linked by a disulfide bond.	Each vial contains 5 and 20 mg drotrecogin alpha and 40.3 and 158.1 mg of sodium chloride, 10.9 and 42.9 mg of sodium citrate, and 31.8 and 124.9 mg of sucrose, respectively.
Efalizumab is humanized IgG1 kappa isotype, monoclonal, and has a MW of approximately 150 kDa.	Each single-use vial contains 150 mg of efalizumab, 123.2 mg of sucrose, 6.8 mg of L-histidine hydrochloride monohydrate, 4.3 mg of L-histidine and, 3 mg of polysorbate 20 and is designed to deliver 125 mg of efalizumab in 1.25 mL.

(Continued)

TABLE 9.3 (*Continued*)

Composition of Approved Biological Products

Product	Composition
Erythropoietin is a glycoprotein (Epoetin alpha), a 165 amino acid glycoprotein with MW of 30,400 Da.	Each 1 mL of single dose solution contains 2000, 3000, 4000 or 10,000 units of Epoetin alpha, 2.5 mg of albumin (human), 5.8 mg of sodium citrate, 5.8 mg of sodium chloride, and 0.06 mg of citric acid in water for injection, USP (pH 6.9 ± 0.3). This formulation contains no preservative. The 2 mL (20,000 units, 10,000 units/mL) multidose vial, each 1 mL of solution contains 10,000 units of Epoetin alpha, 2.5 mg of albumin (human), 1.3 mg of sodium citrate, 8.2 mg of sodium chloride, 0.11 mg of citric acid, and 1% benzyl alcohol as preservative in water for injection, USP (pH 6.1 ± 0.3).
Etanercept is a dimeric fusion protein consisting of the extracellular ligand-binding portion of the human 75 kDa (p75) TNFR linked to the Fc portion of human IgG1. The Fc component of etanercept contains the CH2 domain, the CH3 domain, and hinge region, but not the CH1 domain of IgG1. It consists of 934 amino acids and has an apparent MW of approximately 150 kDa.	After reconstitution with 1 mL of the supplied sterile BWFI, USP (containing 0.9% benzyl alcohol), solution is clear and colorless, with a pH of 7.4 ± 0.3. Each single-use vial of etanercept contains 25 mg of etanercept, 40 mg of mannitol, 10 mg of sucrose, and 1.2 mg of tromethamine.
Filgrastim is a human G-CSF, and is a 175 amino acid protein that has a MW of 18,800 Da.	The single-use 300 mcg prefilled syringe (0.5 mL) contains acetate (0.295 mg), sorbital (25 mg), Tween 80 (0.004%), and sodium (0.0175 mg); higher concentration of 480 mcg contains proportional amounts of additives.
Follicle-stimulating hormone (FSH) consists of two noncovalently linked, nonidentical glycoproteins designated as the (alpha)- and (beta)-subunits. The (alpha)- and (beta)- subunits have 92 and 111 amino acids, respectively.	For subcutaneous injection after reconstitution with SWFI, USP for single-dose ampules or BWFI (0.9% benzyl alcohol), or USP for multiple-dose vials. Each ampule contains 37.5, 75, or 150 IU rFSH, 30 mg of sucrose, 1.11 mg of dibasic sodium phosphate, and 0.45 mg of monobasic sodium phosphate monohydrate. 0-phosphoric acid and/or sodium hydroxide may be used prior to lyophilization for pH adjustment. It may contain up to 15% of oxidized FSH.
hFSH, a glycoprotein hormone, which is manufactured by rDNA technology, a dimeric structure containing two glycoprotein subunits (alpha and beta). Both the 92 amino acid alpha-chain and the 111 amino acid beta-chain have complex heterogeneous structures arising from two N-linked oligosaccharide chains.	Each vial contains 75 IU of FSH activity plus 25.0 mg of sucrose, NF, 7.35 mg of sodium citrate dihydrate, USP, 0.10 mg of polysorbate 20, NF, and hydrochloric acid, NF and/or sodium hydroxide, NF to adjust the pH to a sterile, lyophilized form. The pH of the reconstituted preparation is approximately 7.0.

(*Continued*)

TABLE 9.3 (*Continued*)

Composition of Approved Biological Products

Product	Composition
Galactosidase alpha is an enzyme, which is a homodimeric glycoprotein with a MW of approximately 100 kDa.	Each vial contains 37 mg of alpha-galactosidase beta as well as 222 mg of mannitol, 20.4 mg of sodium phosphate monobasic monohydrate, and 59.2 mg of sodium phosphate dibasic heptahydrate. Following reconstitution as directed, 35 mg of agalactosidase beta (7 mL) may be extracted from each vial.
Gemtuzumab ozogamicin is a humanized IgG4, kappa antibody conjugated with a cytotoxic antitumor or antibiotic, calicheamicin via a bifunctional linker. It has a MW of 151–153 kDa.	Each vial contains 5 mg of drug conjugate (protein equivalent) in a 20 mL amber vial. The inactive ingredients are: dextran 40, sucrose, sodium chloride, monobasic and dibasic sodium phosphate. Light-sensitive.
Glucagon (rDNA origin) has the empirical formula of C153H225 N43O49S, and a MW of 3483. It is a single-chain polypeptide containing 29 amino acid residues and a MW of 3483.	Each vial contains Glucagon as hydrochloride, 1 mg (corresponding to 1 IU). Other ingredient is lactose monohydrate (107 mg).
Hemophilus B conjugate (meningococcal protein conjugate) and Hepatitis B (recombinant) Vaccine is a sterile bivalent vaccine.	Each 0.5 mL contains 7.5 mcg dose conjugated to approximately 125 mcg of outer membrane protein complex, 5 mcg of HBsAg, approximately 225 mcg of aluminum as amorphous aluminum hydroxyphosphate sulfate, and 35 mcg of sodium borate (decahydrate) as a pH stabilizer, in 0.9% sodium chloride. The vaccine contains not more than 0.0004% (w/v) residual formaldehyde.
Hepatitis B (recombinant) vaccine is a noninfectious rDNA hepatitis B vaccine containing purified surface antigen of the virus obtained by culturing genetically engineered Saccharomyces cerevisiae cells, which carry the surface antigen gene of the hepatitis B virus.	Each 0.5 mL of the vaccine consists of 10 mcg of hepatitis B surface antigen adsorbed on 0.25 mg of aluminum as aluminum hydroxide with a trace amount of thimerosal (<0.5 mcg of mercury) from the manufacturing process, sodium chloride (9 mg/mL), and phosphate buffers (disodium phosphate dihydrate, 0.98 mg/mL; sodium dihydrogen phosphate dihydrate, 0.71 mg/mL). Each 1 mL adult dose consists of 20 mcg of hepatitis B surface antigen adsorbed on 0.5 mg of aluminum as aluminum hydroxide. The adult vaccine is formulated without preservatives. The adult formulation contains a trace amount of thimerosal (<1.0 mcg of mercury) from the manufacturing process, sodium chloride (9 mg/mL), and phosphate buffers (disodium phosphate dihydrate, 0.98 mg/mL; sodium dihydrogen phosphate dihydrate, 0.71 mg/mL).

(*Continued*)

TABLE 9.3 (*Continued*)

Composition of Approved Biological Products

Product	Composition
Insulin glargine (rDNA origin) injection is human insulin analog that differs from human insulin in that the amino acid asparagine at position A21 is replaced by glycine and two arginines are added to the C-terminus of the B-chain. Chemically, it is 21 A-Gly-30 B a-L-Arg-30 B b-L-Arg-human insulin and has the empirical formula C267H404N72O78S6 and a MW of 6063.	Each milliliter contains 100 IU (3.6378 mg) of insulin glargine, 30 mcg of zinc, 2.7 mg of m-cresol, 20 mg of glycerol 85%, and water for injection. The pH is adjusted by addition of aqueous solutions of hydrochloric acid and sodium hydroxide and has a pH of approximately 4.
Imiglucerase is an analog of the human enzyme, (beta)-glucocerebrosidase, a monomeric glycoprotein of 497 amino acids, containing four N-linked glycosylation sites (MW = 60,430).	Each vial contains imiglucerase (212 units), mannitol (170 mg), sodium citrates (70 mg), trisodium citrate (52 mg), disodium hydrogen citrate (18 mg), polysorbate 80 (0.53 mg). Citric acid and/or sodium hydroxide may have been added at the time of manufacture to adjust pH. Haemaccel® (cross-linked gelatin polypeptides) is used as a stabilizing agent.
Infliximab is a chimeric IgG1 k MAb with an approximate MW of 149,100 Da. It is composed of human constant and murine variable regions.	Each single-use vial contains 100 mg of infliximab, 500 mg of sucrose, 0.5 mg of polysorbate 80, 2.2 mg of monobasic sodium phosphate, monohydrate, and 6.1 mg of dibasic sodium phosphate, dihydrate. No preservatives are present.
Insulin aspart (rDNA origin) homologous with regular human insulin with the exception of a single substitution of the amino acid proline by aspartic acid in position B28 with the empirical formula C256H381N65O79S6 and a MW of 5825.8.	Each milliliter contains insulin aspart (B28 asp regular human insulin analog), 100 units/mL, glycerin (16 mg/mL), phenol (1.50 mg/mL), metacresol (1.72 mg/mL), zinc (19.6 μg/mL), disodium hydrogen phosphate dihydrate (1.25 mg/mL), and sodium chloride (0.58 mg/mL). It has a pH of 7.2–7.6. Hydrochloric acid 10% and/or sodium hydroxide 10% may be added to adjust pH.
Insulin glulisine (rDNA origin) differs from human insulin in that the amino acid asparagine at position B3 is replaced by lysine and the lysine in position B29 is replaced by glutamic acid. Chemically, it is 3B-lysine-29B-glutamic acid-human insulin, and has the empirical formula C258H384N64O78S6 and a MW of 5823.	Each milliliter of APIDRA (insulin glulisine injection) contains 100 IU (3.49 mg) of insulin glulisine, 3.15 mg of m-cresol, 6 mg of tromethamine, 5 mg of sodium chloride, 0.01 mg of polysorbate 20, and water for injection.

(*Continued*)

TABLE 9.3 (*Continued*)

Composition of Approved Biological Products

Product	Composition
Insulin lispro (rDNA origin) is Lys(B28), Pro(B29) human insulin analog, created when the amino acids at positions 28 and 29 on the insulin B-chain are reversed. It has the empirical formula C257H383N65O77S6 and a MW of 5808, both identical to that of human insulin.	Each milliliter contains insulin lispro 100 units, 16 mg of glycerin, 1.88 mg of dibasic sodium phosphate, 3.15 mg of m-cresol, zinc oxide content adjusted to provide 0.0197 mg of zinc ion, trace amounts of phenol, and water for injection. Insulin lispro has a pH of 7.0–7.8. Hydrochloric acid 10% and/or sodium hydroxide 10% may be added to adjust pH.
Interferon alpha-2a contains 165 amino acids, and it has an approximate MW of 19,000 Da.	Each milliliter contains 3 MIU of interferon alpha-2a, recombinant, 7.21 mg of sodium chloride, 0.2 mg of polysorbate 80, 10 mg of benzyl alcohol as a preservative, and 0.77 mg of ammonium acetate.
Interferon alpha-2b has a MW of 19,271 Da.	Each milliliter contains 3, 5, 18, 25, or 50 MIU and also contains 20 mg of glycine, 2.3 mg of sodium phosphate dibasic, 0.55 mg of sodium phosphate monobasic, and 1.0 mg of human albumin after reconstitution. The solution formulation contains besides the active drug, 7.5 mg of sodium chloride, 1.8 mg of sodium phosphate dibasic, 1.3 mg of sodium phosphate monobasic, 0.1 mg of edetate disodium, 0.1 mg of polysorbate 80, and 1.5 mg of m-cresol as a preservative. The multidose preparations also contain 1.5 mg of cresol as preservative.
Interferon alphacon1 has a 166-amino acid sequence and differs from interferon alpha-2b at 20/166 amino acids (88% homology), and comparison with interferon-beta shows identity over 30% of the amino acid positions and has a MW of 19,434 Da.	Each vial and prefilled syringe contain 0.03 mg/mL of interferon alpha con-1, 5.9 mg/mL of sodium chloride, and 3.8 mg/mL of sodium phosphate in water for injection, USP.
Interferon beta-1a is a 166-amino acid glycoprotein with a MW of approximately 22,500 Da.	Each 0.5 mL contains either 44 mcg or 22 mcg of interferon beta-1a, 4 or 2 mg of albumin (human) USP, 27.3 mg of mannitol USP, 0.4 mg of sodium acetate, and water for injection, USP.
Interferon beta-1a is a 166-amino acid glycoprotein with a predicted MW of approximately 22,500 Da.	Each 1.0 mL (1.0 cc) of reconstituted solution contains 30 mcg of interferon beta-1a, 15 mg of albumin (human), USP, 5.8 mg of sodium chloride, USP, 5.7 mg of dibasic sodium phosphate, USP, and 1.2 mg of monobasic sodium phosphate, USP, at a pH of approximately 7.3.

(Continued)

TABLE 9.3 (Continued)

Composition of Approved Biological Products

Product	Composition
Interferon beta-1b is a protein that has 165 amino acids and an approximate MW of 18,500 Da. It does not include the carbohydrate side-chains found in the natural material.	Dextrose and albumin (human), USP (15 mg each/vial) are added as stabilizers. Lyophilized Betaseron is a sterile, white to off-white powder intended for subcutaneous injection after reconstitution with the diluent supplied (sodium chloride, 0.54% solution).
Interferon gamma-1b is a single-chain polypeptide containing 140 amino acids consisting of noncovalent dimers of two identical 16,465 Da monomers.	Each 0.5 mL contains: 100 mcg (two million IU) of interferon gamma-1b formulated in 20 mg of mannitol, 0.36 mg of sodium succinate, 0.05 mg of polysorbate 20, and SWFI.
Interleukin eleven (IL-11) is a thrombopoietic growth factor, has a molecular mass of approximately 19,000 Da, and is nonglycosylated. The polypeptide is 177 amino acids in length.	Each vial contains 5 mg of IL-11 with 23 mg of glycine, USP, 1.6 mg of dibasic sodium phosphate heptahydrate, USP, and 0.55 mg of monobasic sodium phosphate monohydrate, USP. When reconstituted with 1 mL of SWFI, USP, the resulting solution has a pH of 7.0 and a concentration of 5 mg/mL.
Laronidase is a glycoprotein with a MW of approximately 83 kDa. The recombinant protein is comprised of 628 amino acids after cleavage of the N-terminus and contains six N-linked oligosaccharide modification sites. Two oligosaccharide chains terminate in mannose-6-phosphate sugars.	Must be diluted prior to administration in 0.9% sodium chloride injection, USP containing 0.1% of albumin (human). The solution in each vial contains a nominal laronidase concentration of 0.58 mg/mL and a pH of approximately 5.5. The extractable volume of 5.0 mL from each vial provides 2.9 mg of laronidase, 43.9 mg of sodium chloride, 63.5 mg of sodium phosphate monobasic monohydrate, 10.7 mg of sodium phosphate dibasic heptahydrate, and 0.05 mg of polysorbate 80.
Lepirudin (rDNA) is: [Leu1, Thr2]-63-desulfohirudin, a polypeptide composed of 65 amino acids and has a MW of 6979.5 Da.	Each vial contains 50 mg of lepirudin, 40 mg of mannitol and sodium hydroxide for adjustment of pH to approximately 7.
Muromonab-CD3 is a murine MAb to the CD3 antigen of human T cells. The antibody is a biochemically purified IgG2a with a heavy chain of approximately 50,000 Da and a light chain of approximately 25,000 Da.	Each ampule contains a buffered solution (pH 7.0 + 0.5) of monobasic sodium phosphate (2.25 mg), dibasic sodium phosphate (9.0 mg), sodium chloride (43 mg), and polysorbate 80 (1.0 mg) in water for injection.
Nesiritide is a hBNP with a MW of 3464 g/mol and an empirical formula of $C_{143}H_{244}N_{50}O_{42}S_4$.	Each 1.5 mg vial contains nesiritide (1.58 mg), mannitol (20.0 mg), citric acid monohydrate (2.1 mg), and sodium citrate dihydrate (2.94 mg).

(Continued)

TABLE 9.3 (*Continued*)

Composition of Approved Biological Products

Product	Composition
Omalizumab is a MAb with a MW of approximately 149 kDa.	Each vial contains 202.5 mg of omalizumab, 145.5 mg sucrose, 2.8 mg L-histidine hydrochloride monohydrate, 1.8 mg L-histidine, and 0.5 mg polysorbate 20 and is designed to deliver 150 mg of omalizumab in 1.2 mL after reconstitution with 1.4 mL SWFI, USP.
Palivizumab is a humanized MAb composed of two heavy chains and two light chains and has a MW of approximately 148,000 Da.	Upon reconstitution, it contains the following excipients: 47 mM of histidine, 3.0 mM of glycine and 5.6% mannitol, and the active ingredient, palivizumab, at a concentration of 100 mg/mL solution.
Parathyroid hormone (1–34) has a MW of 4117.8 Da.	Each prefilled delivery device is filled with 3.3 mL to deliver 3 mL. Each milliliter contains 250 mcg of teriparatide (corrected for acetate, chloride, and water content), 0.41 mg of glacial acetic acid, 0.10 mg of sodium acetate (anhydrous), 45.4 mg of mannitol, 3.0 mg of m-cresol, and water for injection. In addition, hydrochloric acid solution 10% and/or sodium hydroxide solution 10% may have been added to adjust the product to pH 4. Each cartridge preassembled into a pen device delivers 20 mcg of teriparatide per dose each day for up to 28 days.
Pegfilgrastim is a covalent conjugate of recombinant methionyl human G-CSF (filgrastim) and monomethoxypolyethylene glycol. Filgrastim is a water-soluble 175 amino acid protein with a MW of approximately 19 kDa. To produce pegfilgrastim, a 20 kDa monomethoxypolyethylene glycol (PEG) molecule is covalently bound to the *N*-terminal methionyl residue of filgrastim. The average MW of pegfilgrastim is approximately 39 kDa.	Each syringe contains 6 mg of pegfilgrastim (based on protein weight), in a sterile, clear, colorless, preservative-free solution (pH 4.0) containing acetate (0.35 mg), sorbitol (30.0 mg), polysorbate 20 (0.02 mg), and sodium (0.02 mg) in water for injection.
Peginterferon alpha-2a is a covalent conjugate of recombinant alpha-2a interferon (approximate MW is 20,000 Da) with a single branched bis-monomethoxy PEG chain (approximate MW is 40,000 Da). Peginterferon alpha-2a has an approximate MW of 60,000 Da.	Each vial contains approximately 1.2 mL of solution to deliver 1.0 mL of DP. Subcutaneous administration of 1.0 mL delivers 180 mcg of DP (expressed as the amount of interferon alpha-2a), 8.0 mg of sodium chloride, 0.05 mg of polysorbate 80, 10.0 mg of benzyl alcohol, 2.62 mg of sodium acetate trihydrate, and 0.05 mg of acetic acid. The solution is colorless to light yellow and the pH is 6.0 ± 0.01.

(*Continued*)

TABLE 9.3 (*Continued*)

Composition of Approved Biological Products

Product	Composition
Peginterferon alpha-2b is a covalent conjugate of recombinant alpha interferon with monomethoxy PEG. The MW of the PEG portion of the molecule is 12,000 Da. The average MW of the PEG-intron molecule is approximately 31,000 Da.	Each vial contains 74, 118.4, 177.6, or 222 μg of PEG-intron, and 1.11 mg of dibasic sodium phosphate anhydrous, 1.11 mg of monobasic sodium phosphate dihydrate, 59.2 mg of sucrose, and 0.074 mg of polysorbate 80. Following reconstitution with 0.7 mL of the supplied diluent (SWFI, USP), each vial contains peginterferon at strengths of 100, 160, 240, or 300 μg/mL.
Pegvisomant is a protein containing 191 amino acid residues to which several PEG polymers are covalently bound (predominantly 4 to 6 PEG/ protein molecule). The MW of the protein of pegvisomant is 21,998 Da. The MW of the PEG portion of pegvisomant is approximately 5000 Da. The predominant MWs of pegvisomant are thus approximately 42,000, 47,000, and 52,000 Da.	Each vial also contains 1.36 mg of glycine, 36.0 mg of mannitol, 1.04 mg of sodium phosphate dibasic anhydrous, and 0.36 mg of sodium phosphate monobasic monohydrate.
Rasburicase is a recombinant urate-oxidase enzyme produced by a genetically modified Saccharomyces cerevisiae strain. It is a tetrameric protein with identical subunits of a molecular mass of about 34 kDa. The molecular formula of the monomer is C1523H2383N417O4625S7. The monomer, made up of a single 301 amino acid polypeptide chain, has no intra- or interdisulfide bridges and is *N*-terminalacetylated.	Each 3 mL vial containing 1.5 mg of rasburicase, 10.6 mg of mannitol, 15.9 mg of L-alanine, and between 12.6 and 14.3 mg of dibasic sodium phosphate. The diluent solution for reconstitution, supplied in a 2 mL clear, glass ampule, is composed of 1.0 mL of SWFI, USP, and 1.0 mg of Poloxamer 188.
Reteplase is a nonglycosylated deletion mutein of tPA, containing the kringle 2 and the protease domains of human tPA. It contains 355 of the 527 amino acids of native tPA (amino acids 1–3 and 176–527). The MW is 39,571 Da.	Each vial contains 10.4 units (18.1 mg), tranexamic acid (8.32 mg), dipotassium hydrogen phosphate (136.24 mg), phosphoric acid (51.27 mg), sucrose (364 mg), and polysorbate 88 (5.2 mg).
Rituximab is a chimeric murine/human MAb composed of two heavy chains of 451 amino acids and two light chains of 213 amino acids.	The product is formulated for intravenous administration in 9.0 mg/mL of sodium chloride, 7.35 mg/mL of sodium citrate dihydrate, 0.7 mg/mL of polysorbate 80, and SWFI. The pH is adjusted to 6.5.

(Continued)

TABLE 9.3 (*Continued*)

Composition of Approved Biological Products

Product	Composition
Sargramostim is a rhu GM-CSF, a glycoprotein of 127 amino acids characterized by three primary molecular species having molecular masses of 19,500, 16,800, and 15,500 Da.	Liquid formulation contains 500 mcg (2.8×10^6 IU/mL) of sargramostim and 1.1% benzyl alcohol in 1 mL solution. Lyophilized vial contains 25 mcg (1.4×10^6 IU/vial) of sargramostim. Both contain 40 mg/mL of mannitol, 10 mg/mL of sucrose, and 1.2 mg/mL of tromethamine.
Sermorelin acetate is the acetate salt of an amidated synthetic 29-amino acid peptide (GRF 1–29 NH2) consisting of 44 amino acid residues. The free base of sermorelin has the empirical formula C 149 H 246 N 44 O 42 S and a MW of 3358 Da.	Each vial contains 0.5 mg of sermorelin (as the acetate) and 5 mg of mannitol. The pH is adjusted with dibasic sodium phosphate and monobasic sodium phosphate buffer. Each 1.0 mL vial contains 1.0 mg of sermorelin (as the acetate) and 5 mg of mannitol. The pH is adjusted with dibasic sodium phosphate and monobasic sodium phosphate buffer.
Somatropin (rDNA origin) is a polypeptide hormone of rDNA origin. It has 191 amino acid residues and a MW of 22,124 Da.	A dose of 1.5 mg is dispensed in a two-chamber cartridge. The front chamber contains recombinant somatropin (1.5 mg) (approximately 4.5 IU), glycine (27.6 mg), sodium dihydrogen phosphate anhydrous (0.3 mg), and disodium phosphate anhydrous (0.3 mg); the rear chamber contains 1.13 mL water for injection. The 5.8 mg dose system has in the rear chamber 0.3% m-cresol (as a preservative) and mannitol, 45 mg in 1.14 mL water for injection. Long acting contains 13.5 mg of somatropin, 1.2 mg of zinc acetate, 0.8 mg of zinc carbonate, and 68.9 mg of poly-L-glutamate. In another formulation, each vial contains 8.8 mg of somatropin (approximately 26.4 IU), 60.2 mg of sucrose and 2.05 mg of O-phosphoric acid. The pH is adjusted with sodium hydroxide or O-phosphoric acid. The diluent is BWFI, USP containing 0.9% benzyl alcohol added as an antimicrobial preservative.
Tenecteplase is a 527-amino acid glycoprotein.	Each vial contains 52.5 mg of Tenecteplase, 0.55 g of L-arginine, 0.17 g of phosphoric acid, and 4.3 mg of polysorbate 20, which includes a 5% overfill.
Thyrotropin alpha is a heterodimeric glycoprotein comprised of two noncovalently linked subunits, an alpha subunit of 92 amino acid residues and a beta subunit of 118 residues containing one *N*-linked glycosylation site.	Each vial contains 1.1 mg thyrotropin alpha (≥4 IU), 36 mg of mannitol, 5.1 mg of sodium phosphate, and 2.4 mg of sodium chloride. After reconstitution with 1.2 mL of SWFI, USP, the thyrotropin alpha concentration is 0.9 mg/mL. The pH of the reconstituted solution is approximately 7.0.

(Continued)

TABLE 9.3 (*Continued*)

Composition of Approved Biological Products

Product	Composition
Tositumomab and iodine I131 Tositumomab. Tositumomab is composed of two murine gamma 2a heavy chains of 451 amino acids each and two lambda light chains of 220 amino acids each. The approximate MW of Tositumomab is 150 kDa.	It is supplied at a nominal concentration of 14 mg/mL Tositumomab in 35 mg and 225 mg single-use vials. The formulation contains 10% (w/v) maltose (145 mM). The formulation for the dosimetric and the therapeutic dosage forms contains 5.0%–6.0% (w/v) of povidone, 1–2 mg/mL of maltose (dosimetric dose) or 9–15 mg/mL of maltose (therapeutic dose), 0.85–0.95 mg/mL of sodium chloride, and 0.9–1.3 mg/mL of ascorbic acid. The pH is approximately 7.0.
Trastuzumab is a rDNA-derived humanized MAb, an IgG1 kappa that contains human framework regions with the complementarity-determining regions of a murine antibody (4D5) that binds to HER2.	Each vial contains 440 mg of Trastuzumab, 9.9 mg of L-histidine HCl, 6.4 mg of L-histidine, 400 mg of (alpha)-trehalose dihydrate, and 1.8 mg of polysorbate 20, USP. Reconstitution with only 20 mL of the supplied BWFI, USP, containing 1.1% of benzyl alcohol as a preservative yields a multidose solution containing 21 mg/mL of Trastuzumab, at a pH of approximately 6.

Abbreviations: AHF, antihemophilic factor; BWFI, bacteriostatic water for injection; DP, drug product; EDTA, ethylenediaminetetraacetic acid; FSH, follicle-stimulating hormone; GCSF, granulocyte colony-stimulating factor; hBNP, human B-type natriuretic peptide; IgG1, immunoglobulin G1; IU, International Unit; MAb, monoclonal antibody; MW, molecular weight; rDNA, recombinant DNA; rhDNase, recombinant human deoxyribonuclease I; rhu GM-CSF, recombinant human granulocyte-macrophage colony-stimulating factor; SWFI, sterile water for injection; TNFR, tumor necrosis factor receptor; tPA, tissue plasminogen activator.

TABLE 9.4

Common Excipients in Biological Products

Albumin, human	Maltose
Aluminum hydroxide	Mannitol
Amorphous aluminum hydroxyphosphate	Parabens
Benzyl alcohol	Polysorbate 80
Cresol	Sodium dodecyl sulphate
Ethylenediamineteraacetic acid	Sucrose
Glutathione	Trehalose dehydrate
Glycerol	Tri-*N*-butyl phosphate
Glycine	Tromethamine
Imidazole	Zinc
L-histidine	

U.S. FDA and their composition. This table should serve as a good source to scout the most common additives found in these formulations.

An early preformulation decision is generally made regarding the final formulation, whether it will be liquid or lyophilized. It is this choice that determines which excipients will be needed (Table 9.4), as liquid and lyophilized products require different excipients. Several products are available in both forms. As clinical supplies will often require a placebo, unless the product is developed as a generic equivalent, these formulations will be made without the active ingredient.

There are common ingredients to specific type of products; for example, vaccines would be stabilized and formulated differently, requiring adsorption ingredients or the use of zinc in insulin to prolong their action, and so on. It is important to know that despite the large number of products available in the market, the formulation of these injectable products includes a rather limited number of components, as anticipated; therefore, any preformulation study may be extended to these interaction studies. As stabilized commercial products have been in use, it becomes easier to select an excipient that would be compatible with packaging commodities, particularly syringes, rubber stoppers, and so on.

Prospective formulations will depend to a great degree on the pharmacokinetics, dosing levels, and indications for use. Unlike other drugs where the pharmacology of the product may be a new discovery, many biological products, especially the recombinant DNA products, focus on providing the endogenous compounds or antigens to promote antibody production. As a result, the indications may well be known at the preformulation stages, and interaction studies to obtain a delivery system can be made by taking into account the pharmacokinetics of the drug. It is also important if the product will be administered daily, weekly, or on longer bases or whether it would be a single-dose packaging or a multiple-dose packaging. Multiple-dose packages require use of preservatives, and there is much disagreement among the regulatory authorities on how the preservative efficacy test should be conducted and also what type of preservatives to use; for example, phenol cannot be used in products destined for Japan.

9.9 Packaging and Materials

Packaging material is an important part of formulation because of possible inter-actions. Protein may stick to the walls of a vial or other containers, particularly in low-concentration formulations. Glass is also reactive; it can be delaminated, for example, through contact with a formulation. Certain kinds of plastic are less reactive than glass. The importance of packaging materials was highlighted in the case of erythropoietin formulation sold outside of the United States under the brand name of Eprex®. Since December 2002, there has been a significant and sustained worldwide decrease in newly reported cases of erythropoietin antibody-positive pure red cell aplasia (PRCA) in patients with chronic renal failure who receive the recombinant erythropoietin medication Eprex (epoetin alpha). The most probable product-specific cause of the increased incidence of PRCA in patients with chronic renal failure being treated with Eprex has been identified as the so-called leach-ates. By 2005, the incidence of PRCA was reduced to its pre-2002 incidence, when steps were taken to remove the causes of PRCA. These included the use of more immune response-causing subcutaneous route in place of intravenous use and the replacement of albumin with Tween 80 in the formulation. An interaction between uncoated rubber stoppers, previously used in prefilled syringes of Eprex, and the stabilizer polysorbate 80 was also identified. This interaction resulted in the pres-ence of organic compounds—called leachates—in prefilled syringes with uncoated rubber stoppers. Coated stoppers, which prevent the interaction with the stabilizer, are now used in all Eprex prefilled syringes. These observations emphasize the need to investigate possible interactions between the formulation and the stopper or elastomer, since such contact could even destroy the protein. To test the reactivity of stoppers, vials are inverted—to give their rubber stoppers total contact with the formulation—and then stored horizontally to create more surface area—and more chances for the protein to degrade. More oxidation of the protein can occur as the surface area grows larger.

The replacement of albumin in Eprex example was made in response to the concern that the human serum albumin used in the manufacture of the drug could transmit a variant of Creutzfeldt–Jakob disease. This example shows remarkably how subtle change in the formulation can produce significant changes in the toxicity of the drug; generally, this would not be the case with small-molecule drugs. Table 9.3 lists eight products wherein human albumin is used as a stabilizer, compared with 31 products wherein polysorbate surfactants are used; it is noteworthy that it was not the surfac-tant but its interaction with the packaging commodity that resulted, at least in part, in the adverse reaction.

9.9.1 Dosage Form and Storage

Storage conditions and handling of product make much difference in how the product is marketed: refrigerated, frozen, freeze-dried, or kept in reduced-light yellow or brown vials, for example. Less stringent storage conditions are preferred. The shelf life of the product is preferably 1–2 years, but it is not possible to wait that long at the prescribed temperature in the early development stage; generally, after 3 months of testing, the data will be sent to the CBER, and it may be necessary to change the formulations as more stability data become available; while formulation changes prove expensive, if these result in extension of the shelf life, it is almost always a good investment.

Proteins are most stable in solid form and show less impact of storage temperature (though they still need to be kept at a cool temperature). The liquid formulations are more advanced formulations that are generally stabilized and must be stored at controlled temperature throughout the use chain. As the bulk manufacturing of proteins results in a concentrated solution state, this must be processed to concentrate and eventually solidify it through such processes as cryopreservation, cryogranulation, spray-drying, undercooling, and lyophilization.

9.9.2 Cryopreservation

Freezing can extend the shelf life of unstable products and improve containment if the freeze–thaw process is consistent. Frozen products can be transported safely for final formulation elsewhere and stockpiled to optimize the fill and finish process, which can reduce the processing costs. Generally, freeze–thaw cycles result in a significant loss of activity, and many believe that proteins cannot be frozen and thawed without damage, because no practical methods exist for doing so on a large scale. The usual method, which is both slow and nonreproducible, involves small volumes in bags, bottles, or vials freezing at $-0°C$ or below. A slow freeze alters the physical properties (pH, diffusion, and reaction rates) of the aqueous solvent medium or mixture, which can denature proteins, particularly over an extended time. The solution is then thawed at room temperature, with some components thawing before others. Ice recrystallization in the thawing process creates mechanical stress.

9.9.2.1 Cryogranulation

It is a frequently used technique for small-molecule drugs, but cryogranulation of proteins using liquid nitrogen has not been very successful.

9.9.2.2 Spray Drying

It is a dehydration process that uses heat from a hot-air stream to evaporate dispersed droplets created by atomization of a continuous liquid feed. Products dry within a few seconds into fine particles (powders). It is similar to freeze-drying. Important data for formulators working with any type of freezing process will be the glass transition temperature (T_g) of each component and the solution. At this temperature, ice crystal formation decreases to undetectable levels, and the freeze is an amorphous glass from which water will sublime. Spray drying offers some advantages over freeze drying: shorter process times, lower capital investment in equipment, and lower energy input to the solution, which can lessen the chances for protein denaturation. Disadvantages include the brief but high air-temperature exposure during the rapid-drying step (around 100°C) and shear stresses caused by spraying a formulation through a nozzle. The product temperature reaches about 80°C but only for a fraction of a second. Particle characteristics and size distribution can be closely controlled in spray drying by changing process variables, such as solution composition and feed rate, atomizing gas pressure, air flow rate, and the inlet and outlet gas temperatures.

Physical characteristics of the final product (size, morphology, surface area, and density of particles), biochemical characteristics (purity, potency, solubility, and stability of the formulation), and process yields may be manipulated. The goal is a dry, free-flowing powder with well-defined particle characteristics and consistent purity and presentation and an active, stable, and acceptable dissolution profile, all obtained by as simple a process as possible.

9.9.2.3 Undercooling

It is another process wherein under certain conditions, a liquid can be cooled to temperatures below its freezing point (supercooling or undercooling). If a solution is separated into droplets, as in a mist or a water-in-oil emulsion, then only those drops with particles in them will freeze if cooled, rather than catalyzing a chain reaction of freezing throughout the solution. For protein formulations, the product in aqueous solution can be dispersed as microparticles through an oil-phase carrier (liquid at the mixing temperature and solid if stored at $-20°C$), so that the drops are locked in as liquid. Reconstitution is easier than with a lyophilized or spray-dried product, as the product is warmed up at the point of use until the phases separate. This undercooling process may be used for even high-concentration protein formulations, requiring no additives like glycerol, which must be filtered out before the product can be used. Undercooling may be a particularly good choice for products that are susceptible to freeze damage.

9.9.2.4 Lyophilization

This technique produces stress conditions that may cause certain stresses on proteins that can result in unfolding (though generally completely refolded when reconstituted); so, specific conditions must be determined, and stabilizing additives must be appropriate for use during both the freezing and drying stages to allow at least 2 years of shelf life, with stable cake morphology, dispersibility, and dissolution. The presence of solutes lowers the freezing temperature of an aqueous solution, making the solution more viscous at even below water's freezing temperature, when the solute becomes supersaturated and releases latent heat; this point is known as the eutectic point, T_e; when the physical state changes from elastic liquid to brittle but amorphous solid glass, this is called glass transition temperature or T_g, at which point ice formation ceases. For pure water, T_g is $-134°C$. The T_g for solutes is generally higher, and for solutions, it is somewhere in between. The T_g is an important temperature, as below this temperature, the mobility of a solution is greatly reduced, and all degradation reactions slow down, except reactions such as oxidation. The presence of some moisture reduces T_g, and the presence of components such as sugar raises it substantially.

Freezing forms an amorphous solid of the protein and excipients with associated water in crystalline form. Annealing, an optional step, increases ice-crystal size and allows crystallization of bulking agents (such as glycine or mannitol), removing them from the amorphous portion and increasing T_g. Primary drying sublimes water ice at temperatures lower than T_g (to avoid collapse of the cake). The higher the T_g, the higher can be the mixture's temperature and sublimation rate. Increasing the protein to the excipient ratio will increase T_g. Secondary drying removes water from the amorphous phase by an increase in the sample temperature, which still may not exceed T_g.

Luckily, as water leaves the amorphous phase, T_g increases. Sample temperatures play a larger role than the duration of secondary drying for determining final water content of the lyophilized cake. Low moisture increases T_g and thus increases the temperature at which the product can be stored.

A drug solution is first frozen at the atmospheric pressure, and then, water is removed by a reduction of pressure in the lyophilizer chamber, collecting the water as ice on a condenser. Samples are placed in glass vials and frozen, either before being put in the lyophilizer or on the lyophilizer shelves. The samples contain ice crystals, unfrozen water, amorphous solids (including the therapeutic protein), and crystalline additives. Pressure is reduced, and the ice crystals sublime. This constitutes the primary drying.

It is harder to remove the unfrozen water trapped in an amorphous solid. So, after primary drying, a secondary drying stage removes that water by increasing the temperature. The final temperature of this secondary process is the key factor in determining the residual moisture in the dried cake. The pressure is kept the same for secondary and primary drying, to avoid protein collapse. The ideal result is a porous cake with little residual moisture. Porosity is important in later reconstituting the product.

Sometimes, an annealing step (in which the product is kept at a set temperature) is added before the primary drying or near the end of secondary drying to crystallize excipients. This assures that crystallization and moisture release do not happen in an uncontrolled fashion later on during shipping and storage. Phase changes (e.g., crystallization of formulation sugars) during shipping or storage can be disastrous. Moisture can even transfer from rubber vial-stoppers during storage, unless savvy formulators plan for and prevent it.

The criteria for dried-protein stability include minimum lyophilization-induced unfolding, with proteins native in the dried solid; a powder with T_g higher than the desired storage temperature; low residual moisture (<1%) in the cake; and formulation conditions (such as pH) that inhibit chemical degradation reactions unaffected by glass transition (such as oxidation). The goal is to design the fastest and most robust (acceptable quality even with variations in operating parameters) processing cycle: one that consumes the least amount of energy, does not compromise product quality, and produces a mechanically strong, rapidly insoluble cake. The cycle must be controlled for reproducibility and rapid correction of any problems that develop.

The use of FT-IR spectroscopy shows that almost all proteins except G-CSF (filgrastim) unfold during lyophilization, and while they do refold upon reconstitution, it is often necessary to add ingredients and stabilizers to keep them from unfolding in the solid state. Some of the ingredients used are listed in Table 9.4. However, the use of additives, when combined, may show unexpected interactions, synergism, enhanced instability, or even altered immunogenicity. For example, sugars (or saccharides) raise T_g and act as stabilizers. Dextran, lactose, maltose, sucrose, and trehalose are used, but the latter two are preferred. Acidic amino acids (glutamic acid, glycine, histidine, and threonine) and alkaline amino acids (arginine and lysine) are used to adjust pH besides the use of buffering systems. A nonionic surfactant (usually a polysorbate) is often added to inhibit protein aggregation in the early stage of processing, and given its innocuous nature, it is left in the formulation, while other contaminants such as the peroxides are removed. Also included in the formulations are other surfactants and bulking agents, such as mannitol and certain biodegradable polymers, mainly in low-concentration formulations.

A patented variation of the classical lyophilization technology is applied as VitriLife (3), wherein the product is lyophilized using a mixture of sugars; this formulation can be prepared in a much shorter time and is different from classic lyophilization in that no sublimation is involved and the product undergoes fast drying; the resultant product can be kept at room temperature, obviating the need for the cold chain for these products. The method has been applied to cholera vaccine and other vaccines and is still under development.

9.9.2.4.1 Stabilization through PEGylation

Where stabilization of native proteins is of great importance while in the formulation, the use of PEGylation is made to prolong the disposition half-lives of proteins in the body. It is a relatively new technique that requires fusing PEG molecule with the drug (Figure 9.15) and features the following:

- Improved bioavailability, including longer circulation time and slower clearance
- Optimized pharmacokinetics, resulting in sustained duration
- Improved safety profile, with lower toxicity, immunogenicity, and antigenicity
- Increased efficacy
- Decreased dosing frequency
- Improved drug solubility and stability
- Reduced proteolysis
- Controlled drug release

There are different types of PEGs. Linear PEGs are straight-chained PEGs that are monofunctional, homobifunctional, or heterobifunctional. Linear monofunctional PEGs (mPEG-X) have one reactive moiety at one end of the PEG, with the other end considered nonreactive (typically end-capped with a methoxy group). Linear homo-bifunctional PEGs (X-PEG-X) contain the same reactive moiety at each end of the PEG. Linear heterobifunctional PEGs (X-PEG-Y) contain a different reactive moiety at each end of the PEG. Branched PEGs (PEG2-X), also referred to as "Y-shaped" branched PEGs, contain two PEGs attached to a central core, from which extends a tethered reactive moiety. Forked PEGs (PEG-X2) contain a PEG whose one end has two or more tethered reactive moieties, extending from a central core. Multiarm PEGs (two-, three-, four-, and eight-arm PEG-Xs) are based on ethyoxylation of either glyc-erin (three-arm), pentaerythritol (four-arm), or hexaglycerin (eight-arm). The two-arm PEG was previously noted under the linear homobifunctional and heterobifunctional PEGs. Each arm has a tethered reactive group on the end. These multifunctional PEGs

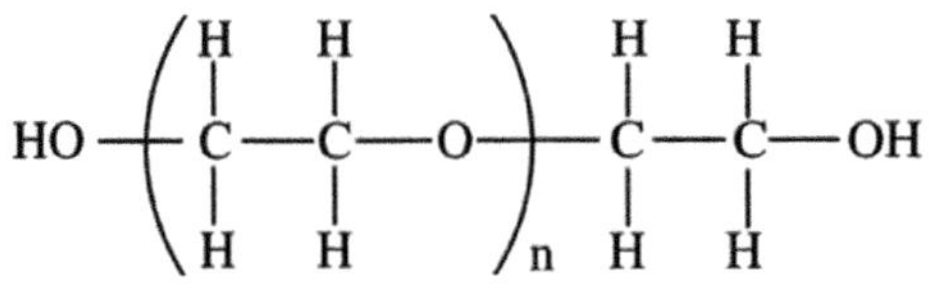

$$HO \left(\begin{array}{c} H \quad H \\ | \quad | \\ C - C - O \\ | \quad | \\ H \quad H \end{array} \right)_n \begin{array}{c} H \quad H \\ | \quad | \\ C - C - OH \\ | \quad | \\ H \quad H \end{array}$$

FIGURE 9.15   Structure of polyethylene glycol.

offer the potential to increase the potency of the resulting conjugate by attaching multiple drug molecules to each arm of the PEG. Multifunctional PEGs have several applications, including linking macromolecules to surfaces (for immunoassays, biosensors, or various probe applications), hydrogel formation, and drug targeting, as well as targeting liposomes and viruses.

All PEGs have some variance in the number of ethylene oxide units; this is a result of anionic polymerization. Polydispersity (PD) is a ratio that represents the broadness of a MW distribution. It is the ratio of the number average MW (M_n) to the weight average MV (M_w) (PD = M_w/M_n). If the PD is equal to one, then M_n equals M_w and the polymer is said to be monodispersed. Typically, polymers are not truly mono-dispersed; however, PEGs made anionically do have a low PD (1.01–1.08). As M_n changes with M_w, the PD changes (PD will always be >1 for polymers).

The process of PEGylation is complex to control the location of the PEGylation bond, requiring detailed studies on the effect of ionic strength, pH; for isotonicity purposes, glycine or sodium chloride is also added; when using cryoprotection, the use of sucrose and mannitol is recommended, and for general purpose, polysorbate 80 works well in most situations. As mPEG fuses to lysine reside on polypeptide chains, the 3D structure of protein must be well understood in native conformation. One of the negative aspects of PEGylation is the heterogeneity of the product that requires more expensive separation procedures, and the final product is more expensive. When the formulation is well-balanced, the in vivo stability is improved and the effect of agitation on the formulation is minimized; how PEGylation protects against agitation is not known. The effect of agitation was noted when the formulations of erythropoietin were changed for protein stabilization using surfactants.

Nektar Advanced PEGylation (4) is a major supplier of activated large PEGs that provide several advantages over early-stage low-MW PEGylation technology. The advanced PEGylation yields single PEGylation, more stable product, higher bioactivity, and high product purity (Figure 9.16).

In an aqueous medium, the long, chain-like PEG molecule is heavily hydrated and in rapid motion. This rapid motion causes the PEG to sweep out a large volume and prevents the approach and interference of other molecules. As a result, when attached to a drug, PEG polymer chains can protect the drug molecules from immune response and other clearance mechanisms, sustaining drug bioavailability. Covalent drug

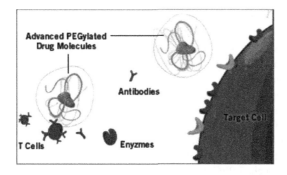

FIGURE 9.16 Improved drug performance using advanced PEGylation. (From http://www.nektar. com.)

modification with PEG enables improved drug performance by optimizing pharmacokinetics, increasing bioavailability, decreasing immunogenicity, and decreasing dosing frequency by using stable PEG linkages. These activated high-MW PEGs can be linked site-specifically to drug molecules. The following is a list of commercial products that were developed in a PEGylated form:

- Neulasta® (pegfilgrastim) by Amgen
- Somavert® (pegvisomant) by Pfizer
- PEGASYS® (peginterferon alpha-2a) by Roche
- PEG-INTRON® (peginterferon alpha-2b) by Schering-Plough
- Definity® (perflutren lipid microsphere) by Bristol-Myers Squibb
- Macugen® (pegabtanib) by Eyetech and Pfizer
- DuraSeal™ (PEG hydrogel) by Confluent Surgical

Numerous studies have demonstrated that PEGylation of biologically active agents is an effective way to prolong the half-life of the drug in the circulation, alter the pattern of drug distribution, and camouflage the drug, thereby reducing immunogenicity and protecting it from biological degradation. The MW of PEG and PEG conjugates, when injected intravenously, has a great effect on the time course of serum circulation. In general, the serum half-life of PEG extends from 18 minutes to 20 hours as the PEG MW increases from 5 to 190 kDa, with a leveling-off of the serum half-life period at 20–24 hours for PEG and PEG conjugates having a MW more than 30 kDa or a molecular size more than 8 nm. Renal clearance rate of PEGs is controlled by the glomerular filtration rate in a normal kidney. The vascular wall of the renal glomeruli functions as a filter for ionic and nonionic substances that may accumulate in the kidney through blood circulation. The excretion of these molecules can be a function of molecular size (3–5 nm) and electric charge. The glomerular filtration for the kidneys is less than 70 kDa for proteins (owing to charge and molecular size) and less than 30 kDa for PEGs (owing to molecular size only for nonionic, randomly coiled molecules). Short linear strands of PEG have a high clearance rate, but large linear PEGs, multiarm PEGs, and PEGylated proteins have a slower clearance rate. This difference in renal clearance rate can be attributed to an increase in structure size and hydrodynamic volume and a change in the total charge of the molecule. In the case of the liver, PEGs with MW less than 50 kDa have decreased hepatic clearance with increasing MW (similar to renal clearance), but the liver clearance increases when the MW is more than 50 kDa.

Amine PEGylation is one of the most common techniques used, and *N*-hydroxysuccinimide (NHS) ester of PEG carboxylic acid remains the most popular derivative for coupling PEG to proteins (Figure 9.17), liposomes, soluble and insoluble polymers, and other biological molecules.

The branched activated PEG ester (mPEG2NHS) has several advantages over linear-based PEGs. First, a branched PEG "acts" as if it were larger than a corresponding linear PEG of the same MW. Second, the compound is purely monofunctional, because the intermediate acid is chromatographically purified. Third, proteins modified with branched PEG possess a greater stability from enzymatic degradation and pH degradation, thereby reducing its antigenicity and likelihood of destruction. Moreover, proteins modified with the branched-PEG reagent may retain more activity

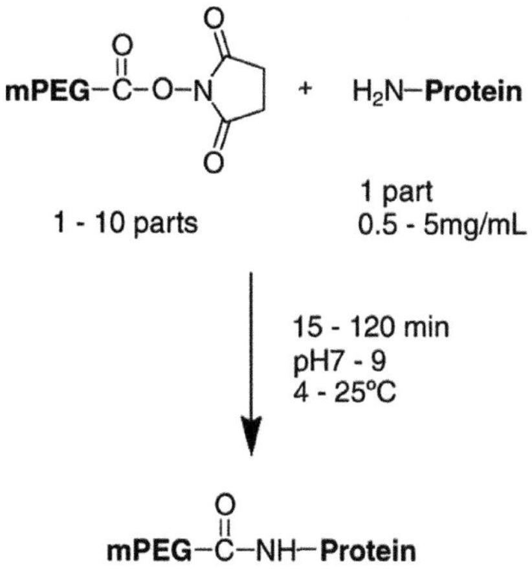

FIGURE 9.17 *m*-PEGylation using *N*-hydroxysuccinimide ester.

when compared with modification with a linear-PEG counterpart. A branched-PEG reagent was used in the creation of PEGASYS (PEGylated-interferon alpha) by Roche and on aptamers. Substitution values are 95% or greater.

9.9.3 Characterization Methods

9.9.3.1 Spectroscopy

Spectrophotometric analyses are the most common methods to characterize proteins. Ultraviolet-visible (UV-VIS) spectroscopy is typically used for the determination of protein concentration by using either a dye-binding assay (e.g., the Bradford or Lowry method) or by determining the absorption of a solution of protein at one or more wavelengths in the near-UV region (260–280 nm). Another spectroscopic method used in the early-phase characterization of biopharmaceuticals is circular dichroism (CD).

The Bradford method, which is more sensitive and less affected by most common detergents or other common biochemicals than the Lowry method, is the most widely used dye-binding method. There are two common Bradford methods: the standard assay Bradford method, with a range of 10–100 mg, and the microassay method, which is linear between 1 and 10 mg. A standard curve is constructed with a common protein that is readily available in pure form, such as bovine serum albumin and bovine gamma globulin. The standards and the sample are then reacted with a solution of Coomassie Brilliant Blue G250 in an acidic solution, and the absorbance is measured at 595 nm. The protein concentration of the sample is then calculated against the constructed curve. This value is an approximation of the protein concentration, because different proteins react differently with the Bradford reagent. Further on in development, the calibration curve should be determined using the protein of interest.

Direct determination of the absorbance of a protein solution requires no other reagents or standards. Two solutions are prepared, one of the samples and one blank solution of water or containing all the buffer components. After zeroing the spectrophotometer at the wavelengths to be measured, using the blank solution, the analyst measures the absorbance of the protein solution. For relatively pure solutions, measuring the absorbance at 280 nm (A280) is usually sufficient. However, for protein solutions containing significant amounts of nucleic acid (as little as a few percent), it is best also to determine the absorbance at 260 nm (A260), to correct for the presence of nucleic acids. The protein concentration is then determined using the following equation:

$$\text{Protein (mg/mL)} = 1.55(\text{A280}) - 0.76(\text{A260}) \qquad (9.1)$$

If the extinction coefficient has not yet been determined, a more absolute concentration is determined using the following equation:

$$\text{A280 (mg/mL)} = (5690 * \text{Trp} + 1280 * \text{Tyr} + 120 * \text{Cys})/\text{protein MW} \qquad (9.2)$$

where Trp is the number of tryptophan residues in the protein, and similarly, Tyr is the number of tyrosines, Cys is the number of cysteine residues, and MW is the molecular weight of the protein.

Spectrophotometric methodologies are used less commonly in late-stage development of proteins but are very helpful in the early development of biopharmaceuticals. For example, CD can be used to study the tertiary structure of proteins. Use of CD does not require the highly pure concentrated protein solutions needed to prepare protein crystals for X-ray crystallography. A protein's specific CD spectrum in the near-UV region (250–340 nm) is determined by its regular 3D structure in solution. By comparing the CD spectra of a protein in both a denaturing and nondenaturing solvent, some estimate can be made regarding the conformational stability of the protein. Because the protein concentration needed to perform CD studies is relatively low, these studies can be undertaken early in development with small amounts of manually purified protein. Because interpretation of the spectra is often difficult, in many cases, CD spectroscopy analyses are sent to laboratories experienced in utilizing these techniques.

The FT-IR can also be used to determine the tertiary structure of a protein. It does not require the protein to be in solution, and it can often be used to support early formulation development for either liquid or lyophilized proteins.

9.9.3.2 Electrophoresis

Electrophoresis is the separation of charged molecules in an electric field. In PAGE, the electric field is formed within the pores of a polyacrylamide gel and are filled with a running buffer. The addition of SDS to the sample preparation buffer as well as to the running buffer is often used to pretreat the protein prior to electrophoresis, hence the term SDS-PAGE. In SDS-PAGE, the SDS molecules interact with the protein, unfolding it and adding multiple charges to the molecule from the associated sulfate groups. Complete unfolding of a protein may require the addition of a reducing agent as well as the SDS. Proteins migrate through the polyacrylamide gel and are separated according to their MW in SDS-PAGE.

Another common technique is to run native or nondenaturing PAGE. In native gel electrophoresis, the migration of the protein through the gel is affected by both the charge and the shape of the protein, as well as the size. While SDS-PAGE is commonly used to determine MW of proteins, it would be incorrect to use native gel PAGE for weight determination. Both methods are used to assess the purity of a protein.

Protein is invisible in the gels and must be stained for detection. The most commonly used visualization techniques are silver and Coomassie blue stains. While silver is more sensitive, the intensity of silver stains is affected by the proteins and is not linear with the concentration of protein, as is Coomassie blue staining. If the intention is to quantify the relative amounts of each protein band, Coomassie blue staining should be used.

In addition to the determination of MW, SDS-PAGE is used to examine the presence of aggregates. Samples can be prepared with and without the reducing agent, either mercaptoethanol or dithiothreitol. Comparison of reduced and nonreduced gel patterns allows the analyst to determine whether the higher-MW aggregates seen are due to intermolecular disulfide bridges. In addition, SDS-PAGE provides information about the purity of the protein. After scanning Coomassie blue-stained gels and calculating the area or relative intensity of each band seen in a sample, the percentage of the total protein can be determined. Most laboratories have scanning software capable of performing both image analysis and quantification. Many software programs can also determine the MW by using results from the standards run on the same gels.

The IEF is another electrophoretic separation method. In this method, the polyacrylamide gel or another support layer also contains a pH gradient. This is a powerful method for investigating the charge differences among proteins. In IEF, each protein migrates through the support layer until it is "trapped" at the point where the pI of the protein is the same as the pH gradient formed in the support media. At this point, the charge on the protein is zero, and it no longer migrates but focuses. Separated proteins need to be stained to be visualized. The pI of a protein can be determined in an IEF separation either by comparison with standards run simultaneously or by measuring the pH of the band with a special pH electrode. In proteins with multiple glycosylated forms, it is often difficult to determine the pI, because the multiple forms may run as a smear across the gel. In such cases, the carbohydrates could be enzymatically removed, yielding a single protein form.

An electrophoretic method used increasingly in the early-stage characterization of proteins is 2D electrophoresis. This method separates the proteins in one dimension based solely on charge (IEF) and in the second dimension based on size (SDS-PAGE). This powerful method can determine whether a protein that is a single band on SDS-PAGE comigrates with another protein. A new use of 2D electrophoresis is for the determination of host-cell proteins. This method can often identify host-cell proteins, which comigrate with the protein of interest in SDS-PAGE gels. The protein is separated in a thin IEF gel; the lane is then placed across the top of an SDS-PAGE gel, and a second electrophoresis is run. After staining, the gel contains one or more spots. The gel can be scanned on a densitometer, and the relative intensity of each spot can be used to determine the percentage of protein that is not the product.

9.9.3.3 Chromatography

High-performance liquid chromatography is a core technique in the characterization of proteins. These separations are coupled with detectors that are sensitive to the proteins eluted during chromatographic separation. The most common detector used in HPLC measures the UV absorption of the elute at one or more wavelengths, or, in the case of a diode array detector, it can scan all the wavelengths simultaneously and provide a clear quantification of each separated protein. Other detection methods sometimes used with HPLC separations are evaporative light scattering and refractive index. The three most common types of HPLC are SEC, which separates based on the size or MW of the protein; ion-exchange (IEX) chromatography, which separates based on the charge of the protein; and reverse-phase (RP) chromatography, which separates based on the hydrophobicity of the protein. The RP is such a common HPLC method that when people do not specify a particular HPLC method, they are usually referring to RP-HPLC.

In RP-HPLC, separation of proteins is accomplished by differential interaction with the column matrix and the column buffer. Two buffers, called the aqueous buffer and the organic buffer (thus identifying the most important attribute of each), are used, and the separation is done with a gradient of these buffers. The most common organic buffers are based on acetonitrile, though other organic solvents, such as methanol and tetrahydrofuran, may be used. The column used for the RP-HPLC separation is most commonly a silica base, coated with hydrocarbon chains of varying sizes, such as C4, C8, and C18. The RP columns built on polymer backbones are becoming more readily available. To minimize any nonspecific interaction between the protein and the column matrix, an ion-pairing component, frequently trifluoroacetic acid, is added to both the aqueous and organic buffers. After the column is equilibrated with either the aqueous buffer or a defined mixture of the aqueous and organic buffers, the sample is loaded onto the column as an aqueous solution. Separation of the varying proteins is done by running a gradient of increasing organic buffer; proteins are resolubilized when the hydrophobic nature of the particular protein partitions into the buffer. The use of highly hydrophobic buffers for RP-HPLC usually precludes the presence of large amounts of salt, which destabilizes some proteins. In addition, proteins are denatured in RP-HPLC, and so, tertiary and quaternary structures are lost. The subunits of multisubunit proteins will usually elute separately. Multiple forms of a protein can usually be separated in RP-HPLC by their small differences of hydrophobicity and sometimes MW. The RP-HPLC is often considered to be a good method to separate related isoforms of a protein.

The IEX-HPLC separates molecules based on charge. The protein interacts with the charged moiety on the column and is then eluted with either salt or pH gradients. Elution from the column is from the weakest to the strongest bound. The protein solution is loaded onto a column that has been charged with the counterion and is then equilibrated with the starting buffer. Proteins are eluted from the column by a gradient of either salt or pH. If the column with a second buffer contains salt, this disrupts the protein interaction with the column and replaces the protein with the counterion. If the second buffer changes the pH, this alters the charge on the protein and decreases the interaction of the protein with the column. The IEX columns can be either anionic or cationic. The most common anion exchangers are quaternary ammonium, diaminoethyl, and quaternary aminoethyl, and the most common cation exchangers are sulfopropyl, methyl sulfonate, and carboxymethyl. By using buffers above or below the protein's pI, the same protein can be analyzed on both anionic and cationic columns. Because of the ionic nature of interaction between the protein and the column, the size of the protein does not affect binding. In addition, because IEX is run in an aqueous environment, the protein is not denatured and maintains its structure, which renders the method to be more sensitive to differences, such as oxidation in surface amino acids. While this method can be used to assess purity, it is generally less sensitive to purity than RP-HPLC, because proteins can remain associated during the separation.

The SEC-HPLC is different from RP-HPLC and IEX in two major ways. The first difference is that separation is based on size only, with a small impact on the shape of the molecule. The second difference is that during SEC, the protein does not adsorb or bind to the separation media. In some cases, a protein will nonspecifically bind to the column. In these instances, it is important to use a different column matrix or to change the composition of the running buffer. The MW of a protein is determined by the comparison of its elution time with the elution time of the standard proteins of known MW. Because there is no binding of the protein with the column matrix, the protein separation is sensitive to the sample's volume. After running a set of known proteins through an SEC column, the protein of interest is loaded onto the column in a small volume and eluted under the same conditions. A standard curve is constructed, based on the MW of the standard proteins and elution time. This curve is used to determine the MW of the eluted sample. Size-exclusion chromatograph columns are available that can separate proteins with MWs as high as 1,000,000, allowing SEC to be used to identify and quantify the size and amount of aggregates in a protein preparation. Unlike SDS-PAGE, the protein is not denatured before separation, so that non–cross-linked aggregates are not disrupted and can be identified. Purity (or percent aggregation) determined by these two methods (SDS-PAGE and SEC) often differs considerably, owing to the detection of the additional aggregate forms in SEC.

9.9.3.4 Mass Spectroscopy

Mass spectroscopy is a method used increasingly to characterize proteins, in the early stages as well as through commercial manufacture. The popularity of this very sensitive technique has increased, as it has become more available in analytical laboratories, and the methods to use it have become more robust. This technique separates proteins based on their mass-to-charge ratio. To separate by MS, a protein is ionized in one of the several ways; then, it is accelerated by the electric or magnetic field. In some cases, the charged protein will break apart to produce ions. The pattern of ions produced is dependent on the structure of the protein, so that they may be used to determine the primary structure of the protein. Most MS instruments in use today ionize proteins in ways that minimize protein fragmentation to allow a true mass determination.

The information lost by reducing fragmentation in standard MS can be determined using MS/MS. In MS/MS, specific ions are subjected to an additional energy by collision, and the resulting daughter ions allow even more structural information to be determined, even to the level of the amino acid sequence. This technique is especially useful for determining posttranslational changes to the protein. The MS/MS can also be used to sequence the structure of carbohydrate side chains on glycosylated proteins and to identify the microheterogeneity that they introduce.

With large proteins, the determination of the primary sequence and PTMs is most efficiently done after digestion with trypsin or another protease to generate smaller peptides. In this case, the peptides are first separated by HPLC, most commonly RP-HPLC, and the column eluant is directed into the MS. In this hyphenated method, known as LC-MS or liquid chromatography-tandem mass spectroscopy (LC-MS/MS), the individual peptides are analyzed, allowing the identification of PTM sites. In some cases, there are potentially multiple sites in a single peptide that may be modified. Absolute identification of the modified amino acids may require more than one enzyme digest to produce different peptides. Some kinds of modifications that are easily identified by MS include phosphorylation of threonine or serine, sulfation or phosphorylation of tyrosine, deamidation of asparagine or glutamine, *O*- or *N*-linked glycosylation, oxidation of methionine or cysteine, and *N*-terminal modification by formylation or prenylation. Combining enzymatic maps (tryptic mapping) with MS/MS may identify single amino acid variants of the protein that cannot be seen otherwise.

Mass spectroscopy is often used as part of hyphenated methods, such as LC-MS, where the proteins are separated by a chromatographic method and the column eluant is then directed to the mass spectrometer for additional characterization. One of the common confusions experienced when evaluating the results of MS analyses of proteins involves equating the observed size of the ion current peak (for a particular ion species) with the amount of the species present. The size of the peak is sensitive to several things and cannot be used for quantification. For this reason, the use of LC separation and quantification "front-end" for the MS allows the relative amounts to be determined.

9.9.3.4.1 Validation

Synthetic drugs are readily characterized by established analytical methods. Biologics, on the other hand, are complex, high-MW products, and analytical methods have limited abilities to completely characterize them and their impurity profiles. Regulation of biologics includes not only final product characterization but also characterization and controls of raw materials and the manufacturing process. The FDA has defined process validation as "establishing documented evidence which provides a high degree of assurance that a specific process will consistently produce a product meeting its predetermined specifications and quality attributes." This involves supporting product and manufacturing process claims with documented scientific studies. Protocols, results with statistical analysis, authorizations, and approvals must be available to regulatory inspectors. Process validation is part of current good manufacturing practices (cGMP) and is required in the United States and Europe for a manufacturing license.

Various types of validation generally required in biopharmaceutical manufacturing include process validation, facility and equipment validation, analytical method validation, software validation, cleaning validation, and expression system characterization. Combined with other elements of cGMP, including lot release testing, raw material testing, vendor quality certifications, and vendor audits, the quality of product can be consistently assured.

9.9.3.5 Process Validation

Process validation involves the identification, monitoring, and control of sources of variation that can contribute to changes in the product. It starts with process characterization studies, using scale-down models for optimization, operating range specification, extractables' and leachables' characterization, and clearance studies. Such work depends on validated assays and representative scale-down models.

Process development normally involves identifying critical variables, defining setpoints for each unit operation, and establishing operating ranges (deviations from the setpoint). Maximum operating range (MOR) limits are typically set during Phase II or III. If they are exceeded, an investigation is necessary to determine if product quality remains acceptable.

Normal operating range (NOR) limits are determined by run-to-run reproducibility with scale-down models and trending with control charts at production scale. The NOR limits lie within the MOR limits, which must allow for normal variability while maintaining acceptable operation.

9.9.3.6 Facility and Equipment Validation

Facility and equipment validation is normally divided into design qualification (DQ), installation qualification (IQ), operational qualification (OQ), and performance qualification (PQ). Equipment validation begins with pilot production of clinical materials for Phase II.

The DQ provides documented evidence that the proposed design of the facilities, equipment, and systems is suitable for the intended purpose. The DQ must compare the design to a set of well-defined user requirements relating to product safety, identity, strength, purity, and quality.

The IQ provides documented evidence that the system is assembled, installed, plumbed, and wired according to the user's design specifications, vendor recommendations, and appropriate codes and standards. Vendors typically provide much of the hardware documentation.

The OQ provides documented evidence that the system performs as expected throughout its intended operating ranges, including all the system's different functions and all its components (hardware, monitoring instruments, controls, alarms, and recorders). Elements of the OQ testing and documentation may be part of the factory acceptance test at the vendor's site. Integration with plant utilities and component installation must be verified at the factory. Hardware cleanliness must also be assessed after cleaning.

The PQ is documented by processing actual feedstock by trained operators by using buffers and utilities at the factory. Full-scale process validation includes testing the consistency of batch production.

9.9.3.7 Analytical Methods

Several methods are used to measure the product characteristics important for therapeutic safety and efficacy during preclinical and early Phase I studies. Additional tests are developed for final product release and in-process sampling of the final manufacturing process. These measure characteristics such as molecular identity, purity, potency, and safety. The number of tests should be sufficient to show manufacturing consistency and the impact of manufacturing changes. Once a test is made a formal part of the manufacturing process, it is almost impossible to remove. Test methods are evaluated for different attributes such as accuracy, precision, range, selectivity, recovery, calibration (detection and quantitation limits), assay sampling, robustness, and stability.

Test method validation is needed to conduct clinical trials. Specifications should start off wide for Phase I and narrow to tighter values in the license application. Relaxing established specifications is very difficult.

9.9.3.8 Software Validation

Software validation operates under the principle that quality should not be diminished if a manual process is replaced with an automated process. Software must be developed and tested under a quality system with defined user requirements, change-control procedures, provisions for authorization of operators for data entry and data checking, data archiving, software backup, provisions for system crashing, and procedures for monitoring and correcting software problems. 21 CFR 11 defines requirements for maintaining the integrity of data and software and handling electronic signatures for traceability.

9.9.3.9 Cleaning Validation

Cleaning validation demonstrates the ability of cleaning procedures to permit the reuse of processing components and equipment, without a concomitant deterioration of product quality. Batch-to-batch carryover is of concern in multiuse plants making more than one product.

Consistency of product quality is demonstrated by showing operating consistency and product quality from batch to batch, processing with only buffer (blank runs) with assays for contaminants, examination of cleaned surfaces and materials, and extended scale-down clearance studies on reused materials. Disposable processing components that eliminate the need for cleaning validation are increasingly used at a small scale.

9.9.3.10 Expression System Characterization

This is performed before Phase I studies in humans to ensure safety. Concerns include the presence of contaminating organisms, tumorigenic cells, proteins, nucleic acids, retroviruses, or other pathogens. Taking tissue culture as an example, characterization includes the source, raw materials used, selection methods, number of generations, transfection or fusion methods used, procedures for establishing working cell banks, facilities, identity, homogeneity, absence of contaminating pathogens, tumorigenicity, and stability.

9.9.4 Stability Considerations

Commercial viability of recombinant production processes depends on the final product yield. This is a particularly more significant issue, as biogeneric manufacturers bring out their line of products that will be sold at a lower price than the innovator's products; the issue of yield becomes more important now. A primary cause of poor yield is neither the quality of the gene construct nor the nature of the molecule but the degradation of the product during the manufacturing process. Protein degradation therefore becomes a key factor that must be thoroughly understood, and steps must be taken to minimize this degradation step, wherever possible. This chapter deals with this significant issue and makes suggestions on how to avoid the degradation of proteins in the downstream processing.

9.9.4.1 Proteolysis

In contrast to the cellular environment, where enzymatic degradation of proteins is highly controlled, extracellular proteases are the cause of uncontrolled protein degradation. The result of this proteolytic attack may vary from complete hydrolysis, single breaks within the peptide chain, or loss of a few *N*- or *C*-terminal amino acid residues. Besides losing the product, the presence of truncated forms may seriously challenge the purification design.

Proteolytic enzymes are released to the medium because of cell death, mechanical stress, or induced cell lysis. Their presence is expected during fermentation and initial downstream unit operations. Most enzymes of the vacuoles and lysosomes are minimally active at a slightly alkaline pH (7–9), a pH interval strongly recommended for the extraction of proteins expressed in bacteria.

Proteins are probably more resistant toward proteolytic attacks in their native state, and stabilizing factors (e.g., cofactor, correct parameter interval, and cosolvent) are always considered optimized. Use of protein inhibitors is not recommended for safety reasons. The primary mechanism of proteolysis is the enzymatic hydrolysis of the peptide bond. The indicators of this reaction taking place in the system include the loss of product or poor yield, lack of expected activity, changes in specific activity, change in MW, high background staining in 1D SDS electrophoresis, smeared bands, many lower-MW bands of poor resolution, disappearance of bands, and discrepancies in MW. The preventive actions taken to prevent proteolysis are listed in Table 9.5.

The use of enzyme inhibitors is not recommended, as they are harmful to human beings. It should be ascertained that the degradation observed is not a function of the analytical assay. Enzyme inhibitors can be used to prevent enzymatic activity in analytical assays. Mild denaturation may accelerate enzymatic digestion. Selective removal (e.g., affinity chromatography) of specific enzymes should also be considered.

9.9.4.2 Deamidation

Two amino acid residues are involved in the deamidation reaction: asparagyl and glutamyl. The conversion to the corresponding carboxylic acid residues results in a shift in net charge of the protein at a pH above the pK_a. As the deamidation may influence the biological activity and the stability of the molecule, the maximal content of des-amido forms in bulk materials and in biopharmaceutical preparations is constantly being debated. The list of proteins that undergo deamidation is comprehensive and includes well-known proteins, such as insulin, human growth hormone, and cytochrome C.

Asparagyl residues tend to be more susceptible to deamidation than glutamyl residues. Further, the deamidation reaction is strongly sequence-specific in model peptides with the half-life of the -Asn-Pro- sequence being 100-fold greater than that of -Asn-Gly-. To some extent, these observations can also be used on proteins that take the structural steric factors and nearby amino acid residues into consideration.

At pH above five, the deamidation of asparagyl or glutamyl occurs via a relatively slow intermediate succinimide formation. The succinimidyl derivative is rapidly

TABLE 9.5

Preventive Actions Against Proteolysis

Factor	Comment
pH	There is no specific pH range in which all enzymes are considered inactive; at slightly alkaline pH, the nonspecific enzymes of the vacuoles and lysosomes are minimally active. Use strong buffers for extraction to prevent unintended shift in pH as a result of cell disruption. Some yeast enzymes are least active in the pH range 4–5 but active in the pH range 7–9. Phosphate may exhibit a stabilizing effect on proteins.
Temperature	Low temperature decreases the proteolytic activity. It is recommended to store harvest at 4°C–8°C or frozen.
Time	Enzymatic protein degradation is a function of time. Lengthy procedures and long storage times should be avoided during harvest, capture, and initial purification steps.
Conductivity	Noncritical.
Redox potential	Reducing and oxidizing conditions may alter the disulfide bridge arrangement and state of free cysteine residues, thus influencing the secondary and tertiary structures of protein.
Cosolvents	Presence of other proteins in excess (e.g., albumin) will reduce the proteolytic damage. Cosolvents, such as glycerol or dimethylsulfoxide, may have a stabilizing effect but will probably be too expensive for large-scale operations.
Low-MW compounds	Substrates, substrate analogs, and cofactors can help in stabilizing the protein. Potential proteinase activators (e.g., divalent metal ions) are excluded from the extraction buffer.
Techniques	Careful cell disruption and specific extraction procedures may lower the enzymatic cleavage.
Denaturation	The proteolytic enzymes lose their biological activity upon denaturation. However, some enzymes are stable under mild denaturing conditions that lead to increased activity if the target protein is partly denatured under the same conditions.

Source: Handbook of Biogeneric Therapeutic Proteins: Regulatory, Manufacturing, Testing and Intellectual Property Issues, Taylor & Francis Group, Boca Raton, FL, 2005.
Abbreviation: MW, molecular weight.

hydrolyzed at either the α- or β-carbonyl group to generate a mixture of normal- and iso-residues. Under strongly acidic conditions, asparagyl or glutamyl residues are hydrolyzed to the corresponding carboxyl residues. The indicators of deamidation include extra bands in electrophoresis and extra peaks in chromatographic recordings. Table 9.6 lists preventive actions against deamidation.

9.9.4.3　Oxidation

The amino acid residues histidyl, methionyl, cysteinyl, tryptophanyl, and tyrosinyl are potential oxidation sites at neutral or at slightly alkaline conditions. Oxidation of the said residues often results in a loss of immunological and/or biological activity. The list of proteins that have been oxidized is comprehensive and includes biopharmaceutical products, such as albumin, growth hormone, glucagons, and interleukin-1b and −2.

TABLE 9.6

Preventive Actions Against Deamidation

Factor	Comment
pH	Deamidation is expected above pH 5. The optimal working range in which to avoid deamidation is probably between 3.0 and 5.0.
Temperature	The deamidation rate increases with increasing temperature.
Time	The deamidation rate is a function of time. Presence of des-amido forms is a marker for drug product stability and shelf life.
Conductivity	The ionic strength of the solution is kept low. At high ionic strength, the deamidation reaction can be fast even at neutral pH.
Redox potential	Nonessential parameter.
Co-solvents	In general, the buffer species and the buffer strength will influence the rate of deamidation. High solvent dielectrics favor deamidation.
	In model peptides, the protein stability was higher in Tris buffer than in phosphate buffer.

Source: Handbook of Biogeneric Therapeutic Proteins: Regulatory, Manufacturing, Testing and Intellectual Property Issues, Taylor & Francis Group, Boca Raton, FL, 2005.

In many cases, the immunological and/or biological activity was only partially lost. In general, the oxidation of methionyl to methionyl sulfoxide does not affect protein antigenicity, probably because the conformational structure of the oxidized protein is close to the native structure. On the other hand, the oxidation of a single amino acid residue often causes changes in the biological activity, and all efforts should be taken to minimize the oxidation reactions.

The mechanism of oxidation involves methionyl residues, which are converted to methionyl sulfoxide residues under mild oxidizing conditions. The most reactive residues are those exposed to the solvent, while those residues buried within the hydrophobic regions are fairly inert to oxidation (e.g., methionine residues in myoglobin and trypsin). Methionyl residues are susceptible to auto-oxidation, chemical oxidation, and photo-oxidation.

The cysteinyl residues are easily oxidized, and the reaction is usually accelerated at an alkaline pH, where the thiol group is deprotonated. Under mild oxidizing conditions, the reactions are oxidation of cysteinyl residues to sulfenic/sulfonic acid (alkaline conditions), cysteinyl residues to dehydroalanyl residues (alkaline conditions), and cysteinyl to cystine residues (neutral to alkaline conditions). In the absence of a thiol reagent or a nearby thiol, the cysteine may instead oxidize to sulfenic acid.

The oxidation reaction is strongly catalyzed by divalent metal ions (e.g., copper). The indicators of oxidation include extra bands in gel electrophoresis and extra peaks in chromatographic recordings. Preventive actions against oxidation are listed in Table 9.7.

The degradation rate is often governed by trace amounts of peroxides, divalent metal ions, and light, base, and free radicals. There are three classes of antioxidants:

- *Phenolic compounds*: Butylated hydroxytoluene (BHT), butylated hydroxyanisole (BHA), propyl gallate, and vitamin E
- *Reducing agents*: Cysteine, dithiothreitol (DTT), methionine, ascorbic acid, sodium sulfite, thioglycolic acid, and thioglycerol
- *Chelating agents*: Ethylenediaminetetraacetic acid (EDTA), citric acid, and thioglycolic acid

TABLE 9.7

Preventive Actions Against Oxidation

Factor	Comment
pH	The oxidation rate is assumed low at slightly acidic pH.
Temperature	Working at low temperatures decreases the rate of oxidation.
Time	The oxidation reaction is a function of time.
Conductivity	No data available.
Redox potential	Disulfide bond formation will take place at a redox potential above 0 mV. A high redox potential indicates presence of oxidizing agents.
Co-solvents	Avoid oxidizing agents and protect against light. Addition of chelating agents (EDTA, citric acid, thioglycolic acid), antioxidants (BHT, BHA, propyl gallate, vitamin E), and/or reducing agents (cysteine, DTT, methionine, ascorbic acid, sodium sulfite, thioglycolic acid, thioglycerol) may reduce oxidation.

Source: *Handbook of Biogeneric Therapeutic Proteins: Regulatory, Manufacturing, Testing and Intellectual Property Issues,* Taylor & Francis Group, Boca Raton, FL, 2005.
Abbreviations: BHA, butylated hydroxyanisole; BHT, butylated hydroxytoluene; DTT, dithiothreitol; EDTA, ethylenediaminetetraacetic acid.

9.9.4.4 Carbamylation

Cyanate is able to react with amino, sulfhydryl, carboxyl, phenolic hydroxyl, imidazole, and phosphate groups in proteins according to the general scheme, $RXH + HNCO = RXCONH_2$. Cyanate is easily soluble in water. Most reactions have a pH optimum around seven. Acidic pH should be avoided, as acidic conditions are ideal for modifications of carboxyl groups. For the same reason, reactions with cyanate should not be terminated with acid. At high concentrations, cyanate may react with itself to form cyanuric acid and cyamelide, and it is recommended to work at concentrations of about 0.2 M. Cyanate reacts rapidly with amino groups. At neutral pH and below, the a-amino group can be expected to react about 100 times faster than the 1-amino group. The resulting carbamoylamino groups are stable, even in dilute NaOH. Typical reaction conditions are 3 mg/mL protein and 0.1 M cyanate at pH 8, at 25°C, for 1 hour. Cyanate also reacts even more rapidly with sulfhydryl groups than amino groups, resulting in the formation of S-carbamylcysteine residues. As cyanate reacts rapidly with sulfhydryl groups, labile disulfide bonds may be ruptured. The resulting carbamylmercaptans decompose readily to free mercaptan and cyanate at alkaline pH. Consequently, cyanate can be used as reversible blocking agent for –SH groups. At acidic pH, cyanate reacts with carboxylic groups, resulting in the formation of a mixed anhydride, which can react with many nucleophiles (e.g., formation of amides). The reaction can be avoided entirely at pH 7–8. Aliphatic hydroxyls are resistant to carbamylation, even at high cyanate concentrations at low pH. However, the reactive hydroxyl groups of chymotrypsin and other proteases react with cyanate to give urethans. Phenolic hydroxyl groups react more readily than aliphatic groups in a reversible reaction that is quite analogous to the one that occurs with –SH groups.

Cyanate present in aqueous urea solutions reacts with the free amino and sulfhydryl groups of proteins. Urea is often tacitly assumed to be a reagent, which alters the structure of the protein and may be used to keep target proteins in their monomeric form during purification. However, at pH 6 and above, urea hydrolyses under the formation of cyanate, leading to carbamylation reactive groups in proteins.

The equilibrium $(NH_2)_2CO=NH_4CNO$ between an undissociated urea and dissociated cyanate in aqueous urea solutions is the main course of unintended carbamylation of primary amino groups in proteins. As the protein concentration normally is from 0.1 to 30 mg/mL, corresponding to the micromolar range, a considerable part of the protein mass is expected to undergo carbamylation under these conditions. Thus, the exposure of ribonuclease to cyanate in an aqueous solution leads to a considerable loss of enzymatic activity. Formation of cyanate is prevented by storage of neutral urea solutions at 4°C or by buffering the solution at pH 4.7. Thus, acidification of urea solutions just before use will decompose any cyanate present. Cyanate can be removed from urea solutions by mixed IEX. The method of Salinas describes a sensitive and specific method for the quantitative estimation of carbamylation in proteins (see Bibliography).

9.9.4.5 β-Elimination

The β-elimination reaction is caused by the abstraction of a β-hydrogen from cysteinyl, seryl, and threonyl residues under alkaline conditions. The cysteinyl residue decomposes as a result of β-elimination under the formation of HS− and free sulfur, thus affecting the redox potential of the solution. Several studies indicate that the rate of the reaction is proportional to the hydroxide ion concentration, and consequently, pH should be kept low (use dilute NaOH solutions to adjust pH preferably below 0.1 M NaOH). In alkaline solutions, the abstraction of β-hydrogen from cysteinyl, seryl, and threonyl residues results in the formation of a carbanion. Depending on the nature of the side-chain, the carbanion can rearrange to form an unsaturated derivative (dehydroalanine or β-methyl-dehydroalanine) or add a proton to give the L- and D-amino acid residues (racemization). The derivatives formed are reactive with a number of nucleophilic protein groups. The reaction is independent of the primary structure of the protein. The indicators of β-elimination include degradation of the protein, cleavage of disulfide bridges, and smell of sulfur. Preventive actions against β-elimination are listed in Table 9.8.

TABLE 9.8

Preventive Actions Against β-Elimination

Factor	Comment
pH	pH is kept below 10. Do not use NaOH solutions above 0.1 M to adjust pH.
Temperature	High temperature even at pH 4–8 results in β-elimination.
Time	The β-elimination reaction is a function of time.
Conductivity	Increased ionic strength increases the rate of β-elimination.
Redox potential	Cystinyl-rich proteins may decompose under formation of HS−, which will lower the redox potential of the solution. Reduction of disulfide bonds may result.
Co-solvents	Removal of divalent metal ions with EDTA.

Source: *Handbook of Biogeneric Therapeutic Proteins: Regulatory, Manufacturing, Testing and Intellectual Property Issues,* Taylor & Francis Group, Boca Raton, FL, 2005.
Abbreviation: EDTA, ethylenediaminetetraacetic acid.

9.9.4.6 Racemization

All amino acid residues except glycine are subject to racemization at an alkaline pH, resulting in the formation of the D-enantiomers of the residue. Racemization is inevitably associated with conformational changes and thereby loss of function. The racemization of proteins has been described in several reports. The initial step of the reaction is abstraction of the β-hydrogen by hydroxide ions. By uptake of a proton, this will result in either the L- or D-amino acid residue. The carbanion formed may also undergo β-elimination. At pH 5–12, Asn, Asp, Gln, and Glu may modify via a succinimidyl intermediate, resulting in both the D- and L-derivatives. The indicators of racemization include change of protein structure and loss of biological activity. The change in optical rotation correlates with the rate of racemization. The amino acid residues undergo racemization at different rates. Preventive actions against racemization are listed in Table 9.9.

9.9.4.7 Cysteinyl Residues

The reactive site of the cysteinyl residue is the thiol group, which is deprotonated at an alkaline pH (pK_a around 8.5). The residue under the oxidizing conditions (and neutral to alkaline pH) is able to react with a similar residue under the formation of a disulfide bond. Many proteins are stabilized by intramolecular disulfide bonds (e.g., insulin, growth hormone, and insulin-like growth factor [IGF]-1), but intermolecular bonds may also result from the reaction under the formation of aggregates. In order to avoid unintended disulfide bond formation and cleavage, the redox potential of the solution must be monitored and controlled. In practice, aqueous buffers contain micromolar amounts of dissolved oxygen, assuring a redox potential of 200–600 mV, which is sufficient to maintain the intramolecular disulfide bonds. Proteins with free cysteines may prefer slightly reducing conditions, which can be obtained by the addition of micromolar amounts of reducing agent (e.g., cysteine and DTT). The number of proteins containing both –SH groups and disulfide bonds are relatively small (e.g., albumin and β-lactoglobulin). In many cases, the disulfide bond stabilization

TABLE 9.9

Preventive Actions Against Racemization

Factor	Comment
pH	High pH will favor abstraction of the β-hydrogen under formation of a carbanion. pH is kept below 10 and use of NaOH in concentration above 0.1 M is avoided when adjusting pH.
Temperature	The temperature is kept low.
Time	The reaction is a function of time.
Conductivity	No data are available.
Redox potential	No data are available.
Co-solvents	No data are available.

Source: Handbook of Biogeneric Therapeutic Proteins: Regulatory, Manufacturing, Testing and Intellectual Property Issues, Taylor & Francis Group, Boca Raton, FL, 2005.

is essential for maintaining the biological activity. Ribonuclease, for example, loses almost all activity when the four disulfide bonds are reduced. The mechanism of reaction involves the cysteinyl and cystinyl residues in the disulfide bond formation by oxidation or reduction, conversion of a cystinyl residue to a cysteinyl residue and a sulfenic/sulfonic acid residue at alkaline pH, and decomposition to a dehydroalanine residue at alkaline pH (β-elimination reaction). Disulfide bond formation is often catalyzed by the presence of a mercapto reagent (e.g., DTT and cysteine) in millimolar concentrations (typically 1–10 mM). Controlled disulfide bond formation has gained much attention in the biopharmaceutical industry in connection with the in vitro folding of proteins expressed in *Escherichia coli*. Presence of divalent metal ions (typically Cu^{2+}) may result in the oxidation of cysteinyl residues by an ill-defined reaction mechanism. Cleavage of the disulfide bond is initiated by an attack on a sulfur atom by a nucleophile reagent (HS−, RS−, CN−, SO_3^-, or OH−). The reaction, which takes place at neutral to alkaline pH, consists of two steps, with a formation of a mixed disulfide as the intermediary step. The indicators of cysteinyl residues include intermolecular disulfide bond formation, resulting in aggregation; under reducing conditions, the disulfide bonds destabilize, resulting in the conversion of cystinyl to cysteinyl residues (in vitro refolding may be the only solution to reestablish the correct disulfide bonds), the presence of scrambled and structural altered forms, and smell of sulfur. Be careful when adjusting pH with high concentrations of NaOH. Locally high pH may facilitate β-elimination. Preventive actions against cysteinyl residue loss are described in Table 9.10.

TABLE 9.10

Preventive Actions Against Cysteinyl Residue Loss

Factor	Comment
pH	Minimum reactivity is expected in the pH range 3–7. The reactivity of the –SH group is at maximum above the pK_a (8.5), where the group is deprotonated. In strongly acidic media the reaction is expected to take place via a sulfenium cation by an electrophile displacement.
Protein concentration	The intramolecular disulfide bond formation is a first-order reaction and thus independent of protein concentration. Intermolecular reactions via the cysteinyl residue may be affected by the protein concentration (aggregation). The aggregation rate is favored by high protein concentration.
Temperature	The temperature is kept low (4°C–20°C) especially at pH above 9.5.
Time	The reaction is a function of time.
Conductivity	No data available.
Redox potential	Reducing conditions favor free cysteinyl residues. Oxidizing conditions favor disulfide bonds. The redox potential is a function of pH (60 mV/pH unit).
Co-solvents	Cysteine (nonanimal origin) is recommended as a reducing agent for large-scale operations. Divalent metal ions are removed by EDTA.

Source: *Handbook of Biogeneric Therapeutic Proteins: Regulatory, Manufacturing, Testing and Intellectual Property Issues*, Taylor & Francis Group, Boca Raton, FL, 2005.
Abbreviation: EDTA, ethylenediaminetetraacetic acid.

9.9.4.8 Hydrolysis

The peptide bond does not undergo significant hydrolysis in the pH interval (3–9.5) and is usually used in industrial downstream processing. However, in dilute acid, where the carboxyl group of aspartyl residues is not dissociated, the peptide bond is cleaved 100 times faster than the other peptide bonds and especially the -Asp-Pro- sequence is prone to degradation. The guanidinium group of arginine is hydrolyzed by OH– to give ornithine and possibly some citrulline, depending on the nature of the protein. The mechanism of hydrolysis includes hydrolysis of the peptide bond, hydrolysis of the amide group of Asn and Gln, and hydrolysis of the guanidine group from Arg residues, resulting in the formation of ornithine residues (hydroxide ion catalyzed). The indicators of hydrolysis include formation of split products of identical MW (the peptide fragments are linked via disulfide bonds). Preventive actions against hydrolysis are described in Table 9.11.

9.9.4.9 Denaturation

The native protein molecule loses its tertiary structure on denaturation, resulting in a population of partially unfolded molecules. In practice, the denaturation process will lead to a mixture of more or less unfolded molecules comprising residual secondary structure elements (helix, β-sheet, β-turn, and *cis–trans* isomers around the prolinyl residue). A population of random coil molecules is not expected even under strong denaturing and reducing conditions. On denaturation, the inner hydrophobic core of the protein molecule is exposed to the hydrophilic environment (solvent water), often resulting in (irreversible) aggregation of the target protein. The cooperativity of the denaturation process results in an abrupt transition from the native to the unfolded state within a narrow range of pH, temperature, ionic strength, and denaturant concentration, meaning that protein denaturation may come fast and unexpected. As globular proteins are only marginally stable in aqueous solutions, parameter interactions should be well understood and described using, for example, factorial design experiments. Proteins with disulfide bonds may undergo unfolding under reducing conditions, where the covalent bond is cleaved.

TABLE 9.11

Preventive Actions Against Hydrolysis

Factor	Comment
pH	The Asp-peptide bonds are prone to degradation at acidic pH. Deamidation of Asn and Gln occurs at pH above 5. Arg is converted to ornithine by OH– in a concentration-dependent manner.
Temperature	The deamidation rate increases with increasing temperature.
Time	The degradation reactions are a function of time.
Conductivity	The ionic strength of the solution is low in order to prevent deamidation. At high ionic strength, the deamidation reaction can be fast even at neutral pH.
Redox potential	No data available.
Co-solvents	No data available.

Source: Handbook of Biogeneric Therapeutic Proteins: Regulatory, Manufacturing, Testing and Intellectual Property Issues, Taylor & Francis Group, Boca Raton, FL, 2005.

A denatured protein may be brought back to its native form by in vitro folding. The folding process is often slow, and yields can be poor. As each protein is unique, the in vitro folding conditions must be determined case by case, often using specific cosolvents as additives. An example is the group of proteins in which disulfide bonds must be reestablished as part of the renaturation process.

Hydrogen bonds and intramolecular interactions (electrostatic and van der Waals) stabilize the native structure of the protein in a cooperative manner. On denaturation, the cooperative effect is lost, resulting in unfolding of the molecule and exposure of the inner hydrophobic core to the hydrophilic aqueous environment. For small globular proteins, denaturation is an almost all-or-none process approximated rather well by the two-state transition. Thermodynamically, the denaturation process can be observed by an increase of molar heat capacity and a rapid enthalpy increase with increasing temperature. The primary structure (amino acid sequence) is not affected by denaturation. The indicators of denaturation include loss of structure and loss of biological activity and aggregation. Preventive actions against denaturation are described in Table 9.12.

TABLE 9.12

Preventive Actions Against Denaturation

Factor	Comment
pH	Loss of tertiary structure is expected at pH above 9.5. Proteins tend to be most stable near the isoelectric point.
Temperature	The unfolding process is a function of temperature. Many proteins have optimal stability in the temperature range 10°C–30°C. Loss of structure is expected both at low temperatures (cold denaturation) and at elevated temperatures. The reason that many protein biopharmaceuticals are stored at low temperatures is to minimize chemical degradation (e.g., deamidation).
Time	The denaturation reaction can be very fast.
Conductivity	No data available.
Redox potential	Cleavage of disulfide bonds is expected under reducing conditions. A redox potential below 100 mV is considered unstable for some proteins (e.g., insulin). Not all proteins undergo conformational changes upon reduction of the disulfide bond(s).
Co-solvents	Sucrose, mannose, glucose, glycine, alanine, glutamine, and ammonium sulfate are examples of compounds acting as protein stabilizers (weak or not binding to the protein surface).
	Magnesium sulfate, guanidinium sulfate, sodium chloride, and other weakly interacting salts exhibit an effect depending on protein charge and concentration.
	PEG and MPD act as stabilizers due to steric exclusion and repulsion from charged groups. Both PEG and MPD may destabilize the protein under certain circumstances, where binding is favored over exclusion.
	Co-solvents, such as urea or guanidinium chloride, which bind strongly to the protein surface, are strong denaturants.

Source: *Handbook of Biogeneric Therapeutic Proteins: Regulatory, Manufacturing, Testing and Intellectual Property Issues,* Taylor & Francis Group, Boca Raton, FL, 2005.
Abbreviations: MPD, 2-methyl-2,4 pentanediol; PEG, polyethylene glycol.

9.9.4.10 Aggregation

Protein aggregation is a major problem in the purification and formulation of protein biopharmaceuticals. Two types of intermolecular reactions dominate: aggregation resulting from hydrophobic interactions and aggregation stemming from intermolecular disulfide bond formation between cysteinyl residues.

Proteins exposed to even mildly denaturing conditions may partially unfold, resulting in the exposure of hydrophobic residues to the aqueous solvent, favoring aggregation. The aggregation process is assumed to be controlled by the initial dimerization step in a second-order reaction. Consequently, high-protein concentrations will increase the aggregation rate.

Intermolecular disulfide bond formation between cysteinyl residues takes place at alkaline pH under oxidizing conditions. Proteins with reactive free thiol groups should be purified under reducing conditions (typically 1–10 mM reducing agent) in the presence of EDTA. Even proteins with disulfide bonds may participate in intermolecular disulfide bond reactions owing to disulfide bond shuffling at neutral and alkaline pH.

Expression of proteins in *E. coli* often results in the formation of insoluble aggregates called inclusion bodies, probably comprising fully or partially unfolded proteins. Inclusion bodies are brought to their monomeric form by extraction with a denaturant (e.g., 8 M urea) under reducing conditions (e.g., 0.1 M cysteine).

The mechanism of the reaction is primarily hydrophobic interaction or interaction via disulfide formation. Exposure of hydrophobic residues to the surface of the molecule leads to disorganization of the surrounding water molecules, thus increasing the entropy of the system. In order to avoid the change of the hydration shell structure, the protein molecules are forced to aggregate. The aggregation reaction can be very fast and will, in severe cases, lead to the formation of insoluble polymers. The dominant mechanism is presumably specific interaction of certain conformations of intermediates rather than nonspecific coaggregation. Proteins comprising free thiol groups may form intermolecular disulfide bonds, leading to aggregation of the protein. The reaction takes place at alkaline pH (presence of $-S-$) under oxidizing conditions. Indicators of aggregation include loss of structure and loss of biological activity, turbid solution, presence of fibrils in the solution, precipitation, and formation of gels. Formation of inclusion bodies in *E. coli* is an example of in vivo protein aggregates. Hydrophobic protein aggregates will often dissolve at high pH (>11). Intermolecular disulfide aggregates may dissolve under reducing conditions (presence of DTT, cysteine, or the like). Preventive actions against aggregation are described in Table 9.13.

9.9.4.11 Precipitation

Protein precipitates are aggregates large enough to be visible. However, in practice, aggregates not visible to the naked eye may result in severe problems, such as filters and chromatographic columns can be blocked.

Protein precipitation is typically observed at high ionic strength, in the presence of organic solvents, or close to the isoelectric point, where solubility is low owing to the zero net charge of the protein. Presence of precipitates is not always easily observed. Typical markers are the presence of large and often white particles or flocculates, a turbid appearance, fibrils, and increased viscosity.

TABLE 9.13

Preventive Actions Against Aggregation

Factor	Comment
pH	High pH is avoided in order to prevent protein unfolding. Some proteins do change conformation as a function of pH and certain pH intervals are avoided. pH < 7 protects the protein from intermolecular disulfide bond formation.
Temperature	The unfolding process is a function of temperature. Many proteins have optimal stability in the temperature range 10°C–30°C. Loss of structure is expected both at low temperatures (cold denaturation) and at elevated temperatures.
Protein concentration	Low protein concentrations are favored.
Time	The aggregation reaction can be very fast.
Conductivity	No data available.
Redox potential	Oxidizing conditions result in formation of disulfide bonds and intermolecular interactions are expected. Reducing conditions will prevent intermolecular disulfide bond formation.
Co-solvents	Denaturing or destabilizing agents (e.g., urea, certain alcohols, and organic solvents) should be used with care. Detergents may prevent aggregation, but they often bind strongly to the protein.

Source: *Handbook of Biogeneric Therapeutic Proteins: Regulatory, Manufacturing, Testing and Intellectual Property Issues*, Taylor & Francis Group, Boca Raton, FL, 2005.

Unintended precipitation can be difficult to predict, as the effect depends on a combination of the distribution of hydrophilic and hydrophobic residues on the protein surface, the pH, ionic strength, protein concentration, temperature, and composition of the aqueous phase. A perfectly clear solution may gradually become turbid during application to a chromatographic column, which results in column blocking.

The mechanism of precipitation involves salting out, isoprecipitation, or the presence of polar solvents. In most cases, high salt concentrations will lead to precipitation of the protein. The process is largely dependent on the hydrophobicity of the protein, and the optimal salts are those favoring dehydration of the nonpolar regions, without binding to the protein. At zero net charge of the protein, the electrostatic repulsion between the molecules is minimal. Therefore, proteins tend to precipitate near the pI of the molecule. Addition of nonpolar organic solvents reduces the water activity. The organic solvent reducing the hydrophobic attraction will displace the water molecules around the hydrophobic areas. The principal forces that lead to precipitation are, therefore, likely to be electrostatic forces and dipolar van der Waals forces. The indicators of precipitation include cloudy solution and precipitation of solid material (the precipitates often appear white). The Hoffmeister series provides the impact of various cations and anions:

Cations:

$$NH_4^+ > K^+ > Na^+ > Li > Mg^2 > Ca^{2+} > Gdn^+ \tag{9.3}$$

Anions:

$$SO_4^- > HPO_4^{-2} > CH_3COO^- > Cl^- > NO_3^- > SCN^- \tag{9.4}$$

The ions to the left in the series exert a stabilizing effect on proteins. The ions to the right may bind to the protein surface and thereby destabilize the protein. The effect of the ions is additive. Ammonium sulfate is a stabilizing salt often used for the precipitation of proteins (2–3 M solution). Gdn-sulfate is a stabilizing salt, while Gdn-chloride is a strong denaturant.

Precipitation is commonly used as a purification tool in downstream processing, as the biological activity is rarely affected by this procedure (organic solvents may result in denaturation). Isoprecipitation becomes more effective by adding alcohols or poly-alcohols to the solvent. pH adjustment may result in unintended isoprecipitation of the protein. Passing the isoelectric point does not affect the biological activity or stability of the protein (in most cases), and the protein will normally enter into solution again, 2–3 pH units from the pI. Precipitates may form hours after the protein solution has been prepared or adjusted. The precipitates are not always visible. As the particles may result in blockage of filters and chromatographic columns, unintended precipitation in application samples constitutes a great problem in downstream processing. Preventive actions taken against precipitation are described in Table 9.14.

The guidance stated in the International Conference on Harmonization (ICH) harmonized tripartite guideline entitled "Stability Testing of New Drug Substances and Products" (issued by the ICH on October 27, 1993) applies in general to biotechnological/biological products. However, biotechnological/biological products have distinguishing characteristics to which consideration should be given in any well-defined testing program designed to confirm their stability during the intended storage period. For such products in which the active components are typically proteins

TABLE 9.14

Preventive Actions Against Precipitation

Factor	Comment
pH	The protein solubility is minimal near the iso-electric point.
	A change in pH may affect the redox potential of the solution, the protein solubility, and the protein stability.
Temperature	High temperature increases the conformational flexibility and, for example, organic solvents may more easily penetrate the internal structure of the protein.
Protein concentration	Low protein concentration protects the protein from precipitation; concentrations below 0.1 mg/mL may be necessary to avoid precipitation.
Time	Precipitation is a function of time. Always determine the holding time for a given sample to assure precipitates are not formed during storage.
Conductivity	High ionic strength normally results in protein precipitation. Keep the salt concentration low to moderate, but at the same time, be aware of the "salting in" effect. Ions such as NH_4^+ do stabilize the protein upon precipitation.
Co-solvents	Typical protein precipitation agents are salts (e.g., ammonium sulfate), PEG (e.g., PEG 20,000), polyelectrolytes (e.g., carboxymethyl cellulose), and organic solvents (e.g., acetone).

Source: *Handbook of Biogeneric Therapeutic Proteins: Regulatory, Manufacturing, Testing and Intellectual Property Issues*, Taylor & Francis Group, Boca Raton, FL, 2005.
Abbreviation: PEG, polyethylene glycol.

and/or polypeptides, maintenance of molecular conformation, and, hence, of biological activity, is dependent on noncovalent and covalent forces. The products are particularly sensitive to environmental factors, such as temperature changes, oxidation, light, ionic content, and shear. To ensure the maintenance of biological activity and to avoid degradation, stringent conditions for their storage are usually necessary.

The evaluation of stability may necessitate complex analytical methodologies. Assays for biological activity, where applicable, should be part of the pivotal stability studies. Appropriate physicochemical, biochemical, and immunochemical methods for the analysis of the molecular entity and the quantitative detection of degradation products should also be part of the stability program, whenever purity and molecular characteristics of the product permit use of these methodologies.

With these concerns in mind, the applicant should develop the proper supporting stability data for a biotechnological/biological product and consider many external conditions that can affect the product's potency, purity, and quality. Primary data to support a requested storage period for either drug substance (DS) or drug product (DP) should be based on long-term, real-time, real-condition stability studies. Thus, the development of a proper long-term stability program becomes critical to the successful development of a commercial product. The purpose of this document is to give guidance to applicants regarding the type of stability studies that need to be provided in support of marketing applications. It is understood that during the review and evaluation process, continuing updates of initial stability data may occur.

Where bulk material is to be stored after manufacture but before formulation and final manufacturing, stability data are provided on at least three batches for which manufacture and storage are representative of the manufacturing scale of production. A minimum of 6-month stability data at the time of submission should be submitted in cases where storage periods greater than 6 months are requested. For DS with storage periods of less than 6 months, the minimum amount of stability data in the initial submission should be determined on a case-by-case basis. Data from pilot plant scale batches of DS produced at a reduced scale of fermentation and purification may be provided at the time the dossier is submitted to the regulatory agencies, with a commitment to place the first three manufacturing scale batches into the long-term stability program after approval.

The quality of the batches of DS placed into the stability program is representative of the quality of the material used in the preclinical and clinical studies and of the quality of the material to be made at the manufacturing scale. In addition, the DS (bulk material) made at pilot plant scale should be produced by a process and stored under conditions representative of that used for the manufacturing scale. The DS entered into the stability program should be stored in containers that properly represent the actual holding containers used during manufacture. Containers of reduced size may be acceptable for DS stability testing, provided that they are constructed of the same material and use the same type of container/closure system that is intended to be used during manufacture.

During manufacture of biotechnological/biological products, the quality and control of certain intermediates may be critical to the production of the final product. In general, the manufacturer should identify intermediates and generate in-house data and process limits that assure their stability within the bounds of the developed process. Although the use of pilot plant scale data is permissible, the manufacturer should establish the suitability of such data by using the manufacturing scale process.

On the whole, there is no single stability-indicating assay or parameter that profiles the stability characteristics of a biotechnological/biological product. Consequently, the manufacturer should propose a stability-indicating profile that provides assurance that changes in the identity, purity, and potency of the product will be detected.

At the time of submission, applicants should have validated the methods that comprise the stability-indicating profile, and the data should be available for review. The determination of tests that should be included will be product-specific. The items emphasized in the following subsections are not intended to be all-inclusive but represent product characteristics that should typically be documented to demonstrate product stability adequately.

For the purpose of stability testing of the products described in this guideline, purity is a relative term. Because of the effect of glycosylation, deamidation, or other heterogeneities, the absolute purity of a biotechnological/biological product is extremely difficult to determine. Thus, the purity of a biotechnological/biological product should be typically assessed by more than one method, and the purity value derived is method dependent. For the purpose of stability testing, tests for purity should focus on the methods for the determination of degradation products.

The degree of purity, as well as the individual and total amounts of degradation products of the biotechnological/biological product entered into the stability studies, should be reported and documented, whenever possible. Limits of acceptable degradation should be derived from the analytical profiles of batches of the DS and DP used in the preclinical and clinical studies.

The use of relevant physicochemical, biochemical, and immunochemical analytical methodologies should permit a comprehensive characterization of the DS and/or DP (e.g., molecular size, charge, and hydrophobicity) and the accurate detection of degradation changes that may result from deamidation, oxidation, sulfoxidation, aggregation, or fragmentation during storage. As examples, methods that may contribute to this include electrophoresis (SDS09Page, immunoelectrophoresis, Western blot, and IEF), high-resolution chromatography (e.g., RP chromatography, gel filtration, IEX, and affinity chromatography), and peptide mapping.

Wherever significant qualitative or quantitative changes indicative of degradation product formation are detected during long-term, accelerated, and/or stress stability studies, consideration should be given to potential hazards and the need for the characterization and quantification of degradation products within the long-term stability program. Acceptable limits should be proposed and justified, taking into account the levels observed in material used in preclinical and clinical studies.

For substances that cannot be properly characterized or products for which an exact analysis of the purity cannot be determined through routine analytical methods, the applicant should propose and justify alternative testing procedures.

9.9.5 Forced Degradation Studies

Stress testing studies are conducted to challenge the specificity of stability-indicating and impurity-monitoring methods as part of the validation protocol. The current regulatory guidances governing forced degradation studies of biological pharmaceuticals are extremely general. They itemize broad principles and approaches with few practical instructions. There is no single document that comprehensively addresses the issues related to stress studies, such as objectives, timing, selection of stress conditions, and extent of degradation. We will attempt to fill this gap by summarizing regulatory guidance for stress studies of biological products and present some examples of their practical applications. Stress-testing studies are conducted to challenge the specificity of stability-indicating and impurity-monitoring methods as part of the validation protocol. Another major goal is to investigate degradation products and pathways. The results of the forced degradation studies are required to be included in a Phase III investigational new drug (IND) filing. It is important to start the study as early as possible to be able to provide valuable information that can be used to improve the formulations and the manufacturing process.

The choice of stress conditions should be consistent with product decomposition under normal manufacturing, storage, and use conditions. Recommended stress factors include high and low pH, elevated temperature, photolysis, and oxidation. The extent of the stress applied in forced degradation studies should ensure the formation of the desired amount (usually 10%–20%) of degradation.

The complexity of biological macromolecules, when compared with small molecule therapeutics; differences in manufacturing; and the broad variety of potential degradation pathways lead to special requirements in the quality assurance and analytical testing of pharmaceutical proteins. The product-related impurities are molecular variants formed during manufacture, storage, or use, and their properties are different from the desired product with respect to activity, efficacy, and safety.

Forced degradation studies are designed to generate product-related variants and develop analytical methods to determine the degradation products formed during accelerated pharmaceutical studies and long-term stability studies. Any significant degradation product should be evaluated for potential hazards and the need for characterization and quantification. Forced degradation or stress-testing studies are part of the development strategy and are also an integral component of validation of analytical methods that indicate stability and detect impurities. This relates to the specificity section of the validation studies. It is important to recognize that forced degradation studies are not designed to establish qualitative or quantitative limits for change in DS or DP. Testing of stressed samples is required to demonstrate the following abilities of analytical techniques employed in stability studies:

- To evaluate the stability of DS and DP in solution
- To determine the structural transformations of the DS and DP
- To detect low concentrations of potential degradation products
- To detect unrelated impurities in the presence of the desired product and product-related degradants
- To separate product-related degradants from those derived from excipients and intact placebo
- To elucidate possible degradation pathways
- To identify degradation products that may be spontaneously generated during drug storage and use
- To facilitate improvements in the manufacturing process and formulations in parallel with accelerated pharmaceutical studies

Stress studies may be useful in determining whether accidental exposures to conditions other than normal ranges (e.g., during transportation) are deleterious to the product and also for evaluating which specific test parameters may be the best indicators of product stability.

9.9.5.1 Stress Testing

This involves the establishment of a stability-indicating analytical procedure that will detect significant changes in the quality of DS at Phase II stage of IND. Stress studies on DS and DP should be completed during Phase III, and significant impurities should be identified, qualified, and quantified. Starting forced degradation experiments before Phase II is highly encouraged and should be conducted on DS, with multiple aims: to provide timely recommendations for improvements in the manufacturing process; to ensure proper selection of stability-indicating analytical techniques; and to assure sufficient time for the identification of degradation product, elucidation of degradation pathways, and optimization of stress conditions.

Every change in stability-indicating analytical methods, manufacturing processes, or formulation requires revalidation of analytical methods; therefore, full validation commences only after the manufacturing process is finalized, formulations are established, and test procedures are developed and qualified. However, method validation must be completed before a formal long-term stability study begins. These limitations impose time constraints on all method-validation activities, including stressed sample development and testing. Consequently, all preliminary work on optimization of stress conditions must be completed at the earlier stages, even though results of forced degradation studies are not required to be reported until Phase III stage of IND application.

The question of how much degradation is sufficient to meet the objectives of stress studies is widely discussed, especially with respect to conventional therapeutics. A degradation level of 10%–15% is considered adequate for validation of a chromatographic purity assay. Chromatographic methods for product-related impurities (including degradants) should be validated by spiking experiments within the range of 0%–20% if the expected range of impurities is 0%–10%. It is also suggested that DS spiked with a mixture of known degradation products can be used to challenge the methods employed for monitoring stability of DP. The apparent consensus among pharmaceutical scientists is that samples degraded ~10% are optimal for use in the validation of analytical method. These considerations apply to small organic pharmaceuticals for which stability is dictated by the typical pharmaceutical limit of 90% of label claim.

No such limits for physicochemical changes, losses of activity, or degradation during shelf life have been established for individual types or groups of biological products. In general, international and national regulations for biological products provide little guidance with respect to stability-related issues. These issues should be considered on a case-by-case basis.

As a group, biological products form a wide variety of product-related degradants under stress conditions. In cases with multiple degradation pathways, it appears to be beneficial to develop multiple product-related variants to challenge the specificity of analytical methods, even when some of the degradants may be present at concentrations that exceed 10%. This is done when accelerated stability studies do not provide clear indication of the degradation pathways. When a stress factor generates only one degradation product, for example, higher-MW noncovalent aggregates, 10%–15%

level of aggregation may be sufficient to challenge the specificity of methods such as SEC or light scattering.

The forced degradation experiments do not necessarily result in product decomposition. The study can be stopped if no degradation is observed after DS or DP has been exposed to a stress that exceeds the conditions of accelerated stability protocol. Protocols for generation of product-related degradation may differ for DS and DP, owing to the differences in matrices and concentrations. For example, sugar additives often present in DP are known to stabilize proteins vis-à-vis denaturing conditions.

9.9.5.2 Selection of Stress Conditions

Forced degradation is normally carried out under more severe conditions than those used for accelerated studies. The choice of stress conditions should be consistent with the product's decomposition under normal manufacturing, storage, and use conditions, which are specific in each case. The ICH guidance recognizes that it is impossible to provide strict degradation guidelines and allows certain freedom in the selection of stress conditions for biologics. The choice of forced degradation conditions should be based on data from accelerated pharmaceutical studies and sound scientific understanding of the product's decomposition mechanism under typical use conditions. A minimal list of stress factors suggested for forced degradation studies must include acid and base hydrolyses, thermal degradation, photolysis, and oxidation and may include freeze–thaw cycles and shear.

Regulatory guidance does not specify pH, temperature ranges, specific oxidizing agents or conditions to use, the number of freeze–thaw cycles, or specific wavelengths and light intensities. The design of photolysis studies is left to the applicant's discretion; however, Q1B recommends that the light source should produce combined VIS and UV (320–400 nm) outputs and that exposure levels should be justified. Consult the appropriate regulatory authorities on a case-by-case basis to determine guidance for light-induced stress.

Degradation products that arise in significant amounts during manufacture and storage should be identified, tested for, and monitored against appropriately established acceptance criteria. Examination of some degradation products generated under stress conditions may not be necessary for certain degradants if it has been demonstrated that they are not formed under accelerated or long-term storage conditions.

The forced degradation studies should be part of impurity characterization. When identification of the impurity is not feasible, incorporate the description of unsuccessful experiments (including those conducted in stress-testing studies) in the text of the application. The most frequently encountered protein variants include truncated fragments, deamidated, oxidized, isomerized, aggregated forms, and mismatched disulfide links.

Degradation pathways for proteins can be separated into two distinct classes that involve chemical and physical instabilities. Chemical instability is any process that yields a new chemical entity, including modification of the protein (via individual amino acid alteration), covalent bond formation, and cleavage. Physical instability refers to changes in the HOSs (secondary and above). Noncovalent aggregation usually results from partial or full unfolding, which enhances the hydrophobic interactions between protein molecules. It may also lead to denaturation, adsorption to surfaces, and precipitation. Aggregation presents a significant patient risk, because protein aggregates are frequently immunogenic; therefore, analytical methods employed in stability testing should detect low concentrations of aggregates. This is generally tested by providing stress conditions in the downstream processing to study if any unusual decomposition products are formed; a placebo is used as control. Potential degradation pathways are extensively researched, and methods for their detection are well established. A number of comprehensive reviews on this topic are available in the literature.

The proposed stability-indicating methodologies should provide assurance that changes in the identity, purity, and potency of the product will be detected. The selection of tests is product-specific. Stability-indicating methods will characterize potency, purity, and biological activity. As examples, stability-indicating methods may include electrophoresis (SDS-PAGE, immunoelectrophoresis, Western blot, and IEF), high-resolution chromatography (e.g., RP chromatography, SEC, gel filtration, IEX, and affinity chromatography), and peptide mapping.

The selected set of methods must be able to detect, separate, and quantify all observed degradation products; however, it is recognized that the identification and characterization of the appropriate variants may require the use of additional analytical methodologies. New analytical technologies and modifications of the existing technologies are continuously being developed and should be utilized when appropriate. The list of assays challenged by stressed samples should include analytical methods employed in the stability program and those monitoring impurities.

9.9.6 Specifications

Specifications are one part of a total control strategy designed to ensure product quality and consistency. Other parts of this strategy include thorough product characterization during development, on which many of the specifications are based; adherence to GMPs; a validated manufacturing process; raw materials testing; in-process testing; stability testing; and so on. Specifications are chosen to confirm the quality of the DS and DP rather than establishing full characterization and should focus on those molecular and biological characteristics found to be useful in ensuring the safety and efficacy of the product.

Characterization of a biotechnological or biological product (which includes the determination of physicochemical properties, biological activity, immunochemical properties, purity, and impurities) by appropriate techniques is necessary to allow relevant specifications to be established. Acceptance criteria should be established and justified based on the data obtained from lots used in preclinical and/or clinical studies, data from lots used for the demonstration of manufacturing consistency, data from stability studies, and relevant development data.

Extensive characterization is performed in the development phase and, where necessary, following significant process changes. At the time of submission, the product should have been compared with an appropriate reference standard, if available. When feasible and relevant, it should also be compared with its natural counterpart. Also, at the time of submission, the manufacturer should have established appropriately characterized in-house reference materials, which will serve for the biological and physicochemical testing of production lots. New analytical technology and modifications to the existing technology are continually being developed and will be utilized when appropriate.

9.9.6.1 Physicochemical Properties

A physicochemical characterization program will generally include the determination of the composition, physical properties, and primary structure of the desired product. In some cases, information regarding the HOS of the desired product (the fidelity of which is generally inferred by its biological activity) may be obtained by appropriate physicochemical methodologies.

An inherent degree of structural heterogeneity occurs in proteins, owing to the biosynthetic processes used by living organisms to produce them; therefore, the desired product can be a mixture of anticipated post-ranslationally modified forms (e.g., glycoforms). These forms may be active, and their presence may have no deleterious effect on the safety and efficacy of the product. The manufacturer should define the pattern of heterogeneity of the desired product and demonstrate consistency with that of the lots used in preclinical and clinical studies. If a consistent pattern of product heterogeneity is demonstrated, an evaluation of the activity, efficacy, and safety (including immunogenicity) of individual forms may not be necessary.

Heterogeneity can also be produced during manufacture and/or storage of the DS or DP. As the heterogeneity of these products defines their quality, the degree and profile of this heterogeneity should be characterized to ensure lot-to-lot consistency. When these variants of the desired product have properties comparable with those of the desired product with respect to activity, efficacy, and safety, they are considered product-related substances. When process changes and degradation products result in heterogeneity patterns that differ from those observed in the material used during the preclinical and clinical development, the significance of these alterations should be evaluated.

9.9.7 Biological Activity

Assessment of the biological properties constitutes an equally essential step in establishing a complete characterization profile. An important property is the biological activity that describes the specific ability or capacity of a product to achieve a defined biological effect.

A valid biological assay to measure the biological activity should be provided by the manufacturer. Examples of procedures used to measure biological activity include the following:

- Animal-based biological assays, which measure an organism's biological response to the product
- Cell culture-based biological assays, which measure biochemical or physiological response at the cellular level
- Biochemical assays, which measure biological activities, such as enzymatic reaction rates and biological responses induced by immunological interactions

Other procedures, such as ligand- and receptor-binding assays, may be acceptable.

Potency (expressed in units) is the quantitative measure of biological activity, based on the attribute of the product that is linked to the relevant biological properties, whereas quantity (expressed in mass) is a physicochemical measure of protein content.

Mimicking the biological activity in the clinical situation is not always necessary. A correlation between the expected clinical response and the activity in the biological assay should be established in pharmacodynamic or clinical studies.

The results of biological assays should be expressed in units of activity calibrated against an international or national reference standard, when available and appropriate for the assay utilized. Where no such reference standard exists, a characterized in-house reference material should be established, and assay results of production lots should be reported as in-house units.

Often, for complex molecules, the physicochemical information may be extensive but is unable to confirm the HOS, which, however, can be inferred from the biological activity. In such cases, a biological assay, with wider confidence limits, may be acceptable when combined with a specific quantitative measure. Importantly, a biological assay to measure the biological activity of the product may be replaced by physicochemical tests only in those instances where:

- Sufficient physicochemical information about the drug, including HOS, can be thoroughly established by such physicochemical methods, and relevant correlation to biologic activity can be demonstrated
- There exists a well-established manufacturing history
- Physicochemical tests alone are used to quantify the biological activity (based on appropriate correlation) (results should be expressed in mass)

For the purpose of lot release, the choice of relevant quantitative assay (biological and/or physicochemical) should be justified by the manufacturer.

9.9.8 Immunochemical Properties

When an antibody is the desired product, its immunological properties should be fully characterized. Binding assays of the antibody to purified antigens and defined regions of antigens should be performed, as feasible, to determine affinity, avidity, and immunoreactivity (including cross-reactivity). In addition, the target molecule bearing the relevant epitope should be biochemically defined and the epitope itself defined, when feasible.

For some DS or DP, the protein molecule may need to be examined using immunochemical procedures (e.g., ELISA and Western blot) and utilizing antibodies that recognize different epitopes of the protein molecule. Immunochemical properties of a protein may serve to establish its identity, homogeneity, or purity or may serve to quantify it.

If immunochemical properties constitute lot release criteria, all relevant information pertaining to the antibody should be made available.

9.9.9 Purity, Impurities, and Contaminants

9.9.9.1 Purity

The determination of absolute, as well as relative, purity presents considerable analytical challenges, and the results are highly method-dependent. Historically, the relative purity of a biological product has been expressed in terms of specific activity (units of biological activity per milligram of product), which is also highly method-dependent. Consequently, the purity of the DS and DP is assessed by a combination of analytical procedures.

Owing to the unique biosynthetic production process and molecular characteristics of biotechnological and biological products, the DS can include several molecular entities or variants. When these molecular entities are derived from anticipated PTM, they are part of the desired product. When variants of the desired product are formed during the manufacturing process and/or storage and have properties comparable with the desired product, they are considered product-related substances and not impurities.

Individual and/or collective acceptance criteria for product-related substances should be set, as appropriate.

For the purpose of lot release, an appropriate subset of methods should be selected and justified to determine purity.

9.9.9.2 Impurities

In addition to the evaluation of the purity of the DS and DP, which may be composed of the desired product and multiple product-related substances, the manufacturer should also assess the impurities, which may be present. Impurities may be either process- or product-related. They may be of known structure, partially characterized, or unidentified. When adequate quantities of impurities can be generated, these materials should be characterized to the extent possible, and, where possible, their biological activities should be evaluated.

Process-related impurities encompass those that are derived from the manufacturing process, that is, cell substrates (e.g., host cell proteins and host cell DNA), cell culture (e.g., inducers, antibiotics, and media components), and downstream processing. Product-related impurities (e.g., precursors and certain degradation products) are molecular variants arising during manufacture and/or storage that do not have properties comparable with those of the desired product with respect to activity, efficacy, and safety.

Further, the acceptance criteria for impurities should be based on the data obtained from lots used in preclinical and clinical studies and manufacturing consistency lots.

Individual and/or collective acceptance criteria for impurities (product-related and process-related) should be set, as appropriate. Under certain circumstances, acceptance criteria for some selected impurities may not be necessary.

9.9.9.3 Contaminants

Contaminants in a product include all adventitiously introduced materials that are not intended to be part of the manufacturing process, such as chemical and biochemical materials (e.g., microbial proteases) and/or microbial species. Contaminants should be strictly avoided and/or suitably controlled with appropriate in-process acceptance criteria or action limits for DS or DP specifications. For the special case of adventitious viral or mycoplasma contamination, the concept of action limits is not applicable, and the strategies proposed in the ICH Guidances *Q5A Quality of Biotechnological/Biological Products: Viral Safety Evaluation of Biotechnology Products Derived from Cell Lines of Human or Animal Origin* and *Q5D Quality of Biotechnological/Biological Products: Derivation and Characterization of Cell Substrates Used for Production of Biotechnological/Biological Products* should be considered.

9.9.10 Quantity

Quantity, usually measured as protein content, is critical for a biotechnological/ biological product and should be determined using an appropriate assay, usually physicochemical in nature. In some cases, it may be demonstrated that the quantity values obtained may be directly related to those found using the biological assay. When this correlation exists, it may be appropriate to use the measurement of quantity rather than the measurement of biological activity in manufacturing processes, such as filling.

9.9.11 Analytical Considerations

9.9.11.1 Reference Standards and Reference Materials

For drug applications of new molecular entities, it is unlikely that an international or national standard will be available. At the time of submission, the manufacturer should have established an appropriately characterized in-house primary reference material, prepared from lot(s) representative of production and clinical materials. In-house working reference material(s) used in the testing of production lots should be calibrated against this primary reference material. Where an international or national standard is available and appropriate, reference materials should be calibrated against it. While it is desirable to use the same reference material for both biological assays and physicochemical testing, in some cases, a separate reference material may be necessary. Also, distinct reference materials for product-related substances, product-related impurities, and process-related impurities may need to be established. When appropriate, a description of the manufacture and/or purification of reference materials should be included in the application. Documentation of the characterization, storage conditions, and formulation supportive of reference material(s) stability should also be provided.

9.9.11.2 Validation of Analytical Procedures

At the time at which the application is submitted to the regulatory authorities, applicants should have validated the analytical procedures used in the specifications in accordance with the ICH Guidances *Q2A Validation of Analytical Procedures: Definitions and Terminology* and *Q2B Validation of Analytical Procedures: Methodology*, except where there are specific issues for unique tests used for analyzing biotechnological and biological products.

9.9.12 Process Controls

Adequate design of a process and knowledge of its capability are parts of the strategy used to develop a manufacturing process that is controlled and reproducible, yielding a DS or DP that meets the specifications. In this respect, limits are justified based on critical information gained from the entire process, spanning the period from early development through commercial-scale production.

For certain impurities, testing of either the DS or the DP may not be necessary and may not need to be included in the specifications if efficient control or removal of acceptable levels is demonstrated by suitable studies. This testing can include verification at the commercial scale, in accordance with regional regulations. It is recognized that only limited data may be available at the time of submission of an application. This concept may, therefore, sometimes be implemented after marketing authorization, in accordance with regional regulations.

In-process tests are performed at critical decision-making steps and at other steps where data serve to confirm consistency of the process during the production of either the DS or the DP. The results of in-process testing may be recorded as action limits or as acceptance criteria. Performing such testing may eliminate the need for testing the DS or DP. In-process testing for adventitious agents at the end of cell culture is an example of testing for which acceptance criteria should be established.

The use of internal action limits by the manufacturer to assess the consistency of the process at less critical steps is also important. Data obtained during development and validation runs should provide the basis for provisional action limits to be set for the manufacturing process. These limits, which are the responsibility of the manufacturer, may be used to initiate investigation or further action. They should be further refined as additional manufacturing experience, and data should be obtained after product approval.

The quality of the raw materials used in the production of the DS (or DP) should meet the standards appropriate for their intended use. Biological raw materials or reagents may require careful evaluation to establish the presence or absence of deleterious endogenous or adventitious agents. Procedures that make the use of affinity chromatography (e.g., employing MAbs) should be accompanied by appropriate measures to ensure that such process-related impurities or potential contaminants arising from their production and use do not compromise the quality and safety of the DS or DP. Appropriate information pertaining to the antibody should be made available.

The quality of the excipients used in the DP formulation (and in some cases, the DS), as well as the container/closure systems, should meet pharmacopoeial standards, where available and appropriate. Otherwise, suitable acceptance criteria should be established for the nonpharmacopoeial excipients.

9.9.13 Release Limits versus Shelf-Life Limits

The concept of release limits versus shelf-life limits may be applied where justified. This concept pertains to the establishment of limits that are tighter for the release than for the shelf life of the DS or DP. Examples where this may be applicable include potency and degradation products. In some regions, the concept of release limits may only be applicable to in-house limits and not to the regulatory shelf-life limits.

Appropriate statistical analysis should be applied, when necessary, to the quantitative data reported. The methods of analysis, including justification and rationale, should be described fully. These descriptions should be sufficiently clear to permit independent calculation of the results presented.

9.9.14 Justification of Specifications

The setting of specifications for DS and DP is part of an overall control strategy, which includes control of raw materials and excipients, in-process testing, process evaluation or validation, adherence to GMPs, stability testing, and testing for the consistency of lots. When combined in total, these elements provide assurance that the appropriate quality of the product will be maintained. As specifications are chosen to confirm the quality rather than to characterize the product, the manufacturer should provide the rationale and justification for including and/or excluding testing for specific quality attributes. The following points should be taken into consideration when establishing scientifically justifiable specifications:

- Specifications are linked to a manufacturing process.
- Specifications should be based on data obtained from lots used to demonstrate manufacturing consistency. Linking specifications to a manufacturing process is important, especially for product-related substances, product-related impurities, and process-related impurities. Process changes and degradation products produced during storage may result in heterogeneity patterns that differ from those observed in the material used during the preclinical and clinical development. The significance of these alterations should be evaluated.
- Specifications should account for the stability of DS and DP.
- Degradation of DS and DP, which may occur during storage, should be considered when establishing specifications. Owing to the inherent complexity of these products, there is no single stability-indicating assay or parameter that profiles the stability characteristics. Consequently, the manufacturer should propose a stability-indicating profile. The result of this stability-indicating profile will then provide assurance that changes in the quality of the product will be detected. The determination of the tests that should be included will be product-specific. The manufacturer is referred to the ICH guidance *Q5C Stability Testing of Biotechnological/Biological Products.*
- Specifications are linked to preclinical and clinical studies.
- Specifications should be based on the data obtained for lots used in preclinical and clinical studies. The quality of the material made at the commercial scale should be representative of the lots used in the preclinical and clinical studies.
- Specifications are linked to analytical procedures.

Critical quality attributes may include items such as potency, the nature and quantity of product-related substances, product-related impurities, and process-related impurities. Such attributes can be assessed by multiple analytical procedures, each yielding different results. In the course of product development, it is not unusual for the analytical technology to evolve in parallel with the product. Therefore, it is important to confirm that the data generated during development correlate with those generated at the time the marketing application is filed.

9.10 Physiochemical Characterization Tests

9.10.1 Structural Characterization and Confirmation

9.10.1.1 Amino Acid Sequence

The amino acid sequence of the desired product should be determined to the extent possible by using customary approaches and then compared with the sequence of the amino acids deduced from the gene sequence of the desired product.

9.10.1.2 Amino Acid Composition

The overall amino acid composition is determined using various hydrolytic and analytical procedures and compared with the amino acid composition deduced from the gene sequence for the desired product, or the natural counterpart, if considered necessary. In many cases, the analysis of amino acid composition provides some useful structural information for peptides and small proteins, but such data are generally less definitive for large proteins. Quantitative amino acid analysis data can also be used to determine protein content in many cases.

9.10.1.3 Terminal Amino Acid Sequence

Terminal amino acid sequence analysis is performed to identify the nature and homogeneity of the amino- and carboxy-terminal amino acids. If the desired product is found to be heterogeneous with respect to the terminal amino acids, the relative amounts of the variant forms should be determined using an appropriate analytical procedure. The sequence of these terminal amino acids should be compared with the terminal amino acid sequence deduced from the gene sequence of the desired product.

9.10.1.4 Peptide Map

Selective fragmentation of the product into discrete peptides is performed using suitable enzymes or chemicals, and the resulting peptide fragments are analyzed by HPLC or other appropriate analytical procedures. The peptide fragments should be identified to the extent possible by using techniques such as amino acid compositional analysis, N-terminal sequencing, and MS. Peptide mapping of the DS or DP using an appropriately validated procedure is a method that is frequently used to confirm the structure of the desired product for lot release purposes.

9.10.2 Sulfhydryl Group(s) and Disulfide Bridges

If, based on the gene sequence for the desired product, cysteine residues are expected, the number and positions of any free sulfhydryl groups and/or disulfide bridges should be determined, to the extent possible. Peptide mapping (under reducing and nonreducing conditions), MS, or other appropriate techniques may be useful for this evaluation.

9.10.3 Carbohydrate Structure

For glycoproteins, the carbohydrate content (neutral sugars, amino sugars, and sialic acids) is determined. In addition, the structure of the carbohydrate chains, the oligo-saccharide pattern (antennary profile), and the glycosylation site(s) of the polypeptide chain are analyzed, to the extent possible.

9.10.4 Physicochemical Properties

9.10.4.1 Molecular Weight or Size

Molecular weight (or size) is determined using SEC, SDS-PAGE (under reducing and/or nonreducing conditions), MS, and other appropriate techniques.

9.10.4.2 Isoform Pattern

This is determined by IEF or other appropriate techniques.

9.10.4.3 Extinction Coefficient (or Molar Absorptivity)

In many cases, it will be desirable to determine the extinction coefficient (or molar absorptivity) for the desired product at a particular UV/VIS wavelength (e.g., 280 nm). The extinction coefficient is determined using UV/VIS spectrophotometry on a solution of the product having a known protein content, as determined by techniques such as amino acid compositional analysis and nitrogen determination. If UV absorption is used to measure the protein content, the extinction coefficient for the particular product should be used.

9.10.4.4 Electrophoretic Patterns

Electrophoretic patterns and data on identity, homogeneity, and purity can be obtained by PAGE, IEF, SDS-PAGE, Western blot, capillary electrophoresis, or other suitable procedures.

9.10.4.5 Liquid Chromatographic Patterns

Chromatographic patterns and data on the identity, homogeneity, and purity can be obtained by SEC, RPLC, IEX-LC, affinity chromatography, or other suitable procedures.

9.11 Spectroscopic Profiles

The UV and VIS absorption spectra are determined, as appropriate. The HOS of the product is examined using procedures such as CD, NMR, and other suitable techniques, as appropriate.

9.11.1 Process-Related Impurities and Contaminants

These are derived from the manufacturing process and are classified into three major categories: cell substrate-derived, cell culture-derived, and downstream-derived.

1. Cell substrate-derived impurities include, but are not limited to, proteins derived from the host organism and nucleic acid (host cell genomic, vector, or total DNA). For host cell proteins, a sensitive assay, for example, immunoassay, capable of detecting a wide range of protein impurities is generally utilized. In the case of an immunoassay, a polyclonal antibody used in the test is generated by immunization with a preparation of a production cell minus the product-coding gene, fusion partners, or other appropriate cell lines. The level of DNA from the host cells can be detected by the direct analysis of the product (such as by hybridization techniques). Clearance studies, which could include spiking experiments at the laboratory scale, to demonstrate the removal of cell substrate-derived impurities, such as nucleic acids and host cell proteins, may sometimes be used to eliminate the need for establishing the acceptance criteria for these impurities.
2. Cell culture-derived impurities include, but are not limited to, inducers, antibiotics, serum, and other media components.
3. Downstream-derived impurities include, but are not limited to, enzymes, chemical and biochemical processing reagents (e.g., cyanogen bromide, guanidine, and oxidizing and reducing agents), inorganic salts (e.g., heavy metals, arsenic, and nonmetallic ion), solvents, carriers, ligands (e.g., MAbs), and other leachables.

For intentionally introduced, endogenous, and adventitious viruses, the ability of the manufacturing process to remove and/or inactivate viruses should be demonstrated, as described in the ICH guidance *Q5A Viral Safety Evaluation of Biotechnology Products Derived from Cell Lines of Human or Animal Origin*.

9.11.2 Product-Related Impurities, Including Degradation Products

The following represents the most frequently encountered molecular variants of the desired product and lists relevant technology for their assessment. Such variants may need considerable effort in isolation and characterization, in order to identify the type of modification(s). Degradation products arising in significant amounts during the manufacture and/or storage should be tested for and monitored against appropriately established acceptance criteria.

9.11.2.1 Truncated Forms

Hydrolytic enzymes or chemicals may catalyze the cleavage of peptide bonds. These may be detected by HPLC or SDS-PAGE. Peptide mapping may be useful, depending on the property of the variant.

9.11.2.2 Other Modified Forms

Deamidated, isomerized, mismatched S–S linked, oxidized, or altered conjugated forms (e.g., glycosylation and phosphorylation) may be detected and characterized by chromatographic, electrophoretic, and/or other relevant analytical methods (e.g., HPLC, capillary electrophoresis, MS, and CD).

9.11.2.3 Aggregates

The category of aggregates includes dimers and higher multiples of the desired product. These are generally resolved from the desired product and product-related substances and quantified by appropriate analytical procedures (e.g., SEC and capillary electrophoresis).

9.12 Design of Preformulation Studies

A typical preformulation study would include a statistical design method to understand the effects of buffer strength, sodium chloride concentration, and pH on conformation and stability of the protein and the related interactions. It is also important to elucidate interactions between these factors. A central composite design (CCD) using a two-level full-factorial study can be used. Secondary structure can be evaluated using CD. Stability toward unfolding is investigated using high-sensitivity differential scanning calorimetry. DePEGylation (where applicable), aggregation, and protein loss are evaluated using SEC-HPLC with online light scattering, at time zero and after a 2-week stability study. Response surface plots are used to show optimal pH, sodium chloride, and buffer conditions. Interactions occur between pH and sodium chloride, as well as between pH and buffer concentration. T_m is predictive of compound stability. Statistical analyses can be performed using standard statistical programs. Generally, a CCD can be set up using a two-level full-factorial design with axial and center points. Factorial design is a statistical tool that allows experimentation on several factors simultaneously. A two-level design involves the evaluation of two or more factors (e.g., sodium chloride concentration, buffer concentration, and pH) at two levels—high and low. A factorial design evaluating three factors at all combinations of high and low levels for each factor will result in a full-factorial design consisting of $2^3 = 8$ runs experiments. Addition of center points allows detection of nonlinearity in the responses. Axial points are also included in the CCD. These points are levels of the factors under investigation, located at a distance outside the original high- and low-factor range. The CCD, therefore, contains five levels of each factor: low-axial, low-factorial, center, high-factorial, and high-axial. With these many levels, enough information is generated to fit second-order polynomials. The total number of runs becomes 2 + 6 runs, with all factors set at the center points + 6 additional runs (one factor set at high- or low-axial condition, with all others set at center points) = 20 runs. Actual fitting of the model is computed using the statistical software.

WEB REFERENCES

1. http://www.gpoaccess.gov/cfr/index.html
2. http://www.fda.gov/cber/transfer/tranfer.htm
3. http://www.avantimmune.com
4. http://www.nektar.com
5. *Handbook of Biogeneric Therapeutic Proteins: Regulatory, Manufacturing, Testing and Intellectual Property Issues.* Boca Raton, FL: Taylor & Francis Group, 2005.

BIBLIOGRAPHY

Anderson CL. Applications of Imaged Capillary Isoelectric Focussing Technique in Development of Biopharmaceutical Glycoprotein-based Products. *Electrophoresis* 2012;33(11):1538–1544.

Bártová E, Krejcí J, Harnicarová A, Galiová G, Kozubek S. Histone Modifications and Nuclear Architecture: A Review. *J Histochem Cytochem.* 2008;56(8):711–721.

Beck A, Sanglier-Cianférani S, Van Dorsselaer A. Biosimilar, Biobetter, and Next Generation Antibody Characterization by Mass Spectrometry. *Anal Chem.* 2012;84(11):4637–4646.

Beck A, Wurch T, Reichert JM. 6th Annual European Antibody Congress 2010: November 29–December 1, 2010, Geneva, Switzerland. *MAbs* 2011;3(2):111–132.

Boubeva R, Reichert C, Handrick R, Müller C, Hannemann J, Borcharda G. Newexpression Method and Characterization of Recombinant Human Granulocyte Colonystimulating Factor in a Stable Protein Formulation. *Chimia (Aarau)* 2012;66(5):281–285.

Brennan DF, Barford D. Eliminylation: A Post-translational Modification Catalyzed by Phosphothreonine Lyases. *Trends Biochem Sci.* 2009;34(3):108–114.

Cantor CR, Schimmel PR. *Biophysical Chemistry Part 1: The Conformation of Biological Macromolecules.* New York: W.H. Freeman & Co., 1980.

Cao J, Sun W, Gong F, Liu W. Charge Profiling and Stability Testing Ofbiosimilar by Capillary Isoelectric Focusing. *Electrophoresis* 2014;35(10):1461–1468.

Chen SL, Wu SL, Huang LJ, Huang JB, Chen SH. A Global Comparability Approach for Biosimilar Monoclonal Antibodies using Lc-Tandem Ms Based Proteomics. *J PharmBiomed Anal.* 2013;80:126–135.

Creighton TE. *Protein Structures and Molecular Properties*, 2nd ed. New York: W. H. Freeman and Co., 1993.

Creighton TE. *The Biophysical Chemistry of Nucleic Acids and Proteins.* New York: Helvetian Press, 2010.

Debaene F, Wagner-Rousset E, Colas O, Ayoub D, Corvaïa N, Van Dorsselaer A, Beck A, Cianférani S. Time Resolved Native Ion-Mobility Mass Spectrometry Tomonitor Dynamics of Igg4 Fab Arm Exchange and "Bispecific" Monoclonal Antibody Formation. *Anal Chem.* 2013;85(20):9785–9792.

Declerck PJ. Biosimilar Monoclonal Antibodies: A Science-Based Regulatory Challenge. *Expert Opin Biol Ther.* 2013;13(2):153–156.

Dorvignit D, Palacios JL, Merino M, Hernández T, Sosa K, Casaco A, López-Requena A, Mateo de Acosta C. Expression and Biological Characterization of an Anti-Cd20 Biosimilar Candidate Antibody: A Case Study. *MAbs* 2012;4(4):488–496.

Eddé B, Rossier J, Le Caer JP, Desbruyères E, Gros F, Denoulet P. Posttranslational Glutamylation of Alpha-tubulin. *Science* 1990;247(4938):83–85.

Eichbaum C, Haefeli WE. Biologics—Nomenclature and Classification. *TherUmsch* 2011;68(11):593–601.

Gadermaier G. Non-specific Lipid Transfer Proteins: A Protein Family in Search of an Allergenic Pattern. *Int Arch Allergy Immunol.* 2014;164(3):169–170.

Gadermaier G, Eichhorn S, Vejvar E, Weilnböck L, Lang R, Briza P, Huber CG, Ferreira F, Hawranek T. Plantago Lanceolata: An Important Trigger of Summerpollinosis with Limited Ige Cross-reactivity. *J Allergy Clin Immunol.* 2014;134(2):472–475.

Glozak MA, Sengupta N, Zhang X, Seto E. Acetylation and Deacetylation of Non-histone Proteins. *Gene* 2005;363:15–23.

Guo Q, Guo H, Liu T, Zheng Y, Gu P, Chen X, Wang H, Hou S, Guo Y. Versatile Characterization of Glycosylation Modification in CTLA4-Ig Fusion Proteins by Liquid Chromatography-mass Spectrometry. *MAbs* 2014;6(6):1474–1485.

Haselberg R, de Jong GJ, Somsen GW. Low-flow Sheathless Capillary Electrophoresis-Mass Spectrometry for Sensitive Glycoform Profiling of Intact Pharmaceutical Proteins. *Anal Chem.* 2013;85(4):2289–2296.

Hashii N, Harazono A, Kuribayashi R, Takakura D, Kawasaki N. Characterization of N-glycan Heterogeneities of Erythropoietin Products by Liquid Chromatography/Mass Spectrometry and Multivariate Analysis. *Rapid Commun MassSpectrom.* 2014;28(8):921–932.

Hassett B, McMillen S, Fitzpatrick B. Characterization and Comparison of Commercially Available TNF Receptor 2-Fc Fusion Protein Products: Letter to the Editor. *MAbs* 2013;5(5):624–625.

Heringa J, Taylor WR. *Computational Protein Science: Methods in Structural Bioinformatics.* New York, NY: John Wiley & Sons, 2016.

Jiang H, Wu SL, Karger BL, Hancock WS. Characterization of the Glycosylation Occupancy and the Active Site in the Follow-on Protein Therapeutic: TNK-tissue Plasminogen Activator. *Anal Chem.* 2010;82(14):6154–6162.

Kessel A, Nir Ben-Tal A. *Introduction to Proteins: Structure, Function, and Motion.* Chapman & Hall/CRC Mathematical and Computational Biology, 2010.

Khoury GA, Baliban RC, Floudas CA. Proteome-wide Post-translational Modification Statistics: Frequency Analysis and Curation of the Swiss-prot Database. *Sci Rep.* 2011;1(90):90.

Li C, Rossomando A, Wu SL, Karger BL. Comparability Analysis of Anti-CD20commercial (rituximab) and RNAi-mediated Fucosylated Antibodies by two LC-MSapproaches. *MAbs* 2013;5(4):565–575.

Lipiäinen T, Peltoniemi M, Sarkhel S, Yrjönen T, Vuorela H, Urtti A, Juppo A. Formulation and Stability of Cytokine Therapeutics. *J Pharm Sci.* 2015;104(2):307–326.

Malakhova OA, Yan M, Malakhov MP, Yuan Y. Ritchie KJ, Kim KI, Peterson LF, Shuai K, Zhang DE. Protein ISGylation Modulates the JAK-STAT Signaling Pathway. *Gene Dev.* 2003;17(4):455–460.

Mueller DA, Heinig L, Ramljak S, Krueger A, Schulte R, Wrede A, Stuke AW. Conditional Expression of Full-length Humanized Anti-prion Protein Antibodies in Chinese Hamster Ovary Cells. *Hybridoma (Larchmt)* 2010;29(6):463–472.

Mydel P, Wang Z, Brisslert M, Hellvard A, Dahlberg LE, Hazen SL, Bokarewa M. Carbamylation-dependent Activation of T Cells: A Novel Mechanism in the Pathogenesis of Autoimmune Arthritis. *J Immunol.* 2010;184(12):6882–6890.

Novo JB, Oliveira ML, Magalhães GS, Morganti L, Raw I, Ho PL. Generation of Polyclonal Antibodies Against Recombinant Human Glucocerebrosidase Produced in Escherichia Coli. *Mol Biotechnol.* 2010;46(3):279–286.

Oh MJ, Hua S, Kim BJ, Jeong HN, Jeong SH, Grimm R, Yoo JS, An HJ. Analytical Platform for Glycomic Characterization of Recombinant Erythropoietin Biotherapeutics and Biosimilars by MS. *Bioanalysis* 2013;5(5):545–559.

Pan J, Borchers CH. Top-down Mass Spectrometry and Hydrogen/Deuterium Exchange for Comprehensive Structural Characterization of Interferons: Implications for Biosimilars. *Proteomics* 2014;14(10):1249–1258.

Parnham MJ, Schindler-Horvat J, Kozlović M. Non-clinical Safety Studies on Biosimilar Recombinant Human Erythropoietin. *Basic Clin Pharmacol Toxicol.* 2007;100(2):73–83.

Polevoda B, Sherman F. N-terminal Acetyltransferases and Sequence Requirements for N-terminal Acetylation of Eukaryotic Proteins. *J Mol Biol.* 2003;325(4):595–622.

Schellekens H. When Biotech Proteins go Off-patent. *Trends Biotechnol.* 2004;22(8):406–410.

Skrlin A, Radic I, Vuletic M, Schwinke D, Runac D, Kusalic T, Paskvan I, Krsic M, Bratos M, Marinc S. Comparison of the Physicochemical Properties of a Biosimilar Filgrastim with those of Reference Filgrastim. *Biologicals* 2010;38(5):557–566.

Sörgel F, Lerch H, Lauber T. Physicochemical and Biologic Comparability of a Biosimilar Granulocyte Colony-stimulating Factor with its Reference Product. *BioDrugs* 2010;24(6):347–357.

Su J, Mazzeo J, Subbarao N, Jin T. Pharmaceutical Development of Biologics: Fundamentals, Challenges and Recent Advances. *Ther Deliv.* 2011;2(7):865–871.

Tan Q, Guo Q, Fang C, Wang C, Li B, Wang H, Li J, Guo Y. Characterization and Comparison of Commercially Available TNF Receptor 2-Fc Fusion Protein Products. *MAbs* 2012;4(6):761–774.

Thelwell C. Biological Standards for Potency Assignment to Fibrinolytic Agents used in Thrombolytic Therapy. *Semin Thromb Hemost.* 2014;40(2):205–213.

Toyama A, Nakagawa H, Matsuda K, Sato TA, Nakamura Y, Ueda K. Quantitative Structural Characterization of Local N-glycan Microheterogeneity in Therapeutic Antibodies by Energy-resolved Oxonium ion Monitoring. *Anal Chem.* 2012;84(22):9655–9662.

Visser J, Feuerstein I, Stangler T, Schmiederer T, Fritsch C, Schiestl M. Physicochemical and Functional Comparability Between the Proposed Biosimilar Rituximab GP2013 and Originator Rituximab. *BioDrugs* 2013;27(5):495–507.

Walsh G. *Post-translational Modification of Protein Biopharmaceuticals.* Wiley-Blackwell, 2009.

Wilson, VG (Ed.). *Sumoylation: Molecular Biology and Biochemistry.* Horizon Bioscience, 2004.

Whiteheart SW, Shenbagamurthi P, Chen L et al. Murine Elongation Factor 1 alpha (EF-1 alpha) is Posttranslationally Modified by Novel Amide-linked Ethanolamine-phosphoglycerol Moieties. Addition of Ethanolamine-phosphoglycerol to Specific Glutamic Acid Residues on EF-1 alpha." *J Biol Chem.* 1989;264(24):14334–14341.

Xie H, Chakraborty A, Ahn J, Yu YQ, Dakshinamoorthy DP, Gilar M, Chen W, Skilton SJ, Mazzeo JR. Rapid Comparison of a Candidate Biosimilar to an Innovator Monoclonal Antibody with Advanced Liquid Chromatography and Mass Spectrometry Technologies. *MAbs* 2010;2(4):379–394.

Yang XJ, Seto E. Lysine Acetylation: Codified Crosstalk with other Posttranslational Modifications. *Mol Cell* 2008;31(4):449–446.

RECOMMENDED READING

Ashrafi, H. et al. (2013). "Nanostructure L-asparaginase-fatty acid bioconjugate: Synthesis, preformulation study and biological assessment." *Int J Biol Macromol* 62:180–187.

The present study aims to develop a novel L-asparaginase fatty acid bioconjugates and characterize their applicability for intravenous delivery of L-asparaginase. These bioconjugates were achieved by covalent linkage of fatty acids having different chain lengths (C12, C16 and C22) to the native enzyme. To determine the optimum conditions of bioconjugation, the effect of lipid:protein ratios, reaction time and medium composition on enzyme activity and conjugation degree were evaluated. The native and bioconjugates have been characterized by activity, conjugation degree, particle size, and zeta potential. The results showed that bioconjugated L-asparaginase were more resistant to proteolysis, more stable at different pH, and had prolonged plasma half-life, compared to the native form. From partition coefficient study, the modified enzymes showed approximately 15-fold increase in hydrophobicity. Secondary structure analysis using circular dichroism revealed alteration after lipid conjugation. In addition, the Michaelis constant of the native enzyme was 3.38 mM, while the bioconjugates showed the higher affinity to the substrate L-asparagine. These findings indicate that new lipid bioconjugation could be a very useful strategy for intravenous delivery of L-asparaginase.

Beg, S. et al. (2015). "QbD-based systematic development of novel optimized solid self-nanoemulsifying drug delivery systems (SNEDDS) of lovastatin with enhanced biopharmaceutical performance." *Drug Deliv* 22(6):765–784.

Of late, solid self-nanoemulsifying drug delivery systems (S-SNEDDS) have been extensively sought-after owing to their superior portability, drug loading, stability and patient compliance. The current studies, therefore, entail systematic development, optimization and evaluation (in vitro, in situ and in vivo) of the solid formulations of (SNEDDS) lovastatin employing rational quality by design (QbD)-based approach of formulation by design (FbD). The patient-centric quality target product profile (QTPP) and critical quality attributes (CQAs) were earmarked. Preformulation studies along with initial risk assessment facilitated the selection of lipid (i.e. Capmul MCM), surfactant (i.e. Nikkol HCO-50) and co-surfactant (i.e. Lutrol F127) as CMAs for formulation of S-SNEDDS. A face-centered cubic design (FCCD) was employed for optimization using Nikkol-HCO50 (X1) and Lutrol-F127 (X2), evaluating CQAs like globule size, liquefaction time, emulsification time, MDT, dissolution efficiency and permeation parameter. The design space was generated using apt mathematical models, and the optimum formulation was located, followed by validation of the FbD methodology. In situ SPIP and in vivo pharmacodynamic studies on the optimized formulation carried out in unisex Wistar rats, corroborated superior drug absorption and enhanced pharmacodynamic potential in regulating serum lipid levels. In a nutshell, the present studies report successful QbD-oriented development of novel oral S-SNEDDS of lovastatin with distinctly improved biopharmaceutical performance.

Beg, S. et al. (2015). "Positively charged self-nanoemulsifying oily formulations of olmesartan medoxomil: Systematic development, in vitro, ex vivo and in vivo evaluation." *Int J Pharm* 493(1–2):466–482.

The current research work explores the potential applications of cationic self-nanoemulsifying oily formulations (CSNEOFs) for enhancing the oral bioavailability of olmesartan medoxomil. Initial preformulation studies, risk assessment and factor screening studies revealed selection of oleic acid, Tween 40 and Transcutol HP as the critical factors. Systematic optimization of SNEOFs was carried out employing D-optimal mixture design and evaluating them for responses viz. emulsification efficiency, globule size and in vitro drug release. The CSNEOFs were prepared from the optimized SNEOFs by adding oleylamine as cationic charge inducer. In vitro cell line studies revealed markedly better drug uptake along with safer and biocompatible nature of CSNEOFs than free drug suspension. In situ perfusion, and in vivo pharmacokinetic and pharmacodynamic studies in Wistar rats revealed significant improvement in the biopharmaceutical performance of the drug from CSNEOFs and SNEOFs vis-à-vis the marketed formulation. Successful establishment of various levels of in vitro/in vivo correlations (IVIVC) substantiated high degree of prognostic ability of in vitro dissolution conditions in predicting the in vivo performance. In a nutshell, the present studies report successful development of CSNEOFs of olmesartan medoxomil with distinctly improved biopharmaceutical performance.

Bergstrom, C. A. et al. (2014). "Early pharmaceutical profiling to predict oral drug absorption: Current status and unmet needs." *Eur J Pharm Sci* 57:173–199.

Preformulation measurements are used to estimate the fraction absorbed in vivo for orally administered compounds and thereby allow an early evaluation of the need for enabling formulations. As part of the Oral Biopharmaceutical Tools (OrBiTo) project, this review provides a summary of the pharmaceutical profiling methods available, with focus on in silico and in vitro models typically used to forecast active pharmaceutical ingredient's (APIs) in vivo performance after oral administration. An overview of the composition of human, animal and simulated gastrointestinal (GI) fluids is provided and state-of-the art methodologies to study API properties impacting on oral absorption are reviewed. Assays performed during early development, i.e. physicochemical characterization, dissolution profiles under physiological conditions, permeability assays and the impact of excipients on these properties are discussed in detail and future demands on pharmaceutical profiling are identified. It is expected that innovative computational and experimental methods that better describe molecular processes involved in vivo during dissolution and absorption of APIs will be developed in the OrBiTo. These methods will provide early insights into successful pathways (medicinal chemistry or formulation strategy) and are anticipated to increase the number of new APIs with good oral absorption being discovered.

Boakye, C. H. et al. (2016). "Lipid-based oral delivery systems for skin deposition of a potential chemopreventive DIM derivative: Characterization and evaluation." *Drug Deliv Transl Res* 6(5):526–539.

The objective of this study was to explore the oral route as a viable potential for the skin deposition of a novel diindolylmethane derivative (DIM-D) for chemoprevention activity. Various lipid-based oral delivery systems were optimized and compared for enhancing DIM-D's oral bioavailability and skin deposition. Preformulation studies were performed to evaluate the log P and solubility of DIM-D. Microsomal metabolism, P-glycoprotein efflux, and caco-2 monolayer permeability of DIM-D were determined. Comparative evaluation of the oral absorption and skin deposition of DIM-D-loaded various lipid-based formulations was performed in rats. DIM-D showed pH-dependent solubility and a high log P value. It was not a strong substrate of microsomal degradation and P-glycoprotein. SMEDDs comprised of medium chain triglycerides, monoglycerides, and kolliphor-HS15 (36.70 ± 0.42 nm). SNEDDs comprised of long chain triglycerides, cremophor RH40, labrasol, and TPGS (84.00 ± 14.14 nm). Nanostructured lipid carriers (NLC) consisted of compritol, miglyol, and surfactants (116.50 ± 2.12 nm). The blank formulations all showed >70% cell viability in caco-2 cells. Differential Scanning Calorimetry confirmed the amorphization of DIM-D within the lipid matrices while Atomic Force Microscopy showed particle size distribution similar to the dynamic light scattering data. DIM-D also showed reduced permeation across caco-2 monolayer that was enhanced ($p < 0.05$) by SNEDDs in comparison to SMEDDs and NLC. Fabsolute for DIM-D SNEDDs, SMEDDs, and NLC was 0.14, 0.04, and 0.007, respectively. SNEDDs caused 53.90, 11.32, and 15.08-fold more skin deposition of DIM-D than the free drug, SMEDDs, and NLC, respectively, at 2 hours following oral administration and shows a viable potential for use in skin cancer chemoprevention. Graphical Abstract.

Bredael, G. M. et al. (2014). "In vitro-in vivo correlation strategy applied to an immediate-release solid oral dosage form with a biopharmaceutical classification system IV compound case study." *J Pharm Sci* 103(7):2125–2130.

The ability to predict in vivo response of an oral dosage form based on an in vitro technique has been a sought-after goal of the pharmaceutical scientist. Dissolution testing that demonstrates discrimination to various critical formulations or process attributes provides a sensitive quality check that may be representative or may be overpredictive of potential in vivo changes. Dissolution methodology with an established in vitro-in vivo relationship or correlation may provide the desired in vivo predictability. To establish this in vitro-in vivo link, a clinical study must be performed. In this article, recommendations are given in the selection of batches for the clinical study followed by potential outcome scenarios. The investigation of a Level C in vitro-in vivo correlation (IVIVC), which is the most common correlation for immediate-release oral dosage forms, is presented. Lastly, an IVIVC case study involving a biopharmaceutical classification system class IV compound is presented encompassing this strategy and techniques.

Budai-Szu Cs, M. et al. (2016). "In vitro testing of thiolated poly(aspartic acid) from ophthalmic formulation aspects." *Drug Dev Ind Pharm* 42(8):1241–1246.

Ocular drug delivery formulations must meet anatomical, biopharmaceutical, patient-driven and regulatory requirements. Mucoadhesive polymers can serve as a better alternative to currently available ophthalmic formulations by providing improved bioavailability. If all requirements are addressed, a polymeric formulation resembling the tear film of the eye might be the best solution. The optimum formulation must not have high osmotic activity, should provide appropriate surface tension, pH and refractive index, must be non-toxic and should be transparent and mucoadhesive. We would like to highlight the importance of in vitro polymer testing from a pharmaceutical aspect. We, therefore, carried out physical-chemical investigations to verify the suitability of certain systems for ophthalmic formulations. In this work, in situ gelling, mucoadhesive thiolated poly(aspartic acid)s were tested from ophthalmic formulation aspects. The results of preformulation measurements indicate that these polymers can be used as potential carriers in ophthalmic drug delivery.

de Kanter, R. et al. (2016). "Physiologically-based pharmacokinetic modeling of macitentan: Prediction of drug-drug interactions." *Clin Pharmacokinet* 55(3):369–380.

INTRODUCTION: Macitentan is a novel dual endothelin receptor antagonist for the treatment of pulmonary arterial hypertension (PAH). It is metabolized by cytochrome P450 (CYP) enzymes, mainly CYP3A4, to its active metabolite ACT-132577. METHODS: A physiological-based pharmacokinetic (PBPK) model was developed by combining observations from clinical studies and physicochemical parameters as well as absorption, distribution, metabolism and excretion parameters determined in vitro. RESULTS: The model predicted the observed pharmacokinetics of macitentan and its active metabolite ACT-132577 after single and multiple dosing. It performed well in recovering the observed effect of the CYP3A4 inhibitors ketoconazole and cyclosporine, and the CYP3A4 inducer rifampicin, as well as in predicting interactions with S-warfarin and sildenafil. The model was robust enough to allow prospective predictions of macitentan-drug combinations not studied, including an alternative dosing regimen of ketoconazole and nine other CYP3A4-interacting drugs. Among these were the HIV drugs ritonavir and saquinavir, which were included because HIV infection is a known risk factor for the development of PAH. CONCLUSION: This example of the application of PBPK modeling to predict drug-drug interactions was used to support the labeling of macitentan (Opsumit).

De Paula, W. X. et al. (2018). "A long-lasting oral preformulation of the angiotensin II AT1 receptor antagonist losartan." *Drug Dev Ind Pharm* 44(9):1498–1505.

Losartan (Los), a non-peptidic orally active agent, reduces arterial pressure through specific and selective blockade of angiotensin II receptor AT1. However, this widely used AT1 antagonist presents low bioavailability and needs once or twice a day dosage. In order to improve its bioavailability, we used the host: guest strategy based on beta-cyclodextrin (betaCD). The results suggest that Los included in betaCD showed a typical pulsatile release pattern after oral administration to rats, with increasing the levels of plasma of Los. In addition, the inclusion compound presented oral efficacy for 72 hours, in contrast to Los alone, which shows antagonist effect for only 6 hours. In transgenic (mREN2)L27 rats, the Los/betaCD complex reduced blood pressure for about 6 d, whereas Los alone reduced blood pressure for only 2 d. More importantly, using this host: guest strategy, sustained release of Los for over a week via the oral route can be achieved without the need for encapsulation in a polymeric carrier. The proposed preformulation increased the efficacy reducing the dose or spacing between each dose intake.

Dorati, R. et al. (2018). "Development of a topical 48-H release formulation as an anti-scarring treatment for deep partial-thickness burns." *AAPS Pharm Sci Tech* 19(5):2264–2275.

The purpose of this study was to develop pirfenidone (PF) ointment formulations for a dose finding study in the prophylactic treatment of deep partial-thickness burns in a mouse model. A preformulation study was performed to evaluate the solubility of PF in buffers and different solvents and its stability. Three different formulations containing 1, 3.5, and 6.5% w/w PF were prepared and optimized for their composition for testing in mice. Optimized formulations showed promising in vitro release profiles, in which 20%–45% of PF was released in the first 7 hours and 70%–90% released within 48 hours. The rheological properties of the ointment remained stable throughout storage at 25°C ± 2°C/60% RH. Animal studies showed treatments of burn wounds during the inflammatory stage of wound healing with PF ointments at different drug concentrations had no adverse effects on reepithelization. Moreover, 6.5% PF ointment (F3) reduced the expression of pro-inflammatory cytokines IL-12p70 and TNFalpha. This study suggests that hydrocarbon base ointment could be a promising dosage form for topical delivery of PF in treatment of deep partial-thickness burns.

Fan, Y. et al. (2015). "Preformulation characterization and in vivo absorption in beagle dogs of JFD, a novel anti-obesity drug for oral delivery." *Drug Dev Ind Pharm* 41(5):801–811.

JFD (*N*-isoleucyl-4-methyl-1,1-cyclopropyl-1-(4-chlorine)phenyl-2-amylamine. HCl) is a novel investigational anti-obesity drug without obvious cardiotoxicity. The objective of this study was to characterize the key physicochemical properties of JFD, including solution-state characterization (ionization constant, partition coefficient, aqueous and pH-solubility profile), solid-state characterization (particle size, thermal analysis, crystallinity and hygroscopicity) and drug-excipient chemical compatibility. A supporting in vivo absorption study was also carried out in beagle dogs. JFD bulk powders are prismatic crystals with a low degree of crystallinity, particle sizes of which are within 2–10 μm. JFD is highly hygroscopic, easily deliquesces to an amorphous glass solid and changes subsequently to another crystal form under an elevated moisture/temperature condition. Similar physical instability was also observed in real-time CheqSol solubility assay. pK(a) (7.49 ± 0.01), log P (5.10 ± 0.02) and intrinsic solubility (S0) (1.75 μg/mL) at 37°C of JFD were obtained using potentiometric titration method. Based on these solution-state properties, JFD was estimated to be classified as BCS II, thus its dissolution rate may be an absorption-limiting step. Moreover, JFD was more chemically compatible with dibasic calcium phosphate, mannitol, hypromellose and colloidal silicon dioxide than with lactose and magnesium stearate. Further, JFD exhibited an acceptable pharmacokinetic profiling in beagle dogs and the pharmacokinetic parameters T(max), C(max), AUC(0-t) and absolute bioavailability were 1.60 ± 0.81 hours, 0.78 ± 0.47 μg/mL, 3.77 ± 1.85 μg.h/mL and 52.30% ± 19.39%, respectively. The preformulation characterization provides valuable information for further development of oral administration of JFD.

Fujimori, M. et al. (2016). "Low hygroscopic spray-dried powders with trans-glycosylated food additives enhance the solubility and oral bioavailability of ipriflavone." *Food Chem* 190:1050–1055.

The improvement in the solubility and dissolution rate may promote a superior absorption property towards the human body. The spray-dried powders (SDPs) of ipriflavone, which was used as a model hydrophobic flavone, with trans-glycosylated rutin (Rutin-G) showed the highest solubilizing effect of ipriflavone among three types of trans-glycosylated food additives. The SDPs of ipriflavone with Rutin-G have both a significant higher dissolution rate and solubility enhancement of ipriflavone. This spray-dried formulation of ipriflavone with Rutin-G exhibited a low hygroscopicity as a critical factor in product preservation. In addition, an improvement in the oral absorption of ipriflavone was achieved by means of preparing composite particles of ipriflavone/Rutin-G via spray drying, indicating a 4.3-fold increase in the area under the plasma concentration-time curve compared with that of untreated ipriflavone. These phenomena could be applicable to food ingredients involving hydrophobic flavones for producing healthy food with a high quality.

Gajdziok, J. and B. Vranikova (2015). "Enhancing of drug bioavailability using liquisolid system formulation." *Ceska Slov Farm* 64(3):55–66.

One of the modern technologies of how to ensure sufficient bioavailability of drugs with limited water solubility is represented by the preparation of liquisolid systems. The functional principle of these formulations is the sorption of a drug in a liquid phase to a porous carrier (aluminometasilicates, microcrystalline cellulose, etc.). After addition of further excipients, in particular a coating material (colloidal silica), a powder is formed with the properties suitable for conversion to conventional solid unit dosage forms for oral administration (tablets, capsules). The drug is subsequently administered to the GIT already in a dissolved state, and moreover, the high surface area of the excipients and their surface hydrophilization by the solvent used, facilitates its contact with and release to the dissolution medium and GI fluids. This technology, due to its ease of preparation, represents an interesting alternative to the currently used methods of bioavailability improvement. The article follows up, by describing the specific aspects influencing the preparation of liquid systems, on the already published papers about the bioavailability of drugs and the possibilities of its technological improvement. Key words: liquisolid systems bioavailability porous carrier coating material preformulation studies.

Gualdesi, M. S. et al. (2014). "Preformulation studies of novel 5'-O-carbonates of lamivudine with biological activity: solubility and stability assays." *Drug Dev Ind Pharm* 40(9):1246–1252.

As a part of preformulation studies, the aim of this work was to examine the solubility and stability of a series of 5′-*O*-carbonates of lamivudine with proven antihuman immunodeficiency virus activity. Solubility studies were carried out using pure solvents (water, ethanol and polyethylene glycol 400 [PEG 400]), as well as cosolvents in binary mixture systems (water-ethanol and water-PEG 400). These ionizable compounds showed that their aqueous solubility is decreasing as the carbon length of the substituent moiety increases but being enhanced as the pH was reduced from 7.4 to 1.2. Thus, 3TC-Metha an active compound of the series, with an intrinsic solubility at 25°C of 17 mg/mL, was about 70 times more soluble than 3TC-Octa (0.24 mg/mL), and at pHs of 1.2, 5.8 and 7.4 had intrinsic solubilities of 36.48, 19.20 and 15.40 mg/mL, respectively. In addition, the solubility was enhanced significantly by using ethanol and PEG 400 as cosolvents. A stability study was conducted in buffer solutions at pH 1.2, 5.8, 7.4 and 13.0 and in human plasma at 37°C. Stability-indicating high-performance liquid chromatography procedure was found to be selective, sensitive and accurate for these compounds and good recovery, linearity and precision were also observed.

Ibrahim, K. A. et al. (2017). "Formulation, evaluation and release rate characteristics of medicated jelly of vitamin C." *Pak J Pharm Sci* 30(2(Suppl.)):579–583.

Medicated jelly formulations are patient friendly dosage form for pediatric, geriatric and dysphagic patients. These formulations offer rapid dissolution and absorption of drugs through oral mucosa therefore show the early onset of action. The objective of the study was to develop and evaluate oral jelly formulations of vitamin C. Slurry method was adopted using glucose 103 gm, sugar 67 gm, gelatin 10 gm and sorbitol 6.56 gm. Preformulation studies were performed including the organoleptic profile, pH, and solubility of both drugs. The medicated jelly of Vitamin C was prepared and evaluated for physical characteristics, weight variation, syneresis, pH, taste and palatability, drug content, release rate characteristics and stability studies. All the jellies were found to have patient welcoming taste and were palatable. All formulations showed more than 50% drug release within 15 minutes, while 93% drug was released in 30 minutes. The results of release kinetics showed that the formulation followed the zero-order release kinetics. Thus, the drug was released at constant rate independent of the drug concentration involved in the process. All the medicated jellies were found to remain stable stored for 60 days at different temperatures. The present study revealed that medicated jellies of vitamin C could be employed orally in an effective form as an alternative solid oral dosage form for special population such as pediatrics, geriatrics and patients with dysphagia.

Kendall, R. et al. (2017). "Using the slug mucosal irritation assay to investigate the tolerability of tablet excipients on human skin in the context of the use of a nipple shield delivery system." *Pharm Res* 34(4):687–695.

PURPOSE: Neonates are particularly challenging to treat. A novel patented drug delivery device containing a rapidly disintegrating tablet held within a modified nipple shield (NSDS) was designed to deliver medication to infants during breastfeeding. However, concerns exist around dermatological nipple tolerability with no pharmaceutical safety assessment guidance to study local tissue tolerance of the nipple and the areola. This is the first Slug Mucosal Irritation (SMI) study to evaluate irritancy potential of GRAS excipients commonly used to manufacture rapidly disintegrating immediate release solid oral dosage form METHODS: Zinc sulphate selected as the antidiarrheal model drug that reduces infant mortality, was blended with functional excipients at traditional levels [microcrystalline cellulose, sodium starch glycolate, croscarmellose sodium, magnesium stearate]. Slugs were exposed to blends slurried in human breast milk to assess their stinging, itching or burning potential, using objective values such as mucus production to categorize irritation potency RESULTS: Presently an in vivo assay, previously validated for prediction of ocular and nasal irritation, was used as an alternative to vertebrate models to anticipate the potential maternal dermatological tolerability issues to NSDS tablet components. The excipients did not elicit irritancy. However, mild irritancy was observed when zinc sulphate was present in blends. CONCLUSION: These promising good tolerability results support the continued investigation of these excipients within NSDS rapidly disintegrating tablet formulations. Topical local tolerance effects being almost entirely limited to irritation, the slug assay potentially adds to the existing preformulation toolbox and may sit in between the in vitro and existing in vivo assays.

Kramer, R. M. et al. (2013). "Development of a stable virus-like particle vaccine formulation against Chikungunya virus and investigation of the effects of polyanions." *J Pharm Sci* 102(12):4305–4314.

Chikungunya virus (CHIKV) is an alphavirus that infects millions of people every year, especially in the developing world. The selective expression of recombinant

CHIKV capsid and envelope proteins results in the formation of self-assembled virus-like particles (VLPs) that have been shown to protect nonhuman primates against infection from multiple strains of CHIKV. This study describes the characterization, excipient screening, and optimization of CHIKV VLP solution conditions toward the development of a stable parenteral formulation. The CHIKV VLPs were found to be poorly soluble at pH 6 and below. Circular dichroism, intrinsic fluorescence, and static and dynamic light scattering measurements were therefore performed at neutral pH, and results consistent with the formation of molten globule structures were observed at elevated temperatures. A library of generally recognized as safe excipients was screened for their ability to physically stabilize CHIKV VLPs using a high-throughput turbidity-based assay. Sugars, sugar alcohols, and polyanions were identified as potential stabilizers and the concentrations and combinations of select excipients were optimized. The effects of polyanions were further studied, and while all polyanions tested stabilized CHIKV VLPs against aggregation, the effects of polyanions on conformational stability varied.

Kumar, V. et al. (2016). "A chromatography-free isolation of rohitukine from leaves of dysoxylum binectariferum: Evaluation for in vitro cytotoxicity, Cdk inhibition and physicochemical properties." *Bioorg Med Chem Lett* 26(15):3457–3463.

Rohitukine is a chromone alkaloid isolated from an Indian medicinal plant Dysoxylum binectariferum. This natural product has led to the discovery of two clinical candidates (flavopiridol and P276-00) for the treatment of cancer. Herein, for the first time we report an efficient protocol for isolation and purification of this precious natural product in a bulk-quantity from leaves (a renewable source) of D. binectariferum (>98% purity) without use of chromatography or any acid-base treatment. Despite of the fact that this scaffold has reached up to clinical stage, particularly for leukemia; however, the antileukemic activity of a parent natural product has never been investigated. Furthermore, rohitukine has never been studied for cyclin-dependent kinase (Cdk) inhibition, kinase profiling and for its experimental physicochemical properties. Thus, herein, we report in vitro cytotoxicity of rohitukine in a panel of 20 cancer cell lines (including leukemia, pancreatic, prostate, breast and CNS) and 2 normal cell lines; kinase profiling, Cdk2/9 inhibition, and physicochemical properties (solubility and stability in biological medias, pKa, LogP, LogD). In cytotoxicity screening, rohitukine displayed promising activity in HL-60 and Molt-4 (leukemia) cell lines with GI50 of 10 and 12 µM, respectively. It showed inhibition of Cdk2/A and Cdk9/T1 with IC50 values of 7.3 and 0.3 µM, respectively. The key interactions of rohitukine with Cdk9 was also studied by molecular modeling. Rohitukine was found to be highly water soluble (Swater = 10.3 mg/mL) and its LogP value was −0.55. The ionization constant of rohitukine was found to be 5.83. Rohitukine was stable in various biological media's including rat plasma. The data presented herein will help in designing better anticancer agents in future.

Kyadarkunte, A. Y. et al. (2015). "Cellular interactions and photoprotective effects of idebenone-loaded nanostructured lipid carriers stabilized using PEG-free surfactant." *Int J Pharm* 479(1):77–87.

In past years, nanostructured lipid carriers (NLCs) have emerged as novel topical antioxidant delivery systems because of combined positive features of liposomes and polymeric nanoparticles. Here, we seek to unlock the possibility of idebenone (IDB;

an antioxidant)-loaded NLCs (IDB-NLCs) cellular interactions such as, viability and uptake, and its photoprotective effects against Ultraviolet-B (UVB)-mediated oxidative stress in immortal human keratinocyte cell line (HaCaT). The two-step preformulation strategy followed by three-level, three-variable, L9 (3(3)) Taguchi robust orthogonal design employed was important in improving IDB-NLCs key physicochemical aspects such as, entrapment efficiency, drug release (sustained), occlusion, skin deposition and physical stability. UV crosslinker, confocal microscopy and flow cytometry techniques were used to (1) mediate oxidative stress in HaCaT cells, (2) study a qualitative cellular uptake, (3) measure intracellular reactive oxygen species (ROS), and mitochondrial membrane potential, respectively. NLCs markedly improved biocompatibility of IDB under normal as well as stress conditions. Quantitative and qualitative cell uptake studies demonstrated a significant uptake of IDB-NLCs (3-fold increase) and nile red-labeled IDB-NLCs (NR-IDB-NLCs) at 2 hours, respectively, hence exerted improved photoprotective effects.

Lee, R. W. and M. Mitchnick (2017). "Early-stage formulation considerations." *Curr Protoc Chem Biol* 9(4):306–314.

When a drug candidate – i.e., a new chemical entity (NCE) or new molecular entity (NME) – is discovered, there is a requirement to identify a vehicle for in vitro and/or in vivo evaluation to assess the activity and/or toxicity of the compound (here we refer to the biologically active compound as the active pharmaceutical ingredient: API). Ideally, this vehicle will not impart any biological activity or any toxicity that would mask or confound the effects of the API. At this early stage in development and given the high attrition rates of drug candidates in discovery, it does not make sense to fully characterize the API-speed and cost are generally the driving factors. This chapter provides guidance for the development of early-stage test articles (i.e., drug products containing APIs intended to be used for the in vitro and/or in vivo evaluation) and not necessarily formulations that are intended to progress into clinical evaluation© 2017 by John Wiley & Sons, Inc.

Leung, D. H. et al. (2017). "Development of a convenient in vitro gel diffusion model for predicting the in vivo performance of subcutaneous parenteral formulations of large and small molecules." *AAPS Pharm Sci Tech* 18(6):2203–2213.

Parenteral delivery remains a compelling drug delivery route for both large- and small-molecule drugs and can bypass issues encountered with oral absorption. For injectable drug products, there is a strong patient preference for subcutaneous administration due to its convenience over intravenous infusion. However, in subcutaneous injection, in contrast to intravenous administration, the formulation is in contact with an extracellular matrix environment that behaves more like a gel than a fluid. This can impact the expected performance of a formulation. Since typical bulk fluid dissolution studies do not accurately simulate the subcutaneous environment, improved in vitro models to help better predict the behavior of the formulation are critical. Herein, we detail the development of a new model system consisting of a more physiologically relevant gel phase to simulate the rate of drug release and diffusion from a subcutaneous injection site using agarose hydrogels as a tissue mimic. This is coupled with continuous real-time data collection to accurately monitor drug diffusion. We show how this in vitro model can be used as an in vivo performance differentiator for different formulations of both large and small molecules. Thus, this model system can be used to improve optimization and understanding of new parenteral drug formulations in a rapid and convenient manner.

Liang, S. et al. (2016). "Solution formulation development and efficacy of MJC13 in a preclinical model of castration-resistant prostate cancer." *Pharm Dev Technol* 21(1):121–126.

MJC13, a novel FKBP52 targeting agent, has potential use for the treatment of castration-resistant prostate cancer. The purpose of this work was to develop a solution formulation of MJC13 and obtain its efficacy profile in a human prostate cancer xenograft mouse model. Preformulation studies were conducted to evaluate the physicochemical properties. Co-solvent systems were evaluated for aqueous solubility and tolerance. A human prostate cancer xenograft mouse model was established by growing 22Rv1 prostate cancer cells in C.B-17 SCID mice. The optimal formulation was used to study the efficacy of MJC13 in this preclinical model of castrate-resistant prostate cancer. We found that MJC13 was stable (at least for 1 month), highly lipophilic (logP = 6.49), poorly soluble in water (0.28 microg/mL), and highly plasma protein bound (>98%). The optimal formulation consisting of PEG 400 and Tween 80 (1:1, v/v) allowed us to achieve a MJC13 concentration of 7.5 mg/mL and tolerated an aqueous environment. After twice weekly intratumoral injection with 10 mg/kg MJC13 in this formulation for four consecutive weeks, tumor volumes were significantly reduced compared to vehicle-treated controls.

Madsen, C. M. et al. (2018). "Effect of composition of simulated intestinal media on the solubility of poorly soluble compounds investigated by design of experiments." *Eur J Pharm Sci* 111:311–319.

The composition of the human intestinal fluids varies both intra- and inter-individually. This will influence the solubility of orally administered drug compounds, and hence, the absorption and efficacy of compounds displaying solubility limited absorption. The purpose of this study was to assess the influence of simulated intestinal fluid (SIF) composition on the solubility of poorly soluble compounds. Using a Design of Experiments (DoE) approach, a set of 24 SIF was defined within the known compositions of human fasted state intestinal fluid. The SIF were composed of phospholipid, bile salt, and different pH, buffer capacities and osmolarities. On a small-scale semi-robotic system, the solubility of 6 compounds (aprepitant, carvedilol, felodipine, fenofibrate, probucol, and zafirlukast) was determined in the 24 SIF. Compound specific models, describing key factors influencing the solubility of each compound, were identified. Although all models were different, the level of phospholipid and bile salt, the pH, and the interactions between these, had the biggest influences on solubility overall. Thus, a reduction of the DoE from five to three factors was possible (11–13 media), making DoE solubility studies feasible compared to single SIF solubility studies. Applying this DoE approach will lead to a better understanding of the impact of intestinal fluid composition on the solubility of a given drug compound.

Manda, S. et al. (2016). "Discovery of a marine-derived bis-indole alkaloid fascaplysin, as a new class of potent P-glycoprotein inducer and establishment of its structure-activity relationship." *Eur J Med Chem* 107:1–11.

The screening of IIIM natural products repository for P-gp modulatory activity in P-gp over-expressing human adenocarcinoma LS-180 cells led to the identification of

7 natural products viz. withaferin, podophyllotoxin, 3-demethylcolchicine, agnuside, reserpine, seseberecine and fascaplysin as P-gp inducers. Fascaplysin (6a), a marine-derived bis-indole alkaloid, was the most potent among all of them, showing induction of P-gp with EC50 value of 25 nM. P-gp induction is one of the recently targeted strategy to increase amyloid-beta clearance from Alzheimer brains. Thus, we pursued a medicinal chemistry of fascaplysin to establish its structure-activity relationship for P-gp induction activity. Four series of analogs viz. substituted quaternary fascaplysin analogs, D-ring opened quaternary analogs, D-ring opened non-quaternary analogs, and beta-carbolinium analogs were synthesized and screened for P-gp induction activity. Among the total of 48 analogs screened, only quaternary nitrogen containing analogs 6a-g and 10a, 10h-l displayed promising P-gp induction activity; whereas non-planar non-quaternary analogs 9a-m, 13a-n, 15a-h were devoid of this activity. The P-gp induction activity of best compounds was then confirmed by western-blot analysis, which indicated that fascaplysin (6a) along with 4,5-difluoro analog of fascaplysin 6f and D-ring opened analog 10j displayed 4–8 fold increase in P-gp expression in LS-180 cells at 1 μM. Additionally, compounds 6a and 6f also showed inhibition of acetylcholinesterase (AChE), an enzyme responsible for neuronal loss in Alzheimer's disease. Thus, fascaplysin and its analogs showing promising P-gp induction along with AChE inhibition at 1 μM, with good safety window (LS-180: IC50 > 10 μM, hGF: 4 μM), clearly indicates their promise for development as an anti-Alzheimer agent.

Mann, A. K. P. et al. (2018). "Producing amorphous solid dispersions via co-precipitation and spray drying: Impact to physicochemical and biopharmaceutical properties." *J Pharm Sci* 107(1):183–191.

Many small-molecule active pharmaceutical ingredients (APIs) exhibit low aqueous solubility and benefit from generation of amorphous dispersions of the API and polymer to improve their dissolution properties. Spray drying and hot-melt extrusion are 2 common methods to produce these dispersions; however, for some systems, these approaches may not be optimal, and it would be beneficial to have an alternative route. Herein, amorphous solid dispersions of compound A, a low-solubility weak acid, and copovidone were made by conventional spray drying and co-precipitation. The physicochemical properties of the 2 materials were assessed via X-ray diffraction, differential scanning calorimetry, thermal gravimetric analysis, and scanning electron microscopy. The amorphous dispersions were then formulated and tableted, and the performance was assessed in vivo and in vitro. In human dissolution studies, the co-precipitation tablets had slightly slower dissolution than the spray-dried dispersion, but both reached full release of compound A. In canine in vitro dissolution studies, the tablets showed comparable dissolution profiles. Finally, canine pharmacokinetic studies showed that the materials had comparable values for the area under the curve, bioavailability, and Cmax. Based on the summarized data, we conclude that for some APIs, co-precipitation is a viable alternative to spray drying to make solid amorphous dispersions while maintaining desirable physicochemical and biopharmaceutical characteristics.

Miao, Y. et al. (2016). "Characterization and evaluation of self-nanoemulsifying sustained-release pellet formulation of ziprasidone with enhanced bioavailability and no food effect." *Drug Deliv* 23(7):2163–2172.

The purpose of this work was to develop self-nanomulsifying drug delivery systems (SNEDDS) in sustained-release pellets of ziprasidone to enhance the oral bioavailability and overcome the food effect of ziprasidone. Preformulation studies including screening of excipients for solubility and pseudo-ternary phase diagrams suggested the suitability of Capmul MCM as oil phase, Labrasol as surfactant, and PEG 400 as co-surfactant for preparation of self-nanoemulsifying formulations. Preliminary composition of the SNEDDS formulations were selected from the pseudo-ternary phase diagrams. The prepared ziprasidone-SNEDDS formulations were characterized for self-emulsification time, effect of pH and robustness to dilution, droplet size analysis and zeta potential. The optimized ziprasidone-SNEDDS were used to prepare ziprasidone-SNEDDS sustained-release pellets via extrusion-spheronization method. The pellets were characterized for SEM, particle size, droplet size distribution and zeta potential. In vitro drug release studies indicated the ziprsidone-SNEDDS sustained-release pellets showed sustained release profiles with 90% released within 10 hours. The ziprsidone-SNEDDS sustained-release pellets were administered to fasted and fed beagle dogs and their pharmacokinetics were compared to commercial formulation of Zeldox as a control. Pharmacokinetic studies in beagle dogs showed ziprasidone with prolonged actions and enhanced bioavailability with no food effect was achieved simultaneously in ziprsidone-SNEDDS sustained-release pellets compared with Zeldox in fed state. The results indicated a sustained release with prolonged actions of schizophrenia and bipolar disorder treatment.

Migoha, C. O. et al. (2015). "Preformulation studies for generic omeprazole magnesium enteric coated tablets." *Biomed Res Int* 2015:307032.

Preformulation is an important step in the rational formulation of an active pharmaceutical ingredient (API). Micromeritics properties: bulk density (BD) and tapped density (TD), compressibility index (Carr's index), Hauser's ratio (H), and sieve analysis were performed in order to determine the best excipients to be used in the formulation development of omeprazole magnesium enteric coated tablets. Results show that omeprazole magnesium has fair flow and compressibility properties (BD 0.4 g mL, TD 0.485 g/mL, Carr's index 17.5%, Hauser's ratio 1.2, and sieve analysis time 5 minutes). There were no significant drug excipient interactions except change in color in all three conditions in the mixture of omeprazole and aerosil 200. Moisture content loss on drying in all three conditions was not constant and the changes were attributed to surrounding environment during the test time. Changes in the absorption spectra were noted in the mixture of omeprazole and water aerosil only in the visible region of 350–2500 nm. Omeprazole magnesium alone and with all excipients showed no significant changes in omeprazole concentration for a 30 day period. Omeprazole magnesium formulation complies with USP standards with regards to the fineness, flowability, and compressibility of which other excipients can be used in the formulation.

Mitra, A. et al. (2016). "Impact of polymer type on bioperformance and physical stability of hot melt extruded formulations of a poorly water soluble drug." *Int J Pharm* 505(1–2):107–114.

Amorphous solid dispersion formulations have been widely used to enhance bioavailability of poorly soluble drugs. In these formulations, polymer is included to physically stabilize the amorphous drug by dispersing it in the polymeric carrier and thus forming a solid solution. The polymer can also maintain supersaturation and promote speciation during dissolution, thus enabling better absorption as compared to crystalline drug substance. In this paper, we report the use of hot melt extrusion

(HME) to develop amorphous formulations of a poorly soluble compound (FaSSIF solubility = 1 µg/mL). The poor solubility of the compound and high dose (300 mg) necessitated the use of amorphous formulation to achieve adequate bioperformance. The effect of using three different polymers (HPMCAS-HF, HPMCAS-LF and copovidone), on the dissolution, physical stability, and bioperformance of the formulations was demonstrated. In this particular case, HPMCAS-HF containing HME provided the highest bioavailability and also had better physical stability as compared to extrudates using HPMCAS-LF and copovidone. The data demonstrated that the polymer type can have significant impact on the formulation bioperformance and physical stability. Thus, a thorough understanding of the polymer choice is imperative when designing an amorphous solid dispersion formulation, such that the formulation provides robust bioperformance and has adequate shelf life.

Muthurania, K. et al. (2015). "Investigation of the sedimentation behavior of aluminum phosphate: Influence of pH, ionic strength, and model antigens." *J Pharm Sci* 104(11):3770–3781.

Evaluation of the physical characteristics of vaccines formulated in the presence of adjuvants, such as aluminum salts (Alum), is an important step in the development of vaccines. Depending on the formulation conditions and the associated electrostatic interactions of the adjuvant particles, the vaccine suspension may transition between flocculated and deflocculated states. The impact of practical formulation parameters, including pH, ionic strength, and the presence of model antigens, has been correlated to the sedimentation behavior of aluminum phosphate suspensions. A novel approach for the characterization of suspension properties of Alum has been developed to predict the flocculated state of the system using a sedimentation analysis-based tool (Turbiscan(R)). Two sedimentation parameters, the settling onset time (Sonset) and the sedimentation volume ratio (SVR) can be determined simultaneously in a single measurement. The results demonstrate the suspension characteristics to be significantly altered by solution conditions (pH and ionic strength) and the charge state of bound antigens. Formulation conditions that promote the flocculated state of the suspension are characterized by faster Sonset and higher SVR and are generally easy to resuspend. The Turbiscan(R) method described herein is a useful tool for the characterization of aluminum-containing suspensions and may be adapted for screening and optimization of suspension-based vaccine formulations in general.

Newman, A. et al. (2018). "Coamorphous active pharmaceutical ingredient-small molecule mixtures: Considerations in the choice of coformers for enhancing dissolution and oral bioavailability." *J Pharm Sci* 107(1):5–17.

In the recent years, coamorphous systems, containing an active pharmaceutical ingredient (API) and a small molecule coformer have appeared as alternatives to the use of either amorphous solid dispersions containing polymer or cocrystals of API and small molecule coformers, to improve the dissolution and oral bioavailability of poorly soluble crystalline API. This Commentary article considers the relative properties of amorphous solid dispersions and coamorphous systems in terms of methods of preparation; miscibility; glass transition temperature; physical stability; hygroscopicity; and aqueous dissolution. It also considers important questions concerning the fundamental criteria to be used for the proper selection of a small molecule coformer regarding its ability to form either coamorphous or cocrystal systems. Finally, we consider various aspects of product development that are specifically associated with the formulation of commercial coamorphous systems as solid oral dosage forms. These include coformer selection; screening; methods of preparation; preformulation; physical stability; bio-availability; and final formulation. Through such an analysis of coamorphous API-small molecule coformer systems, against the more widely studied API-polymer dispersions and cocrystals, it is believed that the strengths and weaknesses of coa-morphous systems can be better understood, leading to more efficient formulation and manufacture of such systems for enhancing oral bioavailability.

Parikh, A. et al. (2016). "Development of a novel oral delivery system of edaravone for enhancing bioavailability." *Int J Pharm* 515(1–2):490–500.

Edaravone (EDR), a strong free radical scavenger, is known for its promising therapeutic potential in oxidative stress (OS) associated diseases, however poor oral bioavail-ability is the major obstacle in its potential use. Oral liquid dosage form is the most preferred delivery method in pediatric, geriatric and specialized therapies. The present research discusses the development of a Novel Oral Delivery System (NODS) of EDR to enhance oral bioavailability. From preformulation study, solubility, and stability were identified as key challenges and the requirement of an acidic environment and protection against oxidation were found to be critical. The NODS made up of a mixture of Labrasol (LBS) and an acidic aqueous system, was optimized on the basis of solubility and sta-bility study. It can be stored $\leq 40°C$ for at least one month. Drug release from NODS was slow, sustained and significantly better as compared to suspension. The significant reduction in metabolism and improvement in permeability across the small intestine were observed with NODS compared to free EDR. The oral pharmacokinetic study showed 571% relative bioavailability with NODS compared to EDR suspension. From the results obtained, NODS is a promising candidate for use in OS associated diseases.

Park, M. H. et al. (2015). "Preformulation studies of bee venom for the preparation of bee nenom-loaded PLGA particles." *Molecules* 20(8):15072–15083.

It is known that allergic people were potentially vulnerable to bee venom (BV), which can induce an anaphylactic shock, eventually leading to death. Up until recently, this kind of allergy was treated only by venom immunotherapy (VIT) and its efficacy has been recognized worldwide. This treatment is practiced by subcuta-neous injections that gradually increase the doses of the allergen. This is inconve-nient for patients due to frequent injections. Poly(D, L-lactide-co-glycolide) (PLGA) has been broadly studied as a carrier for drug delivery systems (DDS) of proteins and peptides. PLGA particles usually induce a sustained release. In this study, the physi-cochemical properties of BV were examined prior to the preparation of BV-loaded PLGA nanoparticles NPs). The content of melittin, the main component of BV, was 53.3%. When protected from the light, BV was stable at 4°C in distilled water, dur-ing 8 weeks. BV-loaded PLGA particles were prepared using dichloromethane as the most suitable organic solvent and two min of ultrasonic emulsification time. This study has characterized the physicochemical properties of BV for the preparation BV-loaded PLGA NPs in order to design and optimize a suitable sustained release system in the future.

Qi, W. et al. (2014). "Preformulation study of highly purified inactivated polio vaccine, serotype 3." *J Pharm Sci* 103(1):140–151.

To improve the effectiveness of the polio vaccination campaign, improvements in the thermal stability of the vaccine are being investigated. Here, inactivated polio vaccine, serotype 3 (IPV3) was characterized via a number of biophysical techniques. The size was characterized by transmission electronic microscopy and light scattering. The capsid protein conformation was evaluated by intrinsic fluorescence and circular dichroism (CD), and the D-antigen content by enzyme-linked immunosorbent assay (ELISA). The pH thermal stability of IPV3 (pH 3.0–8.0; 10°C–87.5°C) was evaluated by fluorescence, CD, and static light scattering. The transition temperatures reflect the responses, respectively, of tertiary structure, secondary structure, and size to applied thermal stress. The data were summarized as empirical phase diagrams, and the most stable conditions were found to be pH 7.0 with temperature lower than 40°C. CD detected a higher transition temperature for capsid protein than that for RNA. The effects of certain excipients on IPV3 thermal stability and antigen content were evaluated. The results of their effects, based on intrinsic fluorescence and ELISA, were in good agreement, suggesting the feasibility of applying intrinsic fluorescence as a high-throughput tool for formulation development. The study improves the understanding of IPV3 thermal stability and provides a starting point for future formulation development of IPV3 and other serotypes.

Raijada, D. et al. (2014). "Miniaturized approach for excipient selection during the development of oral solid dosage form." *J Pharm Sci* 103(3):900–908.

The present study introduces a miniaturized high-throughput platform to understand the influence of excipients on the performance of oral solid dosage forms during early drug development. Wet massing of binary mixtures of the model drug (sodium naproxen) and representative excipients was followed by sieving, drying, and compaction of the agglomerated material. The mini-compacts were subjected to stability studies at 25°C/5% relative humidity (RH), 25°C/60% RH and 40°C/75% RH for 3 months. The physical stability of the drug was affected by the storage condition and by the characteristics of the excipients, whereas all the samples were chemically stable. Force-distance curves obtained during the compression of agglomerated material were used for the comparison of compressibility of different drug-excipient mixtures. The agglomerated drug-excipient mixtures were also subjected to studies of the dissolution trend under sequential pH conditions to simulate pH environment of gastrointestinal tract. Major factors affecting the dissolution behavior were the diffusion layer pH of the binary mixtures and the ability of the excipients to alter the diffusion layer thickness. The proposed approach can be used for excipient selection and for early-stage performance testing of active pharmaceutical ingredient intended for oral solid dosage form.

Sandhu, P. S. et al. (2015). "Novel dietary lipid-based self-nanoemulsifying drug delivery systems of paclitaxel with p-gp inhibitor: Implications on cytotoxicity and biopharmaceutical performance." *Expert Opin Drug Deliv* 12(11):1809–1822.

OBJECTIVES: This work describes the development and characterization of novel self-nanoemulsifying drug delivery systems (SNEDDS) employing polyunsaturated fatty acids for enhancing the oral bioavailability and anticancer activity of paclitaxel (PTX) by coadministration with curcumin (Cu). METHODS: Preformulation studies endorsed sesame oil, labrasol, and sodium deoxycholate as lipid surfactants and cosurfactants based on their solubility for the drugs and spontaneity of emulsification to produce nanoemulsions. Further, phase titration studies were performed to identify a suitable nanoemulsion region for preparing the SNEDDS formulation. RESULTS: The prepared formulations were characterized through in vitro, in situ, and in vivo studies to evaluate the biopharmaceutical performance. In vitro drug release studies showed 2.8- to 3.4-fold enhancement in the dissolution rate of both drugs from SNEDDS as compared with the pure drug suspension. Cell line studies revealed 1.5- to 2.7-fold reduction in the cytotoxicity on MCF-7 cells by plain PTX-SNEDDS and PTX-Cu-SNEDDS vis-à-vis the PTX-suspension. In situ intestinal perfusion studies revealed significant augmentation in permeability and absorption parameters of drug from PTX-Cu-SNEDDS over the plain PTX-SNEDDS and PTX-suspension ($p < 0.001$). In vivo pharmacokinetic studies also showed a remarkable improvement (i.e., 5.8- to 6.3-fold) in the oral bioavailability (Cmax and AUC) of the drug from PTX-SNEDDS and PTX-Cu-SNEDDS vis-à-vis the PTX-suspension. CONCLUSIONS: Overall, the studies corroborated superior biopharmaceutical performance of PTX-Cu-SNEDDS.

Singh, B. et al. (2014). "Synthesis and anti-proliferative activities of new derivatives of embelin." *Bioorg Med Chem Lett* 24(20):4865–4870.

Embelin (1), a benzoquinone isolated from *Embelia ribes*, is known to possess variety of biological activities. Despite of several promising biological activities, preclinical efforts on embelin were hampered because of its poor aqueous solubility. In order to address the solubility issue, herein, we have synthesized a series of Mannich products of embelin by treating it with various secondary amines. The synthesized compounds were screened for antiproliferative and antimicrobial activities. In cytotoxicity screening, the benzyl-piperidine linked derivative 8m was found to possess better antiproliferative activity compared to parent natural product embelin against a panel of cell lines including HCT-116, MCF-7, MIAPaCa-2 and PC-3 with IC50 values of 30, 41, 34 and 36 μM, respectively. The mechanistic study of compound 8m revealed that it exhibits cytotoxicity via induction of apoptosis and mitochondrial membrane potential loss. Further, the compounds were tested for antimicrobial activity where dimethyl-amino-8a and piperidine linked derivative 8b displayed antibacterial activity against *Staphylococcus* aureus with MIC values of 8 and 16 μg/mL, respectively. Mannich derivatives did now show improved aqueous solubility, however their hydrochloride salts 8a. HCl, 8b. HCl and 8m. HCl showed significantly improved aqueous solubility without affecting biological activities of parent Mannich derivatives.

White, J. A. et al. (2017). "Preformulation studies with the Escherichia coli double mutant heat-labile toxin adjuvant for use in an oral vaccine." *J Immunol Methods* 451:83–89.

Double mutant heat-labile toxin (dmLT) is a promising adjuvant for oral vaccine administration. The aims of our study were to develop sensitive methods to detect low concentrations of dmLT and to use the assays in preformulation studies to determine whether dmLT remains stable under conditions encountered by an oral vaccine. We developed a sandwich ELISA specific for intact dmLT and a sensitive SDS-PAGE densitometry method, and tested stability of dmLT in glass and plastic containers, in saliva, at the pH of stomach fluid, and in high-osmolarity buffers. The developed ELISA has a quantification range of 62.5 to 0.9 ng/mL and lower limit of detection of 0.3 ng/mL; the limit of quantification of the SDS-PAGE is 10 μg/mL. This work demonstrates the application of dmLT assays in preformulation studies to development of an oral vaccine containing dmLT. Assays reported here will facilitate the understanding and use of dmLT as an adjuvant.

10

Botanical Drugs

A single rose can be my garden... a single friend, my world.

Leo Buscaglia

10.1 Introduction

Drugs derived from plant sources are generally labeled as phytomedicines, botanical products, natural products, and so on. *Botanical products* are finished, labeled products that contain vegetable matter as ingredients. A botanical product may be a food (including a dietary supplement), a drug (including a biological drug), a medical device (e.g., gutta-percha), or a cosmetic. The term *botanical* includes plant materials, algae, macroscopic fungi, and combinations thereof.

The World Health Organization (WHO) estimates that four billion people—80% of the world population—use herbal medicine for some aspect of primary healthcare. Herbal medicine is a major component in all indigenous peoples' traditional medicine and is a common element in Ayurvedic, homeopathic, naturopathic, traditional oriental, and Native American Indian medicine. Opinions about the safety, efficacy, and appropriateness of medicinal herbs vary widely among medical and health professionals in countries where herbal remedies are used. Some countries' professionals accept historical, empirical evidence as the only necessary criterion for herbal medicine's efficacy. Others would ban all herbal remedies, considering them dangerous or of questionable value.

Early humans recognized their dependence on nature in both health and illness. Led by instinct, taste, and experience, primitive men and women treated illness by using plants, animal parts, and minerals that were not part of their usual diet. Physical evidence of use of herbal remedies goes back some 60,000 years to a burial site of a Neanderthal man uncovered in 1960. All cultures have long folk medicine histories that include the use of plants. The invention of writing was a focus around which herbal knowledge could accumulate and grow. The first written records detailing the use of herbs in the treatment of illness are the Mesopotamian clay tablet writings and the Egyptian papyrus, which contains 876 prescriptions made up of more than 500 different substances, including many herbs. The Middle Eastern era is followed by the Greco-Roman era, which saw the writing of the De Materia Medica, which contains 950 curative substances, of which 600 are plant products and the rest are of animal or mineral origin. The Arab medicine was built on Greco-Roman and the text of Jami of Ibn Baiar (died 1248 AD), which lists more than 2000 substances, including many plant products. India's Ayurvedic book on internal medicine, the *Charaka Samhita*, describes 582 herbs. In China, the *Classic of the Materia Medica*, compiled no earlier than the first-century AD, focuses on the description of individual herbs. It includes 252 botanical substances, 45 mineral substances, and 67 animal-derived substances. Traditional Chinese medicine was brought to Japan via Korea, and Chinese-influenced Korean medicine was adapted by the Japanese during the reign of Emperor Ingyo (411–453 AD).

In North America, early explorers traded knowledge with the Native American Indians. In 1716, French explorer Lafitau found a species of ginseng, *Panax quinquefolius* L., growing in Iroquois territory in the New World. This American ginseng soon became an important item in world herb commerce. The Jesuits dug up the plentiful American ginseng, sold it to the Chinese, and used the money to build schools and churches. Even today, American ginseng is a sizable crude U.S. export. Although herbal medicines played a significant role in the lives of Americans, they have lost touch with it with the onslaught of allopathic medicines. One of the most significant reports on the use of botanical drugs in North America is the Baseline Natural Health Products Survey among consumers, March 2005, conducted by Health Canada. This survey concluded that 71% use botanical—38% use it on a daily basis, 37% seasonally, and 11% weekly—57% use vitamins, 15% use Echinacea, and 11% use other herbal remedies and algal and fungal products. Almost 80% of North Americans believe that botanical drugs are safer, and their use is likely to increase in the future. However, despite a long history of use, botanical drugs are generally considered to be anecdotal and ineffective by the regulatory agencies and allowed for sale only as food supplements. Recently, this trend of rejecting botanical drugs was reversed, mainly owing to pressures from consumers, and the U.S. Food and Drug Administration (FDA) issued its first botanical guideline and established a separate division within the agency to evaluate and approve botanical products as drugs, both prescription and over the counter (OTC).

10.2 Regulatory Status

The legal process of regulation and legislation of herbal medicines changes from country to country (Table 10.1). The reason for this involves mainly cultural aspects and also the fact that herbal medicines are rarely studied scientifically. Thus, few herbal preparations have been tested for safety and efficacy. The WHO has published guidelines to define basic criteria for evaluating the quality, safety, and efficacy of herbal medicines aimed at assisting national regulatory authorities, scientific organizations, and manufacturers in this particular area. Furthermore, the WHO has prepared Pharmacopeia monographs on herbal medicines and the basis of guidelines for the assessment of herbal drugs.

10.2.1 Characteristics of Phytomedicines

Phytotherapeutic agents or phytomedicines are standardized herbal preparations consisting of complex mixtures of one or more plants, which are used in most countries for the management of various diseases. According to the WHO definition, herbal drugs contain as active ingredients plant parts or plant materials in the crude or processed state plus certain excipients, that is, solvents, diluents, or preservatives.

TABLE 10.1

Herbal Drug Approval Rules in Different Countries

Argentina	The Herboristerias are authorized for sale as plant drugs but not as mixtures. Mixtures of plant drugs are controlled (Law No. 16.463). In 1993, a Ministry of Health regulation determined the obligatory registration of medicinal herbs. The Argentinian National Pharmacopeia established control over the existence of crude extracts, extracts, or fractions of complex chemical composition, and pure active principles. About 889 monographs exist in Argentina. About 56 describe crude drugs alone and 33 describe extracts or fractions. However, there is lack of control of raw materials, lack of control over the wild plants, lack of scientific criteria for the collection of plants, and lack of control over methods of drying, conservation, or grinding.
Australia	The Australian Parliament established the Working Party on Natural and Nutritional Supplements to review the quality, safety, efficacy, and labeling of herbal and related products (Therapeutic Good Act, 1990). The act provides "that traditional claims for herbal remedies be allowed, providing general advertising requirements are complied with and providing such claims are justified by literature references."
Brazil	In 1994, the Ministry of Health created a commission to evaluate the situation of phytotherapeutic agents in Brazil. The commission proposed a directive based mainly on German and French regulations and on WHO guidelines for herbal drugs. In 1995, "Directive Number 6" established the legal requirement for the registration of herbal drugs and defined the phytopharmaceutical product as "a processed drug containing as active ingredients exclusively plant material and/or plant drug preparations. They are intended to treat, cure, alleviate, prevent, and diagnose diseases."
Canada	In 1986, the Canadian HPB constituted a special committee (three pharmacists, two herbalists, one nutritionist, and one physician) and classified herbal drugs as "Folk Medicine." The regulation is based on traditional uses, as long as the claim is validated by scientific studies. In 1990, the HPB listed 64 herbs that were considered to be unsafe. In 1992, the HPB submitted a regulatory proposal to the Canadian Parliament and listed another 64 herbs that were considered to be adulterants. The Canadian regulatory system is consistent with the WHO guidelines for the assessment of herbal medicines.
Chile	In 1992, the Unidad de Medicina Tradicional was established with the objective of incorporating traditional medicine with proven efficacy into health programs (Law No. 19.253, October 1993). Directive No. 435/81 defined herbal drugs with therapeutic indication claims and/or dosage recommendations as being drugs restricted for sale in pharmacies and drug stores. Registration for marketing authorization is needed for herbal products. Natural products are legally differentiated as follows: (*i*) drugs intended to cure, alleviate, or prevent disease; (*ii*) food products for medicinal use and with therapeutic properties; and (*iii*) food products for nutritional purposes.
China	In China, until 1984, there was virtually no regulation of pharmaceuticals or herbal preparations. In 1984, the People's Republic implemented the Drug Administration Law, which said that traditional herbal preparations were generally considered "old drugs" and, except for new uses, were exempt from testing for efficacy or side effects. The Chinese Ministry of Public Health would oversee the administration of new herbal products.

(Continued)

TABLE 10.1 (*Continued*)

Herbal Drug Approval Rules in Different Countries

England	England generally follows the rule of prior use, which says that hundreds of years of use with apparent positive effects and no evidence of detrimental side effects are enough evidence—in lieu of other scientific data—that the product is safe. To promote the safe use of herbal remedies, the Ministry of Agriculture, Fisheries, and Food and the Department of Health jointly established a database of adverse effects of nonconventional medicines at the National Poisons Unit. These products are distinguished from approved pharmaceutical drugs by labels stating, "Traditionally used for…" Consumers understand this to mean that indications are based on historical evidence and have not necessarily been confirmed by modern scientific experimentation.
Europe	Drug approval considerations in Europe are the same as those for new drugs in the United States, where drugs are documented for safety, effectiveness, and quality. But historically, Europeans have been more understanding of the value of phytomedicines, and as a result, it is cheaper to secure approval of phytomedicines specially if there is a long history of their anecdotal use. The EEC, recognizing the need to standardize approval of herbal medicines, developed a series of guidelines, The Quality of Herbal Remedies Directive (EEC Directive, 75/318/EEC, adopted in November 1988) outlines standards for quality, quantity, and production of herbal remedies and provides labeling requirements that member countries must meet. The EEC guidelines are based on the principles of the WHO's Guidelines for the Assessment of Herbal Medicines (1991). According to these guidelines, a substance's historical use is a valid way to document safety and efficacy in the absence of scientific evidence to the contrary. The guidelines suggest the following as a basis for determining product safety: A guiding principle should be that if the product has been traditionally used without demonstrated harm, no specific restrictive regulatory action should be undertaken, unless new evidence demands a revised risk-benefit assessment. Prolonged and apparently uneventful use of a substance usually offers testimony of its safety. With regard to efficacy, the guidelines state the following: For treatment of minor disorders and for nonspecific indications, some relaxation is justified in the requirements for proof of efficacy, taking into account the extent of traditional use; the same considerations may apply to prophylactic use (WHO, 1991). The WHO guidelines give further advice for basing approval on existing monographs: If a pharmacopoeia monograph exists, it should be sufficient to make reference to this monograph. If no such monograph is available, a monograph must be supplied and should be set out in the same way as in an official pharmacopoeia. To further the standardization effort and to increase European scientific support, the phytotherapy societies of Belgium, France, Germany, Switzerland, and the United Kingdom founded the ESCOP. ESCOP's approach to eliminating problems of differing quality and therapeutic use within EEC is to build on the German scientific monograph system to create "European" monographs. In Europe, herbal remedies fall into three categories. The most rigorously controlled are the prescription drugs, which include injectable forms of phytomedicines and those used to treat life-threatening diseases. The second category is OTC phytomedicines, similar to American OTC drugs. The third category is traditional herbal remedies, products that typically have not undergone extensive clinical testing but are judged safe on the basis of generations of use without serious incident.

(*Continued*)

TABLE 10.1 (*Continued*)

Herbal Drug Approval Rules in Different Countries

France	Approximately 200 herbs are approved as OTC in France with varying claims. Licensing approval for phytomedicines is subject to regulations generally required for all drugs. There is only one type of license, but for some plant drugs and preparations, this license is granted on the basis of an adapted documentation and an abridged application. In 1990, 115 herbs plus 31 laxatives were involved in this approval procedure. Currently, about 205 herbal drugs are listed. France, where traditional medicines can be sold with labeling based on traditional use, requires licensing by the French Licensing Committee and approval by the French Pharmacopoeia Committee.
Germany	Germany's Commission E (phytotherapy and herbal substances) was established in 1978. It is an independent division of the German Federal Health Agency that collects information on herbal medicines and evaluates them for safety and efficacy. The following methods and criteria are followed by Commission E: (*i*) traditional use; (*ii*) chemical data; (*iii*) experimental, pharmacological, and toxicological studies; (*iv*) clinical studies; (*v*) field and epidemiological studies; (*vi*) patient case records submitted from physician's files; and (*vii*) additional studies, including unpublished proprietary data submitted by manufacturers. Two kinds of monographs are prepared: monopreparations and fixed combinations. The composition of Commission E is as follows: physicians, pharmacists, pharmacologists, toxicologists, industry representatives, and laypersons, for a total of 24 members. Three possibilities for marketing herbal drugs exist: (*i*) temporary marking authorization for old herbal drugs until they are evaluated for safety and efficacy; (*ii*) monographs of standardized marketing authorization; and (*iii*) individual marketing authorization. Evaluations are published in the form of monographs that approve or disapprove the herbal drugs for over-the-counter use. Herbal medicines are sold in pharmacies, drug stores, and health food stores. Some herbal medicines are controlled by a physician's prescription. Commission E has published about 300 monographs: 200 "positives" and 100 "negatives." About 600–700 plants are sold in Germany. Approximately 70% of physicians prescribe registered herbal drugs. Part of the annual sales is paid for by government health insurance. Germany considers whole herbal products as a single active ingredient; this makes it simpler to define and approve the product. The German Federal Health Office regulates such products as ginkgo and milk thistle extracts by using a monograph system that results in products whose potency and manufacturing processes are standardized. The monographs are compiled from scientific literature on a particular herb in a single report and are produced under the auspices of the Ministry of Health Committee for Herbal Remedies (Kommission E). Approval of such remedies requires more scientific documentation than traditional remedies, but less than new pharmaceutical drug approvals.
India	India has thousands of years of history of use of ayurvedic medicine; almost 70%–80% of the rural population of India depends on this mode of traditional medicine; no significant control on quality of drug of botanical origin exists in India.
Japan	Traditional Japanese medicine, called kampo, is similar to and historically derived from Chinese medicine but includes traditional medicines from Japanese folklore. Kampo declined when Western medicine was introduced between 1868 and 1912, but by 1928, it had begun to revive. Today, almost half of Japan's Western-trained medical practitioners prescribe kampo medicines, and Japanese national health insurance pays for these medicines. In 1988, the Japanese herbal medicine industry established regulations to manufacture and control the quality of extract products in kampo medicine. These regulations comply with the Japanese government's Regulations for Manufacturing Control and Quality Control of Drugs.

(Continued)

TABLE 10.1 (*Continued*)

Herbal Drug Approval Rules in Different Countries

U.S.A.	Since 1994, herbal medicines have been regulated under the "Dietary Supplement Health and Education Act of 1994." On the basis of this law, herbal medicines are not evaluated by the FDA, and most important, these products are not intended to diagnose, treat, cure, or prevent diseases. The U.S. FDA issued its first botanical drugs approval guidelines in August 2000. The mission of the NCCAM is, in part, to conduct rigorous research on CAM practices to evaluate the benefits and risks of CAM agents, so as to optimize their effect on human diseases or conditions. NCCAM groups CAM practices in five major domains: biologically based therapies, manipulative and body-based methods, mind-body interventions, energy therapies, and alternative medical systems. Biologically based CAM agents are regulated under the codes of DSHEA 1994. This regulation includes botanicals and their constituents, vitamins, minerals, and amino acids. The U.S. FDA characterizes botanicals and other dietary agents according to their use, not according to their composition. If the intended use is to "promote health," the agent is viewed as a dietary supplement; if the intended use is to treat or prevent a disease, the agent is considered to be a drug.

Abbreviations: CAM, complementary and alternative medicine; DSHEA, Dietary Supplement Health and Education Act; EEC, European Economic Community; ESCOP, European Societies' Cooperative of Phytotherapy; HPB, Health Protection Branch; NCCAM, National Center for Complementary and Alternative Medicine; OTC, over the counter; U.S. FDA, United States Food and Drug Administration; WHO, World Health Organization.

Usually, the active principles responsible for their pharmacological action are unknown. One basic characteristic of phytotherapeutic agents is that they normally do not possess an immediate or strong pharmacological action. For this reason, phytotherapeutic agents are not used for emergency treatment. Other characteristics of herbal medicines are their wide therapeutic use and great acceptance by the population. In contrast to modern medicines, herbal medicines are frequently used to treat chronic diseases. Combinations with chemically defined active substances or isolated constituents are not considered to be herbal medicines. It is important to note that, although homeopathic preparations may frequently contain plants, they are not considered to be herbal medicines.

Compared with well-defined synthetic drugs, herbal medicines exhibit some marked differences, namely:

- The active principles are frequently unknown.
- Standardization, stability, and quality control are feasible but not easy.
- The availability and quality of raw materials are frequently problematic.
- Well-controlled double-blind clinical and toxicological studies to prove their efficacy and safety are rare.
- Empirical use in folk medicine is a very important characteristic.
- They have a wide range of therapeutic use and are suitable for chronic treatments.
- The occurrence of undesirable side effects seems to be less frequent with herbal medicines, but well-controlled randomized clinical trials have revealed that they also exist.
- They usually cost less than the synthetic drugs.

10.2.2 Specifications

The setting of specifications for a herbal preparation (herbal substance) and a herbal medicinal product is part of an overall control strategy, which includes control of raw materials and excipients, in-process testing, process evaluation and validation, stability testing, and testing for consistency of batches. When combined in total, these elements provide assurance that the appropriate quality of the product will be maintained. As specifications are chosen to confirm the quality rather than to characterize the product, the manufacturer should provide the rationale and justification for including and/or excluding testing for specific quality attributes. The following points should be taken into consideration when establishing scientifically justifiable specifications.

Specifications for herbal substances are linked to the following:

- Botanical characteristics of the plant (genus, species, variety, chemotype, and usage of genetically modified organisms) and parts of the plants
- Macroscopical and microscopical characterization, phytochemical characteristics of the plant part constituents with known therapeutic activity or marker substances, and toxic constituents (identity, assay, and limit tests)
- Biological/geographical variation
- Cultivation/harvesting/drying conditions (microbial levels, aflatoxins, heavy metals, and so on)
- Pre-/postharvest chemical treatments (pesticides and fumigants)
- Profile and stability of the constituents

Specifications for herbal preparations are linked to the following:

- Quality of the herbal substance (as discussed previously)
- Definition of the herbal preparation (drug extract ratio, extraction solvent[s])
- Method of preparation from the herbal substance
- Constituents—constituents with known therapeutic activity or marker substances
- Other constituents (identification, assay, and limit tests)
- Drying conditions (e.g., microbial levels and residual solvents in extracts)
- Profile and stability of the constituents and microbial purity on storage
- Batches used in preclinical/clinical testing (safety and efficacy considerations)

Specifications for herbal medicinal products are linked to the following:

- Quality of the herbal substance and/or herbal preparation
- Manufacturing process (temperature effects, and residual solvents)
- Profile and stability of the active constituents/formulation in packaging
- Batches used in preclinical/clinical testing (safety and efficacy considerations)

Specifications should be based on data obtained from lots used to demonstrate manufacturing consistency. Linking specifications to a manufacturing process is important, especially with regard to product-related substances, product-related impurities, and process-related impurities. Historical batch data should be taken into account, where available.

Changes in the manufacturing process and degradation products produced during storage may result in a product that differs from that used in preclinical and clinical development. The significance of these changes should be evaluated.

Because of the inherent complexity of herbal products, there may be no single stability-indicating assay or parameter that profiles the stability characteristics. Consequently, the applicant should propose a series of product-specific, stability-indicating tests, the results of which will provide assurance that changes in the quality of the product during its shelf life will be detected. The determination of the tests that should be included will be product-specific. Applicants are referred to the "Note for guidance on stability testing of new drug substances and products" (committee for proprietary medicinal products [CPMP]/ICH/2736/99), the "Guideline on stability testing of new veterinary drug substances and medicinal products" (Committee for Veterinary Medicinal Products [CVMP]/International Cooperation on Harmonisation of Technical Requirements for Registration of Veterinary Medicinal Products [VICH]/899/99), and the "Note for guidance on stability testing of existing active substances and related finished products" (CPMP/QWP/122/02 rev. 1 and European Agency for the Evaluation of Medicinal Products [EMA]/CVMP/846/99).

10.2.2.1 Standardization

Plants contain several hundred constituents, and some of them are present at very low concentrations. Despite the modern chemical analytical procedures available, only rarely do photochemical investigations succeed in isolating and characterizing all secondary metabolites present in the plant extract. Apart from this, plant constituents vary considerably, depending on several factors that impair the quality control of phototherapeutic agents. Quality control and standardization of herbal medicines involve several steps. However, the source and quality of raw materials play a pivotal role in guaranteeing the quality and stability of herbal preparations. Other factors such as the use of fresh plants; temperature; light exposure; water availability; nutrients; period and time of collection; method of collecting, drying, packing, storage, and transportation of the raw material; age and part of the plant collected; and so on can greatly affect the quality and, consequently, the therapeutic value of herbal medicines. Some plant constituents are heat labile, and the plants containing them need to be dried at low temperatures. Also, other active principles are destroyed by enzymatic processes that continue for long periods of time after plant collection. This explains why frequently the composition of herbal drugs is quite variable. Thus, proper standardization and quality control of raw material and the herbal preparations themselves should be carried out permanently. In cases where the active principles are unknown, marker substance(s) should be established for analytical purposes. However, in most cases, these markers have never been tested to see whether they really account for the therapeutic action reported for the herbal drugs. As pointed out earlier, apart from these variable factors, other factors, such as the method of extraction and contamination with microorganisms, heavy metals, pesticides, and the like, can also interfere with the quality, safety, and efficacy of herbal drugs. For these reasons, pharmaceutical companies prefer using cultivated plants instead of wild-harvested plants, because they show smaller variation in their constituents. Furthermore, and certainly more relevant, when medicinal plants are produced by cultivation, the main secondary metabolites can be monitored, and this permits definition of the best period for harvesting.

The recent advances that occurred in the processes of purification, isolation, and structure elucidation of naturally occurring substances have made it possible to establish appropriate strategies for the analysis of quality and the process of standardization of herbal preparations, in order to maintain as much homogeneity of the plant extract as possible. Among others, thin-layer chromatography (TLC), gas chromatography (GC), high-performance liquid chromatography (HPLC), mass spectrometry (MS), infrared spectrometry (IRS), ultraviolet/visible (UV/VIS) spectrometry, and the like, used alone or in combination, can be used successfully for standardization and control of the quality of both the raw materials and the finished herbal drugs.

10.2.3 Efficacy and Safety

Although clinical trials with herbal drugs are feasible, few well-controlled double-blind (placebo-controlled) trials have been carried out with herbal medicines. Several factors might contribute to the explanation of such discrepancies, for example:

- Lack of standardization and quality control of the herbal drugs used in clinical trials
- Use of different dosages of herbal medicines
- Inadequate randomization in most studies, and patients not properly selected
- Numbers of patients in most trials insufficient for the attainment of statistical significance
- Difficulties in establishing appropriate placebos because of the tastes, aromas, and so on
- Wide variations in the duration of treatments using herbal medicines

However, a large number of clinical trials have been performed with some herbal drugs, including:

- *Ginkgo biloba* (used for the treatment of central nervous system and cardiovascular disorders)
- *Hypericum perforatum* (St. John's wort), used as an antidepressant
- *Panax ginseng* (ginseng) herb, used as a tonic

- *Tanacetum parthenium* (feverfew), used to treat migraine headache
- *Allium sativum* (garlic), used to lower low-density protein cholesterol and some cardiovascular disturbances
- *Matricaria chamomilla* (chamomile), recommended as a carminative, anti-inflammatory, and antispasmodic
- *Silybum marianum* (milk thistle), used for repairing liver function, including cirrhosis
- *Valeriana officinalis* (valerian), used as a sedative and sleeping aid
- *Piper methysticum* (kava kava), used as an anxiolytic
- *Aesculus hippocastanum* (horse chestnut), used for the treatment of chronic venous insufficiency
- *Cassia acutifolia* (senna) and *Rhamnus purshiana* (cascara sagrada), which are used as laxatives
- *Echinacea purpurea* (echinacea), used as an anti-inflammatory and immunostimulant
- *Arnica montana* (arnica), used to treat post-traumatic and postoperative conditions
- *Serenoa repens* (saw palmetto), used for the treatment of benign prostatic hyperplasia

10.2.4 Regulatory Filing Procedure

In general, the chemistry, manufacturing, and control (CMC) requirements for standard synthetic/semisynthetic drugs are as follows:

- Synthesis of the drug
- Manufacturing of the product that is administered to the patient
- Control of these processes

Thus, the drug and the product are made reproducibly to provide assurance that only active ingredients are administered to patients and toxic contaminants are not.

More specific CMC requirements, for example, for a plant substance that is later made into a pure drug (e.g., digitalis for heart failure and artemisinin for malaria), are shown in column 3 of Table 10.2.

10.2.4.1 Plant Substance

- Description of the plant
- Procedure by which a part of the plant is extracted
- Quantity of the active ingredient in the extract
- How the active ingredient is identified
- Stability of the active ingredient (at least over the time of the trial)

TABLE 10.2

Chemistry, Manufacturing, and Control Considerations for National Center for
Complementary and Alternative Medicine Clinical Trials

Subject of Study	Study Parameters	Study Details	Data Required for Proposed NCCAM Trial	
			Phase I/II Trial	Phase III Trial
Plant substance	Starting material	Botanical description	X	Expanded
		Extraction procedure	X	Expanded
		Quantity of active moiety		X
		Identity: chemical/ biologic assay		X
		Stability		X
Plant product	Manufacturing	Reagents/process		X
	Finished product	Quantity of active moiety	X	X
	Product assay	Methods/ specifications		X
		Identity: chemical/ biologic assay	X	X
		Purity		X
	Storage	Describe conditions	X	X
	Stability	Light/heat/time	X	X
	Excipients	List		X
	Impurities	List/analyze	X	X
	Reference standard	Standard batch		X
	In-process controls	Standard operating procedures		X
	Bioavailability	Disintegration/ dissolution rate	X	X
	Microbiology	Contamination		X
	Environmental	Assessment		X

Note: X means applicable.

10.2.4.2 Product (Capsule, Tablet, and Intravenous Formulation)

- How the product is manufactured
- Quantity of the active ingredient in the product
- How the active ingredient is identified
- Impurities in the product, including microbials, pesticides, heavy metals, and adulterants

- Storage conditions and physicochemical stability of the active ingredient during storage
- Specifications of a reference batch and the controls during the manufacturing process, such that each batch is similar to the reference batch
- Bioavailability of the active ingredient (disintegration and dissolution, or breakdown, in physiological solutions in vitro and absorption in vivo)
- Whether the environment is contaminated, for example, with carcinogens, as the product is being made

10.2.5 Overview of Chemistry, Manufacturing, and Control Evidence Needed to Support Clinical Trials for Botanical Drugs

Unlike standard drugs, botanicals have been in use before they were studied in a clinical trial. Prior human use gives some assurance that the product will be safe and effective. Some of the CMC information needed for a standard drug is also needed for botanical drugs.

Unlike synthetic drugs, botanical drugs are mixtures of uncharacterized constituents. It is postulated that a mixture provides a therapeutic advantage. For example, unknown constituents may combine in an additive or synergistic way with the known constituents to provide greater efficacy than would be provided by the known constituent alone. For botanical drugs, the analysis of the active ingredient(s) may be best approached by the analysis of one or more hypothesized active ingredients, such as:

- A chemical constituent that constitutes a sizable percentage of the total ingredients
- A chemical fingerprint of the total ingredients

The two analyses mentioned above are surrogates for the analysis of the unknown constituents that contribute to efficacy.

10.2.6 Information on a Plant Product That Was the Subject of Prior Human Use

Plants are often extracted and processed nonreproducibly. It is important that the product that is produced for a clinical trial is similar in analysis to the original product that has been used in humans.

Consider the following example of a botanical drug with three components. Component 1 is potentially toxic, and components 2 and 3 are potentially effective at low doses but are also potentially toxic at high doses. Table 10.3 shows the number of units of each component for two lots of the drug.

If Lot 1 is administered but the lots previously used were comparable with Lot 2, the participants will suffer toxicity from the higher doses of components 2 and 3. If Lot 2 is administered, but the lots previously used were comparable with Lot 1, the participants will suffer toxicity from the higher dose of component 1, and the efficacy will diminish because of the lower doses of components 2 and 3.

TABLE 10.3

Example of Component Combinations for a Botanical Drug

	Component 1 •Potentially toxic	Component 2 •Low dose: effective •High dose: toxic	Component 3 •Low dose: effective •High dose: toxic
Lot 1	1 unit	122 units	48 units
Lot 2	12 units	11 units	10 units

This example illustrates the wide variation in composition that may be found in the identically labeled botanical products. For this reason, the analysis of the product that is proposed for study in a clinical trial must be performed and shown to be similar to the analysis of the botanical with prior human experience, if prior clinical data are used to justify the proposed trial.

Therefore, the following information is needed for products used previously in humans:

• Plant substance
• Description of the plant
• Genus
• Species (cultivar if appropriate)
• Country(s) of origin
• Plant extraction procedure
• Plant product
• Analysis of commonly accepted or supposed active ingredient(s) via chemical or biological parameters
• Analysis of a sizeable chemical constituent (analytical marker compound)
• Analysis via chemical fingerprint (analytical markers)

10.2.7 Information on the Plant Product Proposed for Phase I/II Studies

10.2.7.1 Plant Substance

This section includes a detailed description of the plant, including genus, species (cultivar if appropriate), country(s) of origin, time of harvest, and plant extraction procedure.

10.2.7.2 Plant Product

• Analysis of commonly accepted or supposed active ingredient(s) via chemical or biological parameters.
• Analysis of a sizeable chemical constituent (analytical marker compound).
• Analysis via chemical fingerprint (analytical markers).

- Analysis for lack of contamination by pesticides, heavy metals, and synthetic drug adulterants.
- The breakdown or dissolution of the analyzed components in physiological solutions.
- List of inert substances (excipients) added to the product.
- Storage conditions and stability over the length of the trial.

10.2.8 Information on the Plant Product Proposed for Phase III Studies

10.2.8.1 Plant Substance

- Botanical description
- Statement that the plant is cultivated according to Good Agricultural Practices or harvested according to Good Wildcrafting Practices
- Extraction procedure
- Quantity and identity of active ingredient(s) and of sizeable chemical constituent
- Statement that extraction and analytic procedures are performed under Good Manufacturing Practices (GMPs) (e.g., that the manufacturing processes and their controls provide the appropriate levels of assurance for the important quality characteristics of the product)

10.2.8.2 Plant Product

- Manufacturing methods
- Analysis of commonly accepted or supposed active ingredient(s) via chemical or biological parameters
- Analysis of a sizeable chemical constituent (analytical marker compound)
- Analysis via chemical fingerprint (analytical markers)
- Analysis for the lack of contamination by pesticides, heavy metals, and synthetic drug adulterants
- The breakdown or dissolution of the analyzed components in physiological solutions
- In-process controls for manufacturing process
- List of inert substances (excipients) added to the product
- Description of the reference batch
- Storage conditions and stability over the length of the trial
- Environmental impact statement
- Statement that the plant product is manufactured and analyzed according to GMP (e.g., that the manufacturing processes and their controls provide appropriate levels of assurance for the important quality characteristics of the product)

10.2.9 Starting Material

Consistent quality of products of herbal origin can be assured only if the starting materials are defined in a rigorous and detailed manner, particularly the specific botanical identification of the plant material used. It is also important to know the geographical source and the conditions under which the herbal substance is obtained to ensure the material of consistent quality.

"Standardized extracts" are herbal preparations adjusted within an acceptable tolerance to a given content of constituents with known therapeutic activity; standardization is achieved by an adjustment of the herbal preparations with inert material or by blending batches of herbal preparations. "Quantified extracts" are herbal preparations adjusted to a defined range of constituents; adjustments are made by blending batches of herbal preparations. "Other extracts" are herbal preparations, essentially defined by their production process and their specifications.

In the case of a herbal substance or a herbal preparation consisting of comminuted or powdered herbal substances, the quantity of the herbal substance or the herbal preparation shall be given as a range corresponding to a defined quantity of constituents with known therapeutic activity, or the quantity of the herbal substance or the quantity of the native herbal preparation shall be stated if constituents with known therapeutic activity are unknown.

Examples of how the composition is listed include *Sennae folium*, 415–500 mg, corresponding to 12.5 mg of hydroxyanthracene glycosides, calculated as Sennoside B or Valerianae radix 900 mg.

In the case of an herbal preparation produced by steps that exceed comminution, the nature and concentration of the solvent and the physical state of the extract have to be given. Furthermore, the following have to be indicated:

- *Standardized extracts*: If the constituents with known therapeutic activity are known, the equivalent quantity or the ratio of the herbal substance to the herbal preparation shall be stated, and the quantity of the herbal preparation may be given as a range corresponding to a defined quantity of these constituents (see example).
- *Quantified extracts*: In the case of quantified extracts, the equivalent quantity or the ratio of the herbal substance to the herbal preparation shall be stated. Furthermore, the content of the quantified substance(s) shall be specified in a range.
- *Other extracts*: The equivalent quantity or the ratio of the herbal substance to the herbal preparation shall be stated if constituents with known therapeutic activity are unknown.

The composition of any solvent or solvent mixture and the physical state of the extract must be indicated. If any other substance is added during the manufacture of the herbal preparation to adjust the preparation to a defined content of constituents with known therapeutic activity, or for any other purpose, the added substance must be mentioned as an "other substance" and the genuine extract must be mentioned as the "active substance." However, where different batches of the same extract are used to adjust constituents with known therapeutic activity to a defined content, or for any other purpose, the final mixture shall be regarded as the genuine extract and listed as the "active substance" in the unit formula. Full details of production and control must, however, be provided in the dossier.

Examples of representation may include the following:

- *Sennae folium* 50–65 mg, corresponding to 12.5 mg of dry extract ethanolic 60% (V/V) hydroxyanthracene glycosides, calculated as ([a–b]: 1) Sennoside B.
- *Ginkgo biloba* L. *folium* 60 mg, containing 13.2–16.2 mg of flavonoid dry extract acetonic 60% (V/V), expressed as flavone glycosides ([a–b]: 1) 1.68–2.04 mg ginkgolides A, B, and C and 1.56–1.92 mg bilobalide.
- *Valerianae radix* 125 mg of dry extract ethanolic 60% (V/V), or *Valerianae radix* 125 mg of dry extract ethanolic 60% (V/V) equivalent to x–y mg *Valerianae radix*.

10.2.9.1 Control of Herbal Substances and of Herbal Preparations

As a general rule, herbal substances must be tested, unless otherwise justified, for microbiological quality and for residues of pesticides and fumigation agents, toxic metals, likely contaminants, adulterants, and so on. The use of ethylene oxide is prohibited for the decontamination of herbal substances in the International Conference on Harmonization (ICH) guidelines. Radioactive contamination should be tested for if there are reasons for concerns. Specifications and descriptions of the analytical procedures must be submitted, together with the limits applied. Analytical procedures not given in a Pharmacopoeia should be validated in accordance with the ICH guideline "Validation of analytical procedures: methodology" (CPMP/ICH/281/95) or the corresponding VICH guideline (CVMP/VICH/591/98).

Reference samples of the herbal substances must be available for use in comparative tests, for example, macroscopic and microscopic examinations, chromatography, and so on.

If the herbal medicinal product contains a preparation, rather than merely the herbal substance, the comprehensive specification for the herbal substance must be followed by a description and validation of the manufacturing process for the herbal preparation. The information may be supplied either as part of the marketing authorization application or by using the European Active Substance Master File procedure. If the latter route is chosen, the documentation should be submitted in accordance with the "Guideline on active substance master file procedure" (EMA/CPMP/QWP/227/02 and EMA/CVMP/134/02).

Where the preparation is the subject of a European Pharmacopoeia monograph, the European Directorate for the Quality of Medicines Certification procedure (for Certificates of Suitability [CEPs]) can be used to demonstrate compliance with the relevant European Pharmacopoeia monograph.

For each herbal preparation, a comprehensive specification is required. This should be established on the basis of recent scientific data and should give particulars of the characteristics, identification tests, and purity tests. Appropriate chromatographic methods should be used. If deemed necessary by analysis of the starting material, tests on microbiological quality, residues of pesticides, fumigation agents, solvents, and toxic metals should be performed. Radioactivity should be tested if there are reasons for concern. A quantitative determination (assay) of markers or of substances with known therapeutic activity is also required. The content should be indicated with the lowest possible tolerance (the narrowest possible tolerance with both upper and lower limits stated). The test methods should be described in detail.

If preparations from herbal substances with constituents of known therapeutic activity are standardized (i.e., adjusted to a defined content of constituents with known therapeutic activity), it should be stated that how such standardization is achieved. If another substance is used for these purposes, it is necessary to specify as a range the quantity that can be added.

10.2.10 Control of Vitamins and Minerals (If Applicable)

Vitamin(s) and mineral(s), which could be ancillary substances in traditional herbal medicinal products for human use, should fulfill the requirements of the "Guideline on summary of requirements for active substances in the quality part of the dossier" (CHMP/QWP/297/97 Rev. 1 corr).

10.2.10.1 Control of Excipients

Excipients, including those added during the manufacture of the herbal preparations, should be described according to the "Note for guidance on excipients in the dossier for application for marketing authorization of a medicinal product" (Eudralex 3AQ 9A) or the "Note for guidance on excipients in the dossier for application for marketing authorisation of veterinary medicinal products" (EMA/CVMP/004/98), as appropriate. For novel excipients, the dossier requirements for active substances apply (refer to Directive 2001/83/EC, as amended for human medicinal products, and Directive 2001/82/EC, as amended for veterinary medicinal products).

The control tests on the finished product should allow the qualitative and quantitative determination of the composition of the active substance(s). A specification should be provided, and this may include the use of markers where constituents with known therapeutic activity are unknown. In the case of herbal substances or herbal preparations with constituents of known therapeutic activity, these constituents should be specified and quantitatively determined. For traditional herbal medicinal products for human use containing vitamins and/or minerals, the vitamins and/or minerals should also be specified and determined quantitatively.

If a herbal medicinal product contains a combination of several herbal substances or preparations of several herbal substances, and if it is not possible to perform a quantitative determination of each active substance, the determination may be carried out jointly for several active substances. The need for this procedure should be justified.

The criteria given by the European Pharmacopoeia to ensure the microbiological quality should be applied, unless justified. The frequency of testing for microbial contamination should be justified.

10.2.11 Stability Testing

As the herbal substance or herbal preparation in its entirety is regarded as the active substance, a mere determination of the stability of the constituents with known therapeutic activity will not suffice. The stability of other substances present in the herbal substance or in the herbal preparation should, as far as possible, also be demonstrated, for example, by means of appropriate fingerprint chromatograms. It should also be demonstrated that their proportional content remains constant.

If a herbal medicinal product contains combinations of several herbal substances or herbal preparations, and if it is not possible to determine the stability of each active substance, the stability of the medicinal product should be determined by appropriate fingerprint chromatograms, appropriate overall methods of assay, and physical and sensory tests or other appropriate tests. The appropriateness of the tests shall be justified by the applicant.

In the case of a herbal medicinal product containing a herbal substance or herbal preparation with constituents of known therapeutic activity, the variation in content during the proposed shelf life should not exceed $\pm 5\%$ of the initial assay value, unless justified. In the case of a herbal medicinal product containing a herbal substance or herbal preparation, where constituents with known therapeutic activity are unknown, a variation in marker content during the proposed shelf life of $\pm 10\%$ of the initial assay value can be accepted, if justified by the applicant.

In the case of traditional herbal medicinal products for human use containing vitamins and/or minerals, the stability of the vitamins and/or minerals should be demonstrated.

10.2.11.1 Testing Criteria

Implementation of the recommendations in the following section should take into account the ICH/VICH guidelines "Validation of analytical methods: definitions and terminology" (CPMP/ICH/381/95 and CVMP/VICH/590/98) and "Validation of analytical procedures: methodology" (CPMP/ICH/281/95 and CVMP/VICH/591/98).

10.2.12 Herbal Substances

Herbal substances are a diverse range of botanical materials, including leaves, herbs, roots, flowers, seeds, bark, and so on. A comprehensive specification must be developed for each herbal substance even if the starting material for the manufacture of the finished product is a herbal preparation. In the case of fatty or essential oils used as active substances of herbal medicinal products, a specification for the herbal substance is required, unless justified. The specification should be established on the basis of recent scientific data and should be set out in the same way as the European Pharmacopoeia monographs. The general monograph "Herbal Drugs" (herbal substances) of the European Pharmacopoeia should be consulted for interpretation of the following requirements.

The following tests and acceptance criteria are considered generally applicable to all herbal substances:

  1. *Definition*: A qualitative statement of the botanical source, plant part used, and its state (e.g., whole, reduced, powdered, fresh, and dry). It is also important to know the geographical source(s) and the conditions under which the herbal substance is obtained.

2. *Characteristics*: A qualitative statement about the organoleptic character(s), including the macro- and microscopic botanic properties of the herbal substance, is described.

3. *Identification*: Identification testing should optimally be able to discriminate between the related species and/or potential adulterants/substitutes, which are likely to be present. Identification tests should be specific for the herbal substance and are usually a combination of three or more of the following: macroscopic, microscopic, chromatographic, and chemical.

4. *Tests*:

- Foreign matter
- Total ash
- Ash insoluble in hydrochloric acid
- Water soluble extractive and
- Extractable matter
- *Particle size*: For some herbal substances intended for use in herbal teas or solid herbal medicinal products, particle size can have a significant effect on dissolution rates, bioavailability, and/or stability. In such instances, testing for particle size distribution should be carried out using an appropriate procedure, and acceptance criteria should be provided. Particle size can also affect the disintegration time of solid dosage forms.
- *Water content*: This test is important when the herbal substances are known to be hygroscopic. For nonpharmacopoeial herbal substances, acceptance criteria should be justified by data on the effects of moisture absorption. A loss on drying procedure may be adequate; however, in some cases (essential oil-containing plants), a detection procedure specific for water is required.
- *Inorganic impurities and toxic metals*: The need for the inclusion of tests and acceptance criteria for inorganic impurities should be studied during development and based on the knowledge of the plant species, its cultivation, and the manufacturing process. Acceptance criteria will ultimately depend on safety considerations. Where justified, procedures and acceptance criteria for sulfated ash/residue on ignition should follow pharmacopoeia precedents; other inorganic impurities may be determined by other appropriate procedures, for example, atomic absorption spectroscopy.
- *Microbial limits*: There may be a need to specify the total count of aerobic microorganisms, the total count of yeasts and molds, and the absence of specific objectionable bacteria. The source of the herbal material should be taken into account when considering the inclusion of other possible pathogens (e.g., *Campylobacter* and *Listeria* species), in addition to those specified in the European Pharmacopoeia. Microbial counts should be determined using pharmacopoeial procedures or other validated procedures. The European Pharmacopoeia gives guidance on the acceptance criteria.

- *Mycotoxins*: The potential for mycotoxins' contamination should be fully considered. Wherever necessary, suitable validated methods should be used to control potential mycotoxins, and the acceptance criteria should be justified.
- *Pesticides, fumigation agents, and the like*: The potential for residues of pesticides, fumigation agents, and the like should be fully considered. Wherever necessary, suitable validated methods should be used to control potential residues, and the acceptance criteria should be justified. In the case of pesticide residues, the method, acceptance criteria, and guidance on the methodology of the European Pharmacopoeia should be applied, unless fully justified.
- Other appropriate tests (e.g., swelling index).

5. *Assay*: In the case of herbal substances with constituents of known therapeutic activity, assays of their content are required with details of the analytical procedure. Wherever possible, a specific, stability-indicating procedure should be included to determine the content of the herbal substance. In cases where use of a nonspecific assay is justified, other supporting analytical procedures should be used to achieve the overall specificity. For example, where determination of essential oils is adopted to assay the herbal substance, the combination of the assay and a suitable test for identification (e.g., fingerprint chromatography) can be used. In the case of herbal substances where the constituents responsible for the therapeutic activity are unknown, assays of marker substances or other justified determinations are required. The appropriateness of the choice of marker substance should be justified. For example, reference to the assay of a marker substance in the relevant monograph of the European Pharmacopoeia is an appropriate justification.

10.2.13 Herbal Preparations

Herbal preparations are also diverse in character, ranging from simple, comminuted plant material to extracts, tinctures, oils, and resins. A comprehensive specification must be developed for each herbal preparation, based on recent scientific data. The general monograph "Herbal Drug Preparations" (herbal preparations) of the European Pharmacopoeia should be consulted for the interpretation of the following requirements.

The following tests and acceptance criteria are considered generally applicable to all herbal preparations:

1. *Definition*: A statement of the botanical source and the type of preparation (e.g., dry or liquid extract). The ratio of the herbal substance to the herbal preparation must be stated.
2. *Characters*: A qualitative statement about the organoleptic characters of the herbal preparation, where characteristic.
3. *Identification*: Identification tests should be specific for the herbal preparation and optimally should be discriminatory with regard to substitutes or adulterants that are likely to occur. Identification solely by

chromatographic retention time, for example, is not regarded as being specific; however, a combination of chromatographic tests (e.g., HPLC and TLC-densitometry) or a combination of tests into a single procedure, such as HPLC/UV-diode array, HPLC/MS, or GC/MS, may be acceptable.

4. *Tests*:
   - *Residual solvents*: Refer to the European Pharmacopoeia general text on residual solvents (01/2005: 50400) for detailed information.
   - *Water content*: This test is important when the herbal preparations are known to be hygroscopic. The acceptance criteria may be justified with data on the effects of hydration or moisture absorption. A loss on drying procedure may be adequate; however, in some cases (essential oil-containing preparations), a detection procedure that is specific for water is required.
   - *Inorganic impurities and toxic metals*: The need for the inclusion of tests and acceptance criteria for inorganic impurities should be studied during development and based on the knowledge of the plant species, its cultivation, and the manufacturing process. The potential for manufacturing process to concentrate toxic residues should be fully addressed. If the manufacturing process will reduce the burden of toxic residues, the tests with the herbal substance may be sufficient. Acceptance criteria will ultimately depend on safety considerations. Where justified, procedures and acceptance criteria for sulfated ash/residue on ignition should follow pharmacopoeial precedents; other inorganic impurities may be determined by other appropriate procedures, for example, atomic absorption spectroscopy.
   - *Microbial limits*: There may be a need to specify the total count of aerobic microorganisms, the total count of yeasts and molds, and the absence of specific objectionable bacteria. These limits should comply with those in the European Pharmacopoeia.
   - *Mycotoxins*: The potential for mycotoxins contamination should be fully considered. Wherever necessary, suitable validated methods should be used to control potential mycotoxins, and the acceptance criteria should be justified.
   - *Pesticides, fumigation agents, and the like*: The potential for residues of pesticides, fumigation agents, and the like should be fully considered. Wherever necessary, suitable validated methods should be used to control potential residues, and the acceptance criteria should be justified. In the case of pesticide residues, the method, acceptance criteria, and guidance on the methodology of the European Pharmacopoeia should be applied, unless fully justified.

5. *Assay*: In the case of herbal preparations with constituents of known therapeutic activity, assays of their content are required, with details of the analytical procedure. Wherever possible, a specific, stability-indicating procedure should be included to determine the content of the herbal substance in the herbal preparation. In cases where use of a nonspecific assay is justified, other supporting analytical procedures should be used to achieve

the overall specificity. For example, where a UV/VIS spectrophotometric assay is used for anthraquinone glycosides, a combination of the assay and a suitable test for identification (e.g., fingerprint chromatography) can be used. In the case of herbal preparations where the constituents responsible for the therapeutic activity are not known, assays of marker substances or other justified determinations are required. The appropriateness of the choice of marker substance should be justified.

RECOMMENDED READING

Barboza, J. L. et al. (2015). "The treatment of gastroparesis, constipation and small intestinal bacterial overgrowth syndrome in patients with Parkinson's disease." *Expert Opin Pharmacother* 16(16):2449–2464.

INTRODUCTION: Parkinson's disease (PD) affects the nerves of the entire gastrointestinal (GI) tract and may result in profound gastrointestinal (GI) dysfunction leading to poor patient outcomes. Common GI disturbances in patients with PD include gastroparesis (GP), constipation and small intestinal bacterial overgrowth syndrome (SIBO). In particular, GP is difficult to treat due to the limited options available and precautions, contraindications and adverse effects associated with the approved treatments. Moreover, some commonly used medications can worsen pre-existing PD. AREAS COVERED: Our review will focus on treatment options for GP and SIBO with motilin agonists, dopamine receptor antagonists, Ghrelin agonists muscarinic agonists, 5-HT4 receptor agonists, antibiotics, probiotics and herbal formulation such as iberogast. Constipation occurs in the majority of patients with PD and fortunately many treatments are now available. Our review is based on original papers or reviews selected from PubMed search and Cochrane reviews. EXPERT OPINION: Motility disorders of the GI tract are found frequently in patients with PD and treating the underlying GI disorders caused by PD with various prokinetics and laxatives is paramount in achieving improvements in patient's motor function. Various prokinetics and laxatives are now available to provide some relief of the GI morbidity caused by PD leading even to better absorption of even the PD treatments.

Celia, C. et al. (2016). "Effect of pre- and post-weaning dietary supplementation with Digestarom(R) herbal formulation on rabbit carcass traits and meat quality." *Meat Sci* 118:89–95.

This study evaluated effects of Digestarom(R) (D) dietary inclusion before weaning (0–5 weeks old; BW) and/or after weaning (5–12 weeks old; AW) on growing rabbit carcass traits and meat quality. During BW, Pannon-Ka rabbits (does, kits) received two diets: a control diet (C) and one supplemented with 300 mg Digestarom(R)/kg (D). At weaning, each group was divided into 3 dietary sub-groups: CC and DD received C and D diets from 5 to 12 weeks of age, whereas DC was fed D from 5 to 8 weeks and C from 8 to 12 weeks of age (54 rabbits/group; AW). Rabbits were slaughtered at 12 weeks of age. Digestarom(R) supplementation improved carcass yield and body mid part proportion only when administered BW. Rabbits fed D BW had higher hind leg meat cooking losses. Loin meat spiciness and rancidity increased with D both BW and AW. In conclusion, Digestarom® herbal formulation was ineffective in improving growing rabbit carcass traits or meat quality.

Cesca, T. G. et al. (2012). "Antinociceptive, anti-inflammatory and wound healing features in animal models treated with a semisolid herbal medicine based on Aleurites moluccana L. Willd. Euforbiaceae standardized leaf extract: semisolid herbal." *J Ethnopharmacol* 143(1):355–362.

ETHNOPHARMACOLOGICAL RELEVANCE: *Aleurites moluccana* L. (Willd) Euforbiaceae is a native tree of Indonesia and India that has become acclimatized and well-adapted to the South and Southwest of Brazil. It is commonly used in traditional medicine to treat pain, fever, inflammation, asthma, hepatitis, headache, gastric ulcer, cuts, skin sores and other ailments. The oral antinociceptive effects of standardized 70:30 (v/v) ethanol:water spray dried extract of A. moluccana leaf, as well as its flavonoids 2″-O-rhamnosylswertisin (I) and swertisin (II), have previously been reported. AIM: The aim of this study was to develop a stable and effective semisolid herbal medicine for topical use in the treatment of pain, inflammation and wound healing, containing 0.5% and 1.0% of standardized dried extract of A. moluccana. MATERIALS AND METHODS: The chemical markers I and II were assayed by HPLC-UV analysis after extraction by matrix solid dispersion phase (MSDP) followed analytical validation as ICH Guidelines. The semisolid preparations of Hostacerin CG® vehicle containing 0.5 and 1.0% of dried extract of A. moluccana were submitted to stability studies (180 day of accelerated and long-term studies). The phytomedicine semisolid was analyzed in croton oil-induced ear oedema model in mice, in the healing process, using the excisional wound model in rats, and to prevent mechanical sensitization following plantar incision in rats in the postoperative model of pain. RESULTS: The MSDP method showed average recovery of 101.6 and 105.7% for I and II, respectively, with good precision (RSD < 2.0%) and selectivity, without interference of the excipients. The formulations were approved in the stability studies, maintaining conformity after 180 day of accelerated and long-term studies, with variation <10% in the analytical parameters. The phytomedicine reduced the ear edema in $37.6\% \pm 5.7\%$ and $64.8\% \pm 6.2\%$, for 0.5 and 1.0% of dried extract, respectively. The formulation also accelerated the healing process by up to $50.8\% \pm 4.1\%$ and $46.0\% \pm 4.0\%$ at 0.5% and 1.0% of extract, respectively, and both amounts were capable of preventing the development of mechanical sensitization following plantar incision in rats. CONCLUSIONS: The MSDP followed by HPLC-UV analytical method was appropriate for the quality control of the topical phytomedicine based on A. moluccana. The formulation developed at 0.5% and 1.0% of A. moluccana dried extract proved to be effective as an analgesic, anti-inflammatory and wound healing in the pre-clinical studies, which is in agreement with the ethnopharmacological data.

Chouhan, N. et al. (2015). "Self emulsifying drug delivery system (SEDDS) for phytoconstituents: A review." *Curr Drug Deliv* 12(2):244–253.

The self-emulsifying drug delivery system (SEDDS) is considered to be the novel technique for the delivery of lipophilic plant actives. The self-emulsifying (SE) formulation significantly enhance the solubility and bioavailability of poorly aqueous soluble phytoconstituents. The self-emulsifying drug delivery system (SEDDS) can be developed for such plant actives to enhance the oral bioavailability using different excipients (lipid, surfactant, co solvent etc.) and their concentration is selected on the basis of pre formulation studies like phase equilibrium studies, solvent capacity of oil for drug and mutual miscibility of excipients. The present review focuses mainly on the development of SEDDS and effect of excipients on oral bioavailability and aqueous solubility of poorly water soluble phytoconstituents/derived products. A recent list of patents issued for self-emulsifying herbal formulation has also been included. The research data for various self-emulsifying herbal formulation and patents issued were reviewed using different databases such as PubMed, Google Scholar, Google patents, Scopus and Web of Science. In a nutshell, we can say that SEDDS was established as a novel drug delivery system for herbals and with the advances in this technique, lots of patents on herbal SEDDS can be translated into the commercial products.

Deng, G. et al. (2011). "A single arm phase II study of a Far-Eastern traditional herbal formulation (sho-sai-ko-to or xiao-chai-hu-tang) in chronic hepatitis C patients." *J Ethnopharmacol* 136(1):83–87.

ETHNOPHARMACOLOGICAL RELEVANCE: Hepatitis C is a major public health problem internationally. Many patients cannot benefit from the current treatment regimen (interferon/ribavirin combinations) due to its side effects or ineffectiveness. Xiao-Chai-Hu-Tang or Sho-sai-ko-to (SST), a compound of seven botanical extracts used for liver diseases traditionally in East Asia, was shown to reduce transaminases and the incidence of hepatocellular carcinoma in hepatitis B patients. We conducted a phase II trial of SST in hepatitis C patients who were not candidates for interferon-based therapy to determine whether this agent is worthy of further study. MATERIALS AND METHODS: Twenty-four chronic hepatitis C patients received SST at 2.5 g per os (p.o.) three times daily (t.i.d.) for 12 months. Liver function, hepatitis C virus (HCV) viral load and liver biopsy histology were assessed before and after the intervention. RESULTS: Improvement of aspartate aminotransferase (AST) was observed in 16 (67%) of study participants. Improvement of alanine aminotransferase (ALT) was seen in 18 (75%) patients. Viral load response was mixed, with 7 patients showing reductions, 10 increases and 7 indeterminate due to assay limitations. Among the 9 (38%) subjects who showed improvement per Knodell's histology activity index (HAI) scores in paired comparison of pre- and post-treatment liver biopsy (the primary endpoints of the study), 5 (21%) showed an improvement of 2 points or greater, meeting the pre-defined criteria for response. CONCLUSIONS: Sho-sai-ko-to (SST or Xiao Chai Hu Tang) may improve liver pathology in selected hepatitis C patients who are not candidates for interferon-based treatment. Larger, controlled studies of this botanical formulation may be warranted.

Devi, A. J. et al. (2014). "Effect of ambrex (a herbal formulation) on oxidative stress in hyperlipidemic rats and differentiation of 3T3-L1 preadipocytes." *Pharmacogn Mag* 10(38):165–171.

BACKGROUND: Ambrex is a polyherbal formulation which consists of *Withania somnifera, Orchis mascula, Cycas circinalis, Shorea robusta* with amber. OBJECTIVE: The present study was designed to explore the potential effects of ambrex on the antioxidant status in high fat diet fed rats and to investigate the possible mechanisms focusing on the gene expression involved in adipogenesis and inflammation in 3T3-L1 cell line. MATERIALS AND METHODS: Male Wistar rats were divided into four groups ($n = 6$); Group A received normal diet, Group B received high fat diet for 30 days, Group C and D received high fat diet for 30 days and treated with ambrex (40 mg/kg b.w) and atorvastatin (10 mg/kg b.w) for successive 15 days respectively. This study also assesses the effect of ambrex on adipogenesis in 3T3-L1 adipocytes.

RESULTS: The serum total cholesterol and triglycerides were significantly decreased in ambrex treated hyperlipidemic animals when compared to untreated animals. The activities of catalase, superoxide dismutase and reduced glutathione were significantly augmented in the serum, liver, and heart of hyperlipidemic rats treated with ambrex when compared to control. Ambrex treated rats had significant reductions in malondialdehyde levels in the serum, liver and heart compared to untreated rats. In addition, we observed that treatment with ambrex resulted in a major inhibition of pre-adipocyte differentiation of 3T3-L1 cells in vitro by suppression of peroxisome proliferator activated receptor gamma, sterol regulatory binding proteins, tumor necrosis factor-alpha, inducible nitricoxide synthase, leptin, and upregulation of thioredoxin 1 (TRX1) and TRX2 mRNA expression. CONCLUSION: Therefore, ambrex may be a potential drug for treatment of hyperlipidemia and related disorders.

Dutta, S. and M. L. Gupta (2014). "Alleviation of radiation-induced genomic damage in human peripheral blood lymphocytes by active principles of *Podophyllum hexandrum*: An in vitro study using chromosomal and CBMN assay." *Mutagenesis* 29(2):139–147.

This study was aimed to evaluate the protection against radiation of human peripheral blood lymphocytic DNA by a formulation of three isolated active principles of *Podophyllum hexandrum* (G-002M). G-002M in various concentrations was administered 1 hour prior to irradiation in culture media containing blood. Radioprotective efficacy of G-002M to lymphocytic DNA was estimated using various parameters such as dicentrics, micronuclei (MN), nucleoplasmic bridges (NPB) and nuclear buds (NuB) in binucleated cells. Certain experiments to ascertain the G2/M arrest potential of G-002M were also conducted. It was effective in arresting the cells even at half of the concentration of colchicine used. Observations demonstrated a radiation-dose-dependent increase in dicentric chromosomes (DC), acentric fragments, MN, NPB and NuB upto 5Gy. These changes were found significantly decreased by pre-administration of G-002M. A highly significant dose modifying factor (DMF) 1.43 and 1.39 based on dicentric assay and cytokinesis block micronuclei assay, respectively, was observed against 5 Gy exposure in the current experiments. G-002M alone in its effective dose did not induct any change in any of the parameters mentioned above. Observations on cell cycle arrest by G-002M showed that the formulation has potential in arresting cells at G2/M, compared with colchicine. Based on significant DMF at highest radiation dose (5Gy) studied currently and meaningful reduction in radiation-induced chromosomal aberrations, we express that G-002M has a potential of minimizing radiation-induced DNA (cytogenetic) damage.

Enioutina, E. Y. et al. (2017). "Phytotherapy as an alternative to conventional antimicrobials: Combating microbial resistance." *Expert Rev Clin Pharmacol* 10(11):1203–1214.

INTRODUCTION: In the modern antimicrobial era, the rapid spread of resistance to antibiotics and introduction of new and mutating viruses is a global concern. Combating antimicrobial resistant microbes (AMR) requires coordinated international efforts that incorporate new conventional antibiotic development as well as development of alternative drugs with antimicrobial activity, management of existing antimicrobials, and rapid detection of AMR pathogens. Areas covered: This manuscript discusses some conventional strategies to control microbial resistance.

The main purpose of the manuscript is to present information on specific herbal medicines that may serve as good treatment alternatives to conventional antimicrobials for infections sensitive to conventional as well as resistant strains of microorganisms. Expert commentary: Identification of potential new antimicrobials is challenging; however, one source for potential structurally diverse and complex antimicrobials are natural products. Natural products may have advantages over other post-germ theory antimicrobials. Many antimicrobial herbal medicines possess simultaneous antibacterial, antifungal, antiprotozoal and/or antiviral properties. Herbal products have the potential to boost host resistance to infections, particularly in immunocompromised patients. Antimicrobial broad-spectrum activity in conjunction with immunostimulatory properties may help to prevent microbial resistance to herbal medicine. As part of the efforts to broaden use of herbal medicines to treat microbial infections, pre-clinical and clinical testing guidelines of these compounds as a whole should be implemented to ensure consistency in formulation, efficacy and safety.

Fatima, S. et al. (2017). "Design and development of Unani anti-inflammatory cream." *J Ayurveda Integr Med* 8(3):140–144.

Inflammation is the symptom of many diseases like rheumatoid arthritis and osteoarthritis. Many side effects are associated with the Non-Steroidal Anti-inflammatory Drugs (NSAIDs) used as conventional treatment for these conditions. In Unani, there are large number of single and compound drugs for inflammatory conditions. One dosage form of Unani system of medicine is named as Zimad in which paste is formed by mixing powder in oil, water, herbal extract. Zimadat is prepared just before application and used in many disease conditions as resolving, styptic, astringent, and antiseptic. As the pre-application procedure is difficult and also complicated for patients, hence, the present study attempted to modify the form of Zimad into cream. Various batches of cream of Zimad Mohallil were prepared by using extracts of the formulation and by adding additives. Various physicochemical parameters of prepared cream were carried and compared with market cream. The optimized cream of Zimad Mohallil (F4) was selected after preliminary tests and evaluated further. The optimized cream showed good results in physicochemical parameters equivalent to market sample. Zimad Mohallil was converted into convenient cream form by adding minimum additives and benefits could be achieved without any hassle and cumbersome work, which is encountered in crude or paste form. The optimized cream was equivalent to standard market cream.

Feher, P. et al. (2016). "Efficacy of pre- and post-treatment by topical formulations containing dissolved and suspended silybum marianum against UVB-induced oxidative stress in guinea pig and on HaCaT Keratinocytes." *Molecules* 21(10).

Plants with high amounts of antioxidants may be a promising therapy for preventing and curing UV-induced oxidative skin damage. The objective of this study was to verify the efficacy of topical formulations containing dissolved and suspended Silybum marianum extract against UVB-induced oxidative stress in guinea pig and HaCaT keratinocytes. Herbal extract was dissolved in Transcutol HP (TC) and sucrose-esters were incorporated as penetration enhancers in creams. Biocompatibility of compositions was tested on HeLa cells and HaCaT keratinocytes as in vitro models. Transepidermal water loss (TEWL) tests were performed to prove the safety of formulations in vivo. Drug release of different compositions was assessed by Franz diffusion methods. Superoxide dismutase (SOD), catalase (CAT), glutathione peroxidase (GPx) and lipid peroxidation (MDA) activities were evaluated before and after UVB irradiation in a guinea pig model and HaCaT cells. Heme oxygenase-1 (HO-1) enzyme activity was measured in the epidermis of guinea pigs treated by different creams before and after UVB irradiation. Treatment with compositions containing silymarin powder (SM) dissolved in TC and sucrose stearate SP 50 or SP 70 resulted in increased activities of all reactive oxygen species (ROS) eliminating enzymes in the case of pre- and post-treatment as well. Reduction in the levels of lipid peroxidation end products was also detected after treatment with these two compositions. Post-treatment was more effective as the increase of the activity of antioxidants was higher. Lower HO-1 enzyme levels were measured in the case of pre- and post-treatment groups compared to control groups. Therefore, this study demonstrates the effectiveness of topical formulations containing silymarin in inhibiting UVB irradiation induced oxidative stress of the skin.

Gao, Y. et al. (2013). "A protocol for the classification of wet mass in extrusion-spheronization." *Eur J Pharm Biopharm* 85(3 Pt B):996–1005.

In this study, a structured protocol for the classification of wet mass in extrusion-spheronization was developed to predict formation and pellet quality. The wet masses of 120 formulae were prepared taking microcrystalline celluloses as pelletization aid and lactose, hydroxypropyl methylcellulose grades, herbal medicines as model drugs. Physical properties of the wet masses such as hardness, adhesiveness, springiness, cohesiveness, chewiness, and resilience were tested, respectively, using a texture analyzer. Particles were produced by spheronization process, and the quality of spherical pellets was also evaluated. Data were analyzed by principal component analysis, factor analysis, and classification analysis. The wet masses could be classified into five groups taking the ratio of hardness to springiness (Ha/Sp) as the first classification index and chewiness, resilience as the second and the third classification index. The wet masses of different classification could correspondingly form the different shapes. So, a new protocol could be devised, for example, if the range of Ha/Sp of the wet masses was 30,992–47,689 g, at the same time, the value of chewiness was less than 4842, and the value of resilience was no more than 0.139; it would form spherical pellets under the experimental condition. These results demonstrate that the proposed protocol could be a valuable asset in a formulation development project to assess the physical properties of wet masses and to predict formation and pellet quality. So, the tedious and expensive pre-production (pre-formulation and optimization) work could be considerably reduced.

Ghosh, A. et al. (2017). "Male contraceptive efficacy of poly herbal formulation, contracept-TM, composed of aqueous extracts of Terminalia chebula fruit and Musa balbisiana seed in rat." *Pharm Biol* 55(1):2035–2042.

CONTEXT: *Terminalia chebula* Retz (Combretaceae) and *Musa balbisiana* Colla (Musaceae) have a traditional reputation as a male contraceptive. OBJECTIVE: To determine the hypo-testicular activity of aqueous extracts of Terminalia chebula (fruit) and Musa balbisiana (seed) separately, and in composite manner at the ratio of 1:1 named as "Contracept-TM" compared to cyproterone acetate (CPA), for developing a polyherbal contraceptive. MATERIALS AND METHODS: The separate extract of above said plants or "Contracept-TM" at the dose of 40 mg/100 g body weight of rat/day or CPA at 2 mg/100 g body weight of rat/day was administered for 28 days. Spermiological, androgenic and oxidative stress sensors, LD50 and ED50/100 g body weight values were measured. RESULTS: Treatment of individual, "Contracept-TM" or CPA resulted significant decrease in the count of spermatogonia A (36.36%– 49.09%), pre-leptotene spermatocyte (19.11%–55.30%), mid-pachytene spermatocyte (28.65%–47.28%) and step 7 spermatid (29.65%–51.59%). Activities of testicular Delta(5), 3beta (21.25%–48.02%),17beta-hydroxysteroid dehydrogenases (29.75%– 55.08%), catalase (19.06%–43.29%) and peroxidase (30.76%–62.82%), levels of testosterone (28.15%–63.44%), testicular cholesterol (19.61%–49.33%), conjugated diene (29.69%–84.99%) and thiobarbituric acid reactive substances (41.25%–86.73%) were elevated compare to the control. The ED50 and LD50 values were 40 mg and 5.8 g (*T. chebula*), 48 mg and 6.3 g (*M. bulbisiana*), 40 mg and 6.0 g ("Contracept-TM"), respectively. DISCUSSION AND CONCLUSION: The said spermiological and androgenic sensors' levels were decreased significantly by "Contracept-TM" than its constitutional individual plant extract and it may be comparable to standard anti-testicular drug like CPA. So, it may be concluded that above polyherbal formulation is potent for inducing hypo-testicular activity.

Gupta, A. et al. (2017). "Ethyl acetate fraction of *Eclipta alba*: A potential phytophar-maceutical targeting adipocyte differentiation." *Biomed Pharmacother* 96:572–583.

Natural products have always fascinated mankind for their miraculous properties. *Eclipta alba* (*E. alba*), a medicinal herb has long been used in traditional medicine for curing several pathologies. It has been shown to have anti-diabetic effect as well as hepato-protective activity. Here, in order to address metabolic derangements, the study was designed to evaluate the efficacy of *E. alba* and its fractions in adipogenesis inhibition and dyslipidemia. Of the crude extract and fractions screened, ethyl acetate fraction of *E. alba* inhibited adipocyte differentiation in 3T3-L1 pre-adipocytes and hMSC derived adipocytes. It inhibited mitotic clonal expansion and caused cell cycle arrest in G1 and S phase as suggested by western blot analysis and flow cytometry. It was also shown to have lipolytic effects. Oral administration of ethyl acetate fraction of *E. alba* to hamsters unveiled its anti-adipogenic as well as anti-dyslipidemic activity in vivo. Mass spectrometry analysis of ethyl acetate fraction confirmed the presence of several bioactive components, projecting it as an effective phytopharma-ceutical agent. In conclusion, ethyl acetate fraction of *E. alba* possesses potent anti-adipogenic as well as anti-dyslipidemic activity and could be projected as an herbal formulation towards obesity.

Kessler, C. S. et al. (2015). "Ayurvedic interventions for osteoarthritis: A systematic review and meta-analysis." *Rheumatol Int* 35(2):211–232.

Ayurveda is one of the fastest growing systems within complementary and alternative medicine. However, the evidence for its effectiveness is unsatisfactory. The aim of this work was to review and meta-analyze the effectiveness and safety of different Ayurvedic interventions in patients with osteoarthritis (OA). 138 electronic databases were searched through August 2013. Randomized controlled trials, randomized crossover studies, cluster-randomized trials, and non-randomized controlled clinical trials were eligible. Adults with pre-diagnosed OA were included as participants. Interventions were included as Ayurvedic if they were explicitly labeled as such. Main outcome measures were pain, physical function, and global improvement. Risk of bias was assessed using the Cochrane risk of bias tool. 19 randomized and 14 non-randomized controlled trials on 12 different drugs and 3 non-pharmaceutical interventions with a total of 2952 patients were included. For the compound preparation, Rumalaya, large and apparently unbiased effects beyond placebo were found for pain (standardized mean difference [SMD] −3.73; 95% confidence interval [CI] −4.97, −2.50; $P < 0.01$) and global improvement (risk ratio 12.20; 95% CI 5.83, 25.54; $P < 0.01$). There is also some evidence that effects of the herbal compound preparation Shunti-Guduchi are comparable to those of glucosamine for pain (SMD 0.08; 95% CI −0.20, 0.36; $P = 0.56$) and function (SMD 0.15; 95% CI −0.12, 0.36; $P = 0.41$). Based on single trials, positive effects were found for the compound preparations RA-11, Reosto, and Siriraj Wattana. For *Boswellia serrata*, *Lepidium sativum*, a *Boswellia serrata* containing multicomponent formulation and the compounds Nirgundi Taila, Panchatikta Ghrita Guggulu, and Rhumayog, and for non-pharmacological interventions like Ayurvedic massage, steam therapy, and enema, no evidence for significant effects against potential methodological bias was found. No severe adverse events were observed in all trials. The drugs Rumalaya and Shunti-Guduchi seem to be safe and effective drugs for treatment of OA-patients, based on these data. However, several limitations relate to clinical research on Ayurveda. Well-planned, well-conducted and well-published trials are warranted to improve the evidence for Ayurvedic interventions.

Kishor, B. et al. (2017). "Adaptogenic potential of Oxitard in experimental chronic stress and chronic unpredictable stress induced dysfunctional homeostasis in rodents." *J Ayurveda Integr Med* 8(3):169–176.

BACKGROUND: Oxitard, a polyherbal formulation comprising the extracts of *Withania somnifera*, *Mangifera indica*, *Glycyrrhiza glabra*, *Daucus carota*, *Vitis vinifera*, powders of *Syzygium aromaticum*, *Yashada bhasma* and *Emblica officinalis*; and oils of *Triticum sativum*. OBJECTIVE: Current study deals with the assessment of Oxitard (a marketed polyherbal formulation) for its adaptogenic potential in chronic unpredictable stress (CUS) and chronic stress (CS) induced dysfunctional homeostasis in rodents. MATERIALS & METHODS: Animals were immobilized for 2 hours every day for ten days to induce CS. In order to induce CUS, animals were employed in a battery of stressors of variable value and duration for 10 days. Following administration of Oxitard, stress was induced in the animals. Stress-induced efficient changes were evaluated by assessing organ (adrenal gland) weights, ulcer index, hematological parameters and biochemical levels of reduced glutathione (GSH), thiobarbituric acid reactive substances (TBARS) and catalase (CAT). RESULTS: CS and CUS significantly modified the oxidative stress parameters (increased MDA and decreased GSH). Furthermore, CS and CUS lead to weight reduction, adrenal hypertrophy and gastric ulceration. Pretreatment with Oxitard (200 and 400 mg/kg, p.o.) significantly modified CS and CUS induced hematological changes, oxidative stress parameters and pathological effects. CONCLUSION: In conclusion, Oxitard-intervened antioxidant actions are accountable for its adaptogenic effects in stress-induced dysfunctional homeostasis.

Liang, S. T. (2017). "Textual research on a prescription, 'Pill of Semen Plantaginis' in the Tangut medical documents unearthed in Khara-Khoto." *Zhonghua Yi Shi Za Zhi* 47(6):369–372.

A prescription, "Pill of Semen Plantaginisfor Treating All Diseases" (capital I, Cyrillic(HB).N(O).4384) carried in the Tangut medical documents unearthed in

Khara-Khoto was published in the 10(th) Volume of Heishuicheng Manuscript Collected in Russia. The prescription is composed of Herba Cistanches, Radix Achyranthis, Semen Plantaginis, white poria, Cortex Cinnamomi, Radix Aconiti preparata, Semen Cuscutae and baked ginger, whose main function is invigorating kidney yang and nourishing kidney essence. This prescription has a close relationship with the Han prescription in central plain of China which may be based on certain lost Chinese medical book.

Liang, W. et al. (2012). "Inhibitory effects of salviae miltiorrhizae radix (danshen) and puerariae lobatae radix (gegen) in carbachol-induced rat detrusor smooth muscle contractility." *Int J Physiol Pathophysiol Pharmacol* 4(1):36–44.

Both danshen (D) and gegen (G) have proven relaxant effects on vascular smooth muscle, thus their potential bladder inhibitory effects have impending interests in urology. The aim of this study was to demonstrate the novel effects of D and G on detrusor smooth muscle contractility. Urothelium-intact (+UE) and urothelium-denuded (−UE) detrusor strips were isolated from the rat. Isometric tension was measured using a myograph system. Carbachol (CCh) was used to pre-contract the detrusor strips prior to stepwise relaxation by adding extracts of D, G, and a DG (7:3) formulation. Tonic relaxation level and phasic contractile activity under the herbal treatments were analyzed. There was no difference in the herbal effects between +UE and −UE strips. D alone induced a much smaller relaxation than G alone or DG. G alone also suppressed phasic amplitude but not phasic frequency while DG suppressed both parameters. D and G acted synergistically to yield the observed effects on detrusor smooth muscle. The findings showed that the DG formulation were able to relax the detrusor as well as suppress phasic contractions, both actions important in maintaining normal bladder filling and urine storage processes. Hence DG may have new application in the management of bladder disorders.

Mao, G. X. et al. (2015). "Salidroside protects against premature senescence induced by ultraviolet B irradiation in human dermal fibroblasts." *Int J Cosmet Sci* 37(3):321–328.

OBJECTIVES: Salidroside, the predominant component of a Chinese herbal medicine, *Rhodiola rosea* L., becomes an attractive bio-agent due to its multifunction. Although it is well proposed that this herbal medicine may have photoprotective effect according to the folk hearsay, the direct supportive experimental evidences linking the drug with skin ageing have rarely been reported so far. The study was conducted to investigate the photoprotective role of salidrosdie and its related mechanisms in vitro. METHODS: First, a premature senescence model induced by UVB irradiation (250 mJ cm(−2)) in human dermal fibroblasts (HDFs) was established, and senescent phenotypes were evaluated by cell morphology, cell proliferation, senescence-associated beta-galactosidase (SA-beta-gal) activity and cell cycle distribution. Then the photoprotective effect of salidroside was investigated. Cells were pre-treated with various doses of salidroside (1, 5 and 10 μM) followed by the sublethal dosage of UVB exposure and then were harvested for various detections, including senescence-associated phenotypes and molecules, alteration of oxidative stress, matrix metalloproteinase-1 (MMP-1) secretion and inflammatory response. RESULTS: Pre-treatment of salidroside dose dependently reversed the senescent state of HDFs induced by UVB as evidenced by elevated cell viability, decreased

SA-beta-gal activity and relieving of G1/G0 cell cycle arrest. UVB-induced increased protein expression of cyclin-dependent kinase (CDK) inhibitors p21(WAF) (1) and p16(INK) (4) was also repressed by salidrosdie treatment in a dose-dependent manner. Meanwhile, the increment of malondialdehyde (MDA) level in UVB-irradiated HDFs was inhibited upon salidroside treatment. Additionally, salidroside significantly attenuated UVB-induced synthesis of MMP-1 as well as the production of IL-6 and TNF-alpha in HDFs. CONCLUSION: Our data provided the evidences for the protective role of salidroside against UVB-induced premature senescence in HDFs probably via its anti-oxidative property and inhibition on production of MMP-1 and pro-inflammatory cytokines, which indicated its potential utilization as an active ingredient in the preparation of photoprotective formulation.

Menghini, L. et al. (2010). "Antiproliferative, protective and antioxidant effects of artichoke, dandelion, turmeric and rosemary extracts and their formulation." *Int J Immunopathol Pharmacol* 23(2):601–610.

Artichoke, dandelion, turmeric extracts and rosemary essential oil are commonly used as ingredients in many herbal preparations to treat hepatic and gallbladder disorders. In the present work we compare the activity of each single extract with a commercial mixture for antiproliferative, antiradical and protective effects against induced oxidant stress effect. In ABTS and DPPH tests, turmeric extract is the most active, followed by artichoke and dandelion. All samples exhibited antiproliferative activity in a dose-dependent manner against HepG2 cells. In the same cell lines, the protective effect of pre-treatment with the extracts were detected by evaluating the prostaglandin E2 release, a marker of oxidative stress induced by hydrogen peroxide. The treatments with the extracts were efficient in reducing the release of PGE2 induced by oxidative stimulus. The positive results of the cell viability test, together with the protective and antiradical activity confirm the rationale for the use of these ingredients in commercial formulations as a health aid tool in modern phytotherapy.

Moon, S. Y. et al. (2014). "Tryptanthrin protects hepatocytes against oxidative stress via activation of the extracellular signal-regulated kinase/NF-E2-related factor 2 pathway." *Biol Pharm Bull* 37(10):1633–1640.

Tryptanthrin [6,12-dihydro-6,12-dioxoindolo-(2,1-b)-quinazoline], originally isolated from Isatidis radix, has been characterized as having anti-microbial and anti-tumor activities. It is well-known that excess oxidative stress is one of the major factors causing cell damage in the liver. This study investigated the cytoprotective effects and molecular mechanism of tryptanthrin against tert-butyl hydroperoxide (tBHP)-induced oxidative stress in human hepatocyte-derived HepG2 cells. Tryptanthrin pretreatment blocked the reactive oxygen species production, mitochondrial dysfunction, and cell death induced by tBHP. Moreover, tryptanthrin reversed tBHP-induced GSH reduction. This study also confirmed the activation of nuclear factor erythroid 2-related factor 2 (Nrf2) by tryptanthrin as a plausible molecular mechanism for its cytoprotective effects. Specifically, tryptanthrin treatment induced nuclear translocation and transactivation of Nrf2 as well as phosphorylation of extracellular signal-regulated kinase (ERK), a potential upstream kinase of Nrf2. Tryptanthrin also up-regulated the expression of the heme oxygenase 1 and glutamate-cysteine ligase catalytic subunits, which are representative target genes of Nrf2. Moreover, inhibitor of ERK was used to verify the important role of the ERK-Nrf2 pathway in the hepatoprotective effects of tryptanthrin. In conclusion, this study demonstrated that tryptanthrin protects hepatocytes against oxidative stress through the activation of the ERK/Nrf2 pathway in HepG2 cells.

More, M. et al. (2017). "A Rosa canina—Urtica dioica—Harpagophytum procumbens/ zeyheri combination significantly reduces gonarthritis symptoms in a randomized, placebo-controlled double-blind study." *Planta Med* 83(18):1384–1391.

The special formulation MA212 (Rosaxan) is composed of rosehip (*Rosa canina* L.) puree/juice concentrate, nettle (*Urtica dioica* L.) leaf extract, and devil's claw (*Harpagophytum procumbens* DC. ex Meisn. or *Harpagophytum zeyheri* Decne.) root extract and also supplies vitamin D. It is a food for special medical purposes ([EU] No 609/2013) for the dietary management of pain in patients with gonarthritis. This 12 week randomized, placebo-controlled double-blind parallel-design study aimed to investigate the efficacy and safety of MA212 versus placebo in patients with gonarthritis. A 3D-HPLC-fingerprint (3-dimensional high-pressure liquid chromatography fingerprint) of MA212 demonstrated the presence of its herbal ingredients. Ninety-two randomized patients consumed 40 mL of MA212 ($n = 46$) or placebo ($n = 44$) daily. The Western Ontario and McMaster Universities Arthritis Index (WOMAC), quality-of-life scores at 0, 6, and 12 weeks, and analgesic consumption were documented. Statistically, the initial WOMAC subscores/scores did not differ between groups. During the study, their means significantly improved in both groups. The mean pre-post change of the WOMAC pain score (primary end-point) was 29.87 in the MA212 group and 10.23 in the placebo group. The group difference demonstrated a significant superiority in favor of MA212 (pU < 0.001; pt < 0.001). Group comparisons of all WOMAC subscores/scores at 6 and 12 weeks reached same significances. Compared to placebo, both physical and mental quality of life significantly improved with MA212. There was a trend towards reduced analgesics consumption with MA212, compared to placebo. In the final efficacy evaluation, physicians (pChi < 0.001) and patients (pChi < 0.001) rated MA212 superior to placebo. MA212 was well tolerated. This study demonstrates excellent efficacy for MA212 in gonarthritis patients.

Patel, M. M. et al. (2013). "Method development for Lawsone estimation in Trichup herbal hair powder by high-performance thin layer chromatography." *J Adv Pharm Technol Res* 4(3):160–165.

A simple, specific, accurate, precise and robust high-performance thin-layer chromatographic method has been developed and validated for estimation of Lawsone in Trichup herbal hair powder (coded as a THHP), polyherbal formulation. The chromatographic development was carried out on aluminum plates pre-coated with silica gel 60F254 and good resolution was achieved with Toluene: Ethyl acetate: Glacial acetic acid (8:1:1 v/v/v) as mobile phase. Lawsone detection was carried out densitometrically at 277 nm and obtained retardation factor value was 0.46 ± 0.02. The method was validated with respect to specificity, linearity, accuracy, precision and robustness. The calibration curve was achieved to be linear over a range of 5–60 µg/mL and regression coefficient was obtained 0.998. Accuracy of chromatographic method was evaluated by standard addition method; recovery was obtained $99.25\% \pm 0.61\%$. The peak purity of Lawsone was achieved 0.999 r. Relative standard deviation for intraday and inter-day precision was 0.37%–0.56% and 0.42%–0.55%, respectively.

The limit of detection and limit of quantification of the Lawsone were found to be 1.08 µg/m land 3.28 µg/mL, respectively. This result shows that the method was well validated. In the present study, the Lawsone content was found 0.322% ± 0.014% in THHP. This study reveals that the proposed high-performance thin layer chromatography method is accurate, fast and cost- effective for routine estimation of Lawsone in polyherbal formulation.

Patra, K. C. et al. (2010). "A validated HPTLC method for determination of trans-caryophyllene from polyherbal formulations." *Nat Prod Res* 24(20):1933–1938.

Formulations of traditional medicines are usually made up of a complex mixture of herbs. However, effective quality control methods in order to select materials of the right quality are lacking. "Amukkara choornam" is a polyherbal Siddha formulation used for gastritis, spleen enlargement, leucorrhoea, hiccups, anaemia, tuberculosis and kappa diseases. Trans-caryophyllene is an important constituent present in the ingredients of this formulation. In a literature survey, it was found that there is no such method for the quantification of trans-caryophyllene except gas chromatography or gas chromatography-mass spectroscopy (GC-MS). So, a high-performance thin layer chromatography (HPTLC) method was developed and validated for the quantification of trans-caryophyllene in amukkara choornam. Pre-coated silica gel 60F-254 plates (10×10 cm(2)) were used for the analysis. The solvent system consisted of toluene-ethyl acetate (9: 3, v/v), and trans-caryophyllene was detected at 260 nm. The developed method was validated for linearity (R(2) = 0.9996 ± 0.0034), limit of detection (LOD) (0.101 ng), limit of quantification (LOQ) (0.639 ng), accuracy (% recovery = 97.19 ± 1.204), and precision (CV < 5%, for both intra-day and inter-day precisions). The levels of trans-caryophyllene were found to be 3.5–4.10 microg per gram of herbal products.

Qiao, X. et al. (2016). "Compound to extract to formulation: A knowledge-transmitting approach for metabolites identification of Gegen-Qinlian Decoction, a traditional Chinese medicine formula." *Sci Rep* 6:39534.

Herbal medicines usually contain a large group of chemical components, which may be transformed into more complex metabolites in vivo. In this study, we proposed a knowledge-transmitting strategy for metabolites identification of compound formulas. Gegen-Qinlian Decoction (GQD) is a classical formula in traditional Chinese medicine (TCM). It is widely used to treat diarrhea and diabetes in clinical practice. However, only tens of metabolites could be detected using conventional approaches. To comprehensively identify the metabolites of GQD, a "compound to extract to formulation" strategy was established in this study. The metabolic pathways of single representative constituents in GQD were studied, and the metabolic rules were transmitted to chemically similar compounds in herbal extracts. After screening diversified metabolites from herb extracts, the knowledge was summarized to identify the metabolites of GQD. Tandem mass spectrometry (MS(n)), fragment-based scan (NL, PRE), and selected reaction monitoring (SRM) were employed to identify, screen, and monitor the metabolites, respectively. Using this strategy, we detected 131 GQD metabolites (85 were newly generated) in rats biofluids. Among them, 112 metabolites could be detected when GQD was orally administered at a clinical dosage (12.5 g/kg). This strategy could be used for systematic metabolites identification of complex Chinese medicine formulas.

Sai Saraswathi, V. et al. (2017). "Solar catalysed activity against methyl orange dye, cytotoxicity activity of MCF-7 cell lines and identification of marker compound by HPTLC of Lagerstroemia speciosa." *J Photochem Photobiol B* 170:263–270.

The investigation was aimed to quantify the Gallic acid present in Lagerstroemia speciosa leaves (Lythraceae). The High-Performance Thin Layer Chromatography (HPTLC) quantification was performed for acetone (AE), methanolic (ME) and chloroform (CE) extract of leaves of L. speciosa. The pre-coated silica gel 60 F254 was used for complete separation of compounds using the mobile phase pet. Ether: ethyl acetate: formic acid (5:5:1v/v). The validation of the extracts was carried out using ICH guidelines for precision, repeatability and accuracy showing the Rf 0.49 against standard Gallic acid. Linearity range for Gallic acid was done from 200 to 1000 ng/spot (AE) and 200 ng to 600 ng/spot (ME), with Correlation, coefficient $r = 0.99$ (AE) and 0.54 (ME) in the said concentrations. The composition in crude leaf extract was determined to be of 49.712 mg (AE) and 20.125 mg (ME), while it was not found in chloroform extract against standard Gallic acid. Hence the proposed method was very simple, precise, accurate and easy for the screening of the bioactive compounds present in the acetone and methanolic extracts of the leaves of L. speciosa. It was observed that the acetone extract subjected to cytotoxicity showed promising activity at higher concentrations (100 and 200 µg/mL) showed 92.9% and 87.13% inhibition against MCF-7 cell lines respectively. The photocatalytic activity of the acetone and methanolic extracts of methyl orange was found to be 90.25% (190 min) and 89.03% (180 min) respectively. Therefore, this can be used as an indicator of purity of herbal drugs and formulation containing L. speciosa.

Saif, M. W. et al. (2010). "Phase I study of the botanical formulation PHY906 with capecitabine in advanced pancreatic and other gastrointestinal malignancies." *Phytomedicine* 17(3–4):161–169.

PURPOSE: The botanical formulation, PHY906, has been used widely in Eastern countries to treat gastrointestinal symptoms including diarrhea, nausea and vomiting. PHY906 may also have anti-tumor properties and may potentiate the action of several chemotherapeutic agents based on pre-clinical studies. We conducted a Phase I study using PHY906 in combination with capecitabine in patients with advanced pancreatic and gastrointestinal malignances to determine the maximum tolerated dose (MTD) of capecitabine in combination with PHY906. PATIENTS AND METHODS: This study was a single institution, open-label, Phase I study of PHY906 800 mg BID on days 1–4 in combination with escalating doses of capecitabine (1000, 1250, 1500, and 1750 mg/m(2)) orally twice daily on days 1–7 of a 14–day cycle (7/7 schedule). Capecitabine was increased until the appearance of dose limiting toxicities (DLTs). Measurements of efficacy included tumor response by Response Evaluation Criteria in Solid Tumors (RECIST). RESULTS: Twenty-four patients with a median age of 67 years (range 40–84) with pancreatic cancer (15), colon cancer (6), cholangiocarcinoma (1), esophageal cancer (1) and unknown primary (1) received a total of 116 cycles (median 5 cycles; range 1–17 cycles) over 4 dose levels of capecitabine. One DLT (Grade 4 AST/ALT, Grade 3 hyponatremia) was observed in the 1000 mg/m(2) cohort of patients. No further DLT was observed in the subsequent cohorts and doses of capecitabine were escalated to 1750 mg/m(2) BID. There were no DLTs at the maximum dose level of 1750 mg/m(2), however, the delivered dose-intensity of capecitabine was similar at the 1750 mg/m(2) dose level as the 1500 mg/m(2) dose level. Therefore, the MTD was defined at 1500 mg/m(2) of capecitabine in this dosing schedule with PHY906. One patient achieved a partial response, and 13 patients had stable disease that lasted more than six weeks. CONCLUSION: The MTD of capecitabine was determined to be 1500 mg/m(2) BID administered in a 7/7 schedule, in combination with PHY906 800 mg BID on days 1–4. This combination was well tolerated and warrants further study.

Shanmugasundaram, D. et al. (2016). "Development of an antidiabetic polyherbal formulation (ADPHF6) and assessment of its antioxidant activity against ROS-induced damage in pUC19 and human lymphocytes—An in vitro study." *J Complement Integr Med* 13(3):267–274.

BACKGROUND: Polyherbalism, an alternative natural-based therapy for various disorders, has been quoted about 1300 years before in Sharangdhar Samhita. Herbal-based combination therapy stages a vital role for the treatment of type 2 diabetes mellitus (T2DM) and associated complications. The present study aims at developing an Ayurvedic-based polyherbal formulation (ADPHF6) and the assessing its antidiabetic and antioxidant property. METHODS: ADPHF6 polyherbal formulation was measured for phytochemical components by qualitative methods. The polyherbal formulation was quantitatively estimated for its phytochemical constituents, i.e. total phenol and flavonoid content. Further, the antioxidant property of ADPHF6 formulation was evaluated by 2,2-diphenyl-1-picryl-hydrazyl-hydrate (DPPH) radical scavenging assay, hydrogen peroxide radical scavenging assay and metal chelating assay. alpha-Amylase and alpha-glucosidase inhibitory activities of polyherbal formulation were also assessed. ADPHF6 was further analyzed for its protective antioxidant property against reactive oxygen species (ROS)-induced damage in human lymphocyte DNA and pUC19 plasmid. RESULTS: ADPHF6 polyherbal formulation revealed the presence of phytochemical constituents such as alkaloids, flavonoids, phenols, tannins, terpenoids, saponins and cardiac glycosides in significant levels. Further, it also measured the higher levels of total phenols (473.3 ± 3.05 mg/g) and flavonoid (664 ± 5.29 mg/g) content. Polyherbal formulation also exhibited IC50 values of 49.9 ± 0.15, 65.1 ± 0.10 and 60.1 ± 0.05 mg/mL for 2,2- diphenyl-1-picryl-hydrazyl-hydrate (DPPH), hydrogen peroxide (H2O2) and Fe2+ radical scavenging activities, respectively. ADPHF6 revealed an inhibitory activity (IC50) of 0.67 ± 0.01 and 0.81 ± 0.01 mg/mL for alpha-amylase and glucosidase, respectively. Pre-treated human peripheral blood lymphocytes with ADPHF6 aqueous extract illustrated enhanced protection against ROS-mediated damage as compared with post-treated groups. DNA nicking assay rendered protective activity against the OH radical-induced DNA damage in supercoiled pUC19 plasmid. CONCLUSIONS: Our present study demonstrates that ADPHF6 offers potent inhibitory activity against free radicals as well as digestive enzymes. However, studies should be conducted using in vivo model to further elucidate the effect against free radicals and its anti-hyperglycemic activity in the management of non-insulin-dependent diabetes.

Shanmugasundaram, S. et al. (2011). "Determination and estimation of pharmacokinetic profile of caffeine in form of extract of green tea leaves and its analogy with synthetic form." *Indian J Pharm Sci* 73(6):649–655.

The aim of the study was to formulate and investigate the pharmacokinetic parameters for the tablets of herbal extract of caffeine with comparison to synthetic formulation. The tablets of the aqueous herbal extract of leaves of Camellia sinensis and synthetic caffeine were formulated by wet granulation technique. The HPLC and HPTLC were applied as analytical tools for estimation of caffeine. The batches of formulation (B1 to B7) were subjected for various pre and post-formulation studies. The pharmacokinetic of the batch B5 was assessed in rabbits, and the results were compared to synthetic batch B7. With the suitable pre and post-formulation results, the B5 showed in vitro release of 90.54% of caffeine at the end of 60 min. The release followed first order kinetics and the plot of Higuchi and Peppas confirms anomalous diffusion as the basic mechanism behind the release. B5 revealed non-significant mean C(max), t(1/2), and AUC of 1.88 μg/mL, 5.52 hours and 9.67 μg.h/mL respectively compared to B7. The study highlights; no significant difference in the pharmacological effect of caffeine when administered in the form of extract. The administration of herbal extract can further provide the other health benefits lacked by synthetic caffeine.

Shen, L. et al. (2012). "Pharmacokinetics of characteristic effective ingredients from individual and combination Shaoyao and Gancao treatment in rats using HPLC fingerprinting." *Eur J Drug Metab Pharmacokinet* 37(2):133–140.

Shaoyao-Gancao decoction, a traditional Chinese formulation composed of Paeoniae Radix and Glycyrrhizae Radix, is commonly used to relieve abdominal pain. In this paper, the compatibility rationality of this decoction was investigated. Shaoyao-Gancao decoction, Shaoyao decoction and Gancao decoction were orally administered to rats, respectively. Blood samples were collected at pre-determined times after administration and analyzed by high-performance liquid chromatography (HPLC). The pharmacokinetic parameters of characteristic peaks were analyzed and the statistical significance of the obtained parameters was determined. Paeoniflorin (12.0 min) and compounds at retention times of 4.7 and 5.2 min were all significantly higher in the Shaoyao-Gancao decoction than in the Shaoyao decoction ($P < 0.05$). In contrast, in the Gancao decoction, the compound at a retention time of 14.6 min was significantly lower than in the Shaoyao-Gancao decoction ($P < 0.01$). However, the compounds at retention times of 17.1 and 18.1 min were significantly higher in the Gancao decoction than in the Shaoyao-Gancao decoction ($P < 0.05$). These results indicate that poor compatibility of the compounds in the Shaoyao-Gancao decoction could result in poor absorption. The compatibility of the component compounds of the Shaoyao-Gancao decoction was revealed in the pharmacokinetic characteristics of the decoction. Generally, the absorption of Shaoyao components was increased in the Shaoyao-Gancao decoction, while the absorption of Gancao components was time dependent. In the Shaoyao-Gancao decoction, the increased absorption of some Shaoyao components may be related to a reduction in absorption of some Gancao components.

Shetty, R. N. et al. (2017). "Comparative evaluation of effect of use of toothbrush with paste and munident on levels of Streptococcus mutans and gingival health in children: An in vivo study." *J Indian Soc Pedod Prev Dent* 35(2):162–166.

AIM: Dental caries is a multifactorial disease which has a deleterious effect on the oral cavity. Improper oral hygiene habits are a cause for the same. The aim of this study was to compare the antibacterial efficacy of Munident, an Ayurvedic (herbal) dentifrice with commercially available toothpaste. MATERIALS AND METHODS: A total of forty subjects between the age group 9 and 12 years, resident of Bala Yeshu

Nilaya Bhavan, Mangalore, Karnataka, India, were chosen for our study. They were divided into two groups containing twenty subjects in each; Group 1 for standard toothpaste and Group 2 for Munident. The decayed, missing, and filled teeth scores were noted from each subject. Group 1 was instructed to brush the teeth using commercially available toothpaste and Group 2 was instructed to brush using commercially available Munident (herbal) dentifrice. Both the groups brushed the teeth using soft variety of tooth brush. The gingival bleeding index and salivary Streptococcus mutans count were noted pre- and post-brushing for both groups. The results obtained were subjected to statistical analysis. RESULTS: Munident (herbal) dentifrice showed better efficacy in comparison to toothpaste in terms of gingival bleeding index and salivary S. mutans count. CONCLUSION: Munident (herbal) dentifrice has better gingival bleeding index compared to standard formulation of toothpaste. Hence, the practice of using herbal dentifrice should be encouraged.

Singh, D. P. et al. (2015). "Hepatoprotective effect of a polyherbal extract containing Andrographis Paniculata, Tinospora Cordifolia and Solanum Nigrum against paracetamol induced hepatotoxicity." *Pharmacogn Mag* 11(Suppl 3):S375–S379.

BACKGROUND: Traditionally, a number of medicinal plants are used to treat various types of hepatic disorders but few of them were pharmacologically evaluated for their safety and efficacy. The combination of Andrographis paniculata (Kalmegha), Tinospora cordifolia (Guduchi), and Solanum nigrum (Kakmachi) was traditionally used in Indian System of Medicine (Ayurveda) for the treatment of various liver-related disorders. OBJECTIVE: In the present study, an attempt was made to substantiate the ethnopharmacological use of a traditional formulation in hepatoprotection against paracetamol-induced hepatotoxicity. SUBJECTS AND METHODS: Swiss albino mice (weight 20–25 g) were used for this study. Intraperitoneal injection of paracetamol (500 mg/kg body weight) was used to induce hepatotoxicity. Serum levels of alanine transaminase, aspartate aminotransferase, bilirubin, alkaline phosphatase, were used as indices of liver injury. In addition, total cholesterol, triglyceride, low-density lipoprotein, high-density lipoprotein and creatinine were also assayed using the standard procedure. RESULTS: Among the two different doses, pretreatment with Polyherbal extract at 500 mg/kg body weight exhibited a significant ($P < 0.05$) hepatoprotective activity as compared to paracetamol group. CONCLUSION: The polyherbal extract exhibits a significant hepatoprotective effect in vivo. The study contributes to its use in traditional Ayurveda system for the management of liver diseases. SUMMARY: Traditionally, a number of medicinal plants are used to treat various types of liver disorders but few of them were pharmacologically evaluated for their safety and efficacy. Combination of Andrographis paniculata (Kalmegha), Tinospora cordifolia (Guduchi), and Solanum nigrum (Kakmachi) was traditionally used in Ayurveda for the treatment of various liver related disorders. In the present study an attempt was made to validate the ethnopharmacological use of a traditional formulation in hepatoprotection against paracetamol induced hepatotoxicity. Swiss albino mice (weight 20–25 g) were used for this study. Intraperitoneal injection (IP) of paracetamol (500 mg/kg body weight) was used to induce hepatotoxicity. Serum levels of Alanine transaminase (ALT), Aspartate Aminotransferase (AST), Bilirubin, and Alkaline phosphatase (ALP) were used as indices of liver injury. In addition, total cholesterol, triglyceride, Low density lipoprotein (LDL), High density lipoprotein (HDL), and creatinine were also assayed using standard procedure.

Among the two different doses, pre-treatment with Polyherbal extract at 500 mg/kg body weight exhibited a significant ($P < 0.05$) hepatoprotective activity as compared to paracetamol group. The polyherbal extract exhibits significant hepatoprotective effect in vivo. The study contributes to its use in traditional Ayurveda system for the management of liver diseases.

Singh, D. P. and D. Mani (2015). "Protective effect of Triphala Rasayana against paracetamol-induced hepato-renal toxicity in mice." *J Ayurveda Integr Med* 6(3):181–186.

BACKGROUND: Paracetamol, a widely used analgesic and antipyretic, is known to cause liver and renal injury in humans when administered in higher and repeated doses that cause acute liver injury. Triphala is a well-known Ayurvedic Rasayana formulation that is prescribed for balancing of Vata, Pitta and Kapha. Traditionally, it is used for the treatment of liver and kidney diseases. OBJECTIVE: The present study was undertaken to examine the protective effect of Triphala extract against paracetamol-induced hepato-renal injury in Swiss albino mice. MATERIALS AND METHODS: Swiss albino mice (weight 20–25 g) were used in this study. The mice were divided into five groups of six animals each. The aqueous extract of Triphala was given orally at two different doses (100 and 300 mg/kg body weight) for seven consecutive days, followed by a single intraperitoneal injection of paracetamol (500 mg/kg body weight) to induce hepato-renal toxicity. Serum levels of liver enzymes, aspartate aminotransferase (AST), alanine aminotransferase (ALT), alkaline phosphatase (ALP), bilirubin, creatinine, urea and uric acid were measured as indices of liver and renal injury. All the statistical analyses were performed with the help of one-way analysis of variance (ANOVA) followed by Student-Newman-Keuls test as post hoc test. Results were considered statistically significant when $P < 0.05$. RESULTS: Pre-treatment with Triphala extract at 100 mg/kg and 300 mg/kg body weight exhibited a significant ($P < 0.01$) hepatoprotective activity. The protective effect of Triphala extract at 300 mg/kg body weight appears more effective than 100 mg/kg body weight. CONCLUSION: The present study gives an evidence of the protective role of Triphala extract against paracetamol-induced hepato-renal toxicity and validates its traditional claim in the Ayurveda system.

Tan, C. S. et al. (2018). "Anti-hypertensive and vasodilatory effects of amended Banxia Baizhu Tianma Tang." *Biomed Pharmacother* 97:985–994.

Although Banxia Baizhu Tianma Tang (BBT) has been long administered for hypertensive treatment in Traditional Chinese Medicine (TCM), the ratio of the herbal components that makes up the formulation has not been optimized with respect to the anti-hypertensive effect that it inherently possesses. A newly amended BBT (ABBT) formulation was developed using the evidence-based approach of orthogonal stimulus-response compatibility model. The ABBT showed enhanced therapeutic effect while maintaining its traditional theoretical approach rooted in TCM. This study was designed to investigate the possible mechanism of actions involved in the vasodilatory activity of ABBT-50 by evaluating its vasodilative effect on isolated Sprague Dawley rats in the presence of absence of various antagonists. When pre-contracted with phenylephrine, relaxation was observed in endothelium intact (EC50 = 0.027 ± 0.003 mg/mL, Rmax = $109.8\% \pm 2.12\%$) and denuded aortic rings (EC50 = 0.409 ± 0.073 mg/mL, Rmax = $63.15\% \pm 1.78\%$), as well as in endothelium intact aortic rings pre-contracted with potassium chloride (EC50 = 32.7 ± 12.16 mg/mL, Rmax = 34.02% ± 3.82%). Significant decrease in the vasodilative effect of ABBT-50 was observed in the presence of Nomega-nitro-l-arginine methyl ester (EC50 = 0.12 ± 0.021 mg/mL, Rmax = 75.33% ± 3.28%), 1H-[1,2,4] Oxadiazolo[4,3-a]quinoxalin-1-one(EC50=0.463±0.18mg/mL,Rmax=54.48%±2.02%), methylene blue (EC50 = 0.19 ± 0.037 mg/mL, Rmax = 83.69% ± 3.19%), indomethacin (EC50 = 0.313 ± 0.046 mg/mL, Rmax = 71.33% ± 4.12%), atropine (EC50 = 0.146 ± 0.013 mg/mL, Rmax = 77.2% ± 3.41%), and 4-aminopyridine (EC50 = 0.045 ± 0.008mg/mL, Rmax = 95.55% ± 2.36%). ABBT-50 was also suppressing Ca(2+) release from sarcoplasmic reticulum and inhibiting calcium channels. Vasodilatory effects of ABBT-50 are mediated through NO/sGC/cGMP cascade and PGI2, followed by muscarinic pathways and calcium channels.

Tan, W. S. D. et al. (2017). "Is there a future for andrographolide to be an anti-inflammatory drug? Deciphering its major mechanisms of action." *Biochem Pharmacol* 139:71–81.

Andrographis paniculata has long been part of the traditional herbal medicine system in Asia and in Scandinavia. Andrographolide was isolated as a major bioactive constituent of A. paniculata in 1951, and since 1984, andrographolide and its analogs have been scrutinized with modern drug discovery approach for anti-inflammatory properties. With this accumulated wealth of pre-clinical data, it is imperative to review and consolidate different sources of information, to decipher the major anti-inflammatory mechanisms of action in inflammatory diseases, and to provide direction for future studies. Andrographolide and its analogs have been shown to provide anti-inflammatory benefits in a variety of inflammatory disease models. Among the diverse signaling pathways investigated, inhibition of NF-kappaB activity is the prevailing anti-inflammatory mechanism elicited by andrographolide. There is also increasing evidence supporting endogenous antioxidant defense enhancement by andrographolide through Nrf2 activation. However, the exact pathway leading to NF-kappaB and Nrf2 activation by andrographolide has yet to be elucidated. Validation and consensus on the major mechanistic actions of andrographolide in different inflammatory conditions are required before translating current findings into clinical settings. There are a few clinical trials conducted using andrographolide in fixed combination formulation which have shown anti-inflammatory benefits and good safety profile. A concerted effort is definitely needed to identify potent andrographolide lead compounds with improved pharmacokinetics and toxicological properties. Taken together, andrographolide and its analogs have great potential to be the next new class of anti-inflammatory agents, and more andrographolide molecules are likely moving towards clinical study stage in the near future.

Tian, J. Y. et al. (2013). "Investigation of a compound, compatibility of Rhodiola crenulata, Cordyceps militaris, and Rheum palmatum on metabolic syndrome treatment III—Controlling blood glucose." *Zhongguo Zhong Yao Za Zhi* 38(10):1570–1576.

Base on the improvement of compound FF16, compatibility of Rhodiola crenulata, Cordyceps militaris, and Rheum palmatum, on both insulin resistance and obesity, its effects on type 2 diabetes (T2DM) was investigated here. The results showed that the levels of fasting and no-fasting blood glucose were controlled in the spontaneous type 2 diabetes KKAy mice; the impaired glucose tolerance (IGT)was improved by decreasing significantly the values of the glucose peaks and the area under the blood glucose-time curve (AUC) after glucose-loading in glucose tolerance test (OGTT) in both high-fat-diet-induced pre-diabetes IRF mice and KKAy mice, respectively. The pancreatic histopathological analysis showed that the increased islet amount, the enlarged islet area, and the lipid accumulation in the pancreas were reversed by FF16 treatment in both IRF mice and KKAy mice. In the palmitate-induced RINm5f cell model, FF16 could effectively reduce the apoptosis and enhance the glucose-stimulated insulin secretion, respectively. In conclusion, FF16 could improve the T2DM by protecting the pancreatic beta-cells.

Wang, N. and X. Yang (2011). "Chemical constitutents from pre-formulation of lonicerae japonicae flos in shuanghuanglian lyophilized powder for injection." *Zhongguo Zhong Yao Za Zhi* 36(12): 1613–1619.

OBJECTIVE: To research the chemical constitutents for the pre-formulation of *Lonicerae japonicae* Flos (the dried buds of *Lonicera japonica*) in Shuanghuanglian lyophilized powder for injection and provide substance foundation for the adverse reaction of Shuanghuanglian lyophilized powder for injection. METHOD: The chemical constituents were isolated by column chromatography and preparative HPLC. All structures were characterized by the spectroscopic methods including ESI-MS, 1H-NMR, 13C-NMR, and compared with data in the literature. RESULT: Twenty compounds were isolated and identified as sophoraricoside(1), luteolin-7-O-beta-D-glucopyranoside(2), rutin(3), quercetin(4), 3,5-*O*-dicaffeoyl quinic acid methyl ester(5), 4,5-*O*-dicaffeoyl quinic acid methyl ester(6), 3,4-*O*-dicaffeoyl quinic acid methyl ester(7), 4,5-dicaffeoyl quinic acid(8), 3,4-dicaffeoyl quinic acid(9), chlorogenic acid(10), epi-vogeloside (11), sweroside(12), vogeloside(13), secoxyloganin(14), macranthoidin A(15), macranthoidin B(16), loniceroside A(17), loniceroside B(18), loniceroside C(19), dipsacoside B(20). CONCLUSION: Compound 1 was identified in genus *Lonicera* for the first time and compounds 1–20 were isolated from the pre-formulation for the first time.

Wells, T. N. (2011). "Natural products as starting points for future anti-malarial therapies: Going back to our roots?" *Malar J* 10(Suppl 1):S3.

BACKGROUND: The discovery and development of new anti-malarials are at a crossroads. Fixed-dose artemisinin combination therapy is now being used to treat a hundred million children each year, with a cost as low as 30 cents per child, with cure rates of over 95%. However, as with all anti-infective strategies, this triumph brings with it the seeds of its own downfall, the emergence of resistance. It takes ten years to develop a new medicine. New classes of medicines to combat malaria, as a result of infection by *Plasmodium falciparum* and *Plasmodium vivax* are urgently needed. RESULTS: Natural product scaffolds have been the basis of the majority of current anti-malarial medicines. Molecules such as quinine, lapachol and artemisinin were originally isolated from herbal medicinal products. After improvement with medicinal chemistry and formulation technologies, and combination with other active ingredients, they now make up the current armamentarium of medicines. In recent years advances in screening technologies have allowed testing of millions of compounds from pharmaceutical diversity for anti-malarial activity in cellular assays. These initiatives have resulted in thousands of new sub-micromolar active compounds—starting points for new drug discovery programmes. Against this backdrop, the paucity of potent natural products identified has been disappointing. Now is a good time to reflect on the current approach to screening herbal medicinal products and suggest revisions. Nearly sixty years ago, the Chinese doctor Chen Guofu, suggested natural products should be approached by dao-xing-ni-shi or "acting in the reversed order," starting with observational clinical studies. Natural products based on herbal remedies are in use in the community and have the potential unique advantage that clinical observational data exist, or can be generated. The first step should be the confirmation and definition of the clinical activity of herbal medicinal products already used by the community. This first step forms a solid basis of observations, before moving to in vivo pharmacological characterization and ultimately identifying the active ingredient. A large part of the population uses herbal medicinal products despite limited numbers of well-controlled clinical studies. Increased awareness by the regulators and public health bodies of the need for safety information on herbal medicinal products also lends support to obtaining more clinical data on such products. CONCLUSIONS: The relative paucity of new herbal medicinal product scaffolds active against malaria results discovered in recent years suggest it is time to re-evaluate the "smash and grab" approach of randomly testing purified natural products and replace it with a patient-data led approach. This will require a change of perspective form many in the field. It will require an investment in standardization in several areas, including: the ethnopharmacology and design and reporting of clinical observation studies, systems for characterizing anti-malarial activity of patient plasma samples ex vivo followed by chemical and pharmacological characterization of extracts from promising sources. Such work falls outside of the core mandate of the product development partnerships, such as MMV, and so will require additional support. This call is timely, given the strong interest from researchers in disease endemic countries to support the research arm of a malaria eradication agenda. Para-national institutions such as the African Network for Drugs and Diagnostics Innovation (ANDi) will play a major role in facilitating the development of their natural products patrimony and possibly clinical best practice to bring forward new therapeutics. As in the past, with quinine, lapinone and artemisinin, once the activity of herbal medicinal products in humans is characterized, it can be used to identify new molecular scaffolds which will form the basis of the next generation of anti-malarial therapies.

Xavier-Santos, J. B. et al. (2018). "Development of an effective and safe topical anti-inflammatory gel containing Jatropha gossypiifolia leaf extract: Results from a pre-clinical trial in mice." *J Ethnopharmacol* 227:268–278.

ETHNOPHARMACOLOGICAL RELEVANCE: *Jatropha gossypiifolia* L. (Euphorbiaceae) is a medicinal plant widely used in traditional medicine as an anti-inflammatory remedy. The topical use of the leaves and/or aerial parts of this plant as anti-inflammatory, analgesic, wound healing and anti-infective in several skin diseases is a common practice in many countries. The use of baths or dressings with this vegetal species is frequently reported in folk medicine. AIM OF THE STUDY: To evaluate the topical anti-inflammatory of aqueous extract from leaves of J. gossypiifolia and to develop a safe and effective herbal gel with anti-inflammatory potential. MATERIAL AND METHODS: First, the topical acute anti-inflammatory activity of J. gossypiifolia extract was evaluated in ear edema induced by single application of croton oil in mice. Then, a polaxamer-based gel containing J. gossypiifolia extract was developed, physicochemically characterized and evaluated in the same model of inflammation to assess whether the extract incorporation in gel would affect its anti-inflammatory potential. The best formulation was then assayed in ear edema induced by multiple applications of croton oil in mice, to evaluate its chronic anti-inflammatory potential. Inflammatory parameters evaluated included edema, nitrite concentration, mieloperoxidase (MPO) activity and oxidative damage in lipids and proteins. Finally, dermal irritation/corrosion test in mice was performed to access the safeness of the developed gel. Phytochemical characterization of J. gossypiifolia extract was performed by high performance liquid chromatography with diode array detector (HPLC-DAD) analysis. RESULTS: J. gossypiifolia showed significant acute anti-inflammatory activity in ear edema model, and this activity was significantly increased when equivalent amounts of extract was applied incorporated in the developed polaxamer gels. The gels containing different amounts of extract reduced significantly the levels of edema, nitrite and MPO enzyme in mice ears, with intensity similar to the anti-inflammatory standard drug dexamethasone. The gel containing 1.0% of extract was further evaluated and also showed significant anti-inflammatory activity in chronic inflammation test, reducing significantly ear edema, lipid peroxidation and depletion of reduced glutathione, similarly to dexamethasone. Placebo formulation as well as gel containing extract showed pH compatible to that of human skin and exhibited absence of signs of toxicity in mice, indicating the safeness of the developed product for topical use. HPLC analysis confirmed the presence of C-glycosylflavonoids (orientin, isoorientin, vitexin, and isovitexin) as the major compounds of J. gossypiifolia aqueous leaf extract. CONCLUSIONS: The results demonstrate the potentiality of J. gossypiifolia gel as a promising safe and effective topical anti-inflammatory agent for treatment of cutaneous inflammatory diseases.

Xu, F. F. et al. (2018). "Applying risk management to analytical methods for the desorbing process of ginkgo diterpene lactone meglumine injection." *Chin J Nat Med* 16(5):366–374.

Analysis errors can occur in the desorbing process of ginkgo diterpene lactone meglumine injection (GDMI) by a conventional analysis method, due to several factors, such as easily crystallized samples, solvent volatility, time-consuming sample pre-processing, fixed method, and offline analysis. Based on risk management, near-infrared (NIR) and mid-infrared (MIR) spectroscopy techniques were introduced to solve the above problems with the advantage of timely analysis and non-destructive nature towards samples. The objective of the present study was to identify the feasibility of using NIR or MIR spectroscopy techniques to increase the analysis accuracy of samples from the desorbing process of GDMI. Quantitative models of NIR and MIR were established based on partial least square method and the performances were calculated. Compared to NIR model, MIR model showed greater accuracy and applicability for the analysis of the GDMI desorbing solutions. The relative errors of the concentrations of Ginkgolide A (GA) and Ginkgolide B (GB) were 2.40% and 2.89%, respectively, which were less than 5.00%. The research demonstrated the potential of the MIR spectroscopy technique for the rapid and non-destructive quantitative analysis of the concentrations of GA and GB.

Yin, H. et al. (2018). "Rapid HPLC Analytical Method Development for Herbal Medicine Formulae Based on Retention Rules Acquired from the Constituting Herbs." *Anal Sci* 34(2):207–214.

Herbal medicine (HM) formulae are the combinations of two or more types of constituting herbs. This study has proposed a novel approach to efficiently develop HPLC methods for HM formulae, which take advantage of the mutual retention rules between HM formulae and their constituting herbs. An HM formula composed of two herbs, Radix Salviae Miltiorrhizae and Rhizoma Chuanxiong, was taken as a case study. Based on design of experiments and stepwise multiple linear regression, models relating the analytical parameters to the chromatographic parameters were built (correlation coefficients >0.9870) for chemical compounds in the two herbs. These models representing the retention rules were utilized to predict the elution profile of the formula. The analytical parameters were numerically optimized to ensure adequate separation of the analytes. In validation experiments, satisfactory separations were achieved without any pre-experiments on the formula. The approach can significantly increase the HPLC method development efficiency for HM formulae.

Zhao, H. et al. (2013). "Development and evaluation of Chinese medicine fire-heat syndrome scale in oral cavity for measuring Chinese herb toothpaste." *Chin J Integr Med* 19(3):192–199.

OBJECTIVE: To formulate the standard measuring tool for the evaluations on fire-heat syndrome in oral cavity by means of Chinese medicine (CM). METHODS: The measuring scale for fire-heat syndrome in the oral cavity by means of CM was investigated by symptom collection, item pool formulation, item selection, pre-investigation, evaluations on the reliability, validity and reactivity of the measuring scale, according to the principles for measuring scale design and under the guidance of CM theories. RESULTS: The measuring scale was composed of two integrative parts: the self-filling section and the interview section. As far as the reliability was concerned, the total Cronbach alpha coefficient of the measuring scale was 0.866, the total test-retest reliability coefficient was 0.726 and the split-half reliability coefficient was 0.851. As far as the validity was concerned, the scores for the subjects of fire-heat syndrome in oral cavity and healthy people in their oral cavity in the items of symptoms were statistically different ($P < 0.01$); three common divisors were extracted according to the theoretical dimensions, the accumulated contribution rate was 63.468%. As far as the reactivity was concerned, the difference between the symptom scores before and after the test in which 31 subjects used the Chinese herb toothpaste was statistically significant ($P < 0.01$). CONCLUSIONS: This measuring scale has relatively good reliability, validity and reactivity, and it can be used in an objective quantitative evaluation on patients suffering from fire-heat syndrome in oral cavity, and thus lay the foundations for the evaluations on the therapeutic effects of Chinese herb toothpaste on fire-heat syndrome in oral cavity.

Zhao, P. et al. (2011). "Analysis on changes of chemical compounds in different processed products of Euodiae fructus." *Zhongguo Zhong Yao Za Zhi* 36(5):559–562.

OBJECTIVE: To study the relationship among processing methods and chemical compounds. METHOD: HPLC was used to compare the difference between pre and post processing. The main peaks in chromatogram were identified and divided into groups of chemical compounds. The contents of identified compounds and groups of chemical compounds were also analyzed. RESULT: The chromatographic peaks were divided into three groups of chemical compounds that were flavonoid glocosides, uinazoline alkaloids and bitter principle, indoloquinazoline alkaloids. The contents of flavonoid glocosides were reduced in each processed product, and that in hot-water processing product were the least. The contents of all three groups of chemical compounds were decreased in Coptidis Rhizoma processing products. The dissolving release of quinolones alkaloids were increased in wine, salt, Glycyrrhizae Radix et Rhizoma and ginger processing products. CONCLUSION: Different processing methods caused different changes of chemical compounds.

Zulkifle, M. et al. (2014). "Management of non-healing leg ulcers in Unani system of medicine." *Int Wound J* 11(4):366–372.

Non-healing leg ulcers are becoming a major public health problem. The high prevalence of leg ulcer directly affects patients' quality of life because it produces psychological (anxiety, depression), social and physical (amputation) handicap. Most leg ulcers become unsightly and they hardly if ever, yield to conventional treatment. Healing of an amputated part may pose a problem; hence, amputation cannot be recommended without extensive pre-operative investigations. Prevalence is high among the poor, for whom expenses of surgery are not affordable. Few surgeons try skin graft but unfavorable local condition of the ulcer leads to rejection and all efforts prove futile. Keeping all these factors in mind, we have tested a Unani formulation for its ulcer healing properties; early results were surprising and in some cases unbelievable.

Index

Note: Page numbers in italic and bold refer to figures and tables, respectively.

abbreviated new drug applications (ANDAs) 175, 186
abciximab **408**
absorption, distribution, metabolism, and excretion (ADME) analysis 128–9, 168
absorptive transporter 192
accelerated stability testing 346–8
ACE-inhibitors (ACEI) 204
acid–base theory: Bronsted–Lowry theory 94–7; definition 94; dissociation 103–4, *104*; Henderson–Hasselbach equation 98–9; Lewis theory 97–8; pH meter 102–3; pH scale 99–102, *101*
acid-catalyzed hydrolysis 340–1
active pharmaceutical ingredients (APIs) 35, 159, 327, 478, 480–1; amorphous form 378; crystalline structure 68; drug products 90; GMP **367**; moisture levels 78; oral absorption 137; OrBiTo 84; PAT 61; physicochemical characteristics 88, 138, 326–7; polymorphic/amorphous forms 91, 378; quality management 368–70; solid oral dosage forms 86; vibrational spectroscopy 86–7
adalimumab **408**
adapalene (ADP) 215
adenylylation 394
ADHD (attention-deficit/hyperactivity disorder) 198–9
ADME analysis *see* absorption, distribution, metabolism, and excretion (ADME) analysis
ADPHF6 polyherbal formulation 519
adsorbate 299
adsorbent 299
adsorption 299, 304; isotherm 300
aerosizer 299
aerosols, VOCs 153–4
AES (Auger Electron Spectroscopy) 75
Aesculus hippocastanum (horse chestnut) 494
aflibercept 220–1
African Network for Drugs and Diagnostics Innovation (ANDi) 525

agarose hydrogels 476
AI (artificial intelligence) 3
aldesleukin **408**
alemtuzumab **408**
Aleurites moluccana 507
aliskiren 5, 204
ALLAI (aripiprazole lauroxil long-acting injectable) 197
Allium sativum (garlic) 494
alpha-galactosidase **413**
alteplase **408**
aluminum phosphate 480
aluminum salts (Alum) 480
Alzheimer's disease 478
ambrex, effect of 508–9
amended BBT (ABBT) 522–3
amide bond formation 394
amino acids: composition 461; oxidation of 407; peptide bond 385–7; properties **384**; sequence 461; structure **383**; terminal sequence 461; translation 382
amorphous forms 249–50
amorphous solid dispersion (ASD) 194–5, 280–1
anakinra **408**
analytical method validation 435–6
Andrographis paniculata 521, 523
andrographolide 523
angiogenic growth factors 197
anhedral 237
animal-based biological assays 455
animal model testing 172
Antibiotic Development to Advance Patient Treatment (ADAPT) Act 3
antibiotics 3
antibody, immunoglobulin (Ig) 379
antidiabetic polyherbal formulation (ADPHF6) 519
anti-fungal agents 231–2
antihemophilic factor (AHF) **409**
anti-HIV microbicides 208, 221
anti-malarial therapy 524–5
antimicrobial resistant microbes (AMR) 509
antimicrobials 509–10

antioxidants 407; ADPHF6 formulation 519;
    classes of 439; flavonoids 154–5;
    melatonin 231; oxidation 314–15;
    rutin 216
anti-scarring treatment 471–2
antivitiligo ointment 223
APIs *see* active pharmaceutical ingredients
    (APIs)
aprepitant (APR) 280
aquatic toxicity, QSARs 150
arcitumomab **409**
aripiprazole lauroxil long-acting injectable
    (ALLAI) 197
Arnica montana (arnica) 494
aroma compounds, partition coefficients 145
Arrhenius equation 346–9
artemisinin combination therapy 524
arthritis 215
artichoke 515
articular cartilage 142–3
artificial intelligence (AI) 3
ASD *see* amorphous solid dispersion (ASD)
asparagyl 437
aspirin 281
assays 165–6; animal model testing 172;
    Caco-2 drug transport 169–72;
    complexity *vs.* correlation with
    human absorption *166*; degradation
    products 333–4; IVIVC 172–5;
    PAMPA 168–9; permeability 166–7
AT1-receptor blockers (ARB) 204
atomic force microscope (AFM) 313, 470
attachment energy model 239
attention-deficit/hyperactivity disorder
    (ADHD) 198–9
Auger Electron Spectroscopy (AES) 75
autoclaving 314
Ayurveda: liver disease treatment 521;
    osteoarthritis, interventions for
    512–13
AZD5329 282
AZD9343 282–3

Banxia Baizhu Tianma Tang (BBT) 522–3
base-catalyzed hydrolysis 340–1
basiliximab **409**
batches, drug substance 353
BBC (bilirubin binding capacity) 131
BCS *see* Biopharmaceutics Classification
    System (BCS)
beagle dogs 472
becaplermin **410**
bee venom (BV) 222, 481
beta-cyclodextrin (betaCD) 471
β-elimination reaction 441, **441**

bevacizumab 220–1
bilirubin binding capacity (BBC) 131
bioaccumulation 156
biochemical assays 455
bioequivalence 213
biological activity 455–6
biological drugs *401*, 407
biological products: composition of **408–20**;
    excipients in **421**; purity of 456–7;
    stability testing 448–50
biologics 6–7
biomedical investigations, electrochemical
    methods 134
Biomek FX Workstation 168–9
biopharmaceuticals: characterization of 379;
    classification system class IV 470;
    products 438; specification of 400;
    stabilization 406
Biopharmaceutics Classification System
    (BCS) 159, 176–7; biowaivers *see*
    biowaivers; class IV drugs 194,
    203–4, 220; dissolution 177, 182–3;
    permeability 177, 179–82; solubility
    177–8
biopharmaceutics drug classification system
    (BDCS) 189–92, **190–1**
biotechnology 448–50
biowaivers: attachment A 188; BCS class 1 and
    3 183, 185; data supporting 186–8;
    excipients 183–4; prodrugs 184;
    regulatory applications of 185–6
bitter taste evaluation 207–8
botanical drugs 7–8; clinical trials 496;
    component combinations for
    496–7, **497**; U.S. Food and Drug
    Administration 486
botanical products 485
Bradford method 429
Bragg's diffraction *262*
branched PEGs (PEG2-X) 426
Braunauer, Emmet, and Teller (BET) method
    299, 301
Bravais lattice system *236*
bronchoalveolar lavage (BAL) 148
Bronsted–Lowry theory 94–6, *97*
Brownian motion 311
Brucker SHellXTL software 237
buccal peptide delivery 223
Butein 155–6

Caco-2 cells 81–2, 169–72
caffeine 519–20
Cambridge Crystallographic Data Centre
    (CCDC) 306
Cambridge Structural Database (CSD) 306

candidate drugs 10–12, 126–7, 310, 339, 350
capecitabine 518
capillary electrophoresis (CE) 128, 132
capromab pendetide **410**
carbachol (CCh) 514
carbamylation 440–1
carrier gas 304
cascara sagrada (*Rhamnus purshiana*) 494
Cassia acutifolia (senna) 494
castration-resistant prostate cancer 477
catalyze hydrolysis reactions 315
cationic self-nanoemulsifying oily formulations
        (CSNEOFs) 469
CD *see* circular dichroism (CD)
CE *see* capillary electrophoresis (CE)
cell culture-based biological assays 455
cell culture/substrate-derived impurity 463
Center for Biologics Evaluation and Research
        (CBER) 401, **401–3**, 403–4
Center for Drug Evaluation and Research
        (CDER) 401, **401–3**, 403
central composite design (CCD) 464
Cerius^2 245–6
chamomile (*Matricaria chamomilla*) 494
chaperones 390
Charaka Samhita (book) 7, 485
chelating agent 316
chemical stability 233
chemistry, manufacturing, and control (CMC):
        for NCCAM **495**; overview of
        496; product 495–6; synthetic/
        semisynthetic drugs 494
CheqSol® (chasing equilibrium solubility) 67,
        69–70, 162
chikungunya virus (CHIKV) 474–5
chimeric antigen receptor (CAR) T-cell therapy
        2
Chinese hamster ovary (CHO) cells 393
Chinese herb toothpaste 527
chirality 332–3
chitin-calcium silicate 269–70
choriogonadotropin alpha **410**
chromatography method 431–3
chronic stress (CS) 513
chronic unpredictable stress (CUS) 513
ciclopirox *vs.* amorolfine 227
Cidara Therapeutics 3
CIMAvax EGF 210
circular dichroism (CD) 134–5
cisplatin loaded protransfersome system 221–2
claims: definiteness 38–9; dependent 39;
        dominant-subservient 39; GAB
        44; Jepson-type 41; Markush
        alternates 41; Markush Group 41;
        means-plus-function clauses 40;

mixed-class 41; narrowing of 39;
        negative limitations 41; process
        40; product-by-process 42; PTA
        42–4; punctuation 38; ranges 40–1;
        reading 38; relative and exemplary
        terminology 41; RRB 45; step-plus-
        function clauses 40
Classic of the Materia Medica (book) 485–6
cleaning validation 436
clinical pharmacokinetic monitoring (CPM)
        148
closed pores 301
C-mannosylation 397
coagulation factor IX (recombinant) **410**
coagulation factor VIIa (rFVIIa) **410**
coamorphous systems 480–1
Code of Federal Regulations (CFR) 47–8,
        400–1, *401*
color measurement 307–8
Combretaceae 511
comparative molecular field analysis
        (CoMFA) 112
compatibility testing 323–4
complementary and alternative medicine
        (CAM) **490**
comprehensive two-dimensional gas
        chromatography 141–2
confirmatory testing 317–18, 359–60
constipation treatment 506
container closure system 354
continuous dissolution–permeation system
        232
contracept-TM 511–12
Cordyceps militaris 523–4
counterion 275–6
Cremophor EL 164–5
CRISPR-Cas9 system 1–2
critical micellar concentration (CMC) 150
critical relative humidity (CRH) 267
cryogranulation: lyophilization 424–9; spray
        drying 423–4; undercooling 424
cryopreservation 423
crystal habit 235–7, *237*, **238**
crystal lattice 234, *234*
crystalline index of refraction 247
crystalline structure 68, 78–89
crystal morphology 234–40, **235**
curcumin 144–5
cyanate 440–1
cyclic voltammetry (CV) 315
cysteine 407
cysteinyl residues 439, 442–3, **443**
cytochrome P4503A4 (CYP3A4) 172, 192
cytochromes P450 134
cytokines 379

daclizumab **411**
dandelion, antioxidant effects of 515
danshen 514
darbepoetin alfa **411**
deacetylation 394
deamidation process 407, 437–8, **439**
degradation, kinetics of 345–9
deliquescence 250–1
DELT *see* DNA-encoded library technology
        (DELT)
De Materia Medica (book) 485
denaturation process 444–5, **445**
denileukin diftitox **411**
dependent claims 39
design of experiments (DoE) approach 477
design qualification (DQ) 370, 435
desorption phase, moisture content 267
development phases, drug discovery: candidate
        drug screening 10–11; candidate
        drug selection 11–12; lead finding/
        establishing directions 9–10; phase
        I clinical studies 12–13; phase II/III
        studies 13; postmarket surveillance
        13–14; preclinical studies 12
diaryltriazines (DATAs) 221
diclofenac 219–20, 229–30
Dietary Supplement Health and Education Act
        (DSHEA) 7, **490**
dietary supplements 7–8
differential scanning calorimetry (DSC) 76, 79,
        89, 256–8, 320, 376
different light scattering (DLS) 297
diffuse reflectance (DR) technique 260–1
Digestarom® herbal formulation 506
digestive tract tumors 201–2
diindolylmethane derivative (DIM-D) 469–70
dimethylsulfoxide (DMSO) 128–30, 138
dimorphism 272
disk intrinsic dissolution rates (DIDR) 270
dispersive liquid–liquid microextraction
        (DLLME) 150
dissolution 160, *160*, 177, 255; acceptance
        criteria 289–91; ASD 194–5; BCS
        class IV drugs 194; diffusion layer
        model 160, *160*; drug 195; HME
        193; oral anticancer drugs 196;
        paediatric oral biopharmaceutics
        192–3; physiologically based
        absorption modeling 195; poorly
        water-soluble drugs 193; testing
        267–8
distribution coefficient 114–16
DLLME *see* dispersive liquid–liquid
        microextraction (DLLME)
DMSO *see* dimethylsulfoxide (DMSO)

DNA-encoded library technology (DELT) 6
DNA structure 398, *398*
dodecyl-L-pyroglutamate (DLP) 215
domain structures, proteins 387–9, *388*
dominant-subservient claims 39
dornase alpha **411**
dosage forms: design and development 135–6,
        324–5, 370–1; dissolution rate 288;
        drug products 138–9; emulsion
        311–19; factors, depend on 287;
        freeze-dried 319–20; general
        compatibility testing 323–4;
        pulmonary delivery 322–3; selection
        criteria 288; solid *see* solid dosage
        forms; solution 310–11; study factors
        for **331**; suspensions 321; topical
        delivery 322
dose limiting toxicities (DLTs) 518
double mutant heat-labile toxin (dmLT) 483
downstream-derived impurity 463
DP *see* drug product (DP)
Dravet syndrome 4
drotrecogin alpha **411**
Drug Administration Law **487**
drug bioavailability 87, 137, 274–5, 326,
        374, 473
drug delivery 151
drug discovery: AI 3; antibiotics 3; biologics
        6–7; botanicals 7–8; DELT 6;
        development phases 9–14; genome
        editing 1–2; HTS 4–5; marijuana
        3–4; microbiome 2–3; phenotype
        6; phytomedicines 14–17, **15–16**;
        preformulation focus 9; protein
        families 5; rational drug design 5;
        recombinant drugs 17–18; target-
        based 4; types of 1, *2*
drug efflux 80–1
drug-excipient compatibility screening 85–6,
        273, 325–6, 372–3
drug product (DP): contaminants 457;
        degradation of 460; development
        90, 138–9, 377; dissolution
        testing 182–3; heterogeneity 455;
        immunochemical procedures 456;
        impurity of 457; peptide mapping of
        461; process controls 458–9; purity
        of 457; release limits *vs.* shelf-life
        limits 459; specifications for 460;
        stability program 449; stress testing
        452–3
drug substance (DS) 329–30; assay 333–4;
        characterization, ICH guidelines
        56, **57–60**; description 66; dosage
        forms, study factors 330, **331**;

and DP *see* drug product (DP); impurities 361–70; NanoCrystal particles 70, *71*; PAT 61, 331–2; physicochemical/biological properties 56, 61, 334–8; properties of 55; solubility class 178; specifications 332–3; stability evaluation 338–52; stability testing 352–60
DS *see* drug substance (DS)
DSC *see* differential scanning calorimetry (DSC)
dye-binding method 429
dynamic DSC (DDSC) 320
dynamic vapor sorption (DVS) 265–7, 292–3; for lactose *294*; for microcrystalline cellulose *293*
dysoxylum binectariferum 475

Echinacea purpurea (echinacea) 494
Eclipta alba 512
edaravone (EDR) 481
EDS *see* energy-dispersive X-ray spectrometry (EDS)
efalizumab **411**
electrochemical biosensors systems 134
electrophoresis method 430–1
electrostaticity 308–9
ELF concentrations *see* epithelial lining fluid (ELF) concentrations
Embelia ribes 483
embelin 483
emulsion formulation 311–14; osmolality 319; oxidation 314–15; particle size *312*; photostability 317–18; stability considerations 314; surface activity 318–19; trace metal 315–17
enantiotropy 240–1, *241*, **242**
endoxifen 225–6
energy-dispersive X-ray spectrometry (EDS) 74–5
Entasis Therapeutics 3
enzyme-linked immunosorbent assay (ELISA) 482
epithelial lining fluid (ELF) concentrations 148
Eprex® 422
erythropoietin (EP) 398, **412**
Escherichia coli 443, 446, 483
ESCOP *see* European Scientific Cooperative on Phytotherapy (ESCOP)
etanercept **412**
ethylenediamine 316
ethylenediaminetetraacetic acid (EDTA) 316–17
euhedral 237
eukaryotes 399–400

eukaryotic cell 28
European Directorate for the Quality of Medicines Certification 500
European Economic Community (EEC) **488**
European Medicines Agency (EMA) 9
European Patent Convention 26
European Pharmacopoeia monograph 500–3
European Scientific Cooperative on Phytotherapy (ESCOP) 14–15, **488**
Euodiae fructus 527–8
eutectic formation 219
exceptional drug solubilization 281
excipients 183–4, 336–8; -induced salt disproportionation 278; NTI drug 185; oral cavity 185; solid oral dosage forms 326, 373
expression system characterization 436
extended release quetiapine fumarate (quetiapine XR) 202
external validation 174
extracellular signal-regulated kinase (ERK) 515–16
extrusion-spheronization process 511
Exubera 323

face-centered cubic design (FCCD) 468
facility and equipment validation 435
fascaplysin 478
FBS (fragment-based screening) 4–5
FCS *see* fluorescence correlation spectroscopy (FCS)
FDA *see* Food and Drug Administration (FDA)
feverfew (*Tanacetum parthenium*) 494
filgrastim **412**, **417**
filter plate method, solubility testing 128–30, *129*
filter probe method 126
fire-heat syndrome 527
flavonoids 154–5
FlowSorb III 304–5
fluorescence correlation spectroscopy (FCS) 76
fluorine 93
folk medicine **487**
follicle-stimulating hormone (FSH) **412**
Food and Drug Administration (FDA) 1; dietary supplements 7–8; and EMA 9; marketing authorization 33–4; patents 45–50
food sensory analysis 141–2
forced degradation studies 317, 359–60, 450–4
Forge Therapeutics 3
forked PEGs (PEG-X2) 426
48-H release formulation 471–2
Fourier transform-infrared (FT-IR) spectroscopy 75, 260, 425
fragment-based screening (FBS) 4–5

Franz diffusion cell approach 230
Fraunhofer theory 298
Freeman Technology 74
freeze-dried drugs 65
freeze-dried formulations 319–20
freeze–thaw test 65, 407, 423
FT4 Powder Rheometer 74
functional groups of drugs **341**
fusion protein 390–1

GAB *see* guaranteed adjustment basis (GAB)
gabapentin 226
garlic (*Allium sativum*) 494
gas physisorption 300
gas pycnometry 305
gastroesophageal reflux disease (GERD) 282–3
gastrointestinal (GI) tract 181–2
gastroparesis (GP) treatment 506
Gegen-Qinlian Decoction (GQD) 517
gelatine co-polymer hydrogel delivery 227–8
gemtuzumab ozogamicin **413**
gene expression system 398, *399*
generic drug 42–3
gene therapy 403–4
genetically engineered crops 53
genetically modified microorganisms 28
genetic engineering (GE) 53
genome editing 1–2
genomics 11
geometric metamerism 308
Germany's Commission E **489**
Ginkgo biloba 493
ginkgo diterpene lactone meglumine injection
     (GDMI) 526
ginseng 486
GI (gastrointestinal) tract 181–2
glucagon **413**
glutamyl 437
glycan 396
glycolipid 229
glycophosphatidylinositol (GPI) anchors 397
glycoproteins 400
glycosylation 394–8, *396*
gonarthritis 516
good manufacturing practice (GMP) 366,
     367, 498
gradient elution 268
gram-positive lactic acid bacteria 81
guaranteed adjustment basis (GAB) 44
guinea pig 510–11

HaCaT keratinocytes 510–11
Haemaccel® **414**
haemophilus B **413**
Hatch-Waxman Act 26, 42

heating experiments 65, 260, 407
heat of hydration 161
Heckel equation 305
heme oxygenase-1 (HO-1) enzyme 511
hemolysis 150
Henderson–Hasselbach equation 98–9, 131
hepatitis B vaccine **413**
hepatitis C 508
herbal drug approval rules **487–9**
herbal medicine (HM): efficacy of 485,
     493–4; excipients, control of 501;
     preparations 499; regulatory filing
     procedure 494–6; safety 493–4;
     specifications 491–2; standardization
     of 492–3; vitamins/minerals 501; *vs.*
     synthetic drugs 490
herbal preparations: control of 500–1; criteria
     504–6; quantified extracts 499;
     stability testing 502; tests 505
herbal substance: control of 500–1;
     criteria 502–4; quantity of 499;
     specifications 491; stability testing
     502; tests 503–4
herboristerias **487**
heterobifunctional PEGs (X-PEG-Y) 426
heterogeneity 455
heterologous proteins 29
hFSH **412**
high-concentration protein formulation 138
higher-order structure (HOS), proteins 385, *386*
high-performance liquid chromatography
     (HPLC) 116, 127, 132, 268–9; for
     HM formulae 527; ion-exchange
     432; reverse-phase 432–3; Shaoyao-
     Gancao decoction 520; size-
     exclusion 433
high-performance thin layer chromatography
     (HPTLC) 517–18
high-pressure homogenization 163
high-throughput screening (HTS) 1, 11,
     17, 129, 140–1; and automated
     synthesis 10; benzodiazepines
     4; crystallization 245–7, 265;
     development of 18; FBS 5;
     natural-compound libraries 5
histaminergic H1/H3 receptors 200
HIV-1 treatment 207
HM *see* herbal medicine (HM)
homobifunctional PEGs (X-PEG-X) 426
homogenization 163–4
hormones 380
horse chestnut (*Aesculus hippocastanum*) 494
host organism 399
hot-melt extrusion (HME) 193, 280, 478–80
hot-stage microscopy 258

HPLC *see* high-performance liquid chromatography (HPLC)
HPTLC (high-performance thin layer chromatography) method 517–18
HSA *see* human serum albumin (HSA)
HTS *see* high-throughput screening (HTS)
human dermal fibroblasts (HDFs) 514–15
human immunodeficiency virus (HIV) infection 131–2
human serum albumin (HSA) 155–6, 422
hydrates **248**, 248–9
hydrocortisone (HC) 216
hydrolysis 339–42, 407, 444, **444**
hydrophobic drugs 146
hygroscopicity 250–1
Hypericum perforatum 493
hyperthyroidism 199–200
hypervariable region 380
hyphenated methods 433–4
hypoxia imaging, nitroimidazole 158

ICH guidelines *see* International Conference on Harmonization (ICH) guidelines
idebenone-loaded nanostructured lipid carriers (IDB-NLCs) 475–6
identification testing, drug substance 332
IGC (inverse gas chromatography) 294–5, *295*
illuminant metamerism 308
imatinib 5
IMHB *see* intramolecular hydrogen bonding (IMHB)
imiglucerase **414**
immunochemical property 456
immunoglobulin (Ig) 28, 379
impurities: decision tree 365; GMP 366, **367**; identification of 361–2; inorganic 362; organic 361; qualification 364; quality management 368–70; specification 363; thresholds of **366**
inactivated polio vaccine, serotype 3 (IPV3) 481–2
inclusion bodies 446
inductively coupled plasma (ICP)-atomic emission spectroscopy 74–5
infliximab **414**
information portals 31–2
infrared spectroscopy (IRS) 259–61
inhaled anesthetics 145–6
inorganic impurities 362
in silico models 166
in situ gel forming system 224
installation qualification (IQ) 370, 435
insulin aspart **414**
insulin glargine **414**
insulin glulisine injection **414**

insulin lispro **415**
intellectual and tangible property (IP/TP) rights 52
interferon alpha-2a/-2b **415**
interferon alphacon1 **415**
interferon beta-1a/-1b **415**
interferon gamma-1b **416**
interleukin eleven (IL-11) **416**
internal validation 174–5
International Conference on Harmonization (ICH) guidelines 63, 65, 457–8, 460, 463, 500; drug substance 56, **57–60**
International Union for Physical and Applied Chemistry (IUPAC) isotherms *300*
Internet search engines 30
interstitial fluid (ISF) 148
intestinal drug absorption 169–70
intestinal permeability methods 179–81
intramolecular hydrogen bonding (IMHB) 141
intravenous formulation development 278
intrinsic dissolution rate 268
inverse gas chromatography (IGC) 294–5, *295*
investigational new drug applications (INDs) 175, 185–6
in vitro gel diffusion model 476–7
in vitro–in vivo correlation (IVIVC) 81, 172, 470; internal validation 174–5; levels 173; lipid-based formulations 149
in vitro solubility assays, drug discovery 88–9, 138, 375–6
ion-associated hydrates 249
ion-exchange (IEX) chromatography method 432
ionization principle *see* acid–base theory
ion pair log *P* 121; CE 128; filter plate method, solubility testing 128–30, *129*; filter probe method 126; HPLC method 127; manual titration 125; shake-flask method 126–7; solubility method 126; spectroscopy 125–6
iontophoretic transport 217–18
ISF *see* interstitial fluid (ISF)
isocratic elution 268
isoelectric focusing (IEF) method 431
isolated lattice sites 249
isoperibol technique 258
isothermal microcalorimetry 259
isothermal solution calorimetry 258–9
Iterum Therapeutics 3
IVIVC *see* in vitro–in vivo correlation (IVIVC)

Japan-specific regulatory aspects 201
Jatropha gossypiifolia 525–6

Jepson-type claims 41
JFD (*N*-isoleucyl-4-methyl-1,1-cyclopropyl-
    1-(4-chlorine)phenyl-2-amylamine
    HCl) 274, 472

kampo medicines **489**
kava kava (*Piper methysticum*) 494
ketoprofen (KTP) 230
kinetic solubility assays 376
KKAy mice, type 2 diabetes 523–4
Kubelka–Munk (K–M) equation 261

labrasol 479
lactose 323
Lagerstroemia speciosa 518
lamivudine 473
lanreotide Autoge® (ATG) 197–8
large-molecule drugs 64–5
laronidase **416**
L-asparaginase 468
Lawsone method 516–17
leachates 422
lead-like libraries 152
lead optimization (LO) 56
Le Chatelier's principle 161
lecithin based nanoemulsions 222–3
leg ulcers, non-healing 528
Lennox-Gastaut syndrome 4
lepirudin **416**
Lewis acid–base theory 97–8
lidocaine carboxymethylcellulose 227–8
light instability 351
light source 359
linkers 387
lipid-based formulations 149
lipid-based oral delivery systems 469–70
lipophilicity 156–7
liposomal drug delivery 54, 205–6
liposomal solubilization 163
liquid chromatography-tandem mass
    spectroscopy (LC-MS) 434
liquid crystalline nanoparticles (LCNPs) 225
liquisolid systems 87, 137, 274–5, 326, 374, 473
Lonicerae japonicae 524
losartan (Los) 471
lyophilization 165, 319; annealing step 424;
    eutectic point 424; FT-IR spectroscopy
    425; glass transition temperature
    424–5; PEGylation 426–9
lyophilized Betaseron **416**
lysozyme transport 217–18

MA212 (Rosaxan) 516
mAbs *see* monoclonal antibodies (mAbs)
macitentan 471

Macrolide Pharmaceuticals 3
macroscopic operations 235
magnesium (II) gluconate 285
magnetic nanoparticles (MNPs) 198
magnetic resonance spectroscopy (MRS)
    133–4
manufacturing 366
marijuana 3–4
Markush Group 41
mass spectroscopy (MS) method 433–4
Matricaria chamomilla (chamomile) 494
matrix metalloproteinase-1 (MMP-1) 514–15
matrix solid dispersion phase (MSDP)
    method 507
maximum likelihood (ML) approach 349
maximum operating range (MOR) 435
MDR *see* multidrug resistance (MDR)
mDSC *see* modulated differential scanning
    calorimetry (mDSC)
measurement strategies: ion pair log *P see* ion
    pair log *P*; pK_a and log *P* 121, **122**;
    preformulation group, limitations
    121; Sirius equipment 121, **123–4**
medicated jelly, vitamin C 473–4
melatonin 214, 231
melittin 222
melting points 91, 139, 255
Mesopotamian clay tablet 485
metal-ion coordinated water 249
metalloproteins 135
metamerism 308
metathesis reactions 344
methicillin-resistant *Staphylococcus aureus*
    (MRSA) 148
methionyl 439
methylphenidate (MPH) 198–9
microbicide 196
microbiology 336
microbiome 2–3
microcrystalline cellulose *293*
micromeritics 304–5
microneedles (MNs) 217, 227–8
micronization 164, 292
microscopic operations 235
microscopy 74–5
microthermal analysis 76
Mie theory 298
milk thistle (*Silybum marianum*) 494, 510
Miniaturized INtrinsic DISsolution Screening
    (MINDISS) assay 270
minisphere emulsion-based formulation 214–15
minoxidil 232
mitoxantrone 143–4
mixed-class claims 41
MJC13 477

MNPs (magnetic nanoparticles) 198
moderately hygroscopic compounds 251
modulated differential scanning calorimetry
        (mDSC) 89, 258, 320, 376
moisture isotherm 78–9
molar refractivity (MR) 112
molecular descriptors (MD): IMHB 141; QSP/
        AR 154
molecular scissors 1
molecular spectroscopy 76–7
molecular transport, articular cartilage 143
monoclonal antibodies (mAbs) 29, 64, 90, 377,
        382, 406
monofunctional PEGs (mPEG-X) 426
mononuclear phagocytic system (MPS)
        infections 165
monotropic system *240*, 240–1, **242**
motifs 387
MRS *see* magnetic resonance spectroscopy
        (MRS)
MRSA *see* methicillin-resistant *Staphylococcus
        aureus* (MRSA)
multiarm PEGs 426
multidomain proteins 387
multidrug resistance (MDR) 80–1
multifunctional PEGs 426–7
multilevel models, laboratory animal research
        152–3
multiple-dose packaging 421
MultiScreen Caco-2 assay system 170, *171*
Munident (herbal) dentifrice 520–1
muromonab-CD3 **416**
Musa balbisiana 511
mycophenolate mofetil (MMF) 218–19
mycophenolic acid (MPA) 218–19
mycotoxins 504–5

N-acetyl acid (NANA) 396
nail disorders 85
naltrexone HCl (NTX-HCl) 228
nanocarriers 147
NanoCrystal® technology 70, *71*, 163
nanoindentation 86, 373
nanonization 164
nanostructured lipid carriers (NLCs) 475–6
nanotherapies, digestive cancers 201–2
National Center for Complementary and
        Alternative Medicine (NCCAM)
        490, **495**
neonatal hyperbilirubinemia 131
nesiritide **416**
new chemical entities (NCEs) 85, 88, 372,
        375, 476
new drug applications (NDAs) 48–50, 175,
        185–6

new molecular entity (NME) 476
N-hydroxysuccinimide (NHS) ester 428, *429*
nicergoline (NIC) 277
nimesulide 272
9-nitrocamptothecin (9NC) 282
96-well permeability testing *167*
nipple shield delivery system (NSDS) 474
nitric oxide, diffusion of 152
nitroimidazole 158
NLCs (nanostructured lipid carriers) 475–6
N-linked glycosylation 397
non-healing leg ulcers 528
nonhygroscopic compounds 251
nonnucleoside reverse transcriptase inhibitors
        (NNRTIs) 221
non–small-cell lung cancer (NSCLC) 210
Non-Steroidal Anti-inflammatory Drugs
        (NSAIDs) 510
normal operating range (NOR) 435
nose-to-brain drug delivery 209–10
novel oral delivery system (NODS) 481
NP-based targeted delivery systems 198
NPC 1161C 273
NSDS (nipple shield delivery system) 474
nuclear factor erythroid 2-related factor 2
        (Nrf2) 515
nucleoside analogs 131–2

OA (osteoarthritis) 512–13
observer metamerism 308
O-linked glycosylation 397
omalizumab **417**
omeprazole magnesium 479
ondansetron hydrochloride (ONH) 272
open pores 301
operational qualification (OQ) 370, 435
ophthalmic drug delivery 470–1
oral anticancer drugs 196, 212–13
oral bioavailability 166, 172, 195, 205
Oral Biopharmaceutical Tools (OrBiTo) 84,
        136–7, 372, 469
oral solid dosage form 86, 326, 373, 482
Orange Book 42–3, 47–8
organic buffers 432
organic impurities 361–2
osmolality 319
osteoarthritis (OA) 512–13
Ostwald ripening 164, 321
over the counter (OTC) **488**
oxidation 314–15, 342–5, 438–40, **440**;
        degradation, kinetics of 345–9;
        number 344, **345**; photostability
        351–2; reduction reactions 343, 345;
        solid-state stability 350–1
Oxitard 513

paclitaxel (PCT/PTX) 226–7, 482–3
paediatric oral biopharmaceutics 192–3
PAGE (polyacrylamide gel electrophoresis) 430
PAHs (polycyclic aromatic hydrocarbons) 147
palatal mucosa 211
palivizumab **417**
Panax ginseng (ginseng) 493
Panax quinquefolius 486
paracetamol 522
parallel artificial membrane permeability
        analysis (PAMPA) 168–9
parathyroid hormone **417**
Parkinson's disease (PD) 506
partial surface area (PSA) 117
particle size: distribution 297–9;
        physicochemical properties 335;
        solid dosage 292–6
partition coefficient (*P*): aroma compounds,
        PRV method 145; distribution
        coefficient 114–16; log *P* values
        113–14; solubility 118–20; solvent
        116–18
passive sampler methods (PSMs) 149
PAT *see* process analytical technology (PAT)
patent application: best mode 37; claims 36,
        38; description 36–7; drawings 36;
        enablement 37; fixed formats 34;
        marketing authorization, FDA 33–4;
        molecular structure 33; specification
        34; statements of invention 34–5;
        utility statement 35
patents: animal and plant varieties 26;
        challenges 21–3; claims *see* claims;
        definitions 24; FDA 45–50; myths
        25–6; systems 23–4
patent search: electronic databases 27;
        information portals 31–2;
        and intellectual property
        services 32–3; Internet search
        engines 30; patent copies and
        search facilities 33; technical
        databases 32; U.S. Patent Office
        Classification 435 27–30
patent term adjustment (PTA) 42–4
PCS (photon correlation spectroscopy) 311–12
PD (Parkinson's disease) 506
pediatric exclusivity 47
pediatric patients 83, 135
PEG *see* polyethylene glycol (PEG)
pegfilgrastim **417**
peginterferon alpha-2a **417**
peginterferon alpha-2b **418**
pegvisomant **418**
PEGylation process *427*, 427–8
penicillin 10

peptide bond: filgrastim structure *387*;
        higher-order structure 385, *386*;
        Ramachandran plot 385, *385*;
        resonance structures *385*
peptide mapping 461
performance qualification (PQ) 370, 435
PerkinElmer Intracooler II 320
permeability assays 166–8
permeability class, drug substance 177; GI
        tract 181–2; intestinal permeability
        methods 179–81; PK studies in
        humans 179
permeation enhancers (PEs) 214, 223, 226
PGDP (propylene glycol dipelargonate) 116
P-glycoprotein (P-gp) 477–8
pharmaceutical profiling methods 136–7
pharmacokinetic (PK) studies 179
phase I and II drugs development 132
phase ratio variation (PRV) method 145
phase solubility analysis 264–5
phenotype 6
pH meter 102–3
phosphopantetheinylation 393
phosphorylation 394
photon correlation spectroscopy (PCS) 311–12
photosensitive pharmaceutical products,
        administration of 371
photosensitive surface active compound 283
photostability testing 83–4, 271, 317–18, 351–2,
        358–60
pH scale 99–102, *101*
pH-solubility profile 178
PHY906 518–19
physicochemical properties 155, 334–5,
        374–5, 455; drug molecules 87;
        electrophoretic patterns 462;
        excipients 336–8; extinction
        coefficient/molar absorptivity
        462; isoform pattern 462; liquid
        chromatographic patterns 462;
        microbiology 336; molecular weight
        462; particle size 335; polymorphic
        forms 335–6
physiochemical characterization tests: amino
        acid 461; carbohydrate structure
        462; peptide mapping 461;
        physicochemical properties 462;
        sulfhydryl groups/disulfide bridges
        461
physiological-based pharmacokinetic (PBPK)
        model 471
physiologically based absorption modeling 195
phytomedicines: antibiotics 14; characteristics
        of 486, 490; cyclosporin A and
        rapamycin 16; ESCOP 14–15;

herbal drugs 62–4; monographs lists 15, **15–16**; natural products and properties 14, 17; quinine and chloroquinine 16; screening systems 17
phytotherapeutic agents 486, 490
phytotherapy 509–10
Pill of Semen Plantaginis 513–14
Piper methysticum (kava kava) 494
piracetam 284–5
pirfenidone (PF) ointment 471–2
plant-derived pharmaceuticals 52–3
plant product 497–8
plant substance 497–8
plasma renin activity (PRA) 204
Plasmodium falciparum 524
Plasmodium vivax 524
platinum formulations, anticancer drugs 208
Podophyllum hexandrum 509
polyacrylamide gel electrophoresis (PAGE) 430
polyamidoamine (PAMAM) dendrimers 210–11
polycyclic aromatic hydrocarbons (PAHs) 147
poly(D, L-lactide-co-glycolide) (PLGA) 481
polyethylene glycol (PEG): drug performance 428; features 426; IDB-NLCs 475–6; NHS ester 428, *429*; rapid motion 427; types of 426–7
polyherbalism 519
polymeric amorphous solid dispersions 84, 136, 271, 325, 371
polymeric micelles 146
polymer screening 194–5
polymorphic transitions, thermodynamic rules for **242**
polymorphism 240–4, 309–10, 335–6
polymorph screening 67–8
polyparameter linear free energy relationship (pp-LFER) model 140
poorly water-soluble drugs 193, 200
porosity 301–2
posttranslational modifications (PTM): amide bond 394; amino acids 395; chemical groups 394–5; common *392*; glycosylation 395–8, *396*; impact of *393*; nonenzymatic additions 395; phosphopantetheinylation 393; of proteins *392*; structural changes 395
powders: caking 309; classification 74; flow and compaction 305–6; nature of 73; packing condition and air content 74; variables 72–3
pravastatin sodium 139
praying mantis model 261

prazosin salts 275–6
PRCA (pure red cell aplasia) 422
prediction errors 174
predictive screening approaches 88, 375
preformulation factors 83
preformulation testing criteria 55–6
preprohormones 380
procaine 342
process analytical technology (PAT) 61, 331–2
process claims 36, 40
process-related impurity 457, 463
process validation method 434–5
prodrugs 146, 184
product-by-process claims 42
product–package interactions 147
product-related impurities 457, 463–4
Prograf® 211–12
prohormones 380
propylene glycol dipelargonate (PGDP) 116
protein(s): aggregation 389–90; amino acids 382–7; bioassays study 406; domain 387–9, *388*; encountered modes 405; expression of 398–400; folding 390; product stabilization 407; storage 423; technical refolding of 51–2; therapeutics 381–2
protein degradation: aggregation 446, **447**; β-elimination 441, **441**; carbamylation 440–1; cysteinyl residue 442–3, **443**; deamidation 437–8, **439**; denaturation 444–5, **445**; hydrolysis 444, **444**; oxidation 438–40, **440**; precipitates 446–50, **448**; proteolysis 437, **438**; racemization 442, **442**
proteolysis 437, **438**
protonation/deprotonation, amine API 277–8
PRV method *see* phase ratio variation (PRV) method
PSA (partial surface area) 117
pseudopolymorphs 247
PSMs *see* passive sampler methods (PSMs)
Psoralea corylifolia (PC) 223
psudopolymorphs 240
PTA (patent term adjustment) 42–4
PTM *see* posttranslational modifications (PTM)
puerariae lobatae radix (gegen) 514
pulmonary delivery 322–3
pure red cell aplasia (PRCA) 422
pyrene fluorescence quenching 152

Q-rule 348
QSARs *see* quantitative structure–activity relationships (QSARs)

QSP/AR *see* quantitative structure–property/
    activity relationships (QSP/AR)
QSurf analyzers 303–4
quality management 368–70
Quality of Herbal Remedies Directive **488**
quantitative structure–activity relationships
    (QSARs): alcohols 105; aquatic
    toxicity 150; benzoic acid 105; dyes
    and fluorescent probes 142; Hammett
    σ constants 109, **109–10**; Hansch
    analysis 110–13; linear free-energy
    relationships *106*, 106–7;
    phenylacetic acids 106; ρ values 107,
    107; σ values 108, **108**, 110
quantitative structure–property/activity
    relationships (QSP/AR) 154
quartz crystal microbalance (QCM)
    technique 134
quetiapine immediate release (quetiapine
    IR) 202

RAAS (renin-angiotensin-aldosterone system)
    204–5
racemization 442, **442**
radioactive contamination 63
radioactivity 63
radio-labeled drug transport 170
radionuclide hypoxia imaging 158
Radix Salviae Miltiorrhizae 514, 527
Ramachandran plot 385, *385*
Raman spectroscopy (RS) 90, 144, 279–80,
    285, 377
Randles–Sevcik equation 315
ranibizumab 220–1
rasburicase **418**
rational drug design 5
recombinant DNA products 65–7
recombinant DNA technology 30
recombinant drugs 17–18
recombinant virus encoding 29
refractive indices, crystals 239–40, 247
regulatory requirements: drug substance *see*
    drug substance (DS); large-molecule
    drugs 64–5; phytomedicines 62–4;
    quality, pharmaceutical products 61;
    recombinant DNA products 65–7
relative humidity (RH) 78–9
release, drug substance 160; ALLAI 197; BCS
    class IV drugs 203–4; Japan-specific
    regulatory aspects 201; lanreotide
    Autoge® (ATG) 197–8; microbicide
    196; MNPs 198; MPH 198–9;
    NPs 198; RAAS 204–5; solubility
    modulation 163–5; 3D models 202–3
release limits *vs.* shelf-life limits 459

renin 5
renin-angiotensin-aldosterone system (RAAS)
    204–5
repackaging/stability, solid oral doses 327,
    376–7
required reduction basis (RRB) 45
reteplase **418**
reverse electro-osmosis 313
reverse-phase (RP) chromatography method
    432–3
Rhamnus purshiana (cascara sagrada) 494
Rheum palmatum 523–4
Rhodiola crenulata 523–4
Rhodiola rosea 514
Rietveld method 246–7
ritonavir 243
rituximab **418**
rofecoxib 14
rohitukine 475
ropinirole 205
Rosa canina 516
rosemary, antioxidant effects of 515
RRB *see* required reduction basis (RRB)
Rubotherm system 266
Rumalaya 513
Rutin-G (transglycosylated rutin) 472–3
rutin-loaded ethosomes 216
rutin with beta-cyclodextrin (RU-beta-CD) 279

safety assessment 364
salidroside 514
salmon calcitonin (sCT) 214–15
salt: disproportionation 278–9, 284; effect
    120; forms 252–4, **254**, 282, 284;
    screening 71–2
sargramostim **419**
saw palmetto (*Serenoa repens*) 494
scale-invariant technologies 51
scanning electron microscopy (SEM) 75
self-emulsifying drug delivery system (SEDDS)
    507–8
self-microemulsifying drug delivery systems 144
self-nanoemulsifying drug delivery systems
    (SNEDDS) 228–9, 468, 478–9,
    482–3
self-nanoemulsifying oily formulations
    (SNEOFs) 469
semivolatile organic compounds (SVOCs)
    153, 157
senna (*Cassia acutifolia*) 494
Sennae folium 499–500
Serenoa repens (saw palmetto) 494
sermorelin **419**
SFOD *see* solidification of floating organic
    droplet (SFOD)

SGA-100 symmetrical gravimetric analyzer 266
shake-flask method 126–7, 132, 139–40
shake test (agitation) 65
Shaoyao-Gancao decoction 520
Sho-sai-ko-to (SST) 508
Shuanghuanglian lyophilized powder 524
significant change 355, 358
Silybum marianum (milk thistle) 494, 510
simulated intestinal fluid (SIF) 477
single-crystal diffraction technique 247
sirolimus 275
size-exclusion chromatography (SEC)
        method 433
skin permeation 155
Skyscan-1172 306
slug mucosal irritation (SMI) 474
slurry method 474
small intestinal bacterial overgrowth syndrome
        (SIBO) 506
small-molecule drugs 400
SNEDDS *see* self-nanoemulsifying drug
        delivery systems (SNEDDS)
sodium dodecyl sulfate-polyacrylamide gel
        electrophoresis (SDS-PAGE) 430–1
software validation 436
Solanum nigrum 521
solid dosage forms 291–2; caking 309;
        color 307–8; electrostaticity
        308–9; excipient stability 326;
        instrumentation 302–5; particle
        size distribution 297–9; particle
        size studies 292–6; polymorphism
        309–10; porosity 301–2; powders,
        flow and compaction of 305–6;
        surface area 299–301; true
        density 305
solidification of floating organic droplet
        (SFOD) 151
solid lipid nanoparticles (SLN) 215
solid self-nanoemulsifying drug delivery
        systems (S-SNEDDS) 468
solid self-nanoemulsifying granules
        (SSNEGs) 272
solid-state characterization: microscopy 74–5;
        molecular spectroscopy 76–7;
        powders 72–4; stability testing
        77–80; thermal analysis 75–6;
        XRD 77
solid-state compatibility 270–1, 276
solid-state properties 233; amorphous forms
        249–50; crystal morphology
        234–40; HT crystal screening
        245–7; hygroscopicity 250–1;
        polymorphism 240–4; solubility
        251–5; solvates 247–9

solid-state stability 350–1
solubility 126, 251–2; additives 120; API 138;
        aprotic solvents 119; behavior
        119; calculation of *162*; class
        boundary 177; classification,
        U.S. Pharmacopeia 118, **119**;
        determination solvents 162–3; dipolar
        aprotic solvents 119; dissolution 255;
        melting point 255; modulation 163–5;
        molecular size 120; permeability 142;
        protic solvents 119; salt forms 252–4;
        temperature 120
Soluplus® (SOL) 280
solution calorimetry 258–9
solution dosage forms 310–11
solvates 247–9
solvents 162–3
somatropin **419**
Sorptomatic 1990 302–3
SPC *see* supplementary protection certificate
        (SPC)
specified impurities 363
spectrophotometer 307–8, 430
spectroscopy 125–6, 429–30
Spero Therapeutics 3
spheronization process 511
spray-dried delivery systems 193, 200
spray-dried powders (SDPs) 472
spray drying method 423–4, 478
stability commitment 356–7
stability evaluation 338–9; hydrolysis 339–42;
        oxidation 342–52
stability-indicating methods 454
stability testing 77, 352–3; batches, selection of
        353; container closure system 354;
        excipient compatibility 80; moisture
        isotherm 78–9; specifications
        354; stability commitment 356–7;
        statements/labeling 358–60; stress
        testing 353; testing frequency 354–6
statements/labeling 358; bracketing 360;
        photostability testing 358–60
static volumetric gas adsorption 302, *303*
storage conditions 354–6, **355, 356**
stress testing 353, 450–4
structurally modified antibodies 28–9
supersaturatable formulations 275
supplementary protection certificate (SPC)
        45–6
surface-active behavior 318–19
surface analysis (AES/XPS) 75
surface area 299–301
Surface Measurement Systems (SMS) 265, 293
surfactant test 65, 407
suspension formulation 321

SVOCs *see* semivolatile organic compounds (SVOCs)
Swiss albino mice 521–2
synchrotron radiation CD (SRCD) 135
synthetic drugs *vs.* herbal medicine 490

tacrolimus 211–12
Tanacetum parthenium (feverfew) 494
target-based drug discovery 4
taste evaluation 207–8
technical databases 32
tenecteplase **419**
terahertz pulsed imaging (TPI)™ 352
Terminalia chebula 511
terpenoid indole alkaloid (TIA) metabolism 53
tert-butyl hydroperoxide (tBHP) 515
testing systems: Caco-2 cells model 67; pK_a, partitioning and solubility 68–71; polymorph screening 67–8; salt screening 71–2; techniques 67
TET-loaded LCNPs (TET-LCNPs) 225
Tetraphase Pharmaceuticals 3
TGA *see* thermogravimetric analysis (TGA)
theranostic nanomedicine 206
thermal activity monitor (TAM) III 352
thermal analysis 75–6, 256, **257**
thermal conductivity detector (TCD) 304
thermodynamic solubility 265
thermogravimetric analysis (TGA) 76, 79, 258
THHP (Trichup herbal hair powder) 516–17
thin-layer chromatography (TLC) method 516
3D cell culture models 203
thyrotropin alpha **419**
Ticagrelor 281
Tinospora cordifolia 521
topical anesthetics, microneedles 217
topical delivery 322
tositumomab **420**
Tourette's syndrome 23
trace metals 315–17
traditional Chinese medicine (TCM) 517, 522
transcription activator-like effector nucleases (TALENs) 2
transdermal drug delivery 147, 157–8
transgenic crops 52
transglycosylated rutin (Rutin-G) 472–3
translational research 53–4
transungual permeation 85
trastuzumab **420**
trichlorofluoromethane 247
Trichup herbal hair powder (THHP) 516–17
Triphala Rasayana 522
TriStar 3000 gas adsorption analyzer 304
tristimulus colorimetry 307

true degradation pattern 346–7
true density 305
tryptanthrin 515–16
tumor necrosis factor (TNF) receptor 391
tumors, drug targeting to 206–7
Turbiscan(R) method 480
turmeric, antioxidant effects of 515
2-methyl cytidine prodrugs 216–17
type 2 diabetes (T2DM) 523–4

UAMC01398, microbicide gel formulation 221
UDPglucuronosyltransferases (UGTs) 192
ultraviolet (UV) spectroscopy 125
ultraviolet-visible (UV-VIS) spectroscopy 429, 462
Unani medicine 510, 528
undercooling process 424
unidentified impurities 363
unit cell 234, 262
Urtica dioica 516
U.S. Food and Drug Administration (FDA) 380, 486, **490**; CBER and CDER 401, **401–3**; CFR 400–1, *401*
U.S. Patent Office Classification 435: enzymes 27; eukaryotic cell 28; genetically modified microorganisms 28; heterologous proteins 29; immunoglobulin 28; monoclonal antibody 29; recombinant DNA technology 30; recombinant virus encoding 29; structurally modified antibody 28–9; viral and bacterial antigens 30
U.S. Pharmacopeia solubility classification 118, **119**
UV spectroscopy *see* ultraviolet (UV) spectroscopy

Valerianae radix 500
Valeriana officinalis (valerian) 494
vancomycin 16
vapor sorption 79
vascularized composite allotransplantation (VCA) 218–19
vibrational spectroscopy 86–7, 273–4, 373–4
Vioxx (rofecoxib) 14
virus-like particles (VLPs) 474–5
Visterra 3
vitamin C, medicated jelly formulations 473–4
vitamin E (VE), analogues of 205–6
VitriLife 426
volatile methylsiloxanes (VMS) 158
volatile organic compounds (VOCs) 153–4

warfarin-beta-cyclodextrin (WAF-beta-CD) 224–5
wavelength-dispersive X-ray spectrometry (WDS) 74–5
WDS *see* wavelength-dispersive X-ray spectrometry (WDS)
Western Ontario and McMaster Universities Arthritis Index (WOMAC) 516
wet mass 511
wistar rats 508
Working Party on Natural and Nutritional Supplements **487**
World Health Organization (WHO) 485–6, **488**

Xiao-Chai-Hu-Tang 508
XPS *see* X-ray Photoelectron Spectroscopy (XPS)

X-ray diffraction (XRD) 75, 77
X-ray microtomography 306
X-ray Photoelectron Spectroscopy (XPS) 75
X-ray powder diffraction (XRPD) 252, 261–4
X-ray powder diffractometer *263*
XRD *see* X-ray diffraction (XRD)

Y-shaped PEGs 426

zafirlukast (ZA) 276–7
zero-background holders (ZBH) 264
zeta potential 312–13, 321
Zimad 510
Zimadat 510
Zimad Mohallil 510
zinc finger nucleases (ZFNs) 2
ziprasidone 478–9

9781032338477